Transfusion Medicine, Hemostasis, and Hemotherapy

D1723943

Progress and Challenges in
Transfusion Medicine, Hemostasis, and Hemotherapy

State of the Art 2008

41th Congress of the German Society for
Transfusion Medicine and Immunohematology

Editor
Rüdiger E. Scharf Düsseldorf

56 figures, 28 in color, 29 tables, 2008

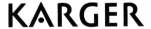

Basel · Freiburg · Paris · London · New York · Bangalore ·
Bangkok · Shanghai · Singapore · Tokyo · Sydney

Prof. Rüdiger E. Scharf, M.D., F.A.H.A.

Department of Experimental and Clinical Hemostasis,
Hemotherapy, and Transfusion Medicine
Heinrich Heine University Medical Center
Moorenstraße 5, 40225 Düsseldorf (Germany)
Tel. +49 211 81-173344, Fax -16221
rscharf@uni-duesseldorf.de

Cover Illustration

Detection of activated tyrosine kinase Src (pTyr418) and $\alpha IIb\beta 3$ in human platelets adherent onto fibrinogen. Immunolabeling of platelets was performed with anti-Src418 (red fluorescence) and anti-$\alpha IIb\beta 3$ (green fluorescence). The left panel documents the co-localization of Src pTyr418 with the integrin.
Taken from the work of Markus Hasse et al. whose paper was one of the 3 top abstracts receiving highest rating by the International Scientific Advisory Board of the Düsseldorf Congress.

Library of Congress Cataloging-in-Publication Data

Progress and Challenges in Transfusion Medicine, Hemostasis, and Hemotherapy / editor, R.E. Scharf.
X + 408 p.; 19 x 25.5 cm.
Includes bibliographical references and index.
ISBN 978-3-8055-8659-7 (soft cover :alk.paper)

Disclaimer. The statements, options and data contained in this publication are solely those of the individual authors and contributors and not of the publisher and the editor. The publisher and the editor disclaim responsibility for any injury to persons or property resulting from any ideas, methods, instructions or products referred to in the content or advertisements.

Drug Dosage. The authors and the publisher have exerted every effort to ensure that drug selection and dosage set forth in this text are in accord with current recommendations and practice at the time of publication. However, in view of ongoing research, changes in government regulations, and the constant flow of information relating to drug therapy and drug reactions, the reader is urged to check the package insert for each drug for any change in indications and dosage and for added warnings and precautions. This is particularly important when the recommended agent is a new and/or infrequently employed drug.

All rights reserved. No part of this publication may be translated into other languages, reproduced or utilized in any form or by any means electronic or mechanical, including photocopying, recording, microcopying, or by any information storage and retrieval system, without permission in writing from the publisher.

© Copyright 2008 by S. Karger Verlag für Medizin und Naturwissenschaften GmbH,
Postfach, 79095 Freiburg (Germany) and S. Karger AG, P.O. Box, 4009 Basel (Switzerland)

www.karger.com
Printed in Germany on acid-free paper by VVA/Konkordia GmbH, 76534 Baden Baden

ISBN 978-3-8055-8659-7

Contents

Stem Cells and Blood Cell Engineering

Molecular Immunohematology

Platelet-Pathogen Interactions

Diagnosis and Management of Bleeding Disorders

Genetic Research and Challenges in Thrombophilia

Novel Cellular Therapeutics

Hemostasis-Navigated Hemotherapy

Demographic Changes and Blood Supply

Λαμπ δια εχοντες διαδ σουσιν αλλ λοις
'Having Light We Pass It On To Others'

Plato, 'The Republic', 328a

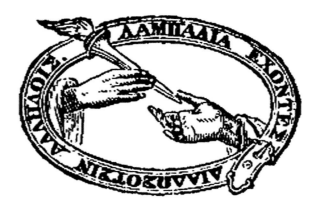

Preface

Conferences come and go. They take more than one year to be prepared but are over within a couple of days. By contrast, research communications and ideas being exchanged among scientists have a longer half-life. Consequently, congress attendees wish to receive take-home messages. To satisfy this demand, this volume gathers the contributions of the Plenary Lectures and State-of-the-Art Symposia speakers who presented at the Joint Congress 2008 of the German Society for Transfusion Medicine and Immunohematology (DGTI) and the Interdisciplinary European Society for Hemapheresis and Hemotherapy (ESFH) in cooperation with the Société Française de Transfusion Sanguine (SFTS), held in Düsseldorf from September 16 through 19, 2008.

The idea of publishing a State-of-the-Art book concomitantly to a congress is not new. It was Professor Marc Verstraete, the doyen among the European scientists in the field of thrombosis and hemostasis, who promoted this activity some 20 years ago at the congress of the International Society of Thrombosis and Hemostasis (ISTH) in Brussels. Since then, a long-standing tradition has been established among the ISTH members. This paragon has now been adapted for the participants of this DGTI-ESFH-SFTS meeting.

In the foreword of the Brussels State-of-the-Art book, Professor Verstraete once wrote, 'A preface is that part of a book that is placed first, written last, and read least'. Since all three statements he made are true, I will be brief. Transfusion medicine, hemostasis, and hemotherapy are relatively 'young' fields. They have in common both the subject 'blood' and the interdisciplinary approach. Thus, it is the translational impact of basic and clinical research that provides progress and challenges in patient care.

I am grateful to the authors, all experts in their field, who provided a chapter to this volume prior to the conference, meeting strict deadlines and accepting inevitable limitations in length, illustrations, and references. The support by our sponsors who made this project possible at all is particularly acknowledged, including CSL Behring, Wyeth, Baxter, NovoNordisk, and Novartis. Special thanks are also extended to the technical editing and production team of Karger publishers who worked hard to deliver this volume in due time. Finally, I would like to thank Uta Vandercappelle for her assistance, Nikola Möller for checking with me all manuscripts, and Anne Scharf for her coordination work as industrial liaison officer.

The editor hopes that the book will be received with the warmth and candor the authors deserve. To quote Professor Verstraete once more, 'History will tell, but obviously, the history we learn depends on who is the historian'.

Rüdiger E. Scharf, Düsseldorf

Social Intelligence and Competence

Scharf RE (ed): Progress and Challenges in Transfusion Medicine, Hemostasis and Hemotherapy.
Freiburg i.Br., Karger, 2008, pp 1–14

Increasing Safety by Implementing Optimized Team Interaction – Experiences of the Aviation Industry

Manfred H. Müller

Lufthansa Flight Safety Department, Frankfurt/Main, Germany

Key Words

Risk management · Optimum team interaction · Optimum hierarchical structure · Nonpunitive error management · Human Factor Research Project · Crew resource management

Summary

The large share of human errors in aviation accidents suggested the solution to replace the fallible human being by an 'infallible' computer. However, even after the introduction of the so-called high-technology (HITEC) airplanes, the factor human error still accounts for 75% of all accidents. Thus, if the computer is ruled out as the ultimate safety system, how else can complex operations involving quick and difficult decisions be controlled? Since a single person is always highly error prone, the principle solution of the problem is to have him/her supported and controlled by a second person. The probability that two persons make exactly the same mistake at the same point within an operating process is relatively low, as long as the two 'thought machines' collect and evaluate the available facts independently from each other before discussing and clarifying the further steps. Optimum team interaction results in a safety network that is able to cushion human errors.   ©2008 S. Karger GmbH, Freiburg i.Br.

Increasing Safety by Implementing Optimized Team Interaction

In times of increasing cost pressure, there is increasing tension between economic efficiency and safety. In numerous economic sectors, product quality is deliberately reduced in order to save costs. The expenses resulting from complaints are set off against the saving potential offered by cheaper production methods. This approach can be optimized by defining specific error or reject rates, e.g. in the production of budget-priced textiles. As long as this approach is used for products with no or few safety requirements, there is no reason to object to the concept, since the customer himself defines the desired quality level by means of the price. In some areas, however, this type of cost optimization cannot be accepted: As soon as life and limb of people are at stake, a management following the above principles can – as soon as the public takes notice – trigger the ruin of the respective company.

The Common Goal of the Medical and the Aviation Industry: Risk Minimization

For this reason, industries sensitive to safety, such as medical or aviation industry, must follow a different principle when defining their quality requirements: Maximum safety and minimum risk must be the topmost corporate objectives – and if it is only for ethic reasons. But there are also economic reasons for this target: The total loss of a large airplane causes an average cost of approx. 0.5 billion Euros. One single accident alone (a 'complete loss of production') can mean the end of an airline, e.g. Birgen Air. The phenomenon having started in the USA, doctors and medical institutions are also increasingly exposed to extremely high financial claims from damaged parties. In the medical field, too, one single human error can trigger a human and a financial catastrophe. So there are also substantial economic interests in avoiding complications and accidents.

Why Do Catastrophes Happen? – A Philosophic Question

Why do disasters and catastrophes happen? Are we unavoidably left unprotected to an unfavorable fate? In the past, efforts to find an answer to these questions inevitably led into the world of metaphysics. Evil spirits, magic, and witchcraft were considered the causes of 'negative events'. And rather unspecific means were used to get rid of possible 'catastrophe triggers': Exorcism and the burning of witches ranked high. According to the understanding of those days, man and his action were hardly responsible for and had little influence on avoiding catastrophes. The power of destiny was the dominating factor. When the ideas of the Enlightenment pushed man's own responsibility into the foreground, safety could be enormously increased in many fields of human life. The plague e.g. is not transmitted by the evil eye, but by fleas.

Acceptance of Self-Determined Risks and of Risks Determined by Others

The personal acceptance of risk, however, is not an objective variable, but highly dependent on the subjectively perceived question in how far the actual risk potential is determined by oneself. A motorcyclist, for example, readily and voluntarily accepts an extremely high risk when exceeding the speed limit on a winding road on his Sunday joyride (self-determined). After an accident caused by the described driving behavior, the motorcyclist's readiness to accept a risk involved in the treatment of a polytrauma tends towards zero (determined by others). For the medical and the aviation industry this means that the 'customer' has extremely high expectations with regard to safety. To identify the respective risk areas in aviation, a detailed error analysis is required. Since aviation catastrophes are of very high public interest, the pressure to identify root causes of accidents is much higher in aviation than it is in many other fields of society. The detailed investigation of more than 500 total losses of large jetliners (takeoff weight >20 tons) since 1960 made it possible to create an extensive database that reveals weak points and system deficits with the largest possible objectivity.

Man: Risk and Rescuer

A detailed investigation of the work environment combined with the analysis of the flight recorder data and the voice recorder in the cockpit provides a clear picture of the working conditions and errors that lead to a catastrophe.

Accident statistics prove that it is the human being in the cockpit who causes about three quarters of all accidents. The large share of human errors suggested the – at first sight brilliant – solution to replace the fallible human being by an 'infallible' digitally operating computer. This measure was meant to eliminate all human insufficiencies from the man/machine control loop. A computer never gets tired, is not emotional, does not need a holiday, has a constant level of motivation, etc. A considerable share of human work has been taken over by robots. In many cases this measure has increased productivity and guarantees unchanged product quality.

Automation and Safety

In aviation, an increased degree of automation has not changed the share of human errors as the cause of accidents. Even after the introduction of the so-called high-technology (HITEC) airplanes, the factor human error still accounts for 75% of all accidents. Up to now, the assumption that an increased degree of automation will necessarily lead to an increase in safety has not come true. In some cases, the human error was simply replaced by a computer error. Experience has shown that the digital computer increases or guarantees safety only in 'trivial' cases. Since even the best programmer is not able to anticipate all possibly occurring situations, the computer frequently 'fails' when unconventional decisions are required or when influencing variables must be weighed and assessed that have not been planned to occur in the respective context by the programmer. Plainly speaking, the machine is an aid as long as support is not really necessary, but it leaves you alone when a demanding decision is required. Extensive and comprehensive research projects have made us recognize that the so-called artificial intelligence (AI) has narrow limits. Even such trivial phenomena as, for example, the healthy common sense cannot be 'imitated' by the computer. The artificial generation of intuition or of ingenious new ideas by digital technology is miles away.

Optimized Team Interaction

If the computer is ruled out as the ultimate safety system, how else can complex operations involving quick and difficult decisions be controlled? We must seek new answers in fields of activity that depend on the smooth, safest possible interactions between man and machine. In this context, findings in biology, psychology, and social sciences are gaining importance. To be able to optimally utilize the capacities of the human brain and to correct potential errors, we have to create operating structures that can identify and correct possible errors. The interdisciplinary exchange of ideas and experience has shown that an optimal interaction between humans (team) and machine(s) in solving complex tasks under time pressure requires the use and observance of rules and standards that are applicable to all systems. In this context, it is of minor importance whether operating procedures in the operating theater, in the cockpit of an airplane, or in the control stand of a power station are considered.

Parallel Connection of Thought Machines

Since a single person is always highly error prone, the principle solution of the problem is to have him/her supported and controlled by a second person with the best possible and most suitable qualification. The probability that two persons working independently of each other make exactly the same mistake at one and the same point within an operating process is relatively low, as long as the two thought machines collect and evaluate the available facts independently from each other before discussing and clarifying the further steps (parallel connection of several independent thought machines). If they have different opinions, the reasons for a decision, as well as its advantages and disadvantages, must be discussed. The independent work of mind of those individuals influencing or controlling the process results in a safety network that is able to cushion human errors. The 'mesh size' is determined by the qualifications of the respective individuals and the quality of cooperation.

Error Omission in the Legal Sense

To develop effective defensive strategies, information on the actually occurring problems must be available. Unfortunately, the 'legal treatment' of human errors according to the principle 'errors must be punished, and errors with severe consequences must be punished severely' has caused much harm. The legislator assumes that threatening with or inflicting a severe penalty can keep people from acting against the rules. This approach might be true with regard to the planning of crimes (bank robbery, shoplifting), but an accidental human error cannot be avoided by the threat of punishment. Possible sanctions prevent an objective investigation and follow-up of an incident and impede the development of effective defensive strategies to avoid similar problems in the future. The fear of punishment leads to hushing up and an incorrect assignment of guilt.

Nonpunitive Error Management

To be able to tackle the actual problems, we have to create an environment characterized by an atmosphere of mutual trust. The open discussion of errors made must not be endangered by the threat of punishment or the fear of a possible career interruption. It should be made clear that the 'real professional' distinguishes him/herself by the fact that he/she addresses errors openly and discusses them. This concept is based on the conviction that even the best expert can make nearly any serious mistake under unfavorable conditions. It is not the mistake itself that is 'reprehensible', but the hiding of valuable information from the colleagues. It has been shown in the past that progress is primarily achieved by investigating and following up mistakes, failures, and catastrophes (that nearly happened). Every pilot has already experienced elements of accident scenarios of others. If we succeed in identifying and eliminating single links of a possibly mortal chain of errors before a catastrophe happens, the system has worked. If the relevant knowledge is only acquired after a catastrophe, the system has failed.

Limits of Confidentiality

To gain the confidence of the colleagues in a nonpunitive reporting system, certain prerequisites are required. The reporting system must be operated independent of the disciplinarian. The relevant incidents must be collected and analyzed by an independent organization unit. Protection of the 'reporting person' must have top priority. Analogous to confession in church, the confessing person must be protected under all circumstances. Serious incidents are reported only if the staff fully trusts the reporting system. If we do not succeed in building up a basis of confidence, only minor incidents are reported, which frequently result in the assignment of guilt to others. Experience with nonpunitive reporting systems has shown that it is usually single persons, not abstract organizations, who enjoy the trust of the staff members. An accepted confidential person is the prerequisite for the system's success. Of course the required basis of confidence cannot be built up over night; rather, it is a time-consuming process. A suitable confidential person is an experienced colleague who is appreciated by everybody and who has already reached his/her own professional goals. This person should be supported by younger colleagues as contact persons for staff members their own age.

Human Factor Research Project

The analysis of accident statistics involves the dilemma that, due to the fortunately low number of catastrophes, it is very difficult to make valid statistical statements. Reference to the number of incidents that have actually occurred is often missing. A comprehensive survey is therefore essential to obtain an objective picture of the safety situation: A well-structured analysis of as many catastrophes that have almost occurred as possible makes visible the part of the 'incident iceberg' that is 'below the waterline', i.e. outside the immediate access of the 'event analysts'. In addition, the question arises, how large is this normally invisible part? In order to get a better idea of potentially safety-critical situations, the aviation industry has conducted a so-called Human Factor Research Project. It has been the most comprehensive study of its kind: 2,070 pilots filled in a 120-page questionnaire. The survey asked for explanations and descriptions of the safety-critical incident that was experienced last. The answers added up to three million two hundred thousand data records. Evaluation of the data took more than two years.

In table 1 the six risk classes established in the Human Factor Research Project are shown. The mean risk value in the above survey is 3.4, i.e. an incident in which the safety-critical impacts could nearly entirely be controlled by the pilots. It is striking that the higher risk classes 4, 5, and 6 together make up for more than 40% of all safety-critical incidents. So the reported events were not just 'peanuts', but a large share of them represent a significant danger potential. Different from a collection of reports on safety-critical incidents, the questionnaires do not, however, reveal how the event developed in detail (no scandalous stories); they only deal with possible influence and disturbance variables, also for reasons of anonymity. Based on the survey data, four main categories have been established, which cover the major aspects of the problems:
- TEC: technical problems, failure of systems;
- HUM: human errors;
- OPS: operational problems, complications;
- SOC: aggravating social factors.

The OPS category refers to influences complicating the operating procedure beyond the standard rate. SOC refers to the team situation in the cockpit: communication deficits, bad crew resource management (CRM; a strategy for optimal utilization of all resources and information that are available to a team), conflicts (which are quite often not openly expressed), a too steep or too flat hierarchy, psychic or psychological problems, etc.

Table 1. The six risk classes established in the Human Factor Research Project

Risk class	Explanation	Description
1	There was an irregular incident. But there was no need to act. It was clear that there would be no safety-relevant impacts.	'No problem'
2	There was a safety-relevant incident. Appropriate actions of the crew made it possible to avoid the building up of any effects that would have impaired safety.	'Routine'
3	There was a safety-relevant incident. The crew was able to control all the effects of the incident completely.	'Well done'
4	There was a safety-relevant incident. The effects of the incident could be controlled only partially by the crew (cockpit, cabin).	'Things turned out all right in the end.'
5	There was a safety-relevant incident. The effects of the incident could not be controlled by the crew (cockpit, cabin). In the end, it was only possible to manage the situation because no further aggravating factors occurred. The last link in the error chain was missing.	'By a hair's breadth ...'
6	There was a safety-relevant incident. The situation got completely out of control, and we survived only by chance or by luck.	'Oh, shit!'

For evaluation, the different risk categories were first considered separately. If the above factors occur alone, the following percentages result (percentage of the total number of incidents): TEC 7.7%, HUM 4.9%, OPS 1.2%, SOC 0.7%. It shows that, when considering individual incidences, TEC are at the top of the scale, followed by HUM. At first sight, this is surprising: How does this figure relate to the fact that 75% of all accidents worldwide are human factor accidents? The analysis shows that cockpit crews are normally well able to manage one single error. The safety network of structured cockpit work eases solitary human errors.

The Effect of Simultaneously Occurring Risk Factors

In a second step the analysis comes closer to the actual risk potential: Now two categories are combined respectively (e.g. TEC + HUM or OPS + SOC, etc.). Here we see that the dangerous impact of the human factor increases when it is combined with other factors. If operational problems (complications) and a human error occur simultaneously, the share of safety-critical incidents increases to 8.3%. Statistics show that a well-organized work environment has considerable risk-reducing influence. The largest risk group with two combined factors is the combination of human factor (HUM) and problematic social climate (SOC). This combination is responsible for

13.7% of all incidents. This shows that the work atmosphere has a much larger influence on risk than complications. All three categories (HUM, HUM + OPS, HUM + SOC) together, however, account for only 26.9% of all safety-critical incidents. What makes up the most important share of the often potentially fatal human factor?

Social Factors – 'Turbofactor' with Regard to Human Error

The next evaluation step gives an answer to this question. When considering combinations of three risk factors (e.g. TEC + OPS + SOC), the following picture develops: By far the most frequent safety-critical situation (37.8% of all events) consists of the following combination: 1. A complication develops (OPS). 2. In this situation of increased stress a human error occurs (HUM). 3. The negative effects of the error cannot be corrected or eased because the working climate (SOC) is not optimal.

This means that a negative social climate has the effect of a 'turbocharger' when a human error occurs: In many cases, tense human relationships turn a 'harmless' error into a potentially life-threatening situation. It needs to be pointed out that a tense atmosphere is usually not identical with a dispute. In many cases, the working climate is burdened without the person responsible for the bad climate noticing it. The others involved in the situation frequently only sense an 'undefined feeling of unease'. A first negative impression, too much or too little respect, contempt, misunderstandings, a bad mood brought from home, lack of motivation, etc. can considerably reduce the efficiency of a team. A first and important step to ease the problem is to clearly express one's own feeling of unease or other personal feelings. Normally, a considerable inner reluctance needs to be overcome to be able to do this. But already statements such as 'I do not feel comfortable in our teamwork' or 'I have the feeling that there are problems nobody addresses' can be a first step to improve the cooperation.

Especially in professions characterized by the picture of brilliant experts who solve any problem without difficulties it is a real challenge to address 'soft' psychosocial factors. Nonetheless, this area must not be neglected or repressed, as this risk potential was not discovered, articulated, and put into the foreground by 'worldly innocent' psychologists, but by those people responsible for the problems.

Working Climate and Safety

Everybody knows that the working climate has an influence on the quality of work and on safety. It is surprising, however, that the impact of 'atmospheric disturbances' is so high. According to the above findings, the fact that colleagues do not get along well with each other ranges highest on the scale of safety problems. Social tensions in the team increase the risk of a safety-critical incident by the factor 5; in other words: An optimal working atmosphere could mitigate or ease 80% of all safety-critical human errors. The study has thus proven a quantitative connection between the 'soft factor' social climate and the risk of dangerous incidents. However, not only the number of incidents increases, but also the risk class! The mean risk of incidents caused by the human factor (HF) amounts to 3.57.

Training for Optimized Teamwork

What does this statement imply for our work organization and for training? The efforts to achieve optimal CRM and optimal team structures must be intensified. In the past, bad team behavior and a miserable atmosphere in the work environment were frequently tolerated with the argument '… but he/she is technically quite competent!' This statement should no longer be accepted. Survey evaluations show that bad team behavior triggers a major share of safety-critical incidents; they are frequently not eased by excellent abilities but simply by good luck. This implies that deficits in team behavior must consequently be addressed by individual colleagues as well as by trainers and superiors. As already mentioned, this is more easily said than done, since the subject often requires more far-reaching discussions. A first reaction to this result of the survey could be to ask not to assign any 'unpleasant' colleagues to the job who do not immediately create a 'great atmosphere' in the team. But in general, this measure would not ease the problem since everybody once in a while – and often unconsciously – burdens the work climate for the colleagues by his/her behavior. Therefore, it will probably be more successful to provide all colleagues with tools that ensure optimal handling of social problems (in a wider sense). Obviously social competence is also important for managing safety problems in technically oriented fields of work, a fact that has been seriously underestimated in the past.

The Various Risk Categories

Figure 1 shows the percentages for the individual risk groups and the frequency distribution by event configurations. The figures reveal that the survey made it possible to break down the fine structure of the safety-relevant human factors: When adding up all categories in which the factor 'human errors' appears, the total is 79.1%. This figure corresponds more or less with the 75% of the IATA (International Air Transport Association) accident statistics.

Social Problems in the Team

What does the term SOC mean if you look at it more closely? The structure of the questionnaire deliberately addressed possible impairments: Approximately 32% of

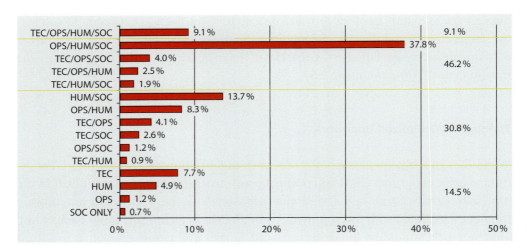

Fig. 1. Possible combinations of the various risk categories. The uppermost line shows the combination of all four groups: Technical problems (TEC), operational problems (OPS), human errors (HUM), and social problems (SOC) account for 9.1% of all incidents. The second data block shows the combinations of three factors. The largest block (37.8%) consists of OPS, HUM, and SOC. In the data block with the combinations of two factors, HUM and SOC show the highest percentage (13.7%). SOC represent with 0.7% the smallest group in the data block with one risk category.

these unfavorable CRM events are triggered by a single-handed action of one pilot. This figure shows that a behavior that is not jointly coordinated and agreed upon poses a safety problem. There is normally no 'ill' will behind such an approach. Time pressure, target fixation, or unexpected complications shortly before the expected completion of a task can turn a good team player into a 'Rambo' in no time. A single-handed attempt of one team member is usually triggered by the captain. Because of the hierarchical structure and the overall responsibility, it is normally a simple matter for the boss to stop a single-handed action of a team member. For a hierarchically subordinate employee, it is much more difficult to convince the boss of the problematic nature of a decision that was made alone, because he/she has to overcome a huge emotional hurdle before expressing criticism from the position of the subordinate. The larger the difference in age or in hierarchy between the team members, the more difficult it can be for the employee to utter criticism.

The fact that approximately one third of all CRM problems is due to 'lone wolfing' shows that there is an urgent need for action in this field and that a team has to make efforts again and again to create a common work basis. A very important preventive measure in this context is the avoidance of any rush. Figure 1 shows that the factor 'SOC only' represents the tail light of the various risk categories with only 0.7%. This clearly tells that social problems, as an isolated factor, are practically irrelevant as the cause of a safety-critical event. Great efforts are being made to create a positive working atmosphere. Existing difficulties become obvious only when additional burdening factors occur.

Who Is Going to Teach Optimized Teamwork?

Who should carry out the relevant training? Basic knowledge of CRM should certainly be taught by psychological experts. However, this method of teaching can be applied to only a relatively limited extent, since the actual knowledge transfer takes place with reference to the personal working situation and must therefore be explained and accompanied by colleagues of the same professional field. In order to be efficient and accepted, the training must be implemented in the specific environment and can, therefore, only be rendered by specialists (pilots, medical doctors) as trainers and multipliers. The results of the survey give additional support to these efforts. More training in this field, however, must never make cutbacks in basic technical training tolerable. CRM training is no substitute for technical knowledge; it is only a necessary supplement.

Communication Deficits

The following figures should illustrate the problems assigned to the field of SOC. It has already been mentioned that 'additional aggravating factors in the field of social interaction' were found in 68.4% of all events described. That this very rarely means a dispute in the common sense or an openly fought conflict has already been explained. In 77.4% of the cases with aggravating factors in the area of social interaction, communication problems were reported. In 48% of all incidents, necessary statements were not made, and corresponding hints were not given; unclear concerns were not expressed; important statements were incomplete, insufficient, or were not heard.

In the above cases, the sender of the message is the one who was negligent, since the quality of communication is entirely determined by whatever arrives at the other end. For this reason, the sender of a message has the obligation to check what information the receiver has actually perceived. The problem, therefore, is not the captain's lack of readiness to put a hint received into the according action, but the missing courage of the first officer to address deviations consequently and clearly.

In only 23% of all communication problems, no corresponding reaction followed a clearly understood hint. But there is a strategy to deal with this type of situation, too. If there is no reaction to a correcting hint, the concern must be repeated. If the first officer does not speak up and the captain is exclusively fixed on the target, this can result in the noncorrection of an error. The worst accident in civil aviation with 583 casualties happened because a young copilot did not have the courage to correct the experienced trainer captain a second time.

Violation of Rules

The so-called violation of rules constitutes a large share of human errors by the cockpit crew. A few years ago, a Boeing taskforce dealt with this phenomenon. The study analyzed accidents. When investigating cases of total loss, the investigating team did not ask what caused the accident, but searched for means that could have prevented it. The survey shows that about 80% of all accidents could have been prevented by strictly observing the rules and regulations. For this reason, the area 'working in accordance with rules' is of special interest to us in the evaluation of the cockpit study, because the statement of the Boeing study means that the number of accidents (at present approx. 18 per year on average) could be reduced by 80% (or approx. 14 total losses per year) at once, if the pilots observed the rules strictly.

Seventy-seven percent (n = 940) of all human errors that trigger a safety-critical incident are nonobservances of rules (omission/violation). The usefulness and protective effect of the rules is not questioned in principle. Nonetheless, violations of fundamental rules obviously occur again and again: time pressure, immense routine, complacency, and the feeling of being invulnerable reduce the threshold to violating rules.

Standard Operating Procedure (SOP)

As a principle rule, there are several procedures to solve a task – all offering the same level of safety. For this reason, it does not necessarily become clear at first glance why they should be limited to a few strictly defined SOPs. There are, however, several reasons for making and observing binding agreements. To be able to control each other and to address deviations from the rules, all cockpit members must be able to refer to commonly accepted procedures. When applying 'personal procedures', the controlling person can no longer determine whether the working step is desired in the way it is implemented or whether an unintentional human error has crept in. If a crew works in this gray zone, it has to rely on its feelings, which are bad or even fatal advisors, as has been documented by many flight accidents.

Failure and Readiness to Take a Risk

Behaviorism presents another important argument for disciplined work. After a tolerated rule violation, the threshold for further, often even more serious violations is reduced. For this reason, deviations from rules must be addressed as soon as they occur, in order to prevent a cascade of violations. The captain is responsible for the observance of binding rules. He or she is assisted by a responsible first officer as a means of support and an additional 'control and redundancy organ'. Thus, a violation of defined rules always means that the redundancy structure in the cockpit has failed. The tolerance threshold accepted by the first officer determines the mesh size of the safety network.

Experience and Adherence to Rules

A high level of self-discipline is required in order to consequently observe rules that are partly considered as inflexible after years of successful work. Training and management personnel is particularly endangered in this respect. A person who has participated in working out the rules and constantly remembers the partially controversial discussion resulting in their implementation sometimes has great difficulty in adhering to these rules. However, because of the trainer's model function, a violation of rules by the trainer has an especially strong negative effect because human errors occurring in this context most probably are corrected by the inexperienced colleague since he/she does not expect this type of rule violation.

Risk and Motivation

In this context, motivation also plays a major role. An investigation of the United States Navy has shown that 90% of the pilots who get involved in a human error accident have serious motivation problems. With fading motivation, the readiness to violate a rule and to accept a higher risk increases. Only those who are highly motivated work carefully and foresightedly and are highly concentrated. The anticipation of possible consequences is the more difficult the more reluctantly a job is done. Apart from discipline and motivation, the readiness to accept one's own imperfection is an imperative prerequisite for good teamwork. Only a person who accepts his/her own weaknesses can convincingly ask for and express criticism (passive and active ability to criticize).

Moral and Values

The personal system of values also plays a decisive role. If we do not show empathy and a certain principal bestowal toward our team members, they will not point out incongruities and possible mistakes with the necessary clarity in a complex critical situation.

Complex Technology as 'Teacher' of Human Interaction

The expectation that a high level of technology will render the technical knowledge of the machine operator and the common sense of man superfluous to a large extent has not been fulfilled. It is almost a paradox of human history that man's efforts to develop machines that compensate human weaknesses have led to the present situation where the inherently human abilities of social competence and optimal teamwork are of utmost importance when dealing with HITEC devices.

Disclosure of Conflict of Interests

The author states that he has no conflict of interest.

Manfred H. Müller
Private Akademie für Risikomanagement
Rudolf-Camerer-Str. 18, 81369 München, Germany
Tel. +49 151 589 34010
E-Mail manfred.mueller@akarisma.de

Scharf RE (ed): Progress and Challenges in Transfusion Medicine, Hemostasis and Hemotherapy.
Freiburg i.Br., Karger, 2008, pp 15–23

Allogeneic Hematopoietic Cell Transplantation – 2008: Achievements and Challenges

Karl G. Blume

Stanford University School of Medicine, Stanford, CA, USA

Key Words

Allogeneic hematopoietic cell transplantation (HCT) · Hematologic malignancies · Bone marrow failure conditions · Graft-versus-host disease · Graft-versus-tumor effect · Quality of life after HCT

Summary

Following the first successful allogeneic hematopoietic cell transplant (HCT) procedures in 1968, the cumulative number of patients treated with HCT has now risen to approximately 850,000 worldwide. Great strides have been made during the past four decades to overcome the major obstacles to make HCT a widely available treatment modality for patients with life-threatening bone marrow disorders – provided a suitable histocompatible donor can be identified. HCT is a paradigm for successful translational research: from curative concept to cure.   ©2008 S. Karger GmbH, Freiburg i.Br.

Introduction to and History of Allogeneic Hematopoietic Cell Transplantation (HCT)

In 1868, two experimental pathologists, Neumann in Königsberg/Prussia and Bizzozero in Pavia/Italy, independently reported that it is the function of bone marrow to generate all types of blood cells [1, 2]. This novel scientific information stimulated the interest of physicians who assumed that one could correct disorders of the blood, such as leukemia, by transferring new bone marrow to the afflicted patients. However, in those years there was no experimental basis for transplanting tissues from one individual to the next and, not surprisingly, all clinical efforts were unsuccessful.

The first observation that bone marrow cells can restore hematopoiesis in lethally irradiated mice was described in 1951 by Lorenz et al. [3]. Again this finding excited clinicians, and the thought of transplanting hematopoietic cells was eagerly pursued [4]. However, during these years essential information was still missing, the most important one being a method to select for a compatible donor. The clinical efforts to res-

Table 1. Clinical use of allogeneic hematopoietic cell transplantation

Disease/Condition	Disease/Condition
Malignant disorders	*Nonmalignant disorders*
Acute leukemia (myeloblastic; lymphoblastic)	Aplastic anemia
Chronic myelogenous leukemia	Fanconi anemia
Chronic lymphocytic leukemia	Thalassemia
Myelodysplastic syndromes	Sickle cell anemia
Myeloproliferative syndromes	Congenital pure red cell aplasia
Non-Hodgkin lymphoma	Paroxysmal nocturnal hemoglobinuria
Hodgkin disease	Severe combined immunodeficiency
Multiple myeloma	Wiskott-Aldrich syndrome
	Congenital leukocyte dysfunction syndromes
	Osteopetrosis
	Familial erythrophagocytic lymphohistiocytosis
	Hereditary storage disorders
	Glanzmann disease
	Selected autoimmune disorders

cue patients with leukemia and other malignancies by transplanting bone marrow from healthy individuals failed again, and it appeared that HCT had no future [5]. Fortunately, in parallel to the clinical transplant attempts, investigators worked to define conditions for successful HCT. The preclinical experiments were mostly performed in mice, rats, monkeys, and dogs. Valuable information was gathered in those years leading to the following milestones: The histocompatibility system was developed, new antibiotics became available, platelet transfusions were standardized, and other supportive care measures such as protective isolation and parenteral nutrition were introduced.

Finally, in 1968, an entire century after the reports by Neumann and Bizzozero had appeared, the time for the first successful HCT procedures had arrived. Independently, three groups of investigators in Madison/WI, in Minneapolis/MN, and in Leiden/Holland, successfully performed HCT procedures in three children who were suffering from severe immunodeficiency disorders [6–8]. All three patients engrafted and became long-term survivors who have now been followed for up to 40 years. In those days, a group of investigators in Seattle/WA, directed by Dr. E. Donnall Thomas, laid the foundation for HCT in patients with leukemia and other hematologic malignancies. During those early years of clinical HCT, only patients with relapsed diseases were transplanted. However, it was possible to save several of these hopelessly ill patients, and approximately 10% of them became disease-free long-term survivors [9, 10]. After it was demonstrated that the concept of HCT was successful in patients in advanced disease stages, the next step was taken, i.e., to explore HCT with better chances for cure in candidates with acute leukemia in first complete remission [11–13]. Since the mid-1970s, based on convincing preclinical and clinical studies,

Table 2. Problems and accomplishments of allogeneic hematopoietic cell transplantation

Recipient age	Graft-versus-host disease
Availability of a suitable donor	Relapse
Regimen-related toxicity	Second and secondary malignancies
Graft failure and rejection	Quality of life issues
Opportunistic infections	Cost and charges

the use of and indications for HCT grew exponentially. A list of diseases now considered curable by HCT includes a broad range of hematologic malignancies, bone marrow failure conditions, hemoglobin disorders, immunodeficiencies, and certain autoimmune diseases (table 1). In 1990, Dr. Thomas was honored for his work by receiving the Nobel Prize in Physiology and Medicine. At the end of the 20th century, several hundred thousand patients had undergone HCT worldwide [14], and by now the estimated cumulative number is approximately 850,000 worldwide.

Achievements and Challenges

With the first patients treated 40 years ago, it became apparent that HCT recipients are facing some formidable challenges, mostly clinical complications related to high-dose therapy, infectious complications, and delayed immune reconstitution aggravated by graft-versus-host disease (GVHD). However, it was also soon recognized that a graft-versus-tumor effect (GVTE) played a beneficial role after HCT. The past four decades have witnessed impressive achievements in the entire field of HCT resulting in an ever increasing number of patients becoming long-term survivors and remaining free of their underlying diseases [14]. Table 2 provides a list of challenges and achievements of HCT. In the following part of this presentation, these areas will be discussed sequentially.

Recipient Age

Initially, most HCT candidates were young patients with end-stage acute leukemia, usually children, adolescents, and young adults. Over time, improvement in conditioning regimens, graft preparation, GVHD prophylaxis, supportive care, antimicrobial drugs, and other supportive care measures have helped raise the patients' age limit to include older adults. Especially, the introduction of reduced-intensity conditioning (RIC) had a major impact on the inclusion of older candidates up to the age of 75 years. It can be stated that in general, younger patients are better able to tolerate high-dose regimens and there is a higher chance of a young person benefiting from HCT compared to older patients.

Availability of a Suitable Donor

In the beginning, HCT was performed exclusively in the 30% of patients who were fortunate enough to have a histocompatible sibling donor. This limitation excluded the majority of HCT candidates, and the need for alternative donors became an urgent problem. For some patients (about 5%), a closely matched alternative related donor could be identified but that still left a vast majority of patients unserved. In the 1980s, the Anthony Nolan Foundation in Great Britain and the National Marrow Donor Program (NMDP) in the United States were started. Other countries followed with similar efforts resulting in a current total pool of approximately 12 million volunteer donors worldwide. It is now possible to find a suitably matched donor for approximately 70% of HCT candidates.

Regimen-Related Toxicity

During the first three decades of HCT, i.e., until the late 1990s, the preparatory conditioning regimens contained mostly high doses of total body irradiation (TBI), delivered since 1980 on a fractionated schedule, combined with high doses of chemotherapeutic drugs, mostly cyclophosphamide (CY), etoposide (VP-16), and other drugs [15–17]. For certain diseases like chronic myelogenous leukemia (CML), busulfan (BU) in combination with CY was found to be as powerful as TBI/CY.

The use of these regimens was based on the concept that high-dose approaches would lead to eradication of all malignant cells (along with the residual healthy hematopoietic cells) and that the graft would serve as the source for all new donor-derived bone marrow and blood cells.

Soon after the first patients were transplanted successfully, the complex interaction between the feared GVHD and the beneficial immunologic activity of the graft against the residual malignant cells (GVTE) was recognized [18]. Several highly informative preclinical studies were performed and served as the basis for clinical trials in which conditioning regimens with reduced intensity (RIC) were explored [19, 20]. A great deal of experience has now been gathered with combinations of low-dose TBI and fludarabine (FLU), or a combination of low-dose total lymphoid irradiation (TLI) and antithymocyte globulin (ATG), or a drug-only combination of BU/FLU [21–23]. These approaches mostly rely on the GVTE mechanism, e.g., TLI/ATG is essentially an immunosuppressive regimen which does not directly kill tumor cells but exploits the GVTE mechanism for tumor ablation.

Graft Failure and Rejection

Through the research of the human leukocyte antigen (HLA) system, it became possible to determine the most compatible donor, both among related and unrelated individuals. Moreover, preclinical studies and clinical observations helped define the minimum number of nucleated cells needed for durable engraftment. Through the introduction of flow cytometric techniques, the precursor cell marker CD34 was found to represent a suitable surrogate for stem cells. A minimum of 2–5 million CD34+ cells/kg recipient body weight have been generally defined as the minimum number of precursor cells in a graft needed for permanent engraftment from a histocompatible sibling donor. The need for more CD34+ cells increases with the degree of HLA incompatibility.

When RIC regimens were first explored, it became clear that peripheral blood grafts obtained through apheresis were more consistently leading to durable donor cell engraftment than the conventional bone marrow grafts [24]. However, since the donor blood cell concentrates contain more T cells, chronic GVHD is seen in a significantly higher number of recipients whose graft is blood derived than in those patients who receive bone marrow cells [25].

Primary graft failure and secondary graft rejection are rare. They occur after approximately 1% of HCT procedures from HLA-identical sibling donors. Before molecular HLA typing was introduced into the selection searches for unrelated donors, the rejection rate of those grafts was about 10%. With markedly improved tissue typing methods, the rejection rate of grafts from unrelated donors is now reduced to low single digit figures.

Opportunistic Infections

The HCT recipient of an allogeneic graft is an immunocompromised host for an extended prior of time – at least for months and often for years. Early after HCT, gramnegative bacteria were the most frequent pathogens leading to overwhelming sepsis. Infections with gram-positive bacteria are most often encountered in patients who are afflicted with chronic GVHD. The introduction of potent broad-spectrum antibiotics reduced bacteria-associated infections to a minimum.

In the 1970s and 1980s, DNA viruses, especially cytomegalovirus (CMV), led to interstitial lung disease in some 15–20% of HCT recipients and proved to be fatal in almost all affected patients. The development of gancyclovir led to successful preventive strategies against CMV [26]. Gancyclovir, in combination with immunoglobulins, proved effective as therapy for those with established CMV pneumonitis and other organ manifestations.

Fungal infections, in particular those with *Aspergillus*, still represent some of the most serious infectious complications after HCT. Newer drugs, the latest being posaconazole, have been introduced, and it appears that the incidence of mold infections is decreasing [27, 28]. Better preventative and therapeutic strategies are still being developed.

Graft-versus-Host Disease

This complication of allogeneic HCT is caused by immunocompetent T cells in the inoculum and by those donor-derived lymphocytes which originate from the transplant. The acute variant of GVHD afflicts to various degrees mostly skin, liver, and the gut, while the chronic manifestations of GVHD resemble autoimmune disorders. Removal of donor T cells from the graft effectively prevents GVHD, however, this manipulation is associated with an increased incidence of graft failure and more relapse of the underlying malignancies. Prevention of GVHD by exposure to combinations of immunosuppressive drugs (methotrexate, cyclosporine, rapamycin, mycophenolate mofetil, tacrolimus, prednisone and others) reduces the incidence of moderate to severe GVHD to about 10–50% of cases. Drug prophylaxis is the most commonly utilized strategy [29]. There is currently no ideal method to prevent GVHD from occurring. Some patients proceed from acute GVHD to the chronic manifestation of this syndrome, while others develop a de novo onset of chronic GVHD. There are limited or extensive manifestations of chronic GVHD which are associated with the benefit of a reduction in disease recurrence, but also may decrease the patient's performance status and affect the quality of life after HCT.

Relapse

Allogeneic HCT procedures are performed most often for patients with hematologic malignancies. A relapse of the underlying disease depends on a number of factors. First, the remission status and the extent of tumor burden at the time of HCT are predictive of relapse-free survival. Second, the response of the malignancy to the various components of the preparatory regimen also affects the outcome, i.e., some malignant cells are more sensitive to a radiation-containing regimen – e.g., acute lymphoblastic leukemia (ALL) responds best to TBI/VP-16 – while other diseases are easier eradicated by chemotherapy-only combinations (CML is best treated with BU/CY).

Data from large clinical trials indicate that the risk of a post-transplant relapse doubles with the event of each disease recurrence prior to HCT, i.e., patients transplanted in first complete remission (CR) of acute leukemia have a chance of 50–80% disease-free survival, while the same procedure performed during second CR results in long-term disease-free survival of only 20–40% of patients. This rule can be applied to the outcomes prediction of HCT for most malignancies.

Second and Secondary Malignancies

Patients who are diagnosed with cancer have an increased risk of later developing a second malignancy, even if the first tumor is surgically removed and there is no exposure to radiation or chemotherapy (second malignancy). Those who are treated with drugs and/or radiation are at an even higher risk for a new tumor later on in life (secondary or treatment-associated malignancy). HCT recipients have usually undergone prior chemotherapy for remission induction and – depending on the underlying disease – have also been exposed to local radiation therapy. These forms of treatment result in cumulative risk of another malignancy, especially if the preparatory regimen contains alkylating agents and TBI. The largest long-term evaluation of over 28 years has captured 19,229 patients who had undergone HCT from allogeneic or syngeneic donors. The risk of a new solid cancer was 8.3 times as high as expected among those who survived ten or more years [30]. The most frequent tumor locations were the bone system and the oral cavity.

Quality of Life

After the first HCT recipients were treated successfully and were followed over time, it became apparent that survival was only one issue on the patient's mind. They wanted to live *and* be reintegrated into their personal and professional lives. Quality of life questionnaires covering the most important domains were developed to quantitate aspects of distress and kinetics of recovery. Self-assessment scores indicate reassuring outcomes results, however, it should be emphasized that the return to pretherapy levels may take years [31].

Cost and Charges

All medical interventions, especially if they require prolonged hospital admissions, are very expensive – even more so in the United States than in Europe. Unfortunately, exact financial data are hard to obtain as they are rarely published. Hospital administrators on both sides of the Atlantic have detected HCT as a lucrative treatment modality, and for a while 'stem cell transplants' were seen as good business. Data from 1999 indicate average HCT charges of USD 232,600 for allogeneic HCT procedures from related donors and USD 293,100 from unrelated volunteer donors, respectively [32]. I do not have access to newer figures, but I suspect that they are considerably higher at this time than those from 9 years ago.

Conclusions and Future Directions

The past four decades have witnessed dramatic improvements in the field of allogeneic HCT. Through the development of new drugs and technologies, the incidence and severity of treatment-related complications have decreased dramatically resulting in an ever increasing number of patients cured of their life-threatening diseases. However, as in all areas of clinical research, progress has been slow to occur. This is not surprising because all new developments must be tested preclinically, need evaluation in exploratory studies, and also require long-term clinical observations under controlled research conditions. It is always a long way from a curative concept to the cure for patients with cancer, and HCT is no exception.

Disclosure of Conflict of Interests

The author states that he has no conflict of interest. He serves as the Chairman of the Advisory Council for Blood Stem Cell Transplantation for the Department of Health and Human Services, USA.

References

1 Neumann E: Ueber die Bedeutung des Knochenmarkes für die Blutbildung. Centralbl Med Wiss 1868;44:44.
2 Bizzozero G: Sulla funzione ematopoetica del midollo delle ossa. Gazz Med Ital Lombardia 1868;46:381.
3 Lorenz E, Uphoff D, Reid TR, Shelton E: Modification of irradiation injury in mice and guinea pigs by bone marrow injections. J Natl Cancer Inst 1951;12:197–201.
4 Thomas ED, Lochte HL Jr., Lu WC, Ferrebee JW: Intravenous infusion of bone marrow in patients receiving radiation and chemotherapy. N Engl J Med 1957;257:491–496.
5 Bortin MM: A compendium of reported human bone marrow transplants. Transplantation 1970;9:571–587.
6 Bach FH, Albertini RJ, Joo P, Anderson JL, Bortin MM: Bone-marrow transplantation in a patient with the Wiskott-Aldrich syndrome. Lancet 1968;2:1364–1366.
7 Gatti RA, Meuwissen HJ, Allen HD, Hong R, Good RA: Immunological reconstitution of sex-linked lymphopenic immunological deficiency. Lancet 1968;2:1366–1369.
8 De Koning J, Van Bekkum DW, Dicke KA, Dooren LJ, Radl J, Van Rood JJ: Transplantation of bone-marrow cells and fetal thymus in an infant with lymphopenic immunological deficiency. Lancet 1969;1:1223–1227.
9 Thomas E, Storb R, Clift RA, Fefer A, Johnson L, Neiman PE, Lerner KG, Glucksberg H, Buckner CD: Bone-marrow transplantation (first of two parts). N Engl J Med 1975;292:832–843.
10 Thomas ED, Storb R, Clift RA, Fefer A, Johnson L, Neiman PE, Lerner KG, Glucksberg H, Buckner CD: Bone-marrow transplantation (second of two parts). N Engl J Med 1975;292:895–902.
11 Thomas ED, Buckner CD, Clift RA, Fefer A, Johnson FL, Neiman PE, Sale GE, Sanders JE, Singer JW, Shulman H, Storb R, Weiden PL: Marrow transplantation for acute nonlymphoblastic leukemia in first remission. N Engl J Med 1979;301:597–599.
12 Blume KG, Beutler E, Bross KJ, Chillar RK, Ellington OB, Fahey JL, Farbstein MJ, Forman SJ, Schmidt GM, Scott EP, Spruce WE, Turner MA, Wolf JL: Bone-marrow ablation and allogeneic marrow transplantation in acute leukemia. N Engl J Med 1980;302:1041–1046.
13 Powles RL, Morgenstern G, Clink HM, Hedley D, Bandini G, Lumley H, Watson JG, Lawson D, Spence D, Barrett A, Jameson B, Lawler S, Kay HE, McElwain TJ: The place of bone-marrow transplantation in acute myelogenous leukaemia. Lancet 1980;1:1047–1050.
14 Thomas ED, Blume KG: Historical markers in the development of allogeneic hematopoietic cell transplantation. Biol Blood Marrow Transplant 1999;5:341–346.

15 Buckner CD, Epstein RB, Rudolph RH, Clift RA, Storb R, Thomas ED: Allogeneic marrow engraftment following whole body irradiation in a patient with leukemia. Blood 1970;35:741–750.

16 Blume KG, Forman SJ, O'Donnell MR, Doroshow JH, Krance RA, Nademanee AP, Snyder DS, Schmidt GM, Fahey JL, Metter GE: Total body irradiation and high-dose etoposide: a new preparatory regimen for bone marrow transplantation in patients with advanced hematologic malignancies. Blood 1987;69:1015–1020.

17 Tutschka PJ, Copelan EA, Klein JP: Bone marrow transplantation for leukemia following a new busulfan and cyclophosphamide regimen. Blood 1987;70:1382–1388.

18 Weiden PL, Flournoy N, Thomas ED, Prentice R, Fefer A, Buckner CD, Storb R: Antileukemic effect of graft-versus-host disease in human recipients of allogeneic-marrow grafts. N Engl J Med 1979;300:1068–1073.

19 Slavin S, Fuks Z, Kaplan HS, Strober S: Transplantation of allogeneic bone marrow without graft-versus-host disease using total lymphoid irradiation. J Exp Med 1978;147:963–972.

20 Storb R, Yu C, Wagner JL, Deeg HJ, Nash RA, Kiem HP, Leisenring W, Shulman H: Stable mixed hematopoietic chimerism in DLA-identical littermate dogs given sublethal total body irradiation before and pharmacological immunosuppression after marrow transplantation. Blood 1997;89:3048–3054.

21 McSweeney PA, Niederwieser D, Shizuru JA, Sandmaier BM, Molina AJ, Maloney DG, Chauncey TR, Gooley TA, Hegenbart U, Nash RA, Radich J, Wagner JL, Minor S, Appelbaum FR, Bensinger WI, Bryant E, Flowers ME, Georges GE, Grumet FC, Kiem HP, Torok-Storb B, Yu C, Blume KG, Storb RF: Hematopoietic cell transplantation in older patients with hematologic malignancies: replacing high-dose cytotoxic therapy with graft-versus-tumor effects. Blood 2001;97:3390–3400.

22 Lowsky R, Takahashi T, Liu YP, Dejbakhsh-Jones S, Grumet FC, Shizuru JA, Laport GG, Stockerl-Goldstein KE, Johnston LJ, Hoppe RT, Bloch DA, Blume KG, Negrin RS, Strober S: Protective conditioning for acute graft-versus-host disease. N Engl J Med 2005;353:1321–1331.

23 Alyea EP, Kim HT, Ho V, Cutler C, Gribben J, DeAngelo DJ, Lee SJ, Windawi S, Ritz J, Stone RM, Antin JH, Soiffer RJ: Comparative outcome of nonmyeloablative and myeloablative allogeneic hematopoietic cell transplantation for patients older than 50 years of age. Blood 2005;105:1810–1814.

24 Maris MB, Niederwieser D, Sandmaier BM, Storer B, Stuart M, Maloney D, Petersdorf E, McSweeney P, Pulsipher M, Woolfrey A, Chauncey T, Agura E, Heimfeld S, Slattery J, Hegenbart U, Anasetti C, Blume K, Storb R: HLA-matched unrelated donor hematopoietic cell transplantation after nonmyeloablative conditioning for patients with hematologic malignancies. Blood 2003;102:2021–2030.

25 Schmitz N, Eapen M, Horowitz MM, Zhang MJ, Klein JP, Rizzo JD, Loberiza FR, Gratwohl A, Champlin RE; International Bone Marrow Transplant Registry; European Group for Blood and Marrow Transplantation: Long-term outcome of patients given transplants of mobilized blood or bone marrow: a report from the International Bone Marrow Transplant Registry and the European Group for Blood and Marrow Transplantation. Blood 2006;108:4288–4290.

26 Schmidt GM, Horak DA, Niland JC, Duncan SR, Forman SJ, Zaia JA: A randomized, controlled trial of prophylactic ganciclovir for cytomegalovirus pulmonary infection in recipients of allogeneic bone marrow transplants; The City of Hope-Stanford-Syntex CMV Study Group. N Engl J Med 1991;324:1005–1011.

27 Ullmann AJ, Lipton JH, Vesole DH, Chandrasekar P, Langston A, Tarantolo SR, Greinix H, Morais de Azevedo W, Reddy V, Boparai N, Pedicone L, Patino H, Durrant S: Posaconazole or fluconazole for prophylaxis in severe graft-versus-host disease. N Engl J Med 2007;356:335–347.

28 Cornely OA, Maertens J, Winston DJ, Perfect J, Ullmann AJ, Walsh TJ, Helfgott D, Holowiecki J, Stockelberg D, Goh YT, Petrini M, Hardalo C, Suresh R, Angulo-Gonzalez D: Posaconazole vs. fluconazole or itraconazole prophylaxis in patients with neutropenia. N Engl J Med 2007;356:348–359.

29 Chao NJ, Sullivan KM: Pharmacologic Prevention of Acute Graft-versus-Host Disease. Oxford, Blackwell Scientific, 2009 (in press).

30 Curtis RE, Rowlings PA, Deeg HJ, Shriner DA, Socíe G, Travis LB, Horowitz MM, Witherspoon RP, Hoover RN, Sobocinski KA, Fraumeni JF Jr, Boice JD Jr: Solid cancers after bone marrow transplantation. N Engl J Med 1997;336:897–904.

31 Syrjala KL, Langer SL, Abrams JR, Storer B, Sanders JE, Flowers ME, Martin PJ: Recovery and long-term function after hematopoietic cell transplantation for leukemia or lymphoma. JAMA 2004;291:2335–2343.

32 Haubolt R: Research Report. *www.milliman.com*.

Prof. Karl G. Blume, M.D.
Stanford University School of Medicine
300 Pasteur Drive, Room H3249
Stanford, CA 94305-5623, USA
E-Mail kgblume@stanford.edu

Scharf RE (ed): Progress and Challenges in Transfusion Medicine, Hemostasis and Hemotherapy.
Freiburg i.Br., Karger, 2008, pp 24–36

Endothelium and Hemostasis in Health and Disease

Jan Steffel · Thomas F. Lüscher

Cardiology, CardioVascular Center, University Hospital Zurich and Cardiovascular Research, Institute of Physiology, University of Zurich, Switzerland

Key Words

Endothelium · Hemostasis · Coagulation · Atherosclerosis · Tissue factor · Coronary artery disease

Summary

The endothelium is critically involved in maintaining vascular homeostasis. In the undiseased state, the endothelium constitutes a nonthrombogenic surface, both regulating vascular tone and preventing activation of platelets and the coagulation cascade. The equilibrium between nitric oxide and reactive oxygen species as well as that between prostacyclin and its endogenous counterplayer thromboxane are pivotal elements in this process. The inflammatory environment of the progressing atherosclerotic plaque, however, leads to a decrease in nitric oxide production and release as well as to a concomitant increase in reactive oxygen species, resulting in a dysfunctional endothelium with augmented vascular tone and increased thrombogenity. There is mounting evidence that the latter is further enhanced by induction of endothelial tissue factor (TF) expression. Indeed, several studies have shown that an increase in TF expression and activity is observed in the presence of all cardiovascular risk factors as well as in established atherosclerosis and in particular in acute coronary syndromes. The exact role of TF as a marker and/or pathogenic player in this context is not entirely resolved and requires further study. This review discusses the role of the endothelium in hemostasis both in the physiologic as well as in the diseased state, with a particular focus on the molecular regulation of TF and its role in thrombotic vascular diseases. ©2008 S. Karger GmbH, Freiburg i.Br.

Introduction

In spite of the progress made in the last decades in diagnosis and treatment, cardiovascular diseases still account for most of the morbidity and mortality in Western countries. Under normal circumstances, the undiseased endothelium constitutes a continuous, uninterrupted, smooth, and nonthrombogenic surface, both regulating vascular tone and preventing activation of intravascular coagulation. The development of atherosclerosis, the underlying cause of most forms of cardiovascular disease, is initiated by endothelial dysfunction followed by intimal thickening with deposition of lipoproteins and invasion of inflammatory cells. In contrast to healthy endothelium, the dysfunctional endothelium promotes vasoconstriction and may locally activate the coagulation cascade through a variety of different pathways. With the progression of atherosclerotic vascular disease, endothelial erosion and eventually plaque rupture may occur, leading to immediate activation of platelets and initiation of the coagulation cascade; as a result, vascular occlusion may ensue, which accounts for most of the morbidity observed in stroke and acute coronary syndromes (ACS). Hence, at every point in the disease process is the endothelium critically involved either in maintaining vascular homeostasis and preventing activation of coagulation or – if dysfunctional – in the initiation of the atherosclerotic process and its clinical complications.

This review updates previous research and publications of the authors in this field; a special focus is set on the molecular regulation of tissue factor, a key enzyme in the initiation of coagulation, and its role in thrombotic vascular diseases.

The Endothelium and Vascular Homeostasis

The uninjured, normal endothelium synthesizes and releases a plethora of vasoactive substances (fig. 1) that are also involved in the regulation of coagulation, inflammation, and smooth muscle function. Functional impairment of the vascular endothe-

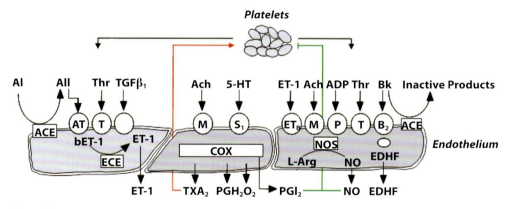

Fig. 1. The uninjured, normal endothelium synthesizes and releases a plethora of vasoactive substances. In response to shear stress and activation of a variety of receptors, nitric oxide (NO) and prostacyclin (PGI$_2$) are released from endothelial cells. They exert vasodilating and antiproliferative effects on smooth muscle cells and inhibit platelet aggregation and leukocyte adhesion (green lines). In contrast, thromboxane is vasoconstrictory and promotes platelet adhesion and aggregation (red arrow). See text for details. ACE = Angiotensin-converting enzyme; Ach = acetylcholine; AI = angiotensin I; AII = angiotensin II; AT1 = angiotensin 1 receptor; B$_2$ = bradykinin receptor; Bk = bradykinin; COX = cyclooxygenase; ECE = endothelin (ET)-converting enzyme; EDHF = endothelium-derived hyperpolarizing factor; ETA and ETB = endothelin A and B receptors; ET-1 = endothelin-1; L-Arg = L-arginine; M = Ach receptor; NOS = NO synthase; P = ADP receptor; PGH$_2$ = prostaglandin H2; S = serotoninergic receptor; T = thromboxane receptor; Thr = thrombin; TGFβ$_1$ = transforming growth factor-b1; TXA$_2$ = thromboxane; 5-HT = 5-hydroxytryptamine (serotonin). Modified from [62].

lium occurs long before the development of visible atherosclerotic changes is noted within the arterial wall. Nitric oxide (NO) is a free radical gas with an in vivo half-life of only a few seconds, which is easily able to cross biological membranes [1–3]. In endothelial cells, NO is synthesized from L-arginine by endothelial NO synthase (eNOS) in presence of the cofactor tetrahydrobiopterin (BH_4) and is released from these cells mainly in response to shear stress produced by blood flow or pharmacological stimulants such as acetylcholine.

NO exerts numerous biological effects, including vasodilation, prevention of leukocyte adhesion and migration into the arterial wall, smooth muscle cell proliferation, and platelet adhesion and aggregation. Both vasodilation as well as inhibition of platelet function is mediated via cyclic guanosine monophosphate (cGMP), while smooth muscle cell proliferation is inhibited via cell cycle regulatory proteins. In patients with atherosclerotic vascular disease, eNOS protein expression and as a consequence NO release are significantly impaired [4]; indeed, an increase in carotid wall thickness (oftentimes used as a surrogate for the general 'atherosclerotic vascular burden') is associated with reduced NO-mediated vasodilation [5].

Furthermore, oxidative stress and generation of reactive oxygen species (ROS) are importantly involved in endothelial dysfunction as well as atherosclerotic plaque progression. The superoxide anion (O_2^-), an oxygen radical, can act as a direct vasoconstrictor [7]. More importantly, however, O_2^- scavenges NO to form the highly reactive ROS intermediate peroxynitrite ($ONOO^-$), which effectively reduces the bioavailability of endothelium-derived NO [7, 8]. Moreover, $ONOO^-$ effectively inhibits the two other major protective endothelial elements, i.e. prostacyclin (PGI_2) and endothelium-derived hyperpolarizing factor (EDHF). Each of the classic atherosclerotic risk factors (diabetes mellitus, hypercholesterolemia, hypertension, tobacco use) is associated with an increase in vascular oxidative stress [6]. Hence, while NO effectively prevents activation of coagulation and, consequently, thrombus formation in the intact endothelium, a decrease in NO (a concomitant increase in ROS) has just the opposite effect in diseased endothelium.

Interaction of Endothelium and Platelets

Platelets are acaryote cellular structures that travel at the periphery of the blood stream in close proximity of the endothelium; they change shape and aggregate when activated with appropriate stimuli (e.g., arachidonic acid, ADP/ATP, thrombin) or when in contact with surface molecules of the subendothelial layer (when those are exposed, e.g. after plaque rupture or endothelial erosion). Under normal circumstances platelet activation is inhibited by NO and PGI_2. Furthermore, NO (through activation of cGMP) and PGI_2 – via cyclic adenosine monophosphate (cAMP) – are in large parts responsible for the antithrombotic properties of the endothelium and potentiate each other's antiaggregatory efficiency.

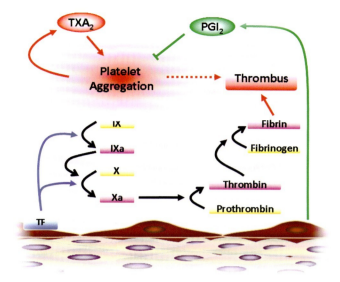

Fig. 2. The equilibrium between prostacyclin (PGI$_2$) and its endogenous counterplayer thromboxane (TXA$_2$) is of pivotal importance in the balance of coagulation. Platelets are activated by TXA$_2$, while they are stabilized by PGI$_2$. Mediators released during platelet activation and aggregation, such as serotonin and histamine, induce endothelial tissue factor (TF) expression; other mediators are cofactors in the conversion of prothrombin to thrombin. TF, the main initiator of the coagulation cascade, activates factor IX and (directly and indirectly) factor X, resulting in the formation of thrombin. Ultimately, thrombus formation results from the initiation of the coagulation cascade in conjunction with platelet activation and aggregation.

Many platelet-derived substances activate receptors on the endothelium leading to the release of NO. Of particular importance, thrombin cleaves a tethered protease-activated receptor (PAR), and ADP activates P$_2$-purinergic receptors (fig. 1). In normal endothelium, this mechanism constitutes an important feedback loop in order to prevent uncontrolled platelet activation. In contrast, after endothelial damage, platelet-derived thromboxane (TXA$_2$) and serotonin lead to vasoconstriction by activating vascular smooth muscle cells (VSMC) and initiation of coagulation. Thus, the endothelium profoundly modulates platelet-vessel wall interaction and normally provides protection.

The equilibrium between PGI$_2$ and its endogenous counterplayer TXA$_2$ is another pivotal element in the homeostasis of coagulation (fig. 2). TXA$_2$ is formed in platelets from arachidonic acid and induces VSMC contraction and platelet aggregation [9], while PGI$_2$, which is continuously released from the endothelium, is a potent vasodilator and possesses antiaggregating properties [10, 11], hence directly counterbalancing the actions of TXA$_2$. Prostaglandins are synthesized by the two isoenzymes of cyclooxygenase (COX), COX-1 and COX-2. COX-1 is constitutively expressed in most cell types and tissues, whereas COX-2 is not; instead, its expression can be induced in most mammalian cells [12]. As such, endothelial cells can induce COX-2 which contributes to PGI$_2$ production, while platelets lack the COX-2 isoenzyme and only synthesize TXA$_2$ via COX-1. It has therefore been proposed that inhibition of COX-2 by selective COX-2 inhibitors (coxibs) may favor a prothrombotic environment by primarily suppressing endothelial PGI$_2$ synthesis leaving COX-1-dependent platelet

TXA$_2$ synthesis unopposed; however, there is increasing evidence that the effect of coxibs on coagulation is dependent on several other variables and cannot be reduced to the alteration of the balance of PGI$_2$ and TXA$_2$ in endothelial cells and platelets, respectively [13]. Nonetheless, any decrease in endothelial PGI$_2$ synthesis (as it occurs in endothelial dysfunction) shifts the balance in favor of TXA$_2$, resulting in a prothrombotic microenvironment.

Tissue Factor and the Coagulation Cascade

Tissue factor (TF), a 47kDa membrane-bound protein, is the key enzyme in the activation of the coagulation cascade. The latter is initiated as soon as TF comes into contact with circulating activated factor VII (VIIa), resulting in the formation of the TF-FVIIa complex (fig. 2). The TF-VIIa complex activates factor IX, which in turn activates factor X (an alternative activation of factor X to Xa can occur through direct conversion by TF-FVIIa). In complex with calcium and factor Va, factor Xa catalyzes the conversion of prothrombin to thrombin, thereby resulting in thrombus formation.

TF is constitutively expressed in subendothelial cells such as VSMC, resulting in rapid initiation of coagulation when vessel injury occurs [14]. While endothelial cells in contrast do not express TF under physiological conditions (resulting in no appreciable contact of vessel-bound TF with the circulating blood) it can be induced in these cells as well in response to numerous stimuli.

Regulation of Endothelial Tissue Factor Expression

Endothelial TF can be induced by a variety of cytokines including tumor necrosis factor-α (TNF-α), interleukin-1β, or CD40 ligand, by biogenic amines such as serotonin or histamine, and by other mediators involved in atherosclerotic disease like thrombin, oxidized low-density lipoproteins (LDL), or vascular endothelial growth factor [15–17]. Despite their diversity, most of these mediators regulate TF induction through similar signal transduction pathways, including the mitogen-activated protein (MAP) kinases p38, p44/42 (ERK), and c-jun terminal NHB$_{2B}$ kinase (JNK), as well as protein kinase C and the PI3 kinase pathway [14].

The extent of TF protein induction in vascular cells does not always correlate well with the biological activity of TF [15, 18]. One possible reason is the concomitant secretion of tissue factor pathway inhibitor (TFPI), the endogenous inhibitor of TF. Another possible explanation is the distribution of TF into several cellular compartments [15, 19]. Indeed, biologically active TF is located at the cell surface, while a 'pool' of intracellular TF is only released upon cell damage. Furthermore, induction of a functionally inactive form of the TF protein at the cell surface has been described, termed encrypted or latent tissue factor. Expression of encrypted TF enables a cell to rapidly increase TF activity in response to certain stimuli without the need for de novo protein synthesis [20]. Hence, the net procoagulant effect elicited by a certain mediator is dependent on the degree of TF protein induction, cellular localization, and structural modification.

Blood-Borne Tissue Factor

Besides in vascular cells or leukocytes, TF can also be detected in the bloodstream, referred to as circulating or blood-borne TF [21], which is mainly associated with microparticles originating from endothelial cells, VSMC, leukocytes, or platelets [23, 24], as well as from atherosclerotic plaques [22].

Interestingly, monocytes and platelets are known to exchange microparticle-bound TF [25], which is likely to represent an important mechanism through which platelets are loaded with TF, as megakaryocytes (the bone marrow sedentary precursors of platelets) do not express TF, and platelets themselves, lacking a cell nucleus, are incapable of de novo protein synthesis. In addition to carrying microparticle-derived TF, activated platelets induce TF expression in endothelial and smooth muscle cells, most likely via the release of soluble mediators such as serotonin and platelet-derived growth factor (PDGF) [26]. Through this positive feedback loop, aggregating platelets thus enhance local TF concentrations via two mechanisms, which may be important for thrombus formation and/or propagation.

Recently, an alternatively spliced form of TF has been discovered, which is soluble, circulates in the blood, and exhibits procoagulant activity [27]. Alternatively spliced TF seems to represent a distinct form of circulating TF and is not bound to microparticles; as such, it may be particularly important in thrombus propagation, as vessel wall-associated TF is immediately separated from the bloodstream by the freshly formed thrombus, thus preventing it from contributing to further thrombus growth [28]. However, the interplay and relative contribution of soluble TF, microparticle-bound TF, and vessel wall-associated TF to initiation and propagation of thrombosis is not yet entirely settled and currently remains a subject of intense debate [28–31].

Tissue Factor in Cardiovascular Diseases

Being a pivotal element in the initiation of coagulation, TF has been implicated in the pathogenesis of several cardiovascular disorders. Indeed, TF is elevated in asymptomatic patients with established atherosclerosis as well as in those with ACS. Interestingly, also in patients with the classic cardiovascular risk factors such as hypertension, diabetes, dyslipidemia, and smoking an elevation of TF can be observed. While a direct effect of each of these risk factors on TF expression appears an appealing and interesting hypothesis, it cannot entirely be ruled out that some of the observed elevations in TF plasma levels occur secondary to TF release from already established atherosclerotic plaques in these subjects.

Cardiovascular Risk Factors

An elevated TF plasma antigen is observed in hypertensive subjects (as compared to normotensive controls), which can be lowered by different classes of antihypertensive drugs [32] such as angiotensin I receptor blockers [33] or angiotensin-converting enzyme (ACE) inhibitors [34]. The latter also reduce endotoxin-induced TF expression in monocytes [35], implying a pleiotropic mechanism of this class of drugs.

High glucose concentrations have been observed to increase thrombin-induced TF expression in human endothelial cells [36], and glucose intake leads to upregulation of TF expression in monocytes of healthy humans. Hyperglycemia leads to the formation of advanced glycation end products (AGE); the latter induce TF expression in endothelial cells via the receptor for advanced glycation end products (RAGE) [37]. Consistently, diabetic ApoE knockout mice display increased vascular expression of RAGE and TF [38]. Increased TF plasma levels are also measured in diabetic patients, even without overt coronary artery disease [39], which can be reduced when glycemic control is improved [40]. Indeed, insulin reduces both monocyte TF expression and TF plasma levels in obese nondiabetic subjects by reducing activation of the proinflammatory transcription factor early growth response gene-1 (Egr-1), implying a beneficial effect of insulin not only via improvement of hyperglycemia [41]. Hence, there is strong evidence that hyperglycemia may have a direct effect on TF expression and activity.

Oxidized LDL increases endothelial TF expression [17], while reconstituted high-density lipoprotein inhibits endothelial TF induction [42]. Consistently, an increased plasma TF activity is observed in patients with elevated LDL levels [40]. In turn, TF expression in endothelial cells, VSMC, and monocytes can be reduced by HMG-CoA reductase inhibitors (statins) [16, 43]. Several beneficial effects of statins in patients appear to be independent of LDL levels, which are believed to occur via pleiotropic anti-inflammatory effects of this class of drugs. Similarly in ApoE knockout mice, simvastatin inhibits TF expression in advanced atherosclerotic lesions independent of plasma lipid levels [44]. Also in healthy human subjects, endotoxin-induced TF expression is blunted after administration of simvastatin [45]. Hence, inhibition of TF induction may in part explain the beneficial, lipid-unrelated effects of HMG-CoA reductase inhibitors.

An increased TF expression in atherosclerotic plaques is observed in ApoE knockout mice exposed to cigarette smoke as compared to mice breathing filtered room air [46]. Similarly in humans, cigarette smoking is associated with increased TF plasma

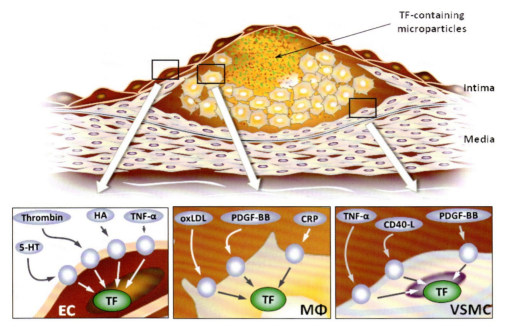

Fig. 3. Tissue factor (TF) is expressed at high levels in the inflammatory environment of atherosclerotic plaques in endothelial cells, vascular smooth muscle cells (VSMC), and macrophages/foam cells, as well as in the necrotic plaque core (where it is mainly associated with microparticles derived from perishing inflammatory cells). Cellular TF induction occurs by a variety of mediators in endothelial cells (EC, left panel), macrophages (MΦ, middle panel), and VSMC (right panel). Upon plaque rupture, the highly procoagulant plaque content (including TF-containing microparticles) is released into the blood, leading to rapid initiation of coagulation. 5-HT = 5-Hydroxytryptamine (serotonin); HA = histamine; TNF-α = tumor necrosis factor-α; oxLDL = oxidized low-density lipoproteins; PDGF-BB = platelet-derived growth factor-BB; CRP = C-reactive protein; CD40-L = CD40-ligand. Modified from [14].

levels (with a strong correlation between the number of cigarettes smoked and the increase in TF plasma levels) [40].

Atherosclerosis

A hallmark of the inflammatory nature of atherosclerosis is the infiltration of monocytes into the intimal layer and the subsequent transformation into macrophages and foam cells [47]. In this inflammatory environment, TF induction is observed in response to a several inflammatory mediators such as TNF-α and interleukins (fig. 3). While during the early stages of atherogenesis, enhanced TF expression is observed in monocytes [48], TF expression is also detected in foam cells, endothelial cells, and smooth muscle cells at later stages [48, 49]. TF is also present in the necrotic core of plaques, mainly associated with microparticles, which are derived from perishing inflammatory cells [22, 49]. Indeed, the major part of the TF activity in atherosclerotic plaques is contained in such microparticles [22].

Rupture of an atherosclerotic plaque exposes its highly procoagulant content to the circulating blood; thereby, TF-laden macrophages as well as TF-containing microparticles originating from the necrotic core initiate thrombus formation and related complications such as acute myocardial infarction. It is well known that in most instances the clinical course of events is not primarily determined by the degree of luminal narrowing, but rather the composition of the atherosclerotic plaque; indeed, large lipid-rich plaques with a thin cap, extensive macrophage infiltration (and abundant TF expression) are more prone to rupture than collagen-rich, fibrous plaques.

Acute Coronary Syndrome and Percutaneous Coronary Intervention

In line with these observations, atherectomy specimens from patients with unstable angina or myocardial infarction show increased levels of TF antigen and activity as compared to those with stable angina [50]. Elevated levels of circulating TF measured in patients with ACS may be derived both from vascular cells (endothelium and smooth muscle cells) as well as from circulating leukocytes and aggregating platelets [51]. Plaque rupture, as mentioned above, leads to exposure of the highly procoagulant plaque content to the circulation and may hence also contribute to elevated TF plasma levels [22]. Consistently, higher TF plasma levels are measured in patients with unstable as compared to those with stable angina [52]. Elevated TF plasma levels may even predict future cardiovascular events in patients with unstable angina, implying a role for TF as a marker of plaque stability. However, plaque rupture is not a 'condition sine qua non' in patients with ACS, as a substantial number of patients rather develop coronary artery thrombi on top just of a superficial erosion, which may nonetheless also lead to increased TF plasma levels in these patients [53].

Antiplatelet agents are a mainstay in the treatment of ACS. Since platelets represent a major source of TF, it is hence conceivable that these drugs may reduce TF plasma levels. The ways in which these drugs affect TF, however, seem to differ substantially: aspirin inhibits endotoxin-induced transcriptional activation of TF expression in monocytes and may hence diminish TF plasma activity by directly interfering with TF regulation on a molecular level [54]. In an animal model of acute myocardial infarction, clopidogrel (an ADP receptor antagonist) reduces TF expression in the ischemic coronary artery, the mechanism of which, however, remains unclear [55]. By reducing platelet-monocyte cross talk, the glycoprotein (GP) IIb/IIIa antagonist abciximab suppresses monocyte TF expression and activity; similarly, abciximab diminishes monocyte TF expression in patients undergoing carotid angioplasty with stenting [56]. In contrast to these agents, long-term treatment with the vitamin K antagonist warfarin increases soluble TF levels, which may be due to decreased TF consumption [57].

After percutaneous coronary intervention, some studies found an increase in TF activity, while others did not [58]. Plaque dissection as a consequence of balloon dilatation may expose the plaque content to the bloodstream (in a similar way as plaque rupture does) and thereby increase TF plasma levels. Drug-eluting stents (DES) are covered with pharmacological agents which, once released into the coronary artery after stent deployment, reduce restenosis as compared to their uncoated counterparts. However, a major controversy is currently ongoing whether or not these stents may be associated with an increase in the rate of stent thrombosis [59]. We were able to demonstrate that rapamycin, a substance used for stent coating, increases endothelial TF expression, suggesting a potential role for this drug in the development of stent thrombosis [60]. Hence, novel coating strategies for DES are being developed; one possible new principle could be dimethyl sulfoxide (DMSO), which prevents VSMC proliferation and migration (just like first-generation substances like rapamycin do), but at the same time inhibits TF upregulation in endothelial cells, VSMC, and monocytes and prevents thrombotic occlusion in a mouse carotid injury model [61]. However, additional studies are needed to assess the implications of these findings in vivo.

Conclusions and Future Directions

The endothelium is critically involved in maintaining vascular homeostasis. While it constitutes a smooth and nonthrombogenic surface in the physiologic, undiseased state, this is drastically changed as a result of the inflammatory processes of atherosclerogenesis. While both the equilibrium between NO and ROS as well as that between PGI_2 and TXA_2 have long been recognized as important elements in the dysfunctional endothelium, increasing evidence also suggests a role for TF in this regard. While the exact role of TF as a marker and/or pathogenic player in this context is not entirely resolved and requires further study, the development of novel antithrombotic therapeutic principles includes strategies aimed directly against TF, several of which are already being investigated in clinical trials [59]. Potentially, targeting TF may even prove to be useful in treating and preventing stent thrombosis, one of the most dreaded complications of interventional cardiology in our day and age.

Disclosure of Conflict of Interests

JS has no conflict of interest to declare. TFL is a coholder of a patent on the potential clinical applications of dimethyl sulfoxide.

Acknowledgements

Original research of the authors was supported by the Swiss National Research Foundation (grant no. 3100-068118.02/1 to TFL) as well as by the European Union (European Vascular Genomics Network; grant no. G5RD-CT-2001-00532 to TFL), the Swiss Heart Foundation, the Wolfermann-Nägeli Foundation, the Bonizzi-Theler Foundation, the Mercator Foundation, and the Center for Integrative Human Physiology of the University of Zurich.

References

1 Furchgott RF, Zawadzki JV: The obligatory role of endothelial cells in the relaxation of arterial smooth muscle by acetylcholine. Nature 1980;288:373–376.

2 Palmer RM, Ashton DS, Moncada S: Vascular endothelial cells synthesize nitric oxide from L-arginine. Nature 1988;333:664–666.

3 Stamler JS, Singel DJ, Loscalzo J: Biochemistry of nitric oxide and its redox-activated forms. Science 1992;258:1898–1902.

4 Oemar BS, Tschudi MR, Godoy N, Brovkovich V, Malinski T, Luscher TF: Reduced endothelial nitric oxide synthase expression and production in human atherosclerosis. Circulation 1998;97:2494–2498.

5 Ghiadoni L, Taddei S, Virdis A, Sudano I, Di Legge V, Meola M, Di Venanzio L, Salvetti A: Endothelial function and common carotid artery wall thickening in patients with essential hypertension. Hypertension 1998;32:25–32.

6 Brunner H, Cockcroft JR, Deanfield J, Donald A, Ferrannini E, Halcox J, Kiowski W, Luscher TF, Mancia G, Natali A, Oliver JJ, Pessina AC, Rizzoni D, Rossi GP, Salvetti A, Spieker LE, Taddei S, Webb DJ; Working Group on Endothelins and Endothelial Factors of the European Society of Hypertension: Endothelial function and dysfunction. Part II: Association with cardiovascular risk factors and diseases. A statement by the Working Group on Endothelins and Endothelial Factors of the European Society of Hypertension. J Hypertens 2005;23:233–246.

7 Rubanyi GM, Vanhoutte PM: Superoxide anions and hyperoxia inactivate endothelium-derived relaxing factor. Am J Physiol 1986;250:H822–827.

8 Katusic ZS, Vanhoutte PM: Superoxide anion is an endothelium-derived contracting factor. Am J Physiol 1989;257:H33–37.

9 Sugimoto Y, Narumiya S, Ichikawa A: Distribution and function of prostanoid receptors: studies from knockout mice. Prog Lipid Res 2000;39:289–314.

10 Whittaker N, Bunting S, Salmon J, Moncada S, Vane JR, Johnson RA, Morton DR, Kinner JH, Gorman RR, McGuire JC, Sun FF: The chemical structure of prostaglandin X (prostacyclin). Prostaglandins 1976;12:915–928.

11 Cheng Y, Austin SC, Rocca B, Koller BH, Coffman TM, Grosser T, Lawson JA, FitzGerald GA: Role of prostacyclin in the cardiovascular response to thromboxane A2. Science 2002;296:539–541.

12 Jones DA, Carlton DP, McIntyre TM, Zimmerman GA, Prescott SM: Molecular cloning of human prostaglandin endoperoxide synthase type II and demonstration of expression in response to cytokines. J Biol Chem 1993;268:9049–9054.

13 Steffel J, Luscher TF, Ruschitzka F, Tanner FC: Cyclooxygenase-2 inhibition and coagulation. J Cardiovasc Pharmacol 2006;47(suppl 1):S15–20.

14 Steffel J, Luscher TF, Tanner FC: Tissue factor in cardiovascular diseases: molecular mechanisms and clinical implications. Circulation 2006;113:722–731.

15 Camera M, Giesen PL, Fallon J, Aufiero BM, Taubman M, Tremoli E, Nemerson Y: Cooperation between VEGF and TNF-alpha is necessary for exposure of active tissue factor on the surface of human endothelial cells. Arterioscler Thromb Vasc Biol 1999;19:531–537.

16 Eto M, Kozai T, Cosentino F, Joch H, Luscher TF: Statin prevents tissue factor expression in human endothelial cells: role of Rho/Rho-kinase and Akt pathways. Circulation 2002;105:1756–1759.

17 Drake TA, Hannani K, Fei HH, Lavi S, Berliner JA: Minimally oxidized low-density lipoprotein induces tissue factor expression in cultured human endothelial cells. Am J Pathol 1991;138:601–607.

18 Steffel J, Akhmedov A, Greutert H, Luscher TF, Tanner FC: Histamine induces tissue factor expression: implications for acute coronary syndromes. Circulation 2005;112:341–349.

19 Schecter AD, Giesen PL, Taby O, Rosenfield CL, Rossikhina M, Fyfe BS, Kohtz DS, Fallon JT, Nemerson Y, Taubman MB: Tissue factor expression in human arterial smooth muscle cells. TF is present in three cellular pools after growth factor stimulation. J Clin Invest 1997;100:2276–2285.

20 Wolberg AS, Monroe DM, Roberts HR, Hoffman MR: Tissue factor de-encryption: ionophore treatment induces changes in tissue factor activ-

ity by phosphatidylserine-dependent and -independent mechanisms. Blood Coagul Fibrinolysis 1999;10:201–210.

21 Giesen PL, Rauch U, Bohrmann B, Kling D, Roque M, Fallon JT, Badimon JJ, Himber J, Riederer MA, Nemerson Y: Blood-borne tissue factor: another view of thrombosis. Proc Natl Acad Sci U S A 1999;96:2311–2315.

22 Mallat Z, Benamer H, Hugel B, Benessiano J, Steg PG, Freyssinet JM, Tedgui A: Elevated levels of shed membrane microparticles with procoagulant potential in the peripheral circulating blood of patients with acute coronary syndromes. Circulation 2000;101:841–843.

23 Llorente-Cortes V, Otero-Vinas M, Camino-Lopez S, Llampayas O, Badimon L: Aggregated low-density lipoprotein uptake induces membrane tissue factor procoagulant activity and microparticle release in human vascular smooth muscle cells. Circulation 2004;110:452–459.

24 Schecter AD, Spirn B, Rossikhina M, Giesen PL, Bogdanov V, Fallon JT, Fisher EA, Schnapp LM, Nemerson Y, Taubman MB: Release of active tissue factor by human arterial smooth muscle cells. Circ Res 2000;87:126–132.

25 Scholz T, Temmler U, Krause S, Heptinstall S, Losche W: Transfer of tissue factor from platelets to monocytes: role of platelet-derived microvesicles and CD62P. Thromb Haemost 2002;88:1033–1038.

26 Cirillo P, Golino P, Calabro P, Ragni M, Forte L, Piro O, De Rosa S, Pacileo M, Chiariello M: Activated platelets stimulate tissue factor expression in smooth muscle cells. Thromb Res 2003;112:51–57.

27 Bogdanov VY, Balasubramanian V, Hathcock J, Vele O, Lieb M, Nemerson Y: Alternatively spliced human tissue factor: a circulating, soluble, thrombogenic protein. Nat Med 2003;9:458–462.

28 Chou J, Mackman N, Merrill-Skoloff G, Pedersen B, Furie BC, Furie B: Hematopoietic cell-derived microparticle tissue factor contributes to fibrin formation during thrombus propagation. Blood 2004;104:3190–3197.

29 Day SM, Reeve JL, Pedersen B, Farris DM, Myers DD, Im M, Wakefield TW, Mackman N, Fay WP: Macrovascular thrombosis is driven by tissue factor derived primarily from the blood vessel wall. Blood 2005;105:192–198.

30 Morrissey JH: Clotting hits the wall. Blood 2005;105:3–4.

31 Butenas S, Bouchard BA, Brummel-Ziedins KE, Parhami-Seren B, Mann KG: Tissue factor activity in whole blood. Blood 2005;105:2764–2770.

32 Felmeden DC, Spencer CG, Chung NA, Belgore FM, Blann AD, Beevers DG, Lip GY: Relation of thrombogenesis in systemic hypertension to angiogenesis and endothelial damage/dysfunction (a substudy of the Anglo-Scandinavian Cardiac Outcomes Trial [ASCOT]). Am J Cardiol 2003;92:400–405.

33 Koh KK, Chung WJ, Ahn JY, Han SH, Kang WC, Seo YH, Ahn TH, Choi IS, Shin EK: Angiotensin II type 1 receptor blockers reduce tissue factor activity and plasminogen activator inhibitor type-1 antigen in hypertensive patients: a randomized, double-blind, placebo-controlled study. Atherosclerosis 2004;177:155–160.

34 Soejima H, Ogawa H, Yasue H, Kaikita K, Takazoe K, Nishiyama K, Misumi K, Miyamoto S, Yoshimura M, Kugiyama K, Nakamura S, Tsuji I: Angiotensin-converting enzyme inhibition reduces monocyte chemoattractant protein-1 and tissue factor levels in patients with myocardial infarction. J Am Coll Cardiol 1999;34:983–988.

35 Napoleone E, Di Santo A, Camera M, Tremoli E, Lorenzet R: Angiotensin-converting enzyme inhibitors downregulate tissue factor synthesis in monocytes. Circ Res 2000;86:139–143.

36 Boeri D, Almus FE, Maiello M, Cagliero E, Rao LV, Lorenzi M: Modification of tissue-factor mRNA and protein response to thrombin and interleukin 1 by high glucose in cultured human endothelial cells. Diabetes 1989;38:212–218.

37 Bierhaus A, Illmer T, Kasper M, Luther T, Quehenberger P, Tritschler H, Wahl P, Ziegler R, Muller M, Nawroth PP: Advanced glycation end product (AGE)-mediated induction of tissue factor in cultured endothelial cells is dependent on RAGE. Circulation 1997;96:2262–2271.

38 Kislinger T, Tanji N, Wendt T, Qu W, Lu Y, Ferran LJ Jr, Taguchi A, Olson K, Bucciarelli L, Goova M, Hofmann MA, Cataldegirmen G, D'Agati V, Pischetsrieder M, Stern DM, Schmidt AM: Receptor for advanced glycation end products mediates inflammation and enhanced expression of tissue factor in vasculature of diabetic apolipoprotein E-null mice. Arterioscler Thromb Vasc Biol 2001;21:905–910.

39 Lim HS, Blann AD, Lip GY: Soluble CD40 ligand, soluble P-selectin, interleukin-6, and tissue factor in diabetes mellitus: relationships to cardiovascular disease and risk factor intervention. Circulation 2004;109:2524–2528.

40 Sambola A, Osende J, Hathcock J, Degen M, Nemerson Y, Fuster V, Crandall J, Badimon JJ: Role of risk factors in the modulation of tissue factor activity and blood thrombogenicity. Circulation 2003;107:973–977.

41 Aljada A, Ghanim H, Mohanty P, Kapur N, Dandona P: Insulin inhibits the pro-inflammatory transcription factor early growth response gene-1 (Egr)-1 expression in mononuclear cells (MNC) and reduces plasma tissue factor (TF) and plasminogen activator inhibitor-1 (PAI-1) concentrations. J Clin Endocrinol Metab 2002;87:1419–1422.

42 Viswambharan H, Ming XF, Zhu S, Hubsch A, Lerch P, Vergeres G, Rusconi S, Yang Z: Reconstituted high-density lipoprotein inhibits thrombin-induced endothelial tissue factor expression through inhibition of RhoA and stimulation of phosphatidylinositol 3-kinase but not Akt/endothelial nitric oxide synthase. Circ Res 2004;94:918–925.

43 Brandes RP, Beer S, Ha T, Busse R: Withdrawal of cerivastatin induces monocyte chemoattractant protein 1 and tissue factor expression in cultured vascular smooth muscle cells. Arterioscler Thromb Vasc Biol 2003;23:1794–1800.

44 Bea F, Blessing E, Shelley MI, Shultz JM, Rosenfeld ME: Simvastatin inhibits expression of tissue factor in advanced atherosclerotic lesions of apolipoprotein E deficient mice independently of lipid lowering: potential role of simvastatin-mediated inhibition of Egr-1 expression and activation. Atherosclerosis 2003;167:187–194.

45 Steiner S, Speidl WS, Pleiner J, Seidinger D, Zorn G, Kaun C, Wojta J, Huber K, Minar E, Wolzt M, Kopp CW: Simvastatin blunts endotoxin-induced tissue factor in vivo. Circulation 2005;111:1841–1846.

46 Matetzky S, Tani S, Kangavari S, Dimayuga P, Yano J, Xu H, Chyu KY, Fishbein MC, Shah PK, Cercek B: Smoking increases tissue factor expression in atherosclerotic plaques: implications for plaque thrombogenicity. Circulation 2000;102:602–604.

47 Hansson GK: Inflammation, atherosclerosis, and coronary artery disease. N Engl J Med 2005;352:1685–1695.

48 Wilcox JN, Smith KM, Schwartz SM, Gordon D: Localization of tissue factor in the normal vessel wall and in the atherosclerotic plaque. Proc Natl Acad Sci U S A 1989;86:2839–2843.

49 Thiruvikraman SV, Guha A, Roboz J, Taubman MB, Nemerson Y, Fallon JT: In situ localization of tissue factor in human atherosclerotic plaques by binding of digoxigenin-labeled factors VIIa and X. Lab Invest 1996;75:451–461.

50 Annex BH, Denning SM, Channon KM, Sketch MH Jr, Stack RS, Morrissey JH, Peters KG: Differential expression of tissue factor protein in directional atherectomy specimens from patients with stable and unstable coronary syndromes. Circulation 1995;91:619–622.

51 Suefuji H, Ogawa H, Yasue H, Kaikita K, Soejima H, Motoyama T, Mizuno Y, Oshima S, Saito T, Tsuji I, Kumeda K, Kamikubo Y, Nakamura S: Increased plasma tissue factor levels in acute myocardial infarction. Am Heart J 1997;134:253–259.

52 Soejima H, Ogawa H, Yasue H, Kaikita K, Nishiyama K, Misumi K, Takazoe K, Miyao Y, Yoshimura M, Kugiyama K, Nakamura S, Tsuji I, Kumeda K: Heightened tissue factor associated with tissue factor pathway inhibitor and prognosis in patients with unstable angina. Circulation 1999;99:2908–2913.

53 Virmani R, Kolodgie FD, Burke AP, Farb A, Schwartz SM: Lessons from sudden coronary death: a comprehensive morphological classification scheme for atherosclerotic lesions. Arterioscler Thromb Vasc Biol 2000;20:1262–1275.

54 Osnes LT, Foss KB, Joo GB, Okkenhaug C, Westvik AB, Ovstebo R, Kierulf P: Acetylsalicylic acid and sodium salicylate inhibit LPS-induced NF-kappa B/c-Rel nuclear translocation, and synthesis of tissue factor (TF) and tumor necrosis factor alfa (TNF-alpha) in human monocytes. Thromb Haemost 1996;76:970–976.

55 Molero L, Lopez-Farre A, Mateos-Caceres PJ, Fernandez-Sanchez R, Luisa Maestro M, Silva J, Rodriguez E, Macaya C: Effect of clopidogrel on the expression of inflammatory markers in rabbit ischemic coronary artery. Br J Pharmacol 2005;146:419–424.

56 Kopp CW, Steiner S, Nasel C, Seidinger D, Mlekusch I, Lang W, Bartok A, Ahmadi R, Minar E: Abciximab reduces monocyte tissue factor in carotid angioplasty and stenting. Stroke 2003;34:2560–2567.

57 Seljeflot I, Hurlen M, Arnesen H: Increased levels of soluble tissue factor during long-term treatment with warfarin in patients after an acute myocardial infarction. J Thromb Haemost 2004;2:726–730.

58 Tutar E, Ozcan M, Kilickap M, Gulec S, Aras O, Pamir G, Oral D, Dandelet L, Key NS: Elevated whole-blood tissue factor procoagulant activity as a marker of restenosis after percutaneous transluminal coronary angioplasty and stent implantation. Circulation 2003;108:1581–1584.

59 Luscher TF, Steffel J, Eberli FR, Joner M, Nakazawa G, Tanner FC, Virmani R: Drug-eluting stent and coronary thrombosis: biological mechanisms and clinical implications. Circulation 2007;115:1051–1058.

60 Steffel J, Latini RA, Akhmedov A, Zimmermann D, Zimmerling P, Luscher TF, Tanner FC: Rapamycin, but not FK-506, increases endothelial tissue factor expression: implications for drug-eluting stent design. Circulation 2005;112:2002–2011.

61 Camici GG, Steffel J, Akhmedov A, Schafer N, Baldinger J, Schulz U, Shojaati K, Matter CM, Yang Z, Luscher TF, Tanner FC: Dimethyl sulfoxide inhibits tissue factor expression, thrombus formation, and vascular smooth muscle cell activation: a potential treatment strategy for drug-eluting stents. Circulation 2006;114:1512–1521.

62 Lüscher TF, Noll G: Endothelial function as an endpoint in interventional trials: concepts, methods and current data. J Hypertens Suppl 1996;14:S111–119.

Prof. Thomas F. Lüscher, M.D., FESC, FRCP
Klinik für Kardiologie
UniversitätsSpital Zürich
Rämistr. 100, 8091 Zürich, Switzerland
E-Mail karlue@usz.unizh.ch

Scharf RE (ed): Progress and Challenges in Transfusion Medicine, Hemostasis and Hemotherapy.
Freiburg i.Br., Karger, 2008, pp 37–47

Intravascular and Extravascular Coagulation and Fibrinolysis in the Diseased Lung

Phillip Markart · Malgorzata Wygrecka · Clemens Ruppert · Martina Korfei · Bhola Dahal · Thorsten Jennes · Klaus T. Preissner · Werner Seeger · Andreas Günther

University of Giessen Lung Center, Giessen, Germany

Key Words

Pulmonary embolism · In situ thrombosis · Chronic thromboembolic pulmonary hypertension (CTEPH) · Acute respiratory distress syndrome (ARDS) · Fibrosis · Interstitial lung disease (ILD)

Summary

Intravascular and extravascular/intra-alveolar fibrin formation is a common observation in a variety of different lung diseases. Among these are primarily vascular entities such as pulmonary thromboembolism, pulmonary arterial hypertension (PAH) or chronic thromboembolic pulmonary hypertension (CTEPH), acute inflammatory diseases affecting all compartments of the lung – e.g. acute respiratory distress syndrome (ARDS), sepsis, pneumonia –, and diffuse parenchymal lung diseases (DPLD) such as idiopathic pulmonary fibrosis (IPF). It has been known for long that fibrin formation within the pulmonary vasculature induces ventilation-perfusion (V/Q) mismatch and propagates pulmonary vascular remodelling. Consequently, anticoagulant strategies are a mainstay of therapy in pulmonary embolism, CTEPH, and PAH. In contrast, the precise contribution of intra-alveolar fibrin formation to V/Q mismatch and fibroproliferative processes in the lung parenchyma is yet unclear and needs to be settled. Drawn against this background, we will review the current understanding of the underlying reasons, pathogenetic role, and therapeutic prospects of intravascular and extravascular/intra-alveolar fibrin generation and the involved coagulation and fibrinolysis factors.   ©2008 S. Karger GmbH, Freiburg i.Br.

Introduction

The deposition of thromboembolic material within the pulmonary vasculature is a frequent phenomenon, and the spectrum of clinical symptoms ranges from slight dyspnea to acute right ventricular failure and the need for immediate cardiopulmonary resuscitation. Still, pulmonary embolism is the third frequent reason for death among cardiovascular diseases, may affect 20–300/100,000 inhabitants, is notoriously underdiagnosed, and may cause most of the deaths of hospitalized patients aged over 65 years [1]. Apart from the mechanical obliteration of the pulmonary vasculature, periembolic events such as in situ activation of coagulation and release of vaso-occlusive mediators such as serotonin, thromboxane, and leukotrienes have been shown to contribute to the increase of pulmonary vascular resistance and maldistribution of perfusion [2–5].

Next to the acute hemodynamic effects of the deposition of thromboembolic material or the in situ generation of fibrin within the pulmonary vasculature, the disturbed local hemostatic balance, in detail the increased procoagulant and antifibrinolytic activities, and the persistence of fibrin may also significantly contribute to vascular remodelling of the pulmonary vasculature, resulting in progressive pulmonary hypertension (chronic thromboembolic pulmonary hypertension, CTEPH). Although clinical data are scarce it has previously been shown that CTEPH patients do have increased type 1 plasminogen activator inhibitor (PAI-1) levels, thereby probably preventing effective clot removal upon embolism or in situ thrombosis [6, 7]. Likewise, patients with pulmonary arterial hypertension (PAH), a form of pulmonary hypertension not primarily triggered by thromboembolism, were reported to have increased circulating PAI-1 levels [8]. In line with the observed improvement of mortality in response to oral anticoagulant treatment [9], increased in situ activation of coagulation and impaired fibrinolysis of intravascular clots may thus contribute to vascular remodelling even in PAH patients in whom no thromboembolism antecedes the development of pulmonary hypertension.

Microthrombosis of the Pulmonary Circulation in Acute Respiratory Distress Syndrome (ARDS)

In situ generation of fibrin within the pulmonary vasculature is also a common finding in patients with acute inflammatory (lung) diseases such as the acute respiratory distress syndrome (ARDS), severe sepsis and vasculitis and may then be described as microembolism/microthrombosis syndrome [10–12]. Under physiological conditions, the pulmonary endothelium contains large amounts of antithrombotic factors. In detail, a high local concentration of glycosaminoglycanes (e.g. heparane sulfate) keeps antithrombin III in an active state and is rich in thrombomodulin, which, upon binding to thrombin, activates protein C and thus induces anticoagulant and profibrinolytic activities. Accordingly, reduction of endothelial expression of thrombomodulin provokes increased fibrin deposition within the pulmonary vasculature [13]. In addition, under normal conditions, the pulmonary endothelium expresses tissue factor pathway inhibitor (TFPI), the physiological antagonist of the extrinsic pathway [14, 15]. In the pulmonary macrocirculation, tissue-type plasminogen activator (t-PA) is highly expressed under normal conditions [15, 16], whereas in the microcirculation, urokinase-type plasminogen activator (u-PA) is increasingly expressed and replaces t-PA [15, 17].

Under acute inflammatory conditions, a marked switch of the pulmonary vascular hemostatic balance can be encountered and includes increased expression of PAI-1 [15, 18] and PAI-2 [15]. Under these conditions, reduced expression of t-PA in the pulmonary macrocirculation and increased expression of u-PA in the macro- and microcirculation was encountered [15, 19], with predominance of PAI activities. In addition, pronounced upregulation (approx. × 30) of tissue factor (TF) [15, 19, 20], combined with unchanged expression of TF pathway inhibitor (TFPI) [15], accounts for the excessive induction of the extrinsic pathway. Furthermore, thrombomodulin [21] and activated protein C (aPC) [22] levels are decreased, and release of free extracellular RNA additionally activates the intrinsic pathway of coagulation [23]. Accordingly, in experimental models of sepsis or endotoxinemia, application of recombinant TFPI [24, 25] or active site-inhibited factor VIIa (FVIIa) [26] resulted in suppression of the extrinsic pathway of coagulation and in a reduction of lung injury scores. Although under debate, the Recombinant Human Protein C Worldwide Evaluation in Severe Sepsis (PROWESS) trial assessing aPC in patients with severe early sepsis also forwarded some evidence for a reduced incidence of pulmonary failure in the treatment arm [27].

Extravascular, Alveolar Deposition of Fibrin Is a Hallmark in ARDS and Other Acute Inflammatory Lung Diseases

Under acute inflammatory conditions, the deposition of fibrin is, however, not restricted to the intravascular space of the lung: hyaline membranes are hallmarks of several acute inflammatory lung diseases and reflect the generation of fibrin in the alveolar compartment. It has been shown that a prominent shift of the hemostatic balance is also found within the alveolar compartment in response to inflammatory stimuli. In bronchoalveolar lavage fluids (BALF) of patients with ARDS or severe pneumonia, but not with cardiogenic (hydrostatic) lung edema, marked upregulation of TF, FVII activities [28–31] and FVII activating protease [32], antigen level of PAI-1 and α-2-antiplasmin [29, 31, 33] was noted. In parallel, the concentration of u-PA, the predominant plasminogen activator in the alveolar space, was found to be greatly depressed [31, 33]. Both, the alveolar macrophages as well as the alveolar type II cells are the predominant source of TF, FVII and factor X (FX) [34, 35] as well as PAI-1 and u-PA [34].

Likewise to the microthrombosis observed in the vascular space, deposition of fibrin in the alveolar compartment seems to contribute to the profound maldistribution of ventilation and perfusion in the acutely inflamed lung. We could show that generation of fibrin in vitro and in vivo would result in a far-reaching incorporation of all hydrophobic surfactant components into the growing fibrin lattice, thereby inducing an increase in alveolar surface tension, alveolar collapse especially at end expiration, and thus pulmonary shunt flow and arterial hypoxemia [36, 37]. A specialized alveolar fibrin lattice evolves, being characterized by reduced stiffness, decreased hydraulic conductivity, increased mean pore size [38], and a higher resistance towards fibrinolysis [39, 40].

Intra-Alveolar Activation of Coagulation and Persistent Alveolar Fibrin Deposition Are Regularly Found in Patients with Diffuse Parenchymal Lung Diseases

Increased procoagulant and depressed fibrinolytic activities are also commonly observed in the lungs of patients with interstitial lung diseases (ILD) such as idiopathic pulmonary fibrosis (IPF) [41, 42]; they are linked to disease severity [43] and result in increased alveolar fibrin deposition due to a local hemostatic imbalance already early in the disease [44, 45]. Similar changes of the alveolar hemostatic balance have been reported in animal models of acute lung injury and pulmonary fibrosis including that of bleomycin-induced lung injury [46, 47]. The underlying changes of coagulation or fibrinolysis factors are more or less the same as encountered in ARDS patients (see above), with TF, FVII, and PAI-1 being the most upregulated factors [41–43, 46, 47] and alveolar type II cells and macrophages serving as major source [48]. In clinical and experimental ILD, such increase of procoagulants is also amplified by unchanged TFPI [49] and suppressed u-PA [43] and aPC levels [50, 51]. It has been reported that epithelial cells of the lung can express and synthesize fibrinogen [52]. Thus, in principle, the lung can regulate generation of procoagulatory factors and deposition of fibrin in an autochthonal manner and independent of the status of barrier function and leakage of plasma proteins.

How Could Procoagulant and/or Antifibrinolytic Pathways Contribute to Lung Fibrosis?

It was previously anticipated that the deposition of fibrin per se may represent an important mechanism in the propagation of lung fibrosis. This was primarily based on the observation that the extent of lung fibrosis was somehow correlated with the severity of procoagulant and antifibrinolytic changes [43]. Next to the induction of ventilation-perfusion (V/Q) mismatch in the lung as outlined above, alveolar fibrin formation was also thought to promote the fibrotic response by providing a provisional matrix capable of fibroblast proliferation and activation. Provisional matrix components such as fibrin and fibronectin have also been recently disclosed to induce epithelial to mesenchymal transition (EMT) in vitro, a pathophysiologically important process in lung and renal fibrosis [53]. Based on these results it was speculated that collapsed, fibrin-glued alveoli may represent the nidus of fibrotic processes in the lung.

 Markart/Wygrecka/Ruppert/Korfei/Dahal/Jennes/Preissner/Seeger/Günther

However, the observation that lung fibrosis may nevertheless develop in fibrinogen knockout mice in response to bleomycin challenge [54, 55], a standard model of lung fibrosis, has raised some doubts in view of the role of fibrin formation per se and has set the stage for the identification of several other, potentially important signalling mechanisms that could additionally contribute to development of organ fibrosis. The first candidate to be mentioned in this context is the protease-activated receptor (PAR)-dependent signalling pathway. PAR 1–4 are a group of 7 transmembrane spanning, G-protein-coupled receptors being found on platelets, endothelial, interstitial and epithelial cells [56, 57]. Upon cleavage of an extracellular, aminoterminal activation domain, the new N-terminus serves as an intramolecular tethered ligand and induces signalling via G-protein-coupled mechanisms. The known 4 PAR differ in protease sensitivity and specificity [58]. Of note, thrombin can activate PAR-1, -3, and -4, FXa mostly PAR-1 and -2, and TF/FVIIa PAR-2 [56–58]. Apart from the pleiotropic effects in the vasculature (regulation of vessel tone, platelet degranulation, induction of endothelial leakage and proliferation, smooth muscle cell proliferation, and matrix production) and immune competent cells (activation of monocytes, T-lymphocytes, and mast cells with release of proinflammatory cytokines), PAR-1 signalling not only induces release of platelet-derived growth factor, connective tissue growth factor, and transforming growth factor-β, but also fibroblast activation, proliferation, myofibroblast transformation, and induction and synthesis of collagen [56–58]. Thus, PAR-mediated signalling could largely influence profibrotic events in the lung.

Moreover, the fibrinolytic system may exert profound influence on lung fibrosis and matrix remodelling independent of the process of fibrin(ogen) cleavage. In detail, it had been shown that u-PA and especially plasmin are capable of directly or indirectly activating different matrix metalloproteases (MMP) such as MMP1 and MMP3 [59, 60]. The u-PA/u-PA receptor system also plays a significant role in pericellular lysis, and thus in cell migration [61]. Finally, u-PA, the predominant plasminogen activator in lung and kidney, has been shown to directly activate hepatocyte growth factor (HGF) [62, 63], a cytokine with distinct antifibrotic and antiapoptotic properties on epithelial cells. In detail, activated HGF has been shown to block transforming growth factor-β-dependent signalling pathways and connective growth factor activation in epithelial cells on the level of signalling proteins Smad 2,3 via upregulation of the Smad transcriptional corepressor SnoN [64–66]; moreover, it is under discussion to represent an important antiapoptotic factor of epithelial cells, being released by the surrounding mesenchymal cells [67–69]. At least in some clinical forms of lung fibrosis such as IPF, the release and the activation of HGF have been found to be greatly reduced in isolated lung fibroblasts [70, 71].

Taken together, there is considerable evidence that the modulation of fibrin deposition per se may play an inferior role as compared to cellular downstream signalling events in the propagation of lung fibrosis by procoagulant or antifibrinolytic factors.

In Vivo Evidence of a Contributing Role of Procoagulant or Antifibrinolytic Factors in Experimental Lung Fibrosis – Therapeutic Prospects

In the past, the respective role of single coagulant or fibrinolytic factors has been assessed in different animal models of lung fibrosis. All available data suggest that in the bleomycin-induced lung injury and fibrosis, being the only model studied up to now, almost any therapeutic modulation of the hemostatic balance in a sense of increased fibrinolytic or suppressed procoagulant activity is followed by an attenuation of the extent of fibrosis [50, 72–77]. As the course of bleomycin-induced lung fibrosis remained largely unchanged in fibrinogen, t-PA, and u-PA receptor (u-PAR) knockout mice [54, 55, 73], it had been suggested that fibrin per se does not play a dominant role. Rather, u-PA/plasmin- or TF/FVII-, FX- or thrombin-elicited downstream signalling pathways may largely determine the magnitude of the fibrotic response. This was reinforced by the observation that gene transfer or protein application of HGF [78–81] as well as use of PAR-1 knockout mice [82] was followed by a far-reaching protection from fibrotic events in the bleomycin model.

Although being fairly reproducible and thereby mimicking the disturbed alveolar coagulatory and fibrinolytic balance observed in ILD, it has to be mentioned that the bleomycin model of lung fibrosis does not represent an optimal model for some of the most aggressive forms of ILD such as IPF. In more depth, the bleomycin model is largely an inflammatory driven lung fibrosis model, whereas IPF is nowadays considered to develop largely independent of inflammatory events. Nevertheless, if the observations made in bleomycin-injured mice could be directly translated to human diseases, this would be very suggestive of a therapeutic efficacy of profibrinolytic or anticoagulatory strategies.

In fact, early clinical trials are either currently performed or planned to assess the role of profibrinolytic or anticoagulatory strategies in IPF. In these trials, systemically applied FXa antagonists, inhalative heparin or warfarin therapies are under investigation. Following the more downstream signalling concept, blockade of PAR signalling as well as administration of HGF may represent alternative approaches, although some mechanistic questions will have to be answered before entering clinical trials. For example, it is currently unclear which type of PAR (PAR-1 or PAR-2 or both) is the most decisive one for development of fibrosis under clinical conditions, and it is also not known if application of u-PA would be more effective as compared to an administration of HGF alone (suggestive of an additional working principle apart from HGF activation).

Conclusions and Future Directions

In summary, activation of coagulation and inhibition of fibrinolysis with consecutive generation of fibrin occurs in the vasculature space as well as in the alveolar compart-

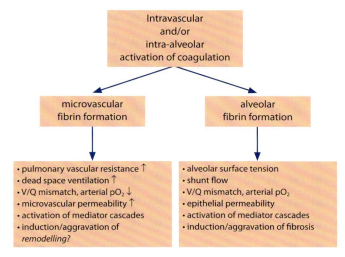

Fig. 1. Pathophysiological consequences of an intravascular (left) and intra-alveolar (right) fibrin formation in the lung in acute inflammatory and chronic interstitial lung diseases. V/Q mismatch = Ventilation-perfusion mismatch.

ment of the lung in a variety of acute inflammatory and diffuse parenchymal lung diseases. In both compartments, the acute generation of fibrin seems to contribute to mismatch of perfusion and ventilation (fig. 1), thereby effecting arterial hypoxemia. In addition, persistent fibrin deposition may also contribute to remodelling processes. Moreover, in diffuse parenchymal lung diseases, downstream signaling pathways elicited by components of the coagulation cascade, especially through PAR-1/-2, or impaired activation of protective factors such as HGF (because of PAI-1-induced u-PA blockade) seem to play an important role in the development of lung fibrosis and thus offer therapeutic targets for future clinical trials.

Disclosure of Conflict of Interests

The authors state that they have no conflict of interest.

Acknowledgement

The authors have been supported by the Deutsche Forschungsgemeinschaft (Clinical Research Group 118 'Pathomechanism and Therapy of Lung Fibrosis'; Excellence Cluster 'Cardiopulmonary System').

References

1 Heit JA, Silverstein MD, Morg DN, Petterson TM, O'Fallon WM, Melton LJ 3rd: Predictors of survival after deep vein thrombosis and pulmonary embolism: a population-based, cohort study. Arch Intern Med 1999;159:445–453.

2 Seeger W, Neuhof H, Hall J, Roka L: Pulmonary vasoconstrictor response to soluble fibrin in isolated lungs: possible role of thromboxane generation. Circ Res 1988;62:651–659.

3 Ge M, Tang G, Ryan TJ, Malik AB: Fibrinogen degradation product fragment D induces endothelial cell detachment by activation of cell-mediated fibrinolysis. J Clin Invest 1992;90:2508–2516.

4 Senior RM, Skogen WF, Griffin GL, Wilner GD: Effects of fibrinogen derivatives upon the inflammatory response. Studies with human fibrinopeptide B. J Clin Invest 1986;77:1014–1019.

5 Perlman MB, Johnson A, Jubiz W, Malik AB: Lipoxygenase products induce neutrophil activation and increase endothelial permeability after thrombin-induced pulmonary microembolism. Circ Res 1989;64:62–73.

6 Lang IM, Moser KM, Schleef RR: Elevated expression of urokinase-like plasminogen activator and plasminogen activator inhibitor type 1 during the vascular remodeling associated with pulmonary thromboembolism. Arterioscler Thromb Vasc Biol 1998;18:808–815.

7 Lang IM, Marsh JJ, Olman MA, Moser KM, Loskutoff DJ, Schleef RR: Expression of type 1 plasminogen activator inhibitor in chronic pulmonary thromboemboli. Circulation 1994;89:2715–2721.

8 Hoeper MM, Sosada M, Fabel H: Plasma coagulation profiles in patients with severe primary pulmonary hypertension. Eur Respir J 1998;12:1446–1449.

9 Rich S, Kaufmann E, Levy PS: The effect of high doses of calcium-channel blockers on survival in primary pulmonary hypertension. N Engl J Med 1992;327:76–81.

10 Saldeen T: Trends in microvascular research. The microembolism syndrome. Microvasc Res 1976;11:227–259.

11 Moalli R, Doyle JM, Tahhan HR, Hasan FM, Braman SS, Saldeen T: Fibrinolysis in critically ill patients. Am Rev Respir Dis 1989;140:287–293.

12 Carvalho AC, DeMarinis S, Scott CF, Silver LD, Schmaier AH, Colman RW: Activation of the contact system of plasma proteolysis in the adult respiratory distress syndrome. J Lab Clin Med 1988;112:270–277.

13 Healy AM, Hancock WV, Christie PD, Rayburn HB, Rosenberg RD: Intravascular coagulation activation in a murine model of thrombomodulin deficiency: effects of lesion size, age, and hypoxia on fibrin deposition. Blood 1998;92:4188–4197.

14 Hara S, Asada Y, Hatakeyama K, Marutsuka K, Sato Y, Kisanuki A, Sumiyoshi A: Expression of tissue factor and tissue factor pathway inhibitor in rats lungs with lipopolysaccharide-induced disseminated intravascular coagulation. Lab Invest 1997;77:581–589.

15 Muth H, Maus U, Wygrecka M, Lohmeyer J, Grimminger F, Seeger W, Günther A: Pro- and antifibrinolytic properties of human pulmonary microvascular versus artery endothelial cells: impact of endotoxin and tumor necrosis factor-alpha. Crit Care Med 2004;32:217–226.

16 Grau GE, de Moerloose P, Bulla O, Lou J, Lei Z, Reber G, Mili N, Ricou B, Morel DR, Suter PM: Haemostatic properties of human pulmonary and cerebral microvascular endothelial cells. Thromb Haemost 1997;77:585–590.

17 Takahashi K, Kiguchi T, Sawasaki Y, Karikusa F, Nemoto N, Matsuoka T, Yamamoto M: Lung capillary endothelial cells produce and secrete urokinase-type plasminogen activator. Am J Respir Cell Mol Biol 1992;7:90–94.

18 Quax PH, van den Hogen CM, Verheijen JH, Padro T, Zeheb R, Gelehrter TD, van Berkel TJ, Kuiper J, Emeis JJ: Endotoxin induction of plasminogen activator and plasminogen activator inhibitor type 1 mRNA in rat tissues in vivo. J Biol Chem 1990;265:15560–15563.

19 van der Poll T, Levi M, Hack CE, ten Cate H, van Deventer SJ, Eerenberg AJ, de Groot ER, Jansen J, Gallati H, Buller HR, Tencate JW, Aarden LA: Elimination of interleukin 6 attenuates coagulation activation in experimental endotoxemia in chimpanzees. J Exp Med 1994;179:1253–1259.

20 Drake TA, Cheng J, Chang A, Taylor FB Jr: Expression of tissue factor, thrombomodulin, and E-selectin in baboons with lethal Escherichia coli sepsis. Am J Pathol 1993;142:1458–1470.

21 Albertson CM, Richter KK, Kudryk BJ, Fink LM, Hauer-Jensen M: Association between decreased pulmonary endothelial cell thrombomodulin and local fibrin deposition in pneumonia. Blood Coagul Fibrinolysis 2001;12:729–733.

22 Fourrier F, Chopin C, Goudemand J, Hendrycx S, Caron C, Rime A, Marey A, Lestavel P: Septic shock, multiple organ failure, and disseminated intravascular coagulation. Compared patterns of antithrombin III, protein C, and protein S deficiencies. Chest 1992;101:816–23.

23 Kannemeier C, Shibamiya A, Nakazawa F, Trusheim H, Ruppert C, Markart P, Song Y, Tzima E, Kennerknecht E, Niepmann M, von Bruehl ML, Sedding D, Massberg S, Günther A, Engelmann B, Preissner KT: Extracellular RNA constitutes a natural procoagulant cofactor in blood coagulation. Proc Natl Acad Sci U S A 2007;104:6388–6393.

24 Creasey AA, Chang AC, Feigen L, Wün TC, Taylor FB Jr, Hinshaw LB: Tissue factor pathway inhibitor reduces mortality from Escherichia coli septic shock. J Clin Invest 1993;91:2850–2860.

25 Enkhbaatar P, Okajima K, Murakami K, Uchiba M, Okabe H, Okabe K, Yamaguchi Y: Recombinant tissue factor pathway inhibitor reduces lipopolysaccharide-induced pulmonary vascular injury by inhibiting leukocyte activation. Am J Respir Crit Care Med 2000;162:1752–1759.

26 Miller DL, Welty-Wolf K, Carraway MS, Ezban M, Ghio A, Suliman H, Piantadosi CA: Extrinsic coagulation blockade attenuates lung injury and proinflammatory cytokine release after intratracheal lipopolysaccharide. Am J Respir Cell Mol Biol 2002;26:650–658.

27 Bernard GR, Vincent JL, Laterre PF, LaRosa SP, Dhainaut JF, Lopez-Rodriguez A, Steingrub JS, Garber GE, Helterbrand JD, Ely EW, Fisher CJ Jr; Recombinant human protein C Worldwide Evaluation in Severe Sepsis (PROWESS) study group: Efficacy and safety of recombinant human activated protein C for severe sepsis. N Engl J Med 2001;344:699–709.

28 Nakstad B, Boye NP, Lyberg T: Procoagulant activities in human alveolar macrophages. Eur J Respir Dis 1987;71:459–471.

29 Idell S, Koenig KB, Fair DS, Martin TR, McLarty J, Maunder RJ: Serial abnormalities of fibrin turnover in evolving adult respiratory distress syndrome. Am J Physiol 1991;261:L240–L248.

30 Seeger W, Hübel J, Klappetek K, Pison U, Obertacke U, Joka T, Roka L: Procoagulant activity in bronchoalveolar lavage of severely traumatized patients – relation to the development of acute respiratory distress. Thromb Res 1991;61:53–64.

31 Günther A, Mosavi P, Heinemann S, Ruppert C, Muth H, Markart P, Grimminger F, Walmrath D, Temmesfeld-Wollbrück B, Seeger W: Alveolar fibrin formation caused by enhanced procoagulant and depressed fibrinolytic capacities in severe pneumonia. Comparison with the acute respiratory distress syndrome. Am J Respir Crit Care Med 2000;161:454–462.

32 Wygrecka M, Markart P, Fink L, Guenther A, Preissner KT: Raised protein levels and altered cellular expression of factor VII activating protease (FSAP) in the lungs of patients with acute respiratory distress syndrome (ARDS). Thorax 2007;62:880–888.

33 Bertozzi P, Astedt B, Zenzius L, Lynch K, LeMaire F, Zapol W, Chapman HA Jr: Depressed bronchoalveolar urokinase activity in patients with adult respiratory distress syndrome. N Engl J Med 1990;322:890–897.

34 Wygrecka M, Markart P, Ruppert C, Kuchenbuch T, Fink L, Bohle RM, Grimminger F, Seeger W, Günther A: Compartment- and cell-specific expression of coagulation and fibrinolysis factors in the murine lung undergoing inhalational versus intravenous endotoxin application. Thromb Haemost 2004;92:529–540.

35 Gross TJ, Simon RH, Sitrin RG: Tissue factor procoagulant expression by rat alveolar epithelial cells. Am J Respir Cell Mol Biol 1992;6:397–403.

36 Seeger W, Elssner A, Günther A, Krämer HJ, Kalinowski HO: Lung surfactant phospholipids associate with polymerizing fibrin: loss of surface activity. Am J Respir Cell Mol Biol 1993;9:213–220.

37 Schermuly RT, Günther A, Ermert M, Ermert L, Ghofrani HA, Weissmann N, Grimminger F, Seeger W, Walmrath D: Conebulization of surfactant and urokinase restores gas exchange in perfused lungs with alveolar fibrin formation. Am J Physiol Lung Cell Mol Physiol 2001;280:L792–800.

38 Günther A, Kalinowski M, Rosseau S, Seeger W: Surfactant incorporation markedly alters mechanical properties of a fibrin clot. Am J Respir Cell Mol Biol 1995;13:712–718.

39 Günther A, Kalinowski M, Elssner A, Seeger W: Clot-embedded natural surfactant: kinetics of fibrinolysis and surface activity. Am J Physiol 1994;267:L618–624.

40 Günther A, Markart P, Kalinowski M, Ruppert C, Grimminger F, Seeger W: Cleavage of surfactant-incorporating fibrin by different fibrinolytic agents. Kinetics of lysis and rescue of surface activity. Am J Respir Cell Mol Biol 1999;21:738–745.

41 Robinson BWS: Production of plasminogen activator by alveolar macrophages in normal subjects and patients with interstitial lung disease. Thorax 1988;43:508–515.

42 Kotani I, Sato A, Hayakawa H, Urano T, Takada Y, Takada A: Increased procoagulant and antifibrinolytic activities in the lungs with idiopathic pulmonary fibrosis. Thromb Res 1995;77:493–504.

43 Günther A, Mosavi P, Ruppert C, Heinemann S, Temmesfeld B, Velcovsky HG, Morr H, Grimminger F, Walmrath D, Seeger W: Enhanced tissue factor pathway activity and fibrin turnover in the alveolar compartment of patients with interstitial lung disease. Thromb Haemost 2000;83:853–860.

44 Kuhn C 3rd, Boldt J, King TE Jr, Crouch E, Vartio T, McDonald JA: An immunohistochemical study of architectural remodeling and connective tissue synthesis in pulmonary fibrosis. Am Rev Respir Dis 1989;140:1693–1703.

45 Imokawa S, Sato A, Hayakawa H, Kotani M, Urano T, Takada A: Tissue factor expression and fibrin deposition in the lungs of patients with idiopathic pulmonary fibrosis and systemic sclerosis. Am J Respir Crit Care Med 1997;156:631–636.

46 Idell S, James KK, Gillies C, Fair DS, Thrall RS: Abnormalities of pathways of fibrin turnover in lung lavage of rats with oleic acid and bleomycin-induced lung injury support alveolar fibrin deposition. Am J Pathol 1989;135:387–399.

47 Olman MA, Mackman N, Gladson CL, Moser KM, Loskutoff DJ: Changes in procoagulant and fibrinolytic gene expression during bleomycin-induced lung injury in the mouse. J Clin Invest 1995;96:1621–1630.

48 Wygrecka M, Markart P, Ruppert C, Petri K, Preissner KT, Seeger W, Guenther A: Cellular origin of pro-coagulant and (anti)-fibrinolytic factors in bleomycin-injured lungs. Eur Respir J 2007;29:1105–1114.

49 de Moerloose P, De Benedetti E, Nicod L, Vifian C, Reber G: Procoagulant activity in bronchoalveolar fluids: no relationship with tissue factor pathway inhibitor activity. Thromb Res 1992;65:507–518.

50 Yasui H, Gabazza EC, Tamaki S, Kobayashi T, Hataji O, Yuda H, Shimizu S, Suzuki K, Adachi Y, Taguchi O: Intratracheal administration of activated protein C inhibits bleomycin-induced lung fibrosis in the mouse. Am J Respir Crit Care Med 2001;163:1660–1668.

51 Kobayashi H, Gabazza EC, Taguchi O, Wada H, Takeya H, Nishioka J, Yasui H, Kobayashi T, Hataji O, Suzuki K, Adachi Y: Protein C anticoagulant system in patients with interstitial lung disease. Am J Respir Crit Care Med 1998;157:1850–1854.

52 Haidaris PJ: Induction of fibrinogen biosynthesis and secretion from cultured pulmonary epithelial cells. Blood 1997;89:873–882.

53 Kim KK, Kugler MC, Wolters PJ, Robillard L, Galvez MG, Brumwell AN, Sheppard D, Chapman HA: Alveolar epithelial cell mesenchymal transition develops in vivo during pulmonary fibrosis and is regulated by the extracellular matrix. Proc Natl Acad Sci U S A 2006;103:13180–13185.

54 Hattori N, Degen J, Sisson TH, Liu H, Moore BB, Pandrangi RG, Simon RH, Drew AF: Bleomycin-induced pulmonary fibrosis in fibrinogen-null mice. J Clin Invest 2000;106:1341–1350.

55 Wilberding JA, Ploplis VA, McLennan L, Liang Z, Cornelissen I, Feldman M, Deford ME, Rosen ED, Castellino FJ: Development of pulmonary fibrosis in fibrinogen-deficient mice. Ann N Y Acad Sci 2001;936:542–548.

56 Leger AJ, Covic L, Kuliopulos A: Protease-activated receptors in cardiovascular diseases. Circulation 2006;114:1070–1077.

57 Chambers RC, Laurent GJ: Coagulation cascade proteases and tissue fibrosis. Biochem Soc Trans 2002;30:194–200.

58 Macfarlane SR, Seatter MJ, Kanke T, Hunter GD, Plevin R: Proteinase-activated receptors. Pharmacol Rev 2001;53:245–282.

59 Murphy G, Stanton H, Cowell S, Butler G, Knäuper V, Atkinson S, Gavrilovic J: Mechanisms for pro matrix metalloproteinase activation. APMIS 1999;107:38–44.

60 Zhang Y, Zhou ZH, Bugge TH, Wahl LM: Urokinase-type plasminogen activator stimulation of monocyte matrix metalloproteinase-1 production is mediated by plasmin-dependent signaling through annexin A2 and inhibited by inactive plasmin. J Immunol 2007;179:3297–3304.

61 Blasi F, Carmeliet P: uPAR: a versatile signalling orchestrator. Nat Rev Mol Cell Biol 2002;3:932–943.

62 Naldini L, Tamagnone L, Vigna E, Sachs M, Hartmann G, Birchmeier W, Daikuhara Y, Tsubouchi H, Blasi F, Comoglio PM: Extracellular proteolytic cleavage by urokinase is required for activation of hepatocyte growth/scatter factor. EMBO J 1992;11:4825–4833.

63 Naldini L, Vigna E, Bardelli A, Follenzi A, Galimi F, Comoglio PM: Biological activation of pro-HGF (hepatocyte growth factor) by urokinase is controlled by a stoichiometric reaction. J Biol Chem 1995;270:603–611.

64 Wahab NA, Mason RM: A critical look at growth factors and epithelial-to-mesenchymal transition in the adult kidney. Interrelationships between growth factors that regulate EMT in the adult kidney. Nephron Exp Nephrol 2006;104:e129–134.

65 Inoue T, Okada H, Kobayashi T, Watanabe Y, Kanno Y, Kopp JB, Nishida T, Takigawa M, Ueno M, Nakamura T, Suzuki H: Hepatocyte growth factor counteracts transforming growth factor-beta1, through attenuation of connective tissue growth factor induction, and prevents renal fibrogenesis in 5/6 nephrectomized mice. FASEB J 2003;17:268–270.

66 Yang J, Dai C, Liu Y: A novel mechanism by which hepatocyte growth factor blocks tubular epithelial to mesenchymal transition. J Am Soc Nephrol 2005;16:68–78.

67 Charbeneau RP, Christensen PJ, Chrisman CJ, Paine R 3rd, Toews GB, Peters-Golden M, Moore BB: Impaired synthesis of prostaglandin E2 by lung fibroblasts and alveolar epithelial cells from GM-CSF –/– mice: implications for fibroproliferation. Am J Physiol Lung Cell Mol Physiol 2003;284:L1103–1111.

68 Kolodsick JE, Peters-Golden M, Larios J, Toews GB, Thannickal VJ, Moore BB: Prostaglandin E2 inhibits fibroblast to myofibroblast transition via E. prostanoid receptor 2 signaling and cyclic adenosine monophosphate elevation. Am J Respir Cell Mol Biol 2003;29:537–544.

69 Moore BB, Peters-Golden M, Christensen PJ, Lama V, Kuziel WA, Paine R 3rd, Toews GB: Alveolar epithelial cell inhibition of fibroblast proliferation is regulated by MCP-1/CCR2 and mediated by PGE2. Am J Physiol Lung Cell Mol Physiol 2003;284:L342–349.

70 Marchand-Adam S, Marchal J, Cohen M, Soler P, Gerard B, Castier Y, Lesèche G, Valeyre D, Mal H, Aubier M, Dehoux M, Crestani B: Defect of hepatocyte growth factor secretion by fibroblasts in idiopathic pulmonary fibrosis. Am J Respir Crit Care Med 2003;168:1156–1161.

71 Marchand-Adam S, Fabre A, Mailleux AA, Marchal J, Quesnel C, Kataoka H, Aubier M, Dehoux M, Soler P, Crestani B: Defect of pro-hepatocyte growth factor activation by fibroblasts in idiopathic pulmonary fibrosis. Am J Respir Crit Care Med 2006;174:58–66.

72   Eitzman DT, McCoy RD, Zheng X, Fay WP, Shen T, Ginsburg D, Simon RH: Bleomycin-induced pulmonary fibrosis in transgenic mice that either lack or overexpress the murine plasminogen activator inhibitor-1 gene. J Clin Invest 1996;97:232–237.

73   Swaisgood CM, French EL, Noga C, Simon RH, Ploplis VA: The development of bleomycin-induced pulmonary fibrosis in mice deficient for components of the fibrinolytic system. Am J Pathol 2000;157:177–187.

74   Sisson TH, Hanson KE, Subbotina N, Patwardhan A, Hattori N, Simon RH: Inducible lung-specific urokinase expression reduces fibrosis and mortality after lung injury in mice. Am J Physiol Lung Cell Mol Physiol 2002;283:L1023–1032.

75   Günther A, Lübke N, Ermert M, Schermuly RT, Weissmann N, Breithecker A, Markart P, Ruppert C, Quanz K, Ermert L, Grimminger F, Seeger W: Prevention of bleomycin-induced lung fibrosis by aerosolization of heparin or urokinase in rabbits. Am J Respir Crit Care Med 2003;168:1358–1365.

76   Howell DC, Johns RH, Lasky JA, Shan B, Scotton CJ, Laurent GJ, Chambers RC: Absence of proteinase-activated receptor-1 signaling affords protection from bleomycin-induced lung inflammation and fibrosis. Am J Pathol 2005;166:1353–1365.

77   Kijiyama N, Ueno H, Sugimoto I, Sasaguri Y, Yatera K, Kido M, Gabazza EC, Suzuki K, Hashimoto E, Takeya H: Intratracheal gene transfer of tissue factor pathway inhibitor attenuates pulmonary fibrosis. Biochem Biophys Res Commun 2006;339:1113–1119.

78   Watanabe M, Ebina M, Orson FM, Nakamura A, Kubota K, Koinuma D, Akiyama K, Maemondo M, Okouchi S, Tahara M, Matsumoto K, Nakamura T, Nukiwa T: Hepatocyte growth factor gene transfer to alveolar septa for effective suppression of lung fibrosis. Mol Ther 2005;12:58–67.

79   Gazdhar A, Fachinger P, van Leer C, Pierog J, Gugger M, Friis R, Schmid RA, Geiser T: Gene transfer of hepatocyte growth factor by electroporation reduces bleomycin-induced lung fibrosis. Am J Physiol Lung Cell Mol Physiol 2007;292:L529–536.

80   Yaekashiwa M, Nakayama S, Ohnuma K, Sakai T, Abe T, Satoh K, Matsumoto K, Nakamura T, Takahashi T, Nukiwa T: Simultaneous or delayed administration of hepatocyte growth factor equally represses the fibrotic changes in murine lung injury induced by bleomycin. A morphologic study. Am J Respir Crit Care Med 1997;156:1937–1944.

81   Dohi M, Hasegawa T, Yamamoto K, Marshall BC: Hepatocyte growth factor attenuates collagen accumulation in a murine model of pulmonary fibrosis. Am J Respir Crit Care Med 2000;162:2302–2307.

82   Howell DC, Goldsack NR, Marshall RP, McAnulty RJ, Starke R, Purdy G, Laurent GJ, Chambers RC: Direct thrombin inhibition reduces lung collagen, accumulation, and connective tissue growth factor mRNA levels in bleomycin-induced pulmonary fibrosis. Am J Pathol 2001;159:1383–1395.

Prof. Dr. med. Andreas Günther
University of Giessen Lung Center (UGLC)
Klinikstr. 36
35392 Giessen, Germany
E-Mail andreas.guenther@uglc.de

Scharf RE (ed): Progress and Challenges in Transfusion Medicine, Hemostasis and Hemotherapy.
Freiburg i.Br., Karger, 2008, pp 48–59

Interaction of Platelets and Inflammatory Endothelium in the Development and Progression of Coronary Artery Disease

Harald F. Langer · Meinrad P. Gawaz

Internal Medicine III, Eberhard Karls University Tübingen, Germany

Key Words

Endothelium · Platelets · Inflammatory response · Atherosclerosis · Coronary artery disease · Athero-thrombosis

Summary

An expanding body of evidence continues to build on the role of platelets as initial actors in the development of atherosclerotic lesions. Platelets bind to leukocytes and endothelial cells and initiate monocyte transformation into macrophages. Thus, platelets can contribute to vascular inflammation. Platelets bind oxidized phospholipids and promote foam cell formation. Platelets also recruit progenitor cells to the scene, which are able to differentiate into foam cells or endothelial cells depending on conditions. Furthermore, platelets are capable of recruiting dendritic cells and influence their functions, presumably modulating immune reactions affecting atherogenesis. Platelets tip the scales in the initiation, development, and total extent of atherosclerotic lesions.   ©2008 S. Karger GmbH, Freiburg i.Br.

Introduction

At the site of vascular lesions, rupture of an atherosclerotic plaque results in discontinuity of the endothelial barrier with exposure of thrombogenic subendothelial matrix proteins such as von Willebrand factor (vWF) and collagen. Platelets are the first cellular components to cover such a defect by a complex cascade with distinct interacting mechanisms. Rupture or erosion of the advanced lesion initiates platelet activation and aggregation on the surface of the disrupted atherosclerotic plaque. Thrombotic vascular occlusion is associated with ischemic episodes, including acute coronary syndromes or cerebral infarction.

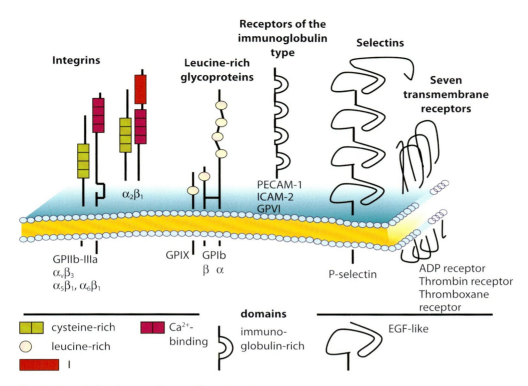

Fig. 1. Central platelet membrane adhesion receptors.

Platelet Adhesion

The adhesion process of platelets is mediated by distinct adhesion receptors (fig. 1). Numerous studies were able to show that the initial contact of circulating platelets with the vascular lesion is mediated via interaction of platelet glycoprotein (GP) Ib-V-IX with collagen-bound vWF. Recent data revealed that a further membrane glycoprotein, the platelet collagen receptor GPVI, plays a critical role for the adhesion process. Fibrillar collagen is the major extracellular matrix protein. Inhibition of interaction of GPVI with collagen by anti-GPVI monoclonal antibodies or soluble dimeric GPVI attenuates thrombosis at arterial lesions in vivo. In contrast to GPIb-V-IX, it directly mediates adhesion to subendothelial collagen and the activation of other adhesion receptors such as $\alpha IIb\beta 3$ (GPIIb-IIIa) and $\alpha 2\beta 1$ (GPIa-IIa). These integrins are essential for firm adhesion of platelets. While $\alpha 2\beta 1$ directly binds to collagen, the GPIIb-IIIa receptor mediates an irreversible adhesion through binding to an RGD sequence in the C1 domain of vWF. The firm integrin-mediated adhesion results in activation and shape change of platelets. During this process, platelets form pseudopodia, which allow an effective sealing of the injured vessel wall. The adhesive and activated platelets produce thromboxane A2 (TxA2) from arachidonic acid (AA), which strengthens the activation process by binding to the specific thromboxane receptor. Next to TxA2, ADP is released from platelets and amplifies the process of adhesion, activation and, finally, aggregation.

Platelet Aggregation and Thrombus Formation

Aggregation is the amplification step that, within minutes, leads to the accumulation of platelets into the hemostatic thrombus. It is mediated by adhesive substrates bound to the membranes of activated platelets. After platelets have established contact with the thrombogenic substrate, the interaction of further platelets from the circulation with already adherent platelets is mediated via the activated GPIIb-IIIa receptor (integrin αIIbβIII). A principal outcome of platelet activation is a change in the ligand-binding function of GPIIb-IIIa. During the initial phase (primary aggregation), platelets are connected to each other only by 'loose' fibrinogen bridges. Seconds to minutes later, this contact is then followed by an irreversible stabilization of the fibrinogen bridges at the GPIIb-IIIa complex. Furthermore, platelets are shedding microparticles from their cell membrane, which catalyze fibrin formation and stabilization of the thrombus. Stability of the aggregate is as important as the rate of growth, deciding whether a thrombus will occlude an artery. CD40 ligand (CD40L), another recently described receptor expressed on platelets, seems to be crucial for the stabilization of the aggregates. Figure 2 gives an overview of the main receptors involved in the process of thrombus formation, from the initiation of adhesion to thrombus formation.

Platelets and Endothelial Inflammation

Atherosclerosis is a systemic inflammatory disease which is characterized by the accumulation of inflammatory cells in the intima of large arteries. These inflammatory cells include monocytes/macrophages, lymphocytes, dendritic cells (DCs), and natural killer cells [1]. While it is widely accepted that platelets play a significant role in thromboembolic complications of advanced atherosclerotic lesions, their involvement in the initiation of the atherosclerotic process has received limited attention.

Governed by disturbed flow, platelets adhere to the arterial wall in vivo, even in the absence of endothelial cell denudation, initiating lesion formation [2, 3]. The intact, nonactivated endothelium normally prevents platelet adhesion to the extracellular matrix. Under inflammatory conditions, however, platelets adhere to the intact, but activated endothelial cell monolayer [4–6]. This adhesion of platelets to the endothelium in vivo under high shear stress conditions, is a distinctly regulated multistep event that involves platelet tethering, followed by rolling and subsequent firm adhesion to the vascular wall [7, 8]. These processes are dependent on receptor interactions via selectins, integrins, and immunoglobulin-like receptors, which induce receptor-spe-

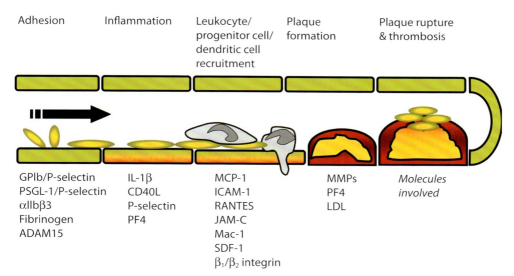

Adhesion	Inflammation	Leukocyte/ progenitor cell/ dendritic cell recruitment	Plaque formation	Plaque rupture & thrombosis

GPIb/P-selectin	IL-1β	MCP-1	MMPs	*Molecules*
PSGL-1/P-selectin	CD40L	ICAM-1	PF4	*involved*
αIIbβ3	P-selectin	RANTES	LDL	
Fibrinogen	PF4	JAM-C		
ADAM15		Mac-1		
		SDF-1		
		β_1/β_2 integrin		

Fig. 2. Model of vascular inflammation and atherogenesis triggered by platelets. Activated platelets roll along the endothelial monolayer via GPIb/platelet selectin (P-selectin) or P-selectin GP ligand-1 (PSGL-1)/P-selectin interaction. Thereafter, platelets firmly adhere to vascular endothelium via β_3 integrins, release proinflammatory compounds – interleukin (IL)-1β, CD40L –, and induce a proatherogenic phenotype of endothelial cells (chemotaxis, MCP-1; adhesion, ICAM-1). Subsequently, adherent platelets recruit circulating leukocytes, progenitor cells, and dendritic cells and interact with them, thereby initiating receptor signals and paracrine pathways. These signals result in leukocyte activation, transmigration, and foam cell formation, but may also provide immunomodulatory effects. Thus, platelets provide the inflammatory basis for plaque formation before physically occluding the vessel by thrombosis upon plaque rupture. ADAM15 = A disintegrin and metalloproteinase; ICAM-1 = intracellular adhesion molecule 1; JAM-C = junctional adhesion molecule-C; LDL = low-density lipoprotein; Mac-1 = integrin αMβ2; MCP-1 = monocyte chemoattractant protein 1; MMPS = matrix metalloproteinases; PF4 = platelet factor 4; SDF-1 = stromal cell-derived factor-1.

cific activation signals in both platelets and the respective partner in cell-cell adhesion, for instance endothelial cells. Inhibition of platelet adhesion to the endothelium resulted in decreased atherogenesis in different studies and animal models. Being a central receptor in this scenario [9–12], disruption of platelet P-selectin resulted in reduced atherosclerotic lesion formation in vivo [13–15]. This effect could be potentiated when both P-selectin (platelet selectin) and E-selectin (endothelial selectin) were knocked out [16].

αIIbβ3 (GPIIb-IIIa) is the major integrin on platelets and plays a key role in platelet accumulation on activated endothelium [6, 17]. Similarly to P-selectin, platelets defective in αIIbβ3 are impaired to adhere to activated endothelial cells [18]. Thus, it is not surprising that a significant contribution of platelet GPIIb to atheroprogression was shown recently in GPIIb/apolipoprotein E (ApoE) double knockout mice [19]. Another central adhesion molecule in platelet-endothelial interaction is the vitronectin receptor (αvβ3), which is upregulated in response to endothelial cell activation, e.g. by interleukin (IL)-1β or thrombin [6, 20]. The field of platelet adhesion is very dynamic and continuously new receptors or ligands are discovered that seem to play a role in platelet adhesion to the endothelium [21, 22].

Platelet Adhesion to the Endothelial Surface Generates Signals for the Recruitment of Monocytes to the Site of Inflammation

After a contact between platelets and the endothelium has been established, transcellular communication via soluble mediators results in proinflammatory signals (for instance the release of chemokines or the upregulation of further receptors mediating downstream events) both within the endothelium and the platelet itself. Between platelets and chemokines an intricate functional relationship exists, that provides a framework of mechanisms for synergistic functions and allows insights into the deleterious basis for proatherogenic, proinflammatory, or thrombogenic effects [23]. Activated platelets can release chemokines and can induce the secretion of chemokines in various cells of the vascular wall including CCL3, RANTES (CCL5), CCL7, CCL17, CXCL1, CXCL5, CXCL8, CXCL12, as well as precursors for CXCL7, such as β-thromboglobulin, from the α-granules [23–25]. In turn, certain chemokines can enhance platelet aggregation and adhesion in combination with primary agonists and can trigger monocyte recruitment [26]. The most important substances involved in platelet-triggered endothelial inflammation are platelet factor 4 (PF4; CXCL4), being the most abundant CXC chemokine released from platelet α-granules [27], CD40 ligand (CD40L, CD154), which shows a strong relation with an acute risk for a coronary event [28], and IL-1β [29]. Recently, a new member of the tumor necrosis factor (TNF) superfamily, LIGHT, has been shown to be involved in platelet-induced vascular inflammation [22]. IL-1β is of particular interest, as it has been recently shown to be one of the proteins actively generated by platelets themselves, a process which is dependent on splicing of pre-mRNA and involves platelet activation and GPIIb-IIIa engagement [30, 31].

Platelet – a Recruitment Factor for Further Circulating Cells

When activated, platelets coaggregate with circulating leukocytes [32, 33]. Once adherent to the vascular wall, platelets also provide a sticky surface to recruit leukocytes to the vessel wall. Recruitment of circulating leukocytes to the vascular wall requires multistep adhesive and signaling events that result in the infiltration of inflammatory cells into the vessel wall, including selectin-mediated attachment and rolling, leukocyte activation, integrin-mediated firm adhesion, and diapedesis [34]. Leukocytes tether to adherent platelets via P-selectin glycoprotein ligand-1 (PSGL-1)/P-selectin interactions and, subsequently, firmly adhere via binding of Mac-1

(CD11b/CD18) to GPIbα [35] and/or other receptors of the platelet membrane, including JAM-C [36] or bridging proteins such as fibrinogen (bound to GPIIb-IIIa) [17, 34]. During this adhesive process, receptor engagement together with platelet-derived inflammatory compounds induces inflammatory cascades in monocytes and endothelial cells and aggravates the inflammatory process leading to atherosclerosis [33, 34].

Platelets Interact with Progenitor Cells: Impact on Atherosclerosis

The first response to vascular injury is platelet adhesion either to the exposed subendothelium or to dysfunctional endothelial cells (see above). We recently showed that platelet adhesion not only triggers vascular atherothrombosis but also represents the essential step for the targeting of progenitor cells to sites of endothelial disruption [24, 37]. Platelets are also believed to have proinflammatory and chemotactic properties that contribute to the progression of atherosclerosis. Activated platelets release a plethora of growth factors, inflammatory mediators, and chemokines into their microenvironment [7]. We found that platelets also secrete the chemokine stromal cell-derived factor-1 (SDF-1), which supports primary adhesion of endothelial progenitor cells to the surface of arterial thrombi in vivo [24, 25]. We [24] and Abi-Younes et al. [38] demonstrated that arterial thrombi isolated from ruptured atherosclerotic plaques of human carotid arteries showed substantial SDF-1 release. Platelet α-granules contain the SDF-1 protein, being released to the platelet surface upon activation [25, 39]. Moreover, cytokine-mediated deployment of platelet-derived SDF-1 induces revascularization through recruitment of CXCR4+ hemangiocytes [40].

We found that human CD34+ progenitor cells adhere to immobilized platelets but not to immobilized collagen type I alone [37], which represents the major extracellular matrix component of the injured arterial wall [41]. Adhesion of CD34+ cells to immobilized platelets was significantly attenuated in the presence of blocking monoclonal antibodies (mAbs) anti-CD162 or anti-CD62P, indicating that platelet P-selectin binds to endothelial progenitor cell PSGL-1 [37, 42]. Moreover, β1-integrin located on the surface of endothelial progenitor cells is involved in the adhesion process between immobilized platelets and human progenitor cells [37, 42].

Using real-time in vivo double fluorescence microscopy of the mouse carotid artery, we demonstrated that CD34+ and c-Kit+ Sca-1+ Lin-1− (KSL) bone marrow-derived progenitor cells directly adhere to platelets after vascular injury in a process that involves platelet P-selectin and the β-subunit of integrin αIIbβ3 [24]. Platelet-endothelial progenitor cell adhesion was proven to be an essential step for the recruitment of endothelial progenitor cells to vascular injury areas because endothelial progenitor cells do not directly adhere to subendothelial matrix proteins under high arterial shear. Flow cytometric experiments showed that endothelial progenitor cells do not express on their surface the respective adhesion receptors to collagen, fibronectin, fibrinogen, and vitronectin, the main components of the extracellular matrix (such as GPIb-V-IX and GPVI). Moreover, in vivo experiments in mice revealed that the absence of adherent platelets in areas of vascular injury through the usage of blocking mAbs to GPIb and GPVI almost completely inhibited the recruitment of CD34[+] progenitor cells [24].

Platelets play a critical part not only in the capture, but also in the subsequent differentiation of murine endothelial progenitor cells, inducing the differentiation of the latter into mature endothelial cells [37, 43]. Endothelial progenitor cells recruited to platelet aggregates give rise to neointimal cells, indicating that accumulation of endothelial progenitor cells in arterial thrombi may contribute to vascular repair and pathological remodelling [24]. Moreover, in the human system, CD34[+] progenitor cells can form colonies on immobilized platelets similar to immobilized fibronectin, indicating differentiation into endothelial cells (fig. 3) [44].

On the other hand, platelets induce distinct morphological changes of human CD34[+] cells and differentiate the subpopulations of these progenitor cells into macrophages and subsequently into foam cells in vitro [44]. After coincubation with platelets for 5–10 days, CD34[+] cells undergo substantial morphological changes. About one third of cells show a 3-fold increase in size with round morphology, high granularity, and a diameter of approximately 25 μm. No change in morphology of CD34[+] cells can be seen within the observation time when platelets are absent. These cells are positive for naphthyl acetate esterase and CD68, indicating differentiation into the macrophage/monocytic lineage. When Sudan Red III staining was performed, we found that a subpopulation of human CD34[+] cells transformed into large granular and lipid-rich cells, a morphology typical for foam cells [44, 45].

Phagocytosis of platelets from CD34[+] progenitor cells results in foam cell formation [44, 45]. Phase contrast microscopy shows that these foam cells are surrounded by a platelet-free zone, indicating enhanced phagocytotic activity of these cells. Transmission electron microscopy of the foam cells revealed the presence of multiple vesicles with phagocytosed platelets or platelet fragments. We found that internalization of platelets occurred rapidly and after 24 hours a substantial number of platelets were internalized by foam cells [44, 45].

Uptake of modified low-density lipoprotein (LDL) by macrophages plays an important role in the formation of foam cells, the early step of atherosclerosis [46, 47]. Platelets bind LDL that, in turn, leads to enhanced platelet responsiveness [44, 46, 47]. We found that platelets bound and internalized substantial amounts of LDL, as verified by fluorescence microscopy and flow cytometry. When LDL-labeled platelets were added to the platelet/CD34[+] cell coculture, a significant uptake of LDL-positive platelets into foam cells was observed, whereas virtually no uptake of LDL-labeled platelets was observed in cells that did not differentiate into foam cells [44]. Thus, platelet-lipoprotein interactions may promote atherosclerosis formation by providing an alternative and probably effective way of transporting lipoproteins into developing foam cells (fig. 3).

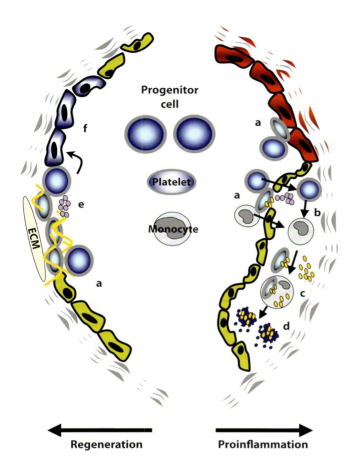

Progenitor cell

Platelet

Monocyte

ECM

Regeneration   Proinflammation

Fig. 3. Platelets serve as a bridging mechanism for circulating endothelial progenitor cells and thereby can contribute to atheroprogression and vascular regeneration. Platelets accumulate at sites of dysfunctional endothelium and disrupted atherosclerotic lesions. By release of proinflammatory molecules they themselves can induce or aggravate endothelial dysfunction. Armed with potent adhesion molecules for circulating cells, platelets are capable of recruiting circulating endothelial progenitor cells. Depending on the surrounding microenvironment, proatherogenetic (for instance the development of foam cells) or vascular reparatory mechanisms (differentiation of progenitor cells towards mature endothelial cells) can be promoted by interaction of platelets with progenitor cells. ECM = Extracellular matrix.

Platelets Recruit Circulating Dendritic Cells

The fact that platelets are significantly involved in atherosclerosis and presumably present for a prolonged time in atherosclerotic plaques is not novel. Already in 1961, Chandler and Hand reported that phagocyted platelets could be a source of lipids in human thrombi and atherosclerotic plaques [48]. Only recently, Jans et al. could show that platelet phagocytosis by macrophages occurs in atherosclerotic plaques and results in foam cell formation involving amyloid-β peptide [49]. Intriguingly, in our investigations we were able to show that also DCs substantially internalize platelets, when coincubated over several days [50]. The prerequisite for this process is that DCs get in contact with platelets at areas of developing or present atherosclerotic plaques. DC progenitors in the bone marrow give rise to circulating precursors that home to tissues, where they reside as immature cells with high phagocytotic capacity [51]. After antigen contact, immature DCs enter the lymph nodes, where they transform to mature DCs capable of interacting with T-cells and to initiate an immune response [51]. It is well known that circulating DCs can adhere to exposed subendothelial matrix proteins of atherosclerotic lesions like fibronectin [52]. Under arterial shear rates in vitro and in vivo, platelets were, however, a prerequisite to mediate substantial adhesion to injured vessels or to exposed collagen, which is the main component of the extracellular matrix [50]. This process was mediated via integrin $\alpha M\beta 2$ (Mac-1) (DC)/junctional adhesion molecule-C (JAM-C) (platelet) interaction [50]. Already earlier, Hagihara et al. could show that shear stress-activated platelets induce maturation of DCs [53]. This may, at least in part, be mediated by platelet heat shock protein [54]. Platelets are furthermore armed with secretory proteins like PF4, which are capable of modulating DCs [55]. According to our investigations, platelet-derived CD40L and PF4 were able to mediate DC activation in a mixed lymphocyte reaction, respectively differentiation of DCs [50]. However, also the direct contact of platelets with DCs alters DC function, as inhibition of Mac-1/JAM-C interaction resulted in decreased apoptosis of DCs [50]. The biological relevance of platelet engulfment by DCs in vivo has not been studied yet. Further in vitro and in vivo studies are needed to understand the role of this observation for atherogenesis. Taken together, platelets present at areas of atherosclerotic tissue can potentially alter DC biology, which could play a significant role in atheroprogression by DC recruitment, activation, differentiation, and induction of apoptosis.

Conclusions and Future Directions

An increasingly persuasive body of evidence indicates that platelets and humoral hemostatic components are important participants in vascular inflammation. These effects are largely mediated by chemokines and cytokines affecting platelets, endothelial cells, and other cells of the vascular wall. An intricate functional relationship exists between platelets and chemokines, which provides a framework of mechanisms for synergistic functions. It has been convincingly shown that platelets can aggravate inflammation by potentiating effects mediated by leukocytes. Now, progenitor cells and DCs come to the scene, giving rise to new theories of atherogenesis and atheroprogression. How progenitor cells and DCs are recruited to sites of vascular injury was poorly understood till recently. We and others were able to show that both human progenitor cells and DCs significantly adhere to platelets, indicating that platelets can be a bridge linking circulating progenitor cells and DCs to areas of inflamed endothelium or vascular injury. This strengthens the role of platelets for central steps involved in endothelial inflammation and the development of early and advanced atherosclerotic lesions. Strikingly, platelets can induce differentiation of progenitor cells to endothelial cells. If this process could be utilized, we may have a therapeutic tool for the treatment of vascular injury. However, also negative effects like the development of foam cells may be mediated. Thus, understanding the exact mechanisms involved is necessary.

Taken together, the platelet seems to be a central regulator in the middle of surrounding cells, including endothelium, macrophages, DCs, and progenitor cells (fig. 3).

Disclosure of Conflict of Interests

The authors state that they have no conflict of interest.

Acknowledgements

The study was supported by grants of the Deutsche Forschungsgemeinschaft (Graduiertenkolleg GK794, MA121/2-1, Li849/3-1), the Wilhelm Sander-Stiftung (Nr. 2003.0601), the Novartis-Stiftung, the Karl und Lore Klein Stiftung (D.30.08886), the Karl-Kuhn-Stiftung (AZ III 1.7-0415.221.18-01/AE04/2005), the Bundesministerium für Bildung, Wissenschaft, Forschung und Technologie, and the fortüne program of the Universitätsklinikum Tübingen (UKT). Dr. Langer received a research grant from the German Cardiac Society (Pfizer-Stipendium).

References

1 Hansson GK, Libby P: The immune response in atherosclerosis: a double-edged sword. Nat Rev Immunol 2006;6:508–519.

2 Jorgensen L: ADP-induced platelet aggregation in the microcirculation of pig myocardium and rabbit kidneys. J Thromb Haemost 2005;3:1119–1124.

3 Theilmeier G, Michiels C, Spaepen E, Vreys I, Collen D, Vermylen J, Hoylaerts MF: Endothelial von Willebrand factor recruits platelets to atherosclerosis-prone sites in response to hypercholesterolemia. Blood 2002;99:4486–4493.

4 Bombeli T, Schwartz BR, Harlan JM: Adhesion of activated platelets to endothelial cells: evidence for a GPIIbIIIa-dependent bridging mechanism and novel roles for endothelial intercellular adhesion molecule 1 (ICAM-1), alphavbeta3 integrin, and GPIbalpha. J Exp Med 1998;187:329–339.

5 Gawaz M, Neumann FJ, Ott I, Schiessler A, Schomig A: Platelet function in acute myocardial infarction treated with direct angioplasty. Circulation 1996;93:229–237.

6 Gawaz M, Neumann FJ, Dickfeld T, Reininger A, Adelsberger H, Gebhardt A, Schomig A: Vitronectin receptor (alpha(v)beta3) mediates platelet adhesion to the luminal aspect of endothelial cells: implications for reperfusion in acute myocardial infarction. Circulation 1997;96:1809–1818.

7 Frenette PS, Johnson RC, Hynes RO, Wagner DD: Platelets roll on stimulated endothelium in vivo: an interaction mediated by endothelial P-selectin. Proc Natl Acad Sci U S A 1995;92:7450–7454.

8 Massberg S, Enders G, Leiderer R, Eisenmenger S, Vestweber D, Krombach F, Messmer K: Platelet-endothelial cell interactions during ischemia/reperfusion: the role of P-selectin. Blood 1998;92:507–515.

9 Frenette PS, Moyna C, Hartwell DW, Lowe JB, Hynes RO, Wagner DD: Platelet-endothelial interactions in inflamed mesenteric venules. Blood 1998;91:1318–1324.

10 Frenette PS, Denis CV, Weiss L, Jurk K, Subbarao S, Kehrel B, Hartwig JH, Vestweber D, Wagner DD: P-Selectin glycoprotein ligand 1 (PSGL-1) is expressed on platelets and can mediate platelet-endothelial interactions in vivo. J Exp Med 2000;191:1413–1422.

11 Johnson RC, Mayadas TN, Frenette PS, Mebius RE, Subramaniam M, Lacasce A, Hynes RO, Wagner DD: Blood cell dynamics in P-selectin-deficient mice. Blood 1995;86:1106–1114.

12 Subramaniam M, Frenette PS, Saffaripour S, Johnson RC, Hynes RO, Wagner DD: Defects in hemostasis in P-selectin-deficient mice. Blood 1996;87:1238–1242.

13 Huo Y, Schober A, Forlow SB, Smith DF, Hyman MC, Jung S, Littman DR, Weber C, Ley K: Circulating activated platelets exacerbate atherosclerosis in mice deficient in apolipoprotein E. Nat Med 2003;9:61–67.

14 Burger PC, Wagner DD: Platelet P-selectin facilitates atherosclerotic lesion development. Blood 2003;101:2661–2666.

15 Manka D, Forlow SB, Sanders JM, Hurwitz D, Bennett DK, Green SA, Ley K, Sarembock IJ: Critical role of platelet P-selectin in the response to arterial injury in apolipoprotein-E-deficient mice. Arterioscler Thromb Vasc Biol 2004;24:1124–1129.

16 Dong ZM, Chapman SM, Brown AA, Frenette PS, Hynes RO, Wagner DD: The combined role of P- and E-selectins in atherosclerosis. J Clin Invest 1998;102:145–152.

17 Gawaz MP, Loftus JC, Bajt ML, Frojmovic MM, Plow EF, Ginsberg MH: Ligand bridging mediates integrin alpha IIb beta 3 (platelet GPIIB-IIIA) dependent homotypic and heterotypic cell-cell interactions. J Clin Invest 1991;88:1128–1134.

18 Massberg S, Enders G, Matos FC, Tomic LI, Leiderer R, Eisenmenger S, Messmer K, Krombach F: Fibrinogen deposition at the postischemic vessel wall promotes platelet adhesion during ischemia-reperfusion in vivo. Blood 1999;94:3829–3838.

19 Massberg S, Schurzinger K, Lorenz M, Konrad I, Schulz C, Plesnila N, Kennerknecht E, Rudelius M, Sauer S, Braun S, Kremmer E, Emambokus NR, Frampton J, Gawaz M: Platelet adhesion via glycoprotein IIb integrin is critical for atheroprogression and focal cerebral ischemia: an in vivo study in mice lacking glycoprotein IIb. Circulation 2005;112:1180–1188.

20 Gawaz M, Brand K, Dickfeld T, Pogatsa-Murray G, Page S, Bogner C, Koch W, Schomig A, Neumann F: Platelets induce alterations of chemotactic and adhesive properties of endothelial cells mediated through an interleukin-1-dependent mechanism. Implications for atherogenesis. Atherosclerosis 2000;148:75–85.

21 Langer H, May AE, Bultmann A, Gawaz M: ADAM 15 is an adhesion receptor for platelet GPIIb-IIIa and induces platelet activation. Thromb Haemost 2005;94:555–561.

22 Celik S, Langer H, Stellos K, May AE, Shankar V, Kurz K, Katus HA, Gawaz MP, Dengler TJ: Platelet-associated LIGHT (TNFSF14) mediates adhesion of platelets to human vascular endothelium. Thromb Haemost 2007;98:798–805.

23 Weber C: Platelets and chemokines in atherosclerosis: partners in crime. Circ Res 2005;96:612–616.

24 Massberg S, Konrad I, Schurzinger K, Lorenz M, Schneider S, Zohlnhoefer D, Hoppe K, Schiemann M, Kennerknecht E, Sauer S, Schulz C, Kerstan S, Rudelius M, Seidl S, Sorge F, Langer H, Peluso M, Goyal P, Vestweber D, Emambokus NR, Busch DH, Frampton J, Gawaz M: Platelets secrete stromal cell-derived factor 1alpha and recruit bone marrow-derived progenitor cells to arterial thrombi in vivo. J Exp Med 2006;203:1221–1233.

25 Stellos K, Langer H, Daub K, Schoenberger T, Gauss A, Geisler T, Bigalke B, Mueller I, Schumm M, Schaefer I, Seizer P, Kraemer BF, Siegel-Axel D, May AE, Lindemann S, Gawaz M: Platelet-derived stromal cell-derived factor-1 regulates adhesion and promotes differentiation of human CD34+ cells to endothelial progenitor cells. Circulation 2008;117:206–215.

26 von Hundelshausen P, Weber KS, Huo Y, Proudfoot AE, Nelson PJ, Ley K, Weber C: RANTES deposition by platelets triggers monocyte arrest on inflamed and atherosclerotic endothelium. Circulation 2001;103:1772–1777.

27 Scheuerer B, Ernst M, Durrbaum-Landmann I, Fleischer J, Grage-Griebenow E, Brandt E, Flad HD, Petersen F: The CXC-chemokine platelet factor 4 promotes monocyte survival and induces monocyte differentiation into macrophages. Blood 2000;95:1158–1166.

28 Heeschen C, Dimmeler S, Hamm CW, van den Brand MJ, Boersma E, Zeiher AM, Simoons ML; CAPTURE Study Investigators: Soluble CD40 ligand in acute coronary syndromes. N Engl J Med 2003;348:1104–1111.

29 Gawaz M, Neumann FJ, Dickfeld T, Koch W, Laugwitz KL, Adelsberger H, Langenbrink K, Page S, Neumeier D, Schomig A, Brand K: Activated platelets induce monocyte chemotactic protein-1 secretion and surface expression of intercellular adhesion molecule-1 on endothelial cells. Circulation 1998;98:1164–1171.

30 Lindemann S, Tolley ND, Dixon DA, McIntyre TM, Prescott SM, Zimmerman GA, Weyrich AS: Activated platelets mediate inflammatory signaling by regulated interleukin 1beta synthesis. J Cell Biol 2001;154:485–490.

31 Denis MM, Tolley ND, Bunting M, Schwertz H, Jiang H, Lindemann S, Yost CC, Rubner FJ, Albertine KH, Swoboda KJ, Fratto CM, Tolley E, Kraiss LW, McIntyre TM, Zimmerman GA, Weyrich AS: Escaping the nuclear confines: signal-dependent pre-mRNA splicing in anucleate platelets. Cell 2005;122:379–391.

32 Gawaz M, Reininger A, Neumann FJ: Platelet function and platelet-leukocyte adhesion in symptomatic coronary heart disease. Effects of intravenous magnesium. Thromb Res 1996;83:341–349.

33 Gawaz M, Langer H, May AE: Platelets in inflammation and atherogenesis. J Clin Invest 2005;115:3378–3384.

34 Gawaz M: Do platelets trigger atherosclerosis? Thromb Haemost 2003;90:971–972.

35 Ehlers R, Ustinov V, Chen Z, Zhang X, Rao R, Luscinskas FW, Lopez J, Plow E, Simon DI: Targeting platelet-leukocyte interactions: identification of the integrin Mac-1 binding site for the platelet counter receptor glycoprotein Ibalpha. J Exp Med 2003;198:1077–1088.

36 Santoso S, Sachs UJ, Kroll H, Linder M, Ruf A, Preissner KT, Chavakis T: The junctional adhesion molecule 3 (JAM-3) on human platelets is a counterreceptor for the leukocyte integrin Mac-1. J Exp Med 2002;196:679–691.

37 Langer H, May AE, Daub K, Heinzmann U, Lang P, Schumm M, Vestweber D, Massberg S, Schonberger T, Pfisterer I, Hatzopoulos AK, Gawaz M: Adherent platelets recruit and induce differentiation of murine embryonic endothelial progenitor cells to mature endothelial cells in vitro. Circ Res 2006;98:e2–10.

38 Abi-Younes S, Sauty A, Mach F, Sukhova GK, Libby P, Luster AD: The stromal cell-derived factor-1 chemokine is a potent platelet agonist highly expressed in atherosclerotic plaques. Circ Res 2000;86:131–138.

39 Stellos K, Gawaz M: Platelets and stromal cell-derived factor-1 in progenitor cell recruitment. Semin Thromb Hemost 2007;33:159–164.

40 Jin DK, Shido K, Kopp HG, Petit I, Shmelkov SV, Young LM, Hooper AT, Amano H, Avecilla ST, Heissig B, Hattori K, Zhang F, Hicklin DJ, Wu Y, Zhu Z, Dunn A, Salari H, Werb Z, Hackett NR, Crystal RG, Lyden D, Rafii S: Cytokine-mediated deployment of SDF-1 induces revascularization through recruitment of CXCR4+ hemangiocytes. Nat Med 2006;12:557–567.

41 Ruggeri ZM: Platelets in atherothrombosis. Nat Med 2002;8:1227–1234.

42 Langer HF, May AE, Vestweber D, de Boer HC, Hatzopoulos AK, Gawaz M: Platelet-induced differentiation of endothelial progenitor cells. Semin Thromb Hemost 2007;33:136–143.

43 Gawaz M, Stellos K, Langer HF: Platelets modulate atherogenesis and progression of atherosclerotic plaques via interaction with progenitor and dendritic cells. J Thromb Haemost 2008;6:235–242.

44 Daub K, Langer H, Seizer P, Stellos K, May AE, Goyal P, Bigalke B, Schonberger T, Geisler T, Siegel-Axel D, Oostendorp RA, Lindemann S, Gawaz M: Platelets induce differentiation of human CD34+ progenitor cells into foam cells and endothelial cells. FASEB J 2006;20:2559–2561.

45 Daub K, Lindemann S, Langer H, Seizer P, Stellos K, Siegel-Axel D, Gawaz M: The evil in atherosclerosis: adherent platelets induce foam cell formation. Semin Thromb Hemost 2007;33:173–178.

46 Lindemann S, Kramer B, Daub K, Stellos K, Gawaz M: Molecular pathways used by platelets to initiate and accelerate atherogenesis. Curr Opin Lipidol 2007;18:566–573.

47 Lindemann S, Kramer B, Seizer P, Gawaz M: Platelets, inflammation and atherosclerosis. J Thromb Haemost 2007;5(suppl 1):203–211.

48 Chandler AB, Hand RA: Phagocytized platelets: a source of lipids in human thrombi and atherosclerotic plaques. Science 1961;134:946–947.

49 Jans DM, Martinet W, Fillet M, Kockx MM, Merville MP, Bult H, Herman AG, De Meyer GR: Effect of non-steroidal anti-inflammatory drugs on amyloid-beta formation and macrophage activation after platelet phagocytosis. J Cardiovasc Pharmacol 2004;43:462–470.

50 Langer HF, Daub K, Braun G, Schonberger T, May AE, Schaller M, Stein GM, Stellos K, Bueltmann A, Siegel-Axel D, Wendel HP, Aebert H, Roecken M, Seizer P, Santoso S, Wesselborg S, Brossart P, Gawaz M: Platelets recruit human dendritic cells via Mac-1/JAM-C interaction and modulate dendritic cell function in vitro. Arterioscler Thromb Vasc Biol 2007;27:1463–1470.

51 Banchereau J, Briere F, Caux C, Davoust J, Lebecque S, Liu YJ, Pulendran B, Palucka K: Immunobiology of dendritic cells. Annu Rev Immunol 2000;18:767–811.

52 Saint-Vis B, Bouchet C, Gautier G, Valladeau J, Caux C, Garrone P: Human dendritic cells express neuronal Eph receptor tyrosine kinases: role of EphA2 in regulating adhesion to fibronectin. Blood 2003;102:4431–4440.

53 Hagihara M, Higuchi A, Tamura N, Ueda Y, Hirabayashi K, Ikeda Y, Kato S, Sakamoto S, Hotta T, Handa S, Goto S: Platelets, after exposure to a high shear stress, induce IL-10-producing, mature dendritic cells in vitro. J Immunol 2004;172:5297–5303.

54 Hilf N, Singh-Jasuja H, Schwarzmaier P, Gouttefangeas C, Rammensee HG, Schild H: Human platelets express heat shock protein receptors and regulate dendritic cell maturation. Blood 2002;99:3676–3682.

55 Xia CQ, Kao KJ: Effect of CXC chemokine platelet factor 4 on differentiation and function of monocyte-derived dendritic cells. Int Immunol 2003;15:1007–1015.

Prof. Dr. med. Meinrad Gawaz
Medizinische Klinik III
Eberhard-Karls-Universität Tübingen
Otfried-Müller-Str. 10, 72076 Tübingen, Germany
Tel. +49 7071 29-83688, Fax -5749
E-Mail meinrad.gawaz@med.uni-tuebingen.de

Scharf RE (ed): Progress and Challenges in Transfusion Medicine, Hemostasis and Hemotherapy.
Freiburg i.Br., Karger, 2008, pp 60–70

Infectious Agents, the Contact System, and Innate Immunity

Inga-Maria Frick · Heiko Herwald

Department of Clinical Sciences, Division of Infection Medicine, Lund University, Lund, Sweden

Key Words

Coagulation · Contact system · Inflammation · Infectious diseases · Innate immunity

Summary

The early host response to an infection is dependent on an efficient innate immune system. The human contact system once activated at a bacterial surface results in the induction of proinflammatory reactions and the release of antimicrobial peptides. However, under severe conditions its systemic activation may evoke the generation of pathologic levels of kinins and a consumption of contact factors, which can both contribute to the progression of the disease and cause life-threatening complications. The present review aims to give an update on the role of the contact system in infectious diseases.

©2008 S. Karger GmbH, Freiburg i.Br.

Introduction

Over the last decades there has been a considerable increase in our knowledge of the innate immunity system. This immediate host response provides the first line of defense at biological boundaries prone to infection. Besides the physical barriers provided by epithelial surfaces, elements involved in the nonspecific response against invading pathogens are both cellular components and soluble components, such as antimicrobial peptides (AMPs), chemokines, complement and coagulation systems [1]. Neutrophils, monocytes, and macrophages are critical cellular components specialized in phagocytosis, that upon recognition of microbial pathogens rapidly triggers an innate immune response. This quick action depends on recognition of distinct microbial products by for instance Toll-like receptors (TLRs) [2], which are constitutively expressed on phagocytic cells.

Innate Immunity

One of the most evolutionarily ancient parts of innate immunity is represented by AMPs, molecules providing a soluble barrier against a broad range of microorganisms (for a review see [3]). The diversity of AMPs is great, and the number of isolated and characterized peptides is continuously increasing. The most prominent families of AMPs are the defensins and cathelicidins [4, 5], that in response to infection and inflammation are released from epithelial cells or from recruited circulating neutrophils. In addition, these AMPs possess chemotactic activity against a variety of cells, thereby bridging the innate and adaptive immune systems.

Complement represents yet another link between innate and adaptive responses [6]. This system is activated via a proteolytic cascade resulting in release of multiple active products, including the anaphylatoxin C3a [7]. C3a has structural features resembling those of AMPs, and indeed, C3a has been found to exert antimicrobial activity against a broad range of microorganisms [8, 9]. Situations that trigger an activation of the complement system, for instance infection or tissue damage, are generally also associated with an increased propensity for coagulation [10]. Based on accumulating evidence over the last years it is now believed that coagulation and innate immunity are closely linked and function as highly integrated defense systems against infections [7, 11]. An essential feature of innate immunity is the detection of conserved microbial structures. Interestingly, contact factors of the intrinsic clotting system, the focus of this review, function in a similar manner to pattern recognition molecules of the innate immune system, emphasizing the close relation between these systems.

Pattern Recognition

Pattern recognition is an important element in innate immunity [12]. Previously considered as a nonspecific defense mechanism, it is now clear that pattern recognition molecules interact in a very specific manner with various structures from the invading pathogen, so-called pathogen-associated molecular patterns or PAMPs. The mode of action of pattern recognition molecules is manifold and can in general be divided into three groups based on their function and manner of interaction. The first group consisting of so-called pattern recognition receptors (PRRs), such as TLRs and Nod-like receptors (NLRs), is involved in evoking inflammatory reactions in the host, which is often followed by a cellular response, for instance the recruitment of phagocytic cells [13, 14]. The second group also comprises cell wall-anchored proteins, including scavenger receptors. However, these receptors are involved in an active uptake of the microorganism or products thereof and have therefore an important function in clearance rather than inflammation [15]. Finally, there are soluble pattern recognition molecules such as complement and contact factors, which are able to opsonize a foreign particle and induce thereby its uptake, destruction, or recognition by the immune system [16, 17].

The variety of PAMPs is substantial and includes almost all kinds of substances including small molecules, such as bacterial lipopeptides, proteins, for instance viral envelope proteins from respiratory syncytial virus (RSV) and mouse mammary tumor virus (MMTV), or ligands of complex nature such as bacterial flagellin or DNA [12]. Even though most ligands are derived from intruders, it is now clear that the discrimination between self and nonself PAMPs in innate immunity is not as strict as it was believed some five years ago. Thus, the list of host-derived PAMPs is constantly growing, and it includes proteins such as β-defensin-3, heat shock protein 70, and fibrinogen [18–20]. However, whether or not this leads to serious pathological complications is not completely understood. Although some pattern recognition molecules, such as TLR3 and Nod1, have recently been crystallized (at least in parts) [21, 22], there is still limited structural information available on how PAMPs interact with their respective counterparts. Moreover, it is still obscure by which pattern PAMPs can be classified and why some pattern recognition molecules are able to interact with a broad arsenal of PAMPs, while others are more selective. Notably, a great deal of effort has been undertaken to identify novel PAMPs that bind to PRRs belonging to the family of TLRs and Nod proteins, whereas not much work has lately been investigated to find novel PAMPs that interact with other pattern recognition molecules such as complement or contact systems.

The Contact System

The human contact system is built up by three serine proteinases, namely plasma kallikrein (PK) and factors X (F X) and XI (F XI) as well as by high molecular weight kininogen (HK), a nonenzymatic cofactor [23]. These factors normally circulate as zymogens in the bloodstream or are assembled at the many cellular surfaces, including endothelial cells, polymorphonuclear neutrophils, or platelets, whereby HK is in complex with either PK or F XI. Apart from eukaryotic cell surfaces, also many nonphysiological materials, such as kaolin, glass, ellagic acid, and silica are able to bind and activate the contact system. At these surfaces, activation starts with an autocatalytically driven activation of F XII. This leads to a subsequent conversion of PK to its active form (PKa) by activated F XII (F XIIa) and eventually results in an amplification of F XIIa activity by PKa and the induction of the intrinsically driven pathway of coagulation via activation of F XI by F XIIa. Concurrently, PKa acts on HK, and this leads to the liberation of bradykinin (BK), a potent peptide hormone that is considered as a locally acting proinflammatory agent [24]. The activation of the contact system on eukaryotic surfaces is currently controversially discussed, and it seems to be more complex than on nonphysiological materials.

When the contact system was described for the first time in the 1950's [25] and its mode of action was unraveled, it was believed that it had a primary role in hemostasis. However, this point of view changed some forty years ago, when the first patients with contact factor deficiencies were reported and it was found that these patients do not suffer from severe bleeding disorders [26]. Based on these observations, the scientific interest in the contact system dropped, and it was only recently that the contact system has undergone a renaissance, when it has been reported that mice deficient in F XII or F XI do not show signs of abnormal hemostasis but are protected from thrombus formation in arterial injury models [27, 28]. Moreover, evidence is nowadays accumulating that the contact system has an important function in inflammation [29].

The induction of inflammatory reactions due to contact activation is mainly caused by the release of BK from the HK precursor. BK like other kinins are extremely short-lived peptides, as they are degraded within seconds, for instance by membrane-bound carboxypeptidases [30]. Once released from their precursor, kinins bind to two types of receptors, termed B1 (B1R) and B2 receptor (B2R), respectively. Both receptors belong to the group of seven-membrane G protein-coupled receptors that are typically G_q sensitive [31]. However, the two receptors share little homology in their amino acid composition and have different pharmacological profiles. While activation of B2R gives rise to a transient inflammatory response, stimulation of B1R is involved in sustained inflammatory reactions [24].

Infectious Agents in Relation to the Contact System

Since the discovery that bacterial elements, like lipopolysaccharides (LPS) of Gram-negative bacteria and peptidoglycan and teichoic acid of Gram-positive bacteria, could activate the contact system [32], an increasing number of reports have shown efficient activation of contact factors by microbial products. Several bacterial proteinases are able to activate F XII and/or PK, leading to the release of kinins (table 1). Also, a direct kinin release through degradation of kininogens has been described for many microbial proteinases (table 2). As mentioned above, kinins are inflammatory mediators causing an increase in vascular permeability. Thus, microbial release of these potent peptides will promote plasma exudation into the site of infection, providing opportunities for bacterial growth and spread of the infection through the circulation. For instance, *Staphylococcus aureus* (*S. aureus*), which is a frequent causative agent of Gram-positive sepsis, secretes two cysteine proteinases that induce vascular leakage through the release of BK [33]. Furthermore, in mice models of infection, bacterial dissemination of *Vibrio vulnificus* and *Porphyromonas gingivalis* was shown to be dependent on activation of the contact system and BK release [34, 35].

Adsorption of HK and/or other contact components to the microbial surface is another mechanism by which pathogenic organisms can initiate contact activation. Important virulence factors, such as curli fibers expressed at the surface of *Escherichia*

Bacterial species	Target	Reference
Aeromonas sobria	PK	[61]
Aspergillus melleus	F XII	[62]
Bacillus stearothermophilus	F XII/PK	[62]
Bacillus subtilis	F XII/PK	[62]
Clostridium histolyticum	PK/F XII	[63]
Porphyromonas gingivalis	PK/HK	[64, 65]
Pseudomonas aeruginosa	F XII	[62, 66]
Serratia marcescens	F XII	[62]
Vibrio cholerae	not known	[67]
Vibrio parahaemolyticus	F XII/PK	[68]
Vibrio vulnificus	F XII/PK	[62, 68]

Table 1. Bacterial proteinases that activate contact factors

PK = Plasma kallikrein; F XII = factor XII; HK = high molecular weight kininogen.

coli (*E. coli*) and *Salmonella* and M proteins of *Streptococcus pyogenes*, are able to bind and assemble all four contact factors leading to release of BK [36–39]. In the case of *S. aureus*, contact activation on the bacterial surface resulted in a massive release of BK and in plasma, activation could be blocked by a specific F XII inhibitor or fragments of HK [40]. Binding of HK to the surface of *Candida* species was recently described [41]; interestingly, invasive fungi presented a higher affinity for HK as compared to less pathogenic yeast forms, suggesting a role for contact activation in *Candida* infection. Studies have shown that contact activation triggered by peptidoglycan preparations induces both local and systemic inflammation in rats [42], findings that further underline the significance of the system in relation to inflammation. LPS, that elicit inflammatory responses and are capable of contact activation, have a negatively charged moiety. Recently, binding of LPS to HK was localized to the cell-binding site in domain D5 [43]. It has also been demonstrated that activation of the contact system on the surface of several important pathogens results in further processing of HK with the release of potent AMPs derived from domain D3 [44]. In addition, in a mouse model of infection blocking of contact activation leads to enhanced dissemination of bacteria to the spleens of infected animals, demonstrating an important function for the system in bacterial elimination [44].

Local Effects of Contact Activation

Local lesions of the epithelial barriers will allow pathogens as well as bacteria of the normal flora to enter the microcirculation. In the initial protection against invasive bacteria the innate immune system plays a crucial role. The local inflammatory responses induced by infectious agents lead to enhanced vascular permeability and plasma leak-

Table 2. Bacterial proteinases that trigger the release of kinins from kininogens

Bacterial species	Enzyme	Reference
Porphyromonas gingivalis	Lys-gingivain	[69]
Staphylococcus aureus	staphopain	[33]
Streptococcus pyogenes	SpeB	[70]
Streptomyces caespitosus	Streptomyces proteinase	[62]

SpeB = Streptococcal pyrogenic exotoxin B.

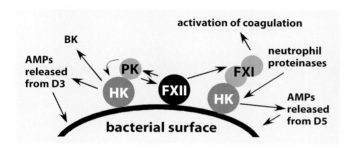

Fig. 1. Contact activation on bacterial surfaces. Upon binding and assembly of contact factors on the bacterial surface, the autocatalytically driven activation of factor XII (F XII) triggers the activation of high molecular weight kininogen (HK)-bound plasma kallikrein (PK), which in turn can increase the activity of F XII. Active F XII then converts F XI into its active form, whereby the intrinsic pathway of coagulation is activated, while HK is cleaved by PK under the release of bradykinin (BK). In addition, HK becomes processed and releases antimicrobial peptides (AMPs) from domain D3. AMPs from HK domain D5 can also be released through the action of neutrophil proteinases.

age, and components of the contact system will then be present at the infectious site. At this stage, a local and rapid contact activation at bacterial surfaces generate AMPs from domain D3 of HK [44]. The simultaneous release of BK can also be regarded as part of the innate response as kinins are reported to induce migration of neutrophils, involving both B1R and B2R [45, 46]. Furthermore, alveolar macrophages release chemotactic substances as a result of BK interaction, leading to neutrophil migration [47]. Thus, kinin generation at the site of infection may result in the recruitment of large numbers of neutrophils. In addition, proteolytic degradation of HK by elastase, released from activated neutrophils, will generate AMPs from domain D3 and domain D5 of HK (fig. 1) [44, 48]. An antimicrobial activity of BK has been found in vitro, although high concentrations were required [49]. Exogenous BK was also reported to induce dendritic cell maturation through activation of B2R [50]. This observation was recently confirmed using a mouse model of *Trypanosoma cruzi* infection [51], suggesting that kininogen proteolysis modulates mechanisms linking the innate and adaptive immune systems. On the other hand, a local release of BK, causing plasma exudation, will provide pathogens with nutrients and may promote bacterial dissemination.

Apart from initiating the release of BK from HK, contact activation also triggers the intrinsic pathway of coagulation leading to thrombin generation. Locally, in the microvasculature at the site of infection, the formation of thrombi provides an efficient barrier preventing microbial spread. Contact activation on the surface of *Salmonella* leads to the generation of active thrombin [39]. Thus, clot formation on a bacterial surface should play a pivotal role in host defense against invasive infection. However, when the inflammatory response is not limited to the primary site of infection, the detrimental effects of systemic contact activation constitute a serious threat to the host.

Contact Activation in Severe Infectious Diseases

As early as in the 1970's, Manson et al. showed that patients with hypotensive septicemia have significantly decreased levels of contact factors [52]. More recently, it was reported that systemic contact activation in patients suffering from severe infectious diseases triggers the generation of pathological levels of kinins and leads to a consumption of contact factors. Both conditions would explain complications such as hypovolemic hypotension and coagulopathy in patients suffering from sepsis or septic shock [53]. In particular low levels of F XII and HK in patients with SIRS (systemic inflammatory response syndrome) correlate with a fatal outcome of the disease [53]. Notably, pronounced contact activation has also been reported in children with meningococcal septic shock [54, 55] and in patients with streptococcal toxic shock syndrome [56]. Other studies have shown that the systemic activation of the contact system is, however, not necessarily combined with severe bleeding disorders, but rather with irreversible hypotension as seen in an *E. coli* sepsis model in baboons [57]. Similar findings were also made when analyzing patients suffering from streptococcal toxic shock syndrome; Sriskandan and Cohen found that these patients have prolonged clotting times of contact system-driven, but normal tissue factor-driven clotting times and they do not suffer from bleeding disorders [56]. These findings suggest that the generation of kinins has an important role in hemodynamic rearrangements during sepsis [57] and are in line with reports that kinin concentrations in septic patients can reach levels that exceed the lower nanomolar range [40] which are pathophysiologically relevant concentrations [24]. There are several reports on the regulation of kinin receptors in infectious diseases. These studies revealed that for instance stimulation of human fibroblasts with *Burkholderia cenocepacia* leads to an upregulation of B1R, but not B2R [58]; similar findings were reported when tissue biopsies from patients with soft tissue infections caused by *S. aureus* were examined by immunohistochemistry [59]. Other studies have shown that B1R and B2R are upregulated in murine tracheal muscle cells upon stimulation of TLR4 and TLR3 [60]. Thus, the regulation of kinin receptors appears to be an important regulatory moment that can trigger an amplification of the inflammatory response due to activation of the contact system and the subsequent release of kinins.

Conclusions and Future Directions

The contact system has lately undergone a renaissance, and it is now clear that it acts as a double-edged sword in infectious diseases. On the one hand it has an important role in the innate immune system when activated locally, but on the other hand it contributes to severe and life-threatening complications under systemic conditions. As contact activation is initiated at an early stage of an infection and acts as an inflammatory amplification cascade when activated systemically, it presents an interesting target for the development of novel antimicrobial therapies.

Disclosure of Conflict of Interests

The authors state that they have no conflict of interest.

Acknowledgements

This work was supported in part by the foundations of Alfred Österlund, Crafoord, Greta and Johan Kock, the Royal Physiographic Society, the Medical Faculty of Lund University, the Swedish Research Council (project 13413, 7480), the Blood and Defence Network at Lund University, and Hansa Medical AB.

References

1 Suckale J, Sim RB, Dodds AW: Evolution of innate immune systems. Biochem Mol Biol Educ 2005;33:177–183.
2 Takeda K, Akira S: Toll-like receptors in innate immunity. Int Immunol 2005;17:1–14.
3 Zasloff M: Antimicrobial peptides of multicellular organisms. Nature 2002;415:389–395.
4 Selsted ME, Ouellette AJ: Mammalian defensins in the antimicrobial immune response. Nat Immunol 2005;6:551–557.
5 Bals R, Wilson JM: Cathelicidins – a family of multifunctional antimicrobial peptides. Cell Mol Life Sci 2003;60:711–720.
6 Morgan BP, Marchbank KJ, Longhi MP, Harris CL, Gallimore AM: Complement: central to innate immunity and bridging to adaptive responses. Immunol Lett 2005;97:171–179.
7 Markiewski MM, Nilsson B, Ekdahl KN, Mollnes TE, Lambris JD: Complement and coagulation: strangers or partners in crime? Trends Immunol 2007;28:184–192.
8 Nordahl EA, Rydengård V, Nyberg P, Nitsche DP, Mörgelin M, Malmsten M, Björck L, Schmidtchen A: Activation of the complement system generates antibacterial peptides. Proc Natl Acad Sci U S A 2004;101:16879–16884.
9 Pasupuleti M, Walse B, Nordahl EA, Mörgelin M, Malmsten M, Schmidtchen A: Preservation of antimicrobial properties of complement peptide C3a, from invertebrates to humans. J Biol Chem 2007;282:2520–2528.
10 Esmon CT: The impact of the inflammatory response on coagulation. Thromb Res 2004;114:321–327.
11 Opal SM, Esmon CT: Bench-to-bedside review: functional relationships between coagulation and the innate immune response and their respective roles in the pathogenesis of sepsis. Crit Care 2003;7:23–38.
12 Lee MS, Kim YJ: Signaling pathways downstream of pattern-recognition receptors and their cross talk. Annu Rev Biochem 2007;76:447–480.
13 Kawai T, Akira S: Signaling to NF-kappaB by Toll-like receptors. Trends Mol Med 2007;13:460–469.

14 Carneiro LA, Travassos LH, Girardin SE: Nod-like receptors in innate immunity and inflammatory diseases. Ann Med 2007;39:581–593.

15 Peiser L, Mukhopadhyay S, Gordon S: Scavenger receptors in innate immunity. Curr Opin Immunol 2002;14:123–128.

16 Rus H, Cudrici C, Niculescu F: The role of the complement system in innate immunity. Immunol Res 2005;33:103–112.

17 Frick IM, Björck L, Herwald H: The dual role of the contact system in bacterial infectious disease. Thromb Haemost 2007;98:497–502.

18 Funderburg N, Lederman MM, Feng Z, Drage MG, Jadlowsky J, Harding CV, Weinberg A, Sieg SF: Human β-defensin-3 activates professional antigen-presenting cells via Toll-like receptors 1 and 2. Proc Natl Acad Sci U S A 2007;104:18631–18635.

19 Zhou J, An H, Xu H, Liu S, Cao X: Heat shock up-regulates expression of Toll-like receptor-2 and Toll-like receptor-4 in human monocytes via p38 kinase signal pathway. Immunology 2005;114:522–530.

20 Kuhns DB, Priel DA, Gallin JI: Induction of human monocyte interleukin (IL)-8 by fibrinogen through the toll-like receptor pathway. Inflammation 2007;30:178–188.

21 Sun J, Duffy KE, Ranjith-Kumar CT, Xiong J, Lamb RJ, Santos J, Masarapu H, Cunningham M, Holzenburg A, Sarisky RT, Mbow ML, Kao C: Structural and functional analyses of the human Toll-like receptor 3. Role of glycosylation. J Biol Chem 2006;281:11144–11151.

22 Coussens NP, Mowers JC, McDonald C, Nunez G, Ramaswamy S: Crystal structure of the Nod1 caspase activation and recruitment domain. Biochem Biophys Res Commun 2007;353:1–5.

23 Colman RW, Schmaier AH: Contact system: a vascular biology modulator with anticoagulant, profibrinolytic, antiadhesive, and proinflammatory attributes. Blood 1997;90:3819–3843.

24 Leeb-Lundberg LMF, Marceau F, Müller-Esterl W, Pettibone DJ, Zuraw BL: International union of pharmacology. XLV. Classification of the kinin receptor family: from molecular mechanisms to pathophysiological consequences. Pharmacol Rev 2005;57:27–77.

25 Roberts HR: Oscar Ratnoff: his contributions to the golden era of coagulation research. Br J Haematol 2003;122:180–192.

26 Ratnoff OD: A quarter century with Mr. Hageman. Thromb Haemost 1980;43:95–98.

27 Renné T, Pozgajová M, Grüner S, Schuh K, Pauer HU, Burfeind P, Gailani D, Nieswandt B: Defective thrombus formation in mice lacking coagulation factor XII. J Exp Med 2005;202:271–281.

28 Kleinschnitz C, Stoll G, Bendszus M, Schuh K, Pauer HU, Burfeind P, Renné C, Gailani D, Nieswandt B, Renné T: Targeting coagulation factor XII provides protection from pathological thrombosis in cerebral ischemia without interfering with hemostasis. J Exp Med 2006;203:513–518.

29 Costa-Neto CM, Dillenburg-Pilla P, Heinrich TA, Parreiras-e-Silva LT, Pereira MG, Reis RI, Souza PP: Participation of kallikrein-kinin system in different pathologies. Int Immunopharmacol 2008;8:135–142.

30 Skidgel RA, Erdös EG: Cellular carboxypeptidases. Immunol Rev 1998;161:129–141.

31 Kang DS, Leeb-Lundberg LMF: Negative and positive regulatory epitopes in the C-terminal domains of the human B1 and B2 bradykinin receptor subtypes determine receptor coupling efficacy to G(q/11)-mediated [correction of G(9/11)-mediated] phospholipase Cbeta activity. Mol Pharmacol 2002;62:281–288.

32 Kalter ES, van Dijk WC, Timmerman A, Verhoef J, Bouma BN: Activation of purified human plasma prekallikrein triggered by cell wall fractions of *Escherichia coli* and *Staphylococcus aureus*. J Infect Dis 1983;148:682–691.

33 Imamura T, Tanase S, Szmyd G, Kozik A, Travis J, Potempa J: Induction of vascular leakage through release of bradykinin and a novel kinin by cysteine proteinases from *Staphylococcus aureus*. J Exp Med 2005;201:1669–1676.

34 Maruo K, Akaike T, Ono T, Maeda H: Involvement of bradykinin generation in intravascular dissemination of *Vibrio vulnificus* and prevention of invasion by a bradykinin antagonist. Infect Immun 1998;66:866–869.

35 Hu SW, Huang CH, Huang HC, Lai YY, Lin YY: Transvascular dissemination of *Porphyromonas gingivalis* from a sequestered site is dependent upon activation of the kallikrein/kinin pathway. J Periodontal Res 2006;41:200–207.

36 Ben Nasr AB, Herwald H, Müller-Esterl W, Björck L: Human kininogens interact with M protein, a bacterial surface protein and virulence determinant. Biochem J 1995;305:173–180.

37 Ben Nasr AB, Olsén A, Sjöbring U, Müller-Esterl W, Björck L: Assembly of human contact phase factors and release of bradykinin at the surface of curli-expressing *Escherichia coli*. Mol Microbiol 1996;20:927–935.

38 Herwald H, Mörgelin M, Olsén A, Rhen M, Dahlbäck B, Müller-Esterl W, Björck L: Activation of the contact-phase system on bacterial surfaces – a clue to serious complications in infectious diseases. Nat Med 1998;4:298–302.

39 Persson K, Mörgelin M, Lindbom L, Alm P, Björck L, Herwald H: Severe lung lesions caused by *Salmonella* are prevented by inhibition of the contact system. J Exp Med 2000;192:1415–1424.

40 Mattsson E, Herwald H, Cramer H, Persson K, Sjöbring U, Björck L: *Staphylococcus aureus* induces release of bradykinin in human plasma. Infect Immun 2001;69:3877–3882.

41 Rapala-Kozik M, Karkowska J, Jacher A, Golda A, Barbasz A, Guevara-Lora I, Kozik A: Kininogen adsorption to the cell surface of *Candida* spp. Int Immunopharmacol 2008;8:237–241.

42 Isordia-Salas I, Pixley RA, Sainz IM, Martinez-Murillo C, Colman RW: The role of plasma high molecular weight kininogen in experimental intestinal and systemic inflammation. Arch Med Res 2005;36:87–95.

43 Perkins R, Ngo MD, Mahdi F, Shariat-Madar Z: Identification of lipopolysaccharide binding site on high molecular weight kininogen. Biochem Biophys Res Commun 2008;366:938–943.

44 Frick IM, Åkesson P, Herwald H, Mörgelin M, Malmsten M, Nägler DK, Björck L: The contact system – a novel branch of innate immunity generating antibacterial peptides. EMBO J 2006;25:5569–5578.

45 Ehrenfeld P, Millan C, Matus CE, Figueroa JE, Burgos RA, Nualart F, Bhoola KD, Figueroa CD: Activation of kinin B1 receptors induces chemotaxis of human neutrophils. J Leukoc Biol 2006;80:117–124.

46 Paegelow I, Trzeczak S, Bockmann S, Vietinghoff G: Migratory responses of polymorphonuclear leukocytes to kinin peptides. Pharmacology 2002;66:153–161.

47 Sato E, Koyama S, Nomura H, Kubo K, Sekiguchi M: Bradykinin stimulates alveolar macrophages to release neutrophil, monocyte, and eosinophil chemotactic activity. J Immunol 1996;157:3122–3129.

48 Nordahl EA, Rydengård V, Mörgelin M, Schmidtchen A: Domain 5 of high molecular weight kininogen is antibacterial. J Biol Chem 2005;280:34832–34839.

49 Kowalska K, Carr DB, Lipkowski AW: Direct antimicrobial properties of substance P. Life Sci 2002;71:747–750.

50 Aliberti J, Viola JP, Vieira-de-Abreu A, Bozza PT, Sher A, Scharfstein J: Cutting edge: bradykinin induces IL-12 production by dendritic cells: a danger signal that drives Th1 polarization. J Immunol 2003;170:5349–5353.

51 Scharfstein J, Schmitz V, Svensjo E, Granato A, Monteiro AC: Kininogens coordinate adaptive immunity through the proteolytic release of bradykinin, an endogenous danger signal driving dendritic cell maturation. Scand J Immunol 2007;66:128–136.

52 Mason JW, Kleeberg U, Dolan P, Colman RW: Plasma kallikrein and Hageman factor in Gram-negative bacteremia. Ann Intern Med 1970;73:545–551.

53 Pixley RA, Colman RW: The kallikrein-kinin system in sepsis syndrome; in Farmer SG (ed): Handbook of Immunopharmacology – The Kinin System. New York, Academic Press, 1997, pp 173–186.

54 Wuillemin WA, Fijnvandraat K, Derkx BH, Peters M, Vreede W, ten Cate H, Hack CE: Activation of the intrinsic pathway of coagulation in children with meningococcal septic shock. Thromb Haemost 1995;74:1436–1441.

55 van Deuren M, Brandtzaeg P, van der Meer JW: Update on meningococcal disease with emphasis on pathogenesis and clinical management. Clin Microbiol Rev 2000;13:144–166.

56 Sriskandan S, Cohen J: Kallikrein-kinin system activation in streptococcal toxic shock syndrome. Clin Infect Dis 2000;30:961–962.

57 Pixley RA, De La Cadena R, Page JD, Kaufman N, Wyshock EG, Chang A, Taylor FB Jr, Colman RW: The contact system contributes to hypotension but not disseminated intravascular coagulation in lethal bacteremia. In vivo use of a monoclonal anti-factor XII antibody to block contact activation in baboons. J Clin Invest 1993;91:61–68.

58 Phagoo SB, Reddi K, Silvallana BJ, Leeb-Lundberg LM, Warburton D: Infection-induced kinin B1 receptors in human pulmonary fibroblasts: role of intact pathogens and p38 mitogen-activated protein kinase-dependent signaling. J Pharmacol Exp Ther 2005;313:1231–1238.

59 Bengtson SH, Phagoo SB, Norrby-Teglund A, Påhlman L, Mörgelin M, Zuraw BL, Leeb-Lundberg LM, Herwald H: Kinin receptor expression during *Staphylococcus aureus* infection. Blood 2006;108:2055–2063.

60 Bachar O, Adner M, Uddman R, Cardell LO: Toll-like receptor stimulation induces airway hyper-responsiveness to bradykinin, an effect mediated by JNK and NF-kappa B signaling pathways. Eur J Immunol 2004;34:1196–1207.

61 Imamura T, Kobayashi H, Khan R, Nitta H, Okamoto K: Induction of vascular leakage and blood pressure lowering through kinin release by a serine proteinase from *Aeromonas sobria*. J Immunol 2006;177:8723–8729.

62 Molla A, Yamamoto T, Akaike T, Miyoshi S, Maeda H: Activation of Hageman factor and prekallikrein and generation of kinin by various microbial proteinases. J Biol Chem 1989;264:10589–10594.

63 Vargaftig BB, Giroux EL: Mechanism of clostripain-induced kinin release from human, rat and canine plasma. Adv Exp Med Biol 1976;70:157–175.

64 Imamura T, Pike RN, Potempa J, Travis J: Pathogenesis of periodontitis: a major arginine-specific cysteine proteinase from *Porphyromonas gingivalis* induces vascular permeability enhancement through activation of the kallikrein/kinin pathway. J Clin Invest 1994;94:361–367.

65 Imamura T, Potempa J, Pike RN, Travis J: Dependence of vascular permeability enhancement on cysteine proteinases in vesicles of *Porphyromonas gingivalis*. Infect Immun 1995;63:1999–2003.

66 Sakata Y, Akaike T, Suga M, Ijiri S, Ando M, Maeda H: Bradykinin generation triggered by *Pseudomonas* proteases facilitates invasion of the systemic circulation by *Pseudomonas aeruginosa*. Microbiol Immunol 1996;40:415–423.

67 Sakata Y, Akaike T, Khan MM, Ichinose Y, Hirayama H, Suga M, Ando M, Maeda H: Activation of bradykinin generating cascade by *Vibrio cholerae* protease. Immunopharmacology 1996;33:377–379.

68 Miyoshi S, Watanabe H, Kawase T, Yamada H, Shinoda S: Generation of active fragments from human zymogens in the bradykinin-generating cascade by extracellular proteases from *Vibrio vulnificus* and *V. parahaemolyticus*. Toxicon 2004;44:887–893.

69 Scott CF, Whitaker EJ, Hammond BF, Colman RW: Purification and characterization of a potent 70-kDa thiol lysyl-proteinase (Lys-gingivain) from *Porphyromonas gingivalis* that cleaves kininogens and fibrinogen. J Biol Chem 1993;268:7935–7942.

70 Herwald H, Collin M, Müller-Esterl W, Björck L: Streptococcal cysteine proteinase releases kinins: a novel virulence mechanism. J Exp Med 1996;184:665–673.

Prof. Heiko Herwald, Ph.D.
Clinical and Experimental Infection Medicine
Department of Clinical Sciences BMC, B14
Lund University, Tornavägen 10, 22184 Lund, Sweden
Tel. +46 46-2224182, Fax -157756
E-Mail Heiko.Herwald@med.lu.se

Scharf RE (ed): Progress and Challenges in Transfusion Medicine, Hemostasis and Hemotherapy.
Freiburg i.Br., Karger, 2008, pp 71–88

Fibrinolysis and Host Response in Bacterial Infections

Simone Bergmann · Sven Hammerschmidt

Max von Pettenkofer Institute, Ludwig Maximilians University Munich, Germany

Key Words

Plasminogen · Bacterial infection · Fibrinolysis · Inflammation · Urokinase · Plasminogen activator inhibitor

Summary

The plasminogen activation system is part of the fibrinolysis, which is tightly regulated and protected against dysfunction by various activators and inhibitors. However, microorganisms including bacteria, fungi, and also parasites have been proven to interact in a specific manner with components of the fibrinolytic pathways. Pathogenic bacteria are capable of subverting the function of proteases, activators or inhibitors for their own benefits including dissemination within the host and evasion of host inflammatory immune response. In this report, we provide a state of the art overview of the diverse strategies employed by bacteria to interact with components of the fibrinolytic system and to exploit the system for invasion. Moreover, the role of factors of the fibrinolytic cascade in inflammatory host response due to different bacterial infections will be presented.   ©2008 S. Karger GmbH, Freiburg i.Br.

Introduction

Invasive bacterial pathogens have developed a variety of strategies to subvert homeostatic processes like blood coagulation and its counterpart fibrinolysis by endogenous proteolytic mechanisms and by exploitation of enzymatic activities of host-derived proteases. Fibrin clots are formed during coagulation and immediately close injured micro- and macrovascular blood vessel walls. These clots are later degraded to enable structured tissue regeneration. The activation of coagulation and fibrin deposition is one of the consequences of inflammation and is implicated in different vascular diseases. In bacterial pathogenesis the interplay between blood coagulation and inflammation is considered to be an essential part of the host defense against infectious agents. This host defense strategy may concentrate the invaders and directed inflammatory host response to a protected and focused area within the host [1].

A key component of the fibrinolysis system is the 92-kDa glycoprotein human plasminogen, which is present in high concentrations within human plasma as precursor of the serine protease plasmin [2]. Plasminogen is converted into the two-chained enzymatically active plasmin by host plasminogen activators such as the tissue-type plasminogen activator (tPA) and the urokinase-type plasminogen activator (uPA). The fibrinolytic system comprises an anticoagulative protease cascade which is integrated into the wound healing process. This cascade is highly regulated by activators and inhibitors such as plasminogen activator inhibitors (PAI) 1–3 and plasmin inhibitors such as α_2-antiplasmin and α_2-macroglobulin [2, 3]. Moreover, the broad substrate spectrum of plasmin includes the extracellular matrix (ECM) glycoproteins fibronectin, laminin, vitronectin and precursors of degradative matrix metalloproteases (MMPs) like procollagenases [4]. The host components are target molecules for the proteolytic activity of plasmin and are degraded in processes of tissue renewal or angiogenesis [5, 6]. The number of bacteria, fungi, and parasites which were identified to recruit and exploit plasmin(ogen) for degradative processes has increased substantially in the last decade.

Interference of bacteria with plasminogen occurs in general via two distinct mechanisms (fig. 1). Firstly, bacteria produce plasminogen receptors which activate plasminogen by complex formation or by proteolysis. Secondly, plasminogen is recruited to the bacterial cell surface by plasminogen receptors. The immobilized form of plasminogen is then converted into plasmin by host-derived activators. Cell-surface bound plasmin is exploited by bacteria for proteolytic degradation of components of the ECM, basal membrane, and host tissues [7]. It is thought that this destruction facilitates bacterial translocation and dissemination within the host. By using animal infection models, a direct impact on bacterial pathogenesis and induction of inflammatory immune response of the host, respectively, was demonstrated for several of the identified bacterial plasminogen receptors and activators. This report provides an overview of principle strategies of how bacteria interact with key elements of the host fibrinolytic system and, thus, subvert inflammatory defense mechanisms of the host.

Impact of Bacterial Plasminogen Activators on Inflammatory Host Response and Fibrinolysis

The Versatile Plasminogen Activators Streptokinase and Staphylokinase

The streptokinase, produced by group A, C, and G streptococci, is the prototype of bacterial plasminogen activators. The crystal structure of the three-domain protein streptokinase from *Streptococcus pyogenes* (*S. pyogenes)* is solved in a complex with the katalytic unit of plasmin (microplasmin) [8]. The structural analysis depicted the interaction sites with microplasmin in loops of the α-domain and the γ-domain of the streptokinase [9]. The formation of the complex induces conformational changes, so

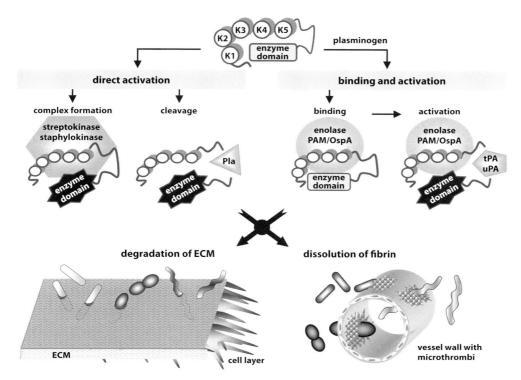

Fig. 1. Schematic model of bacterial plasminogen activation mechanisms and pathophysiological consequences. A direct activation of plasminogen occurs by complex formation of plasminogen with secreted or surface-bound proteases like streptokinase or staphylokinase. Alternatively, plasminogen is cleaved by bacterial proteases such as Pla from *Yersinia pestis* or members of the omptin family. A two-step mechanism of plasminogen activation involves in a first step the recruitment of plasminogen to the bacterial cell surface; in a second step surface-bound plasminogen is activated by host-derived plasminogen activators such as tissue-type plasminogen activator (tPA) or urokinase-type plasminogen activator (uPA). Prototypes of these surface-exposed bacterial plasminogen receptors are enolases, the lipoproteins OspA and OspC from *Borrelia burgdorferi*, and PAM from *Streptococcus pyogenes*. ECM = Extracellular matrix. Reproduced with permission from reference [127].

that the plasminogen molecule is converted into plasmin [10, 11]. The conversion by streptokinase protects plasmin against enzymatic inactivation by the plasmin-specific inhibitor α_2-antiplasmin [12]. In contrast to mammalian plasminogen activators like uPA, which is able to activate plasminogen from all species, activation of plasminogen by streptokinase is a species-specific trait [13]. In a humanized plasminogen mice model, Sun et al. cross-linked the infectivity of group A streptococci with the species-specific activation of plasminogen by the secreted streptokinase [14].

A similar mechanism of plasminogen activation was identified for the staphylokinase, even though there is no primary structural homology between streptokinase and staphylokinase from *Staphylococcus aureus* [15]. Staphylokinase requires fibrin as cofactor. Contrary to the streptokinase, the staphylokinase-plasmin complex is efficiently inhibited by α_2-antiplasmin. However, binding of plasminogen to fibrin or bacterial cell surfaces protects against inactivation by α_2-antiplasmin and, more important, enhances the staphylokinase-induced plasminogen activation [16]. Interestingly, staphylokinase induces immunogenic antibody responses and provokes proliferation of staphylokinase-specific T-lymphocytes [17]. Furthermore, staphylokinase interacts directly with the host innate immune system by diminishing the bactericidal effect of α-defensins [18]. Under physiological conditions, defensins enhance specific antibody production and promote maturation of dendritic cells [19]. Staphylokinase induces a fast release of defensins from the granules of polymorphonuclear cells (PMNs), which is followed by a rapid binding and efficient neutralization of the short peptides by the staphylokinase [18]. This inhibits the bactericidal effect of the defensins and reduces the rate of plasminogen activation. As a result, the functional activity of staphylokinase promotes the bacterial infection process [18].

Staphylokinase and streptokinase are applied as thrombolytic pharmaceuticals in clinical treatments of acute myocardial infarctions and arterial thromboses [20, 21]. A frequent problem in thrombolytic therapy is the reocclusion of the injured vessel walls due to the lack of pharmaceuticals that promote tissue regeneration. An eminent drug for thrombolytic therapy is proposed to contain a plasminogen activator domain derived from staphylokinase, a fibrin affinity domain containing a kringle 2 motif derived from tPA, an antiplatelet domain with an Arg-Gly-Asp (RGD) peptide, and finally an anticoagulant domain derived from hirudin [22]. This drug will facilitate rapid clot lysis and exhibit antiplatelet and anticoagulant activity as well. Hence, a drug with these features will represent an auspicious solution for effective thrombolytic therapies.

Intermediate Streptococcal Plasminogen Activators

PauA and PauB were identified as plasminogen activators of *Streptococcus uberis* [23, 24]. The mechanism of plasminogen activation via PauA has similarities to the mechanisms of staphylokinase and streptokinase, respectively. PauA activates plasminogen in a streptokinase-like manner, however, plasmin remains susceptible to α_2-antiplasmin like the staphylokinase-activated plasminogen [25]. Other examples for members of the streptokinase family are the plasminogen activators Esk [26] from the equine pathogen *Streptococcus equisimilis* and PadA from *Streptococcus dysgalactiae* [27]. These plasminogen activators interact preferentially with nonhuman plasminogen [27].

Pla, Member of the Omptin Family Plasminogen Activators and Mediator of Invasion

Pla of *Yersinia pestis (Y. pestis)* activates plasminogen by proteolysis like tPA and uPA [28] (fig. 1). Pla is a prominent member of the omptin family including OmpT of

Escherichia coli and PgtE of *Salmonella enterica (S. enterica)*, which in general convert plasminogen by peptide bond hydrolysis into plasmin. However, the enzymatic activities are considerably different. OmpT is less active in plasminogen activation compared to Pla and PgtE and, moreover, OmpT is not able to inhibit α_2-antiplasmin [29, 30]. Pla and OmpT also differ in their substrate specificity. Pla degrades complement proteins including C3, C3b, and C4b [31, 32], which results in reduced bacterial opsonophagocytosis and declined chemotaxis of phagocytes into infected host niches. In contrast, OmpT and PgtE degrade cationic antimicrobial peptides [33–36], which promotes bacterial survival and resistance against the innate immune defense mechanism of the host. Strikingly, plasminogen activation via PgtE of *S. enterica* or Pla of *Y. pestis* is diminished in the presence of O-antigen repeats. The O-antigens also prevent PgtE- or Pla-mediated bacterial adhesion to basement membranes and invasion into endothelial cells [37]. Moreover, O-antigens in *Yersinia pseudotuberculosis* inhibit Pla-mediated cleavage and inhibition of α_2-antiplasmin [38]. The concerted action of bacteria to recruit plasminogen and to bind in parallel plasmin-specific substrates may represent a high level of bacterial adaptation to the host environment. The intrinsic adhesive properties of Pla were shown for laminin, collagen type IV, and reconstituted basement membrane [39–41]. The Pla-mediated adhesion of *Yersinia* to proteins of human ECM promotes the focusing of the acquired serine protease activity to target sites of bacterial colonization and subsequent dissemination. In addition, intracellular signalling cascades are induced in response to Pla-expressing *Y. pestis*. Pla is involved in tyrosine kinase phosphorylation and Rho-dependent signalling and, hence, contributes significantly to bacterial internalization [42].

Disease-Specific Effects of Pla in Mice Infection Models

Pla enables dissemination of *Y. pestis* from the subdermal infection site into the lymph nodes and blood circulation in mice infected subcutaneously with *Y. pestis* [32]. However, when using the intravenous route, Pla did not alter the morbidity of mice [32]. Further insights into the role of Pla in virulence were demonstrated when pla-knockout strains were employed in subcutaneous and intradermal mouse infection models. Here, Pla-deficient strains were avirulent in both infection models. Nevertheless, pla-knockout strains were able to cause fatal septicemic plague after transmission by fleas. In addition to fatal septicemic plague infections, Pla-expressing *Yersinia* strains caused bubonic plague [43]. These differences in virulence potential are probably due to an evolutionary epidemic disease development. It is hypothesized that after horizontal pla gene transfer the flea-transmitted septicemic plague developed into the highly infectious bubonic form of disease [43]. Moreover, Pla is essential for the development of primary pneumonic plague but is less important for dissemination during pneumonic plague than during bubonic plague [44]. In the absence of Pla an anti-inflammatory state is maintained in the lungs, so that the infection is not able to progress. Although inflammations in the lungs occur, these were restricted to small lesions in the absence of the Pla surface protease [44]. Hence, the Pla-mediated virulence of *Y. pestis* is a suitable example of the variable but at the same time highly specific bacterial adaptation to different infection strategies and disease outcome. These data are supported by a study that indicates the essential role of Pla during the induction of pulmonary plague, whereas Pla is less important for dissemination during pulmonary plague [44]. These different effects of Pla on virulence open several questions. It remains open whether the unbalanced fibrinolysis due to the Pla-mediated activation of plasminogen is required to cause bubonic plague or pneumonic plague, respectively. A future aspect will be the comparison of pathophysiological effects after infections of plasminogen-knockout mice with Pla-expressing *Yersinia* versus infections with Pla-deficient *Yersinia*.

Interference of Bacteria with the Fibrinolytic Cascade via Plasminogen Receptors

Table 1 shows the interference of bacterial proteins with components of the fibrinolytic system.

Several, if not all, bacteria recruit plasminogen to their cell surface. The acquisition of plasminogen occurs via surface-exposed plasminogen-binding proteins, which have been reviewed recently [45]. Therefore, we will not specify all the plasminogen-binding proteins known to date. Instead, we will focus on the influence of plasminogen-binding proteins and plasminogen acquisition on fibrinolysis, ECM degradation, and induction of inflammatory host responses. In general, immobilization of plasminogen on cellular surfaces causes conformational opening of plasminogen, which in turn enhances its activation to plasmin by uPA or tPA [46, 47]. This endows the bacteria with host-derived proteolytic activity (fig. 1). In addition, the immobilized form of plasmin is protected against the serine protease inhibitor α_2-antiplasmin [48]. The tPA is a major activator of intrinsic fibrinolysis and possesses fibrin-binding activity. In contrast, uPA is recognized by a specific cell surface receptor, the urokinase-type plasminogen activator receptor (uPAR), and is mainly involved in processes of cellular adhesion and migration, tissue reconstruction, and protection against apoptosis [49–51]. Urokinase PAR is a glycosylphosphatidylinositol (GPI)-anchored glycoprotein [52], which was initially identified on monocytic cells [53] but is also present on many leukocytic blood cells [54–56]. Binding of the uPA-plasminogen complex to uPAR concentrates plasmin activity on cell surfaces and promotes cell migration.

Subversion of the Fibrinolytic System by Bacterial Glycolytic Enzymes

Remarkably, several glycolytic enzymes including the glyceraldehyde-3-phosphate dehydrogenase (GAPDH) and enolase from different bacterial species interact spe-

Table 1. Interference of bacterial proteins with components of the fibrinolytic system

Bacterial protein	Physiological consequence	Reference
Plasminogen activators		
Streptokinase	plasminogen activation, fibrinolytic activity	[10, 11, 13]
	inhibition of α_2-antiplasmin	[12]
	streptococcal virulence determinant	[14]
Staphylokinase	plasminogen activation, fibrinolytic activity	[16]
	neutralization of bactericidal defensins	[18]
	induction of specific antibody response	[17]
	proliferation of staphylokinase-specific T-lymphocytes	[17]
Plasminogen activator Pla	plasminogen activation, fibrinolytic activity	[28]
	inhibition of α_2-antiplasmin	[29]
	degradation of complement factors	[31, 32]
	reduction of opsonophagocytosis	[31, 32]
	induction of tyrosine phosphorylation and	[42]
	Rho-dependent signalling	[43, 44]
	required for induction of bubonic and pneumonic plague adhesion to ECM proteins (laminin, collagen type IV, matrigel)	[39–41]
OmpT, PgtE	plasminogen activation, degradation of cationic bactericidal peptides	[33–36]
Plasminogen receptors		
SDH/Plr	plasminogen binding to SDH and activation via uPA/tPA	[16, 57–62]
	enhancement of bacterial adherence and invasion	[67, 68]
	induction of histone H3-specific signal transduction cascade	[65, 70]
Enolase	plasminogen binding to enolase and activation via uPA/tPA	[60, 64]
		[74]
	promotes fibrinolysis, mediates degradation and transmigration of basal membrane, involved in pneumococcal virulence	[75]
PAM	cofactor for plasminogen activation via uPA/tPA	[76]
	enhancement of streptococcal virulence	[14]
OspA/OspC	cofactor for plasminogen activation via uPA/tPA	[81]
	proteolytic activity for soluble and insoluble ECM components	[78–84]
	transmigration of endothelial monolayers including blood-brain barrier	
HP-NAP	inhibition of fibrinolysis, stabilization of fibrin	[91]
	stimulation of PAI-2 and tissue factor synthesis	[91, 92]

ECM = Extracellular matrix; uPA = urokinase-type plasminogen activator; tPA = tissue-type plasminogen activator; PAI = plasminogen activator inhibitor.

cifically with plasmin(ogen) [57–62]. The GAPDH of *S. pyogenes*, referred to as Plr or SDH, and the GAPDH of pneumococci possess a lower affinity for the zymogen plasminogen than for plasmin. The C-terminal lysine residue of Plr/SDH has been demonstrated to be essential for plasmin binding, whereas the two lysine residues at the C-terminus of the enolases of *S. pyogenes* and *Streptococcus pneumoniae* have no direct role in plasmin(ogen) binding. For the pneumococcal enolase a nine-residue plasminogen-binding motif was localized between amino acids 248–256 and has been proven to be essential for the enolase-plasminogen interaction under physiologically relevant conditions [60, 63, 64]. This motif is highly conserved among several enolases which have been shown to bind plasminogen. The implication of glycolytic enzymes in plasminogen acquisition and subversion of the host fibrinolytic system is intriguing. Despite the lack of typical signal peptides required for surface export and the absence of a membrane anchorage motif required for cell wall anchorage, the GAPDHs and enolases as well as other glycolytic enzymes were discovered on microbial cell surfaces [60, 62, 65, 66]. In addition to their housekeeping functions, these enzymes are involved in bacterial-induced fibrinolysis and inflammation through their ability to interact with plasminogen and/or host cell receptors.

In addition to its plasminogen-binding activity, the Plr/SDH binds to the ectodomain D1 of uPAR/CD87, which is expressed on human pharyngeal cells [65]. Under physiological conditions, the interaction of uPA with its receptor uPAR promotes pericellular fibrinolysis, adhesion of leukocytes and contributes to cell migration and inflammation [67, 68]. Interestingly, the kinase phosphorylation pattern induced in pharyngeal cells in response to treatment with purified SDH was similar to that induced by viable streptococci [69]. Urokinase PAR is a highly potent mediator of signalling and cell-cell communications. It has been demonstrated that the specific interaction between the bacterial SDH and uPAR upregulates uPAR, which induces a tyrosine kinase-dependent phosphorylation of histone H3 kinases [70]. Taken together, this interaction is an example that the binding of a bacterial protein to a receptor of the pericellular fibrinolysis contributes to an intracellular reprogramming of host cell-cell communication.

The enolase is another example of proteins possessing multiple functions. In addition to plasminogen-binding activity [60, 69, 71, 72], the involvement in autoimmune diseases, hypoxic stress response, and tumor formation has been shown in particular for the enolase of *S. pyogenes* [73]. The detailed molecular and functional characterization of the pneumococcal enolase indicated a novel plasmin(ogen)-binding motif [60, 63, 64]. Strikingly, the nine-amino acid plasminogen-binding peptide FYDKERKVYD of the enolase is a key cofactor in pneumococcal plasminogen binding and plasmin-mediated degradation of ECM proteins (fig. 2) [74]. Similarly, the nonameric plasminogen-binding peptide is pivotal for dissolution and transmigration of pneumococci through a fibrin matrix [74]. The functional inactivation of the motif significantly impairs virulence of pneumococci in an intranasal mouse infection model [75]. However, the pathophysiological consequences of plasmin acquisi-

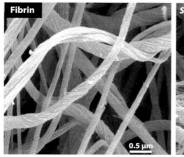 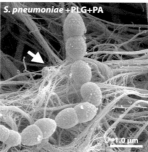

Fig. 2. Degradation of fibrin clots by *Streptococcus pneumoniae*. Field emission electron microscopy illustrates that the fibrin matrix exhibits thick bundles, each consisting of several fibrin fibrils twisted around each other. A fibrin matrix generated on a transwell filter and incubated with plasminogen-coated pneumococci is completely degraded after activation of the bacterial-bound plasminogen with uPA. Reproduced with permission from reference [74].

tion in the lung and the impact of plasmin on induced inflammatory host responses and pneumococcal dissemination within the host are yet unknown.

Fibrillar and Nonfibrillar Plasminogen Receptors: Players for Plasmin-Mediated Bacterial Penetration of Tissue Barriers

S. pyogenes produces several plasminogen-binding proteins. A high-affinity plasmin(ogen) receptor is the M-like protein PAM [76]. In contrast to the streptokinase, PAM (plasminogen-binding group A streptococcal M protein) binds in a non human-specific manner plasminogen, which has to be activated by host PA. Although the streptokinase is a key factor for plasmin-mediated virulence, the concerted action of PAM and streptokinase improves significantly the ability of streptococci to overcome microvascular occlusions and, hence, enhances streptococcal virulence [14]. The importance of plasmin acquisition for tissue penetration has been demonstrated in particular for the vector-borne spirochetes *Borrelia burgdorferi (B. burgdorferi)*. These bacteria are transmitted by ticks and have to traverse the human skin layers and disseminate in the blood to cause e.g. Lyme disease [77]. *Borrelia* recruit plasminogen via surface proteins OspA and OspC [78–80]. The acquired and surface-bound proteolytic activity enables the bacterium to degrade soluble and insoluble components of the ECM [81] and to penetrate endothelial monolayers including the blood-brain barrier [82–84] (fig. 1). The plasmin-mediated penetration of tissue barriers is in accordance with reports of bacterial invasion of brain and heart in murine relapsing borreliosis [85]. Interestingly, the plasminogen-binding proteins OspA and OspC are differentially expressed in the tick and e.g. human host. OspA is abundantly expressed on the surface of spirochetes within unfed ticks [86]. Feeding of the nymphs induces OspC expression, while OspA expression is downregulated. After transmission of *Borrelia* to mammals, OspC is constitutively produced and stimulates antibody development [86–88]. These data reveal that host-derived proteolytic activity and its subversion of the fibrinolysis are important in both the tick and the infected host.

Helicobacter pylori Stabilizes Fibrin Clot Formation

Binding of plasminogen was also reported for *Helicobacter pylori (H. pylori)* isolates, which are able to cause a variety of gastric diseases and chronic ulcers [89, 90]. In addition to two plasminogen-binding proteins, *H. pylori* produce a dodecameric neutrophil-activating protein (HP-NAP) that is able to increase the procoagulant potential of *H. pylori* by inhibiting fibrinolytic activities. HP-NAP stimulates PAI-2 synthesis and tissue factor expression in monocytes. In contrast, uPA expression is not changed. As a result, the uPA-induced plasma clot lysis is inhibited and the fibrinolysis is shifted towards a stabilization of fibrin clot formation. This in turn is probably beneficial for the bacteria by protecting them against phagocytosis [91]. The increased levels of PAI-2 were also demonstrated in gastric biopsies of *H. pylori*-positive patients and in gastric cancer cells after *H. pylori* infection [92]. The detection of elevated levels of PAI-2 and tissue factor expression in monocytes of patients suffering from *H. pylori* infection supported these data and suggests that the pathogen is involved in the regulation of the fibrinolytic balance and, hence, disease development [93].

Role of PAI-1 in Bacterial Pneumonia

Coagulation and fibrin deposition as a result of inflammation are an essential part of the host defense system. Fibrinogen and fibrin stimulate expression of proinflammatory cytokines in mononuclear cells and chemokines in endothelial cells and fibroblasts [94]. Activation of coagulation is regulated by three major procoagulant pathways, and the key components of these pathways are antithrombin, protein C, and tissue factor protein 1 [95]. In contrast, tPA and uPA are mainly released from vascular endothelial cells in fibrinolytic response to acute inflammations and activate plasminogen. The serpin (serine protease inhibitor) PAI-1, which acts as acute phase protein in periods of acute inflammation during sepsis and trauma, counteracts the fibrinolytic activity of plasmin [96, 97]. Inhibition of plasmin by PAI-1 results in an inadequate fibrin removal inducing microvascular thrombosis [1]. Intra-alveolar fibrin deposition is frequently found during acute lung diseases [98]. Importantly, fibrin deposition in mice deficient for plasminogen activators is more extensive after challenge with endotoxin (lipopolysaccharide, LPS), whereas PAI-1-knockout mice develop no vascular thrombosis after administration of LPS [99]. Taken together, these data demonstrate the significant influence of individual fibrinolytic components on endotoxin-induced fibrin generation. The procoagulatory activity of PAI-1 is elevated in patients with severe pneumonia and sepsis. PAI-1 competes with vitronectin for binding to uPAR and integrins and, thus, affects leukocyte migration during pneumonia [100–102]. However, recent data of mice infection experiments with Gram-positive pneumococci using PAI-1-deficient mice suggest that the host response against pulmonary infections is regulated predominantly by uPA and uPAR, but not PAI-1 [103, 104].

In contrast, pneumonia caused by Gram-negative *Klebsiella pneumoniae (K. pneumoniae)* is associated with increased production of PAI-1 in the lungs. PAI-1 deficiency resulted in reduced accumulation levels of neutrophils in the lung, similar to uPAR deficiency in pneumococcal pneumonia infection model [104, 105]. As a result, PAI-1-deficient mice have an impaired host defense against *K. pneumoniae*, resulting in higher bacterial loads, increased bacterial dissemination and, hence, in reduced survival rates of the mice [105]. PAI-1 overexpression in the lung of mice induced higher infiltration of neutrophils in the lungs and improved host defense against *K. pneumoniae*-induced sepsis [105].

Induction of Host Responses by tPA, uPA, and its Receptor uPAR during Pneumonia and Bacterial Meningitis

As mentioned above, host response against pneumococcal pneumonia is regulated predominantly by uPA and uPAR. Urokinase PAR-deficient mice showed reduced granulocyte accumulation in alveoli, indicating that leukocyte trafficking is strongly dependent on uPAR expression [104]. In contrast to the increased susceptibility of uPAR-knockout mice, uPA-knockout mice show an enhanced host defense [104, 106]. The lack of uPA in pulmonary infections increased leukocyte influx into the inflamed area and lowered amounts of pneumococci in the lungs [104].

Bacterial meningitis is associated with an infiltration of leukocytes into the subarachnoidal space, production of cytokines, chemokines, and proteases including MMPs. The induced inflammatory responses lead to a breakdown of the blood-brain barrier and formation of brain edema [107, 108]. This results in a higher expression of PAI-1, PAI-2, and uPAR, whereas the uPA level was only slightly increased during pneumococcal meningitis in mice. However, in patients suffering from pneumococcal meningitis, increased levels of tPA, uPAR, PAI-1, PAI-2, and also uPA were indicated in the cerebrospinal fluid (CSF) [109]. When using tPA-deficient mice in experimental meningitis, no differences in inflammatory host responses were demonstrated compared to wild-type mice, suggesting that tPA is not predominantly involved in the pathophysiology of pneumococcal meningitis [110]. Leukocyte infiltration in the subarachnoidal space was significantly increased in uPAR-knockout mice, indicating that uPAR participates in the recruitment of leukocytes to the CSF space [110]. These results are similar to the pathophysiology of pneumococcal pneumonia [104].

The Plasminogen Activation System and Infectious Diseases by *Borrelia*

Viable *B. burgdorferi* but also purified lipoproteins induce elevated levels of cell-anchored and soluble uPAR in monocytic cells [111], which are accumulated in inflammatory infiltrates during Lyme disease [112]. Toll-like receptor 2 (TLR2) and CD14, which represent key elements of the innate immunity and pattern recognition receptors, are at least partially involved in *B. burgdorferi*-induced uPAR expression [113]. Only the combined blockage of CD14 and TLR2 diminished the *Borrelia*-mediated uPAR induction, whereas the individual deficiency in CD14 or TLR2 in peritoneal exudate macrophages was not sufficient to inhibit induction of uPAR expression. On the one hand this demonstrates a new link between the innate immunity and plasminogen activation system, but on the other hand these data suggest the presence of additional pathways [113]. Infection experiments with plasminogen-knockout mice indicated that plasminogen is required for migration of spirochetes through microvessels and efficient dissemination of *Borrelia* in mice [114]. Moreover, these studies demonstrated that plasminogen is also essential for transmigration of *B. burgdorferi* to the salivary glands of the ticks [114].

Cell culture infections with *B. burgdorferi* increased the expression of MMPs including MMP-1, MMP-3, and MMP-9 in neural cells [115–119]. In addition, *B. burgdorferi* stimulates the expression of uPA and PAI-2 in monocytic cells in an in vitro transmigration model system which mimics physiological tissue barriers. Tissue PA expression was not induced [120]. Finally, elevated uPA production promotes transmigration of *B. burgdorferi* through a fibronectin-coated barrier independent of PAI-2 [120]. In contrast, PAI-2 induction by *Borrelia* reduced transmigration of monocytic cells through a matrigel [120]. In conclusion, *B. burgdorferi* subvert the plasminogen activation system in two ways. First, bacterial dissemination is facilitated and second, the inflammatory migration of phagocytic cells is decreased.

Conclusions and Future Directions

In humans, homozygous deficiencies of plasminogen activation system factors or of other components of the fibrinolytic system are rare. Transgenic mice overexpressing components of the plasminogen system and mice with single or combined gene deficiencies in fibrinolytic factors were employed to study the effects on vessel formation, tumor cell invasion, metastasis, and bacterial infections, respectively [121–124]. To date, we know that individual fibrinolytic factors accelerate the inflammatory responses against bacterial infections and contribute significantly to the elimination of the bacteria from host tissues. However, several pathogens have developed strategies to manipulate the host defense by interfering with factors of the plasminogen activation cascade and thereby reprogramming the immune protection machinery. Hence, the balance between repression of host inflammatory responses by bacterial mechanisms and induction of host defense mechanisms upon bacterial infections is the critical point which determines the progression of a bacterial infection within the host. Interestingly, recent data demonstrate that in addition to pathogenic bacteria also commensal and probiotic bacteria exploit the host-derived proteolytic activity of plasmin [125, 126]. However, the beneficial effects on colonization or immune evasion are not known. The identification of the bacterial factors manipulating the fibrinolytic cascade and their host receptor molecules provides targets for novel therapeutic treatments. Finally, the induced signal transduction cascade upon sensing of receptors of the fibrinolytic cascade such as the uPAR is of pivotal interest in order to identify novel strategies to combat infectious diseases.

Disclosure of Conflict of Interests

The authors state that they have no conflict of interest.

Acknowledgements

Our apologies to the authors of primary articles we have failed to discuss in detail or to cite due to limitations on space. The work in the group is supported by grants of the German Research Foundation (DFG-SFB 479 to S.H.) and Federal Ministry of Education and Research (grant 01KI0430 to S.H., Competence Network CAPNETZ).

References

1 Levi M, van der Poll T, Buller HR: Bidirectional relation between inflammation and coagulation. Circulation 2004;109:2698–2704.

2 Miyashita C, Wenzel E, Heiden M: Plasminogen: a brief introduction into its biochemistry and function. Haemostasis 1988;18(suppl 1):7–13.

3 Collen D, De Cock, Verstraete M: Immunochemical distinction between antiplasmin and alpha-antitrypsin. Thromb Res 1975;7:245–249.

4 Chu CT, Howard GC, Misra UK, Pizzo SV: Alpha 2-macroglobulin: a sensor for proteolysis. Ann N Y Acad Sci 1994;737:291–307.

5 Duval-Jobe C, Parmely MJ: Regulation of plasminogen activation by human U937 promonocytic cells. J Biol Chem 1994;269:21353–21357.

6 Hantai D, Festoff BW: Degradation of muscle basement membrane zone by locally generated plasmin. Exp Neurol 1987;95:44–55.

7 Wong AP, Cortez SL, Baricos WH: Role of plasmin and gelatinase in extracellular matrix degradation by cultured rat mesangial cells. Am J Physiol 1992;263: F1112–1118.

8 Wang X, Lin X, Loy JA, Tang J, Zhang XC: Crystal structure of the catalytic domain of human plasmin complexed with streptokinase. Science 1998;281:1662–1665.

9 Lahteenmaki K, Edelman S, Korhonen TK: Bacterial metastasis: the host plasminogen system in bacterial invasion. Trends Microbiol 2005;13:79–85.

10 Wang H, Lottenberg R, Boyle MD: Analysis of the interaction of group A streptococci with fibrinogen, streptokinase and plasminogen. Microb Pathog 1995;18:153–166.

11 Lottenberg R, Broder CC, Boyle MD, Kain SJ, Schroeder BL, Curtiss R 3rd: Cloning, sequence analysis, and expression in *Escherichia coli* of a streptococcal plasmin receptor. J Bacteriol 1992;174:5204–5210.

12 Wiman B: On the reaction of plasmin or plasmin-streptokinase complex with aprotinin or alpha 2-antiplasmin. Thromb Res 1980;17:143–152.

13 Gladysheva IP, Turner RB, Sazonova IY, Liu L, Reed GL: Coevolutionary patterns in plasminogen activation. Proc Natl Acad Sci U S A 2003;100:9168–9172.

14 Sun H, Ringdahl U, Homeister JW, Fay WP, Engleberg NC, Yang AY, Rozek LS, Wang X, Sjöbring U, Ginsburg D: Plasminogen is a critical host pathogenicity factor for group A streptococcal infection. Science 2004;305:1283–1286.

15 Rabijns A, De Bondt HL, De Ranter C: Three-dimensional structure of staphylokinase, a plasminogen activator with therapeutic potential. Nat Struct Biol 1997;4:357–360.

16 Molkanen T, Tyynela J, Helin J, Kalkkinen N, Kuusela P: Enhanced activation of bound plasminogen on Staphylococcus aureus by staphylokinase. FEBS Lett 2002;517:72–78.

17 Warmerdam PA, Vanderlick K, Vandervoort P, De Smedt H, Plaisance S, De Maeyer M, Collen D: Staphylokinase-specific cell-mediated immunity in humans. J Immunol 2002;168:155–161.

18 Jin T, Bokarewa M, Foster T, Mitchell J, Higgins J, Tarkowski A: Staphylococcus aureus resists human defensins by production of staphylokinase, a novel bacterial evasion mechanism. J Immunol 2004;172:1169–1176.

19 Yang D, Biragyn A, Kwak LW, Oppenheim JJ: Mammalian defensins in immunity: more than just microbicidal. Trends Immunol 2002;23:291–296.

20 Sakharov DV, Lijnen HR, Rijken DC: Interactions between staphylokinase, plasmin(ogen), and fibrin. Staphylokinase discriminates between free plasminogen and plasminogen bound to partially degraded fibrin. J Biol Chem 1996;271:27912–27918.

21 Collen D: Staphylokinase: a potent, uniquely fibrin-selective thrombolytic agent. Nat Med 1998;4:279–284.

22 Szemraj J, Walkowiak B, Kawecka I, Janiszewska G, Buczko W, Bartkowiak J, Chabielska E: A new recombinant thrombolytic and antithrombotic agent with higher fibrin affinity – a staphylokinase variant. I. In vitro study. J Thromb Haemost 2005;3:2156–2165.

23 Leigh JA: Purification of a plasminogen activator from Streptococcus uberis. FEMS Microbiol Lett 1994;118:153–158.

24 Johnsen LB, Poulsen K, Kilian M, Petersen TE: Purification and cloning of a streptokinase from Streptococcus uberis. Infect Immun 1999;67:1072–1078.

25 Johnsen LB, Rasmussen LK, Petersen TE, Etzerodt M, Fedosov SN: Kinetic and structural characterization of a two-domain streptokinase: dissection of domain functionality. Biochemistry 2000;39:6440–6448.

26 Nowicki ST, Minning-Wenz D, Johnston KH, Lottenberg R: Characterization of a novel streptokinase produced by Streptococcus equisimilis of non-human origin. Thromb Haemost 1994;72:595–603.

27 Leigh JA, Hodgkinson SM, Lincoln RA: The interaction of Streptococcus dysgalactiae with plasmin and plasminogen. Vet Microbiol 1998;61:121–135.

28 Sodeinde OA, Sample AK, Brubaker RR, Goguen JD: Plasminogen activator/coagulase gene of Yersinia pestis is responsible for degradation of plasmid-encoded outer membrane proteins. Infect Immun 1988;56:2749–2752.

29 Kukkonen M, Korhonen TK: The omptin family of enterobacterial surface proteases/adhesins: from housekeeping in Escherichia coli to systemic spread of Yersinia pestis. Int J Med Microbiol 2004;294:7–14.

30 Kukkonen M, Lahteenmaki K, Suomalainen M, Kalkkinen N, Emody L, Lang H, Korhonen TK: Protein regions important for plasminogen activation and inactivation of alpha2-antiplasmin in the surface protease Pla of Yersinia pestis. Mol Microbiol 2001;40:1097–1111.

31 Holmberg SR: Thrombolysis in acute myocardial infarction. Br J Hosp Med 1992;47:572–576, 578–580.

32 Sodeinde OA, Subrahmanyam YV, Stark K, Quan T, Bao Y, Goguen JD: A surface protease and the invasive character of plague. Science 1992;258:1004–1007.

33 Stumpe S, Schmid R, Stephens DL, Georgiou G, Bakker EP: Identification of OmpT as the protease that hydrolyzes the antimicrobial peptide protamine before it enters growing cells of Escherichia coli. J Bacteriol 1998;180:4002–4006.

34 Sugimura K, Nishihara T: Purification, characterization, and primary structure of Escherichia coli protease VII with specificity for paired basic residues: identity of protease VII and OmpT. J Bacteriol 1988;170:5625–5632.

35 Guina T, Yi EC, Wang H, Hackett M, Miller SI: A PhoP-regulated outer membrane protease of Salmonella enterica serovar typhimurium promotes resistance to alpha-helical antimicrobial peptides. J Bacteriol 2000;182:4077–4086.

36 Boyle MD, Lottenberg R: Plasminogen activation by invasive human pathogens. Thromb Haemost 1997;77:1–10.

37 Kukkonen M, Suomalainen M, Kyllonen P, Lahteenmaki K, Lang H, Virkola R, Helander IM, Holst O, Korhonen TK: Lack of O-antigen is essential for plasminogen activation by Yersinia pestis and Salmonella enterica. Mol Microbiol 2004;51:215–225.

38 Pouillot F, Derbise A, Kukkonen M, Foulon J, Korhonen TK, Carniel E: Evaluation of O-antigen inactivation on Pla activity and virulence of *Yersinia pseudotuberculosis* harbouring the pPla plasmid. Microbiology 2005;151:3759–3768.

39 Lobo LA: Adhesive properties of the purified plasminogen activator Pla of *Yersinia pestis*. FEMS Microbiol Lett 2006;262:158–162.

40 Benedek O, Bene J, Melegh B, Emody L: Mapping of possible laminin binding sites of *Y. pestis* plasminogen activator (Pla) via phage display. Adv Exp Med Biol 2003;529:101–104.

41 Benedek O, Khan AS, Schneider G, Nagy G, Autar R, Pieters RJ, Emody L: Identification of laminin-binding motifs of *Yersinia pestis* plasminogen activator by phage display. Int J Med Microbiol 2005;295:87–98.

42 Benedek O, Nagy G, Emody L: Intracellular signalling and cytoskeletal rearrangement involved in *Yersinia pestis* plasminogen activator (Pla) mediated HeLa cell invasion. Microb Pathog 2004;37:47–54.

43 Sebbane F, Jarrett CO, Gardner D, Long D, Hinnebusch BJ: Role of the *Yersinia pestis* plasminogen activator in the incidence of distinct septicemic and bubonic forms of flea-borne plague. Proc Natl Acad Sci U S A 2006;103:5526–5530.

44 Lathem WW, Price PA, Miller VL, Goldman WE: A plasminogen-activating protease specifically controls the development of primary pneumonic plague. Science 2007;315:509–513.

45 Lahteenmaki K, Kuusela P, Korhonen TK: Bacterial plasminogen activators and receptors. FEMS Microbiol Rev 2001;25:531–552.

46 Miles LA, Plow EF: Binding and activation of plasminogen on the platelet surface. J Biol Chem 1985;260:4303–4311.

47 Plow EF, Freaney DE, Plescia J, Miles LA: The plasminogen system and cell surfaces: evidence for plasminogen and urokinase receptors on the same cell type. J Cell Biol 1986;103:2411–2420.

48 Rouy D, Angles-Cano E: The mechanism of activation of plasminogen at the fibrin surface by tissue-type plasminogen activator in a plasma milieu in vitro. Role of alpha 2-antiplasmin. Biochem J 1990;271:51–57.

49 Plow EF, Ploplis VA, Busuttil S, Carmeliet P, Collen D: A role of plasminogen in atherosclerosis and restenosis models in mice. Thromb Haemost 1999;82(suppl 1):4–7.

50 Lijnen HR, Collen D: Fibrinolytic agents: mechanisms of activity and pharmacology. Thromb Haemost 1995;74:387–390.

51 Crippa MP: Urokinase-type plasminogen activator. Int J Biochem Cell Biol 2007;39:690–694.

52 Ploug M, Behrendt N, Lober D, Dano K: Protein structure and membrane anchorage of the cellular receptor for urokinase-type plasminogen activator. Semin Thromb Hemost 1991;17:183–193.

53 Cubellis MV, Nolli ML, Cassani G, Blasi F: Binding of single-chain prourokinase to the urokinase receptor of human U937 cells. J Biol Chem 1986;261:15819–15822.

54 Miles LA, Plow EF: Receptor mediated binding of the fibrinolytic components, plasminogen and urokinase, to peripheral blood cells. Thromb Haemost 1987;58:936–942.

55 Nykjaer A, Kjoller L, Cohen RL, Lawrence DA, Garni-Wagner BA, Todd RF 3rd, van Zonneveld AJ, Gliemann J, Andreasen PA: Regions involved in binding of urokinase-type-1 inhibitor complex and pro-urokinase to the endocytic alpha 2-macroglobulin receptor/low density lipoprotein receptor-related protein. Evidence that the urokinase receptor protects pro-urokinase against binding to the endocytic receptor. J Biol Chem 1994;269:25668–25676.

56 Nykjaer A, Petersen CM, Moller B, Andreasen PA, Gliemann J: Identification and characterization of urokinase receptors in natural killer cells and T-cell-derived lymphokine activated killer cells. FEBS Lett 1992;300:13–17.

57 Bernal D, de la Rubia JE, Carrasco-Abad AM, Toledo R, Mas-Coma S, Marcilla A: Identification of enolase as a plasminogen-binding protein in excretory-secretory products of *Fasciola hepatica*. FEBS Lett 2004;563:203–206.

58 Fox D, Smulian AG: Plasminogen-binding activity of enolase in the opportunistic pathogen *Pneumocystis carinii*. Med Mycol 2001;39:495–507.

59 Ge J, Catt DM, Gregory RL: *Streptococcus mutans* surface alpha-enolase binds salivary mucin MG2 and human plasminogen. Infect Immun 2004;72:6748–6752.

60 Bergmann S, Rohde M, Chhatwal GS, Hammerschmidt S: Alpha-enolase of *Streptococcus pneumoniae* is a plasmin(ogen)-binding protein displayed on the bacterial cell surface. Mol Microbiol 2001;40:1273–1287.

61 Pancholi V, Fischetti VA: Alpha-enolase, a novel strong plasmin(ogen) binding protein on the surface of pathogenic streptococci. J Biol Chem 1998;273:14503–14515.

62 Schaumburg J, Diekmann O, Hagendorff P, Bergmann S, Rohde M, Hammerschmidt S, Jänsch L, Wehland J, Kärst U: The cell wall subproteome of *Listeria monocytogenes*. Proteomics 2004;4:2991–3006.

63 Bergmann S, Rohde M, Chhatwal GS, Hammerschmidt S: Characterization of plasmin(ogen) binding to *Streptococcus pneumoniae*. Indian J Med Res 2004;119:29–32.

64 Ehinger S, Schubert WD, Bergmann S, Hammer-schmidt S, Heinz DW: Plasmin(ogen)-binding alpha-enolase from *Streptococcus pneumoniae*: crystal structure and evaluation of plasmin(ogen)-binding sites. J Mol Biol 2004;343:997–1005.

65 Jin H, Song YP, Boel G, Kochar J, Pancholi V: Group A streptococcal surface GAPDH, SDH, recognizes uPAR/CD87 as its receptor on the human pharyngeal cell and mediates bacterial adherence to host cells. J Mol Biol 2005;350:27–41.

66 Bergmann S, Rohde M, Hammerschmidt S: Glyceraldehyde-3-phosphate dehydrogenase of *Streptococcus pneumoniae* is a surface-displayed plasminogen-binding protein. Infect Immun 2004;72:2416–2419.

67 Blasi F: uPA, uPAR, PAI-1: key intersection of proteolytic, adhesive and chemotactic highways? Immunol Today 1997;18:415–417.

68 Blasi F, Carmeliet P: uPAR: a versatile signalling orchestrator. Nat Rev Mol Cell Biol 2002;3:932–943.

69 Pancholi V, Fischetti VA: A novel plasminogen/plasmin binding protein on the surface of group A streptococci. Adv Exp Med Biol 1997;418:597–599.

70 Boel G, Jin H, Pancholi V: Inhibition of cell surface export of group A streptococcal anchorless surface dehydrogenase affects bacterial adherence and antiphagocytic properties. Infect Immun 2005;73:6237–6248.

71 Jolodar A, Fischer P, Bergmann S, Buttner DW, Hammerschmidt S, Brattig NW: Molecular cloning of an alpha-enolase from the human filarial parasite *Onchocerca volvulus* that binds human plasminogen. Biochim Biophys Acta 2003;1627:111–120.

72 Jong AY, Chen SH, Stins MF, Kim KS, Tuan TL, Huang SH: Binding of *Candida albicans* enolase to plasmin(ogen) results in enhanced invasion of human brain microvascular endothelial cells. J Med Microbiol 2003;52:615–622.

73 Pancholi V: Multifunctional alpha-enolase: its role in diseases. Cell Mol Life Sci 2001;58:902–920.

74 Bergmann S, Rohde M, Preissner KT, Hammer-schmidt S: The nine residue plasminogen-binding motif of the pneumococcal enolase is the major cofactor of plasmin-mediated degradation of extracellular matrix, dissolution of fibrin and transmigration. Thromb Haemost 2005;94:304–311.

75 Bergmann S, Wild D, Diekmann O, Frank R, Bracht D, Chhatwal GS, Hammerschmidt S: Identification of a novel plasmin(ogen)-binding motif in surface displayed alpha-enolase of *Streptococcus pneumoniae*. Mol Microbiol 2003;49:411–423.

76 Berge A, Sjobring U: PAM, a novel plasminogen-binding protein from *Streptococcus pyogenes*. J Biol Chem 1993;268:25417–25424.

77 Benach JL, Bosler EM, Hanrahan JP, Coleman JL, Habicht GS, Bast TF, Cameron DJ, Ziegler JL, Barbour AG, Burgdorfer W, Edelman R, Kaslow RA: Spirochetes isolated from the blood of two patients with Lyme disease. N Engl J Med 1983;308:740–742.

78 Fuchs H, Wallich R, Simon MM, Kramer MD: The outer surface protein A of the spirochete *Borrelia burgdorferi* is a plasmin(ogen) receptor. Proc Natl Acad Sci U S A 1994;91:12594–12598.

79 Klempner MS, Noring R, Epstein MP, McCloud B, Hu R, Limentani SA, Rogers RA: Binding of human plasminogen and urokinase-type plasminogen activator to the Lyme disease spirochete, *Borrelia burgdorferi*. J Infect Dis 1995;171:1258–1265.

80 Hu LT, Perides G, Noring R, Klempner MS: Binding of human plasminogen to *Borrelia burgdorferi*. Infect Immun 1995;63:3491–3496.

81 Coleman JL, Roemer EJ, Benach JL: Plasmin-coated *Borrelia burgdorferi* degrades soluble and insoluble components of the mammalian extracellular matrix. Infect Immun 1999;67:3929–3936.

82 Coleman JL, Benach JL: The generation of enzymatically active plasmin on the surface of spirochetes. Methods 2000;21:133–141.

83 Coleman JL, Sellati TJ, Testa JE, Kew RR, Furie MB, Benach JL: *Borrelia burgdorferi* binds plasminogen, resulting in enhanced penetration of endothelial monolayers. Infect Immun 1995;63:2478–2484.

84 Grab DJ, Perides G, Dumler JS, Kim KJ, Park J, Kim YV, Nikolskaia O, Choi KS, Stins MF, Kim KS: *Borrelia burgdorferi*, host-derived proteases, and the blood-brain barrier. Infect Immun 2005;73:1014–1022.

85 Gebbia JA, Monco JC, Degen JL, Bugge TH, Benach JL: The plasminogen activation system enhances brain and heart invasion in murine relapsing fever borreliosis. J Clin Invest 1999;103:81–87.

86 Schwan TG, Piesman J, Golde WT, Dolan MC, Rosa PA: Induction of an outer surface protein on *Borrelia burgdorferi* during tick feeding. Proc Natl Acad Sci U S A 1995;92:2909–2913.

87 Liang FT, Nelson FK, Fikrig E: Molecular adaptation of *Borrelia burgdorferi* in the murine host. J Exp Med 2002;196:275–280.

88 de Silva AM, Telford SR 3rd, Brunet LR, Barthold SW, Fikrig E: *Borrelia burgdorferi* OspA is an arthropod-specific transmission-blocking Lyme disease vaccine. J Exp Med 1996;183:271–275.

89 Pantzar M, Ljungh A, Wadstrom T: Plasminogen binding and activation at the surface of *Helicobacter pylori* CCUG 17874. Infect Immun 1998;66:4976–4980.

90 Ringner M, Valkonen KH, Wadstrom T: Binding of vitronectin and plasminogen to *Helicobacter pylori*. FEMS Immunol Med Microbiol 1994;9:29–34.

91 Montemurro P, Barbuti G, Dundon WG, Del Giudice G, Rappuoli R, Colucci M, De Rinaldis P, Montecucco C, Semeraro N, Papini E: *Helicobacter pylori* neutrophil-activating protein stimulates tissue factor and plasminogen activator inhibitor-2 production by human blood mononuclear cells. J Infect Dis 2001;183:1055–1062.

92 Varro A, Noble PJ, Pritchard DM, Kennedy S, Hart CA, Dimaline R, Dockray GJ: *Helicobacter pylori* induces plasminogen activator inhibitor 2 in gastric epithelial cells through nuclear factor-kappaB and RhoA: implications for invasion and apoptosis. Cancer Res 2004;64:1695–1702.

93 Colucci M, Rossiello MR, Pentimone A, Berloco P, Russo F, Di Leo A, Semeraro N: Changes in coagulation-fibrinolysis balance in blood mononuclear cells and in gastric mucosa from patients with *Helicobacter pylori* infection. Thromb Res 2005;116:471–477.

94 Szaba FM, Smiley ST: Roles for thrombin and fibrin(ogen) in cytokine/chemokine production and macrophage adhesion in vivo. Blood 2002;99:1053–1059.

95 van der Poll T, Levi M: Mechanisms of action of activated protein C: an evolving story. Crit Care Med 2004;32:1086–1087.

96 Brodsky SV, Malinowski K, Golightly M, Jesty J, Goligorsky MS: Plasminogen activator inhibitor-1 promotes formation of endothelial microparticles with procoagulant potential. Circulation 2002;106:2372–2378.

97 Hermans PW, Hazelzet JA: Plasminogen activator inhibitor type 1 gene polymorphism and sepsis. Clin Infect Dis 2005;41(suppl 7):S453–458.

98 Abraham E: Coagulation abnormalities in acute lung injury and sepsis. Am J Respir Cell Mol Biol 2000;22:401–404.

99 Yamamoto K, Loskutoff DJ: Fibrin deposition in tissues from endotoxin-treated mice correlates with decreases in the expression of urokinase-type but not tissue-type plasminogen activator. J Clin Invest 1996;97:2440–2451.

100 Waltz DA, Natkin LR, Fujita RM, Wei Y, Chapman HA: Plasmin and plasminogen activator inhibitor type 1 promote cellular motility by regulating the interaction between the urokinase receptor and vitronectin. J Clin Invest 1997;100:58–67.

101 Kjoller L, Kanse SM, Kirkegaard T, Rodenburg KW, Ronne E, Goodman SL, Preissner KT, Ossowski L, Andreasen PA: Plasminogen activator inhibitor-1 represses integrin- and vitronectin-mediated cell migration independently of its function as an inhibitor of plasminogen activation. Exp Cell Res 1997;232:420–429.

102 Deng G, Curriden SA, Wang S, Rosenberg S, Loskutoff DJ: Is plasminogen activator inhibitor-1 the molecular switch that governs urokinase receptor-mediated cell adhesion and release? J Cell Biol 1996;134:1563–1571.

103 Rijneveld AW, Florquin S, Bresser P, Levi M, De Waard V, Lijnen R, Van Der Zee JS, Speelman P, Carmeliet P, Van Der Poll T: Plasminogen activator inhibitor type-1 deficiency does not influence the outcome of murine pneumococcal pneumonia. Blood 2003;102:934–939.

104 Rijneveld AW, van den Dobbelsteen GP, Florquin S, Standiford TJ, Speelman P, van Alphen L, van der Poll T: Roles of interleukin-6 and macrophage inflammatory protein-2 in pneumolysin-induced lung inflammation in mice. J Infect Dis 2002;185:123–126.

105 Renckens R, Roelofs JJ, Bonta PI, Florquin S, de Vries CJ, Levi M, Carmeliet P, van't Veer C, van der Poll T: Plasminogen activator inhibitor type 1 is protective during severe Gram-negative pneumonia. Blood 2007;109:1593–1601.

106 Gyetko MR, Sud S, Kendall T, Fuller JA, Newstead MW, Standiford TJ: Urokinase receptor-deficient mice have impaired neutrophil recruitment in response to pulmonary *Pseudomonas aeruginosa* infection. J Immunol 2000;165:1513–1519.

107 Scheld WM, Koedel U, Nathan B, Pfister HW: Pathophysiology of bacterial meningitis: mechanism(s) of neuronal injury. J Infect Dis 2002;186(suppl 2): S225–233.

108 Koedel U, Scheld WM, Pfister HW: Pathogenesis and pathophysiology of pneumococcal meningitis. Lancet Infect Dis 2002;2:721–736.

109 Winkler F, Kastenbauer S, Koedel U, Pfister HW: Role of the urokinase plasminogen activator system in patients with bacterial meningitis. Neurology 2002;59:1350–1355.

110 Paul R, Angele B, Sporer B, Pfister HW, Koedel U: Inflammatory response during bacterial meningitis is unchanged in Fas- and Fas ligand-deficient mice. J Neuroimmunol 2004;152:78–82.

111 Coleman JL, Gebbia JA, Benach JL: *Borrelia burgdorferi* and other bacterial products induce expression and release of the urokinase receptor (CD87). J Immunol 2001;166:473–480.

112 Salazar JC, Pope CD, Sellati TJ, Feder HM Jr, Kiely TG, Dardick KR, Buckman RL, Moore MW, Caimano MJ, Pope JG, Krause PJ, Radolf JD; Lyme Disease Network: Coevolution of markers of innate and adaptive immunity in skin and peripheral blood of patients with erythema migrans. J Immunol 2003;171:2660–2670.

113 Coleman JL, Benach JL: The urokinase receptor can be induced by *Borrelia burgdorferi* through receptors of the innate immune system. Infect Immun 2003;71:5556–5564.

114 Coleman JL, Gebbia JA, Piesman J, Degen JL, Bugge TH, Benach JL: Plasminogen is required for efficient dissemination of *B. burgdorferi* in ticks and for enhancement of spirochetemia in mice. Cell 1997;89:1111–1119.

115 Gebbia JA, Coleman JL, Benach JL: *Borrelia* spirochetes upregulate release and activation of matrix metalloproteinase gelatinase B (MMP-9) and collagenase 1 (MMP-1) in human cells. Infect Immun 2001;69:456–462.

116 Hu LT, Eskildsen MA, Masgala C, Steere AC, Arner EC, Pratta MA, Grodzinsky AJ, Loening A, Perides G: Host metalloproteinases in Lyme arthritis. Arthritis Rheum 2001;44:1401–1410.

117 Hu LT, Pratt SD, Perides G, Katz L, Rogers RA, Klempner MS: Isolation, cloning, and expression of a 70-kilodalton plasminogen binding protein of *Borrelia burgdorferi*. Infect Immun 1997;65:4989–4995.

118 Kirchner A, Koedel U, Fingerle V, Paul R, Wilske B, Pfister HW: Upregulation of matrix metalloproteinase-9 in the cerebrospinal fluid of patients with acute Lyme neuroborreliosis. J Neurol Neurosurg Psychiatry 2000;68:368–371.

119 Perides G, Tanner-Brown LM, Eskildsen MA, Klempner MS: *Borrelia burgdorferi* induces matrix metalloproteinases by neural cultures. J Neurosci Res 1999;58:779–790.

120 Haile WB, Coleman JL, Benach JL: Reciprocal upregulation of urokinase plasminogen activator and its inhibitor, PAI-2, by *Borrelia burgdorferi* affects bacterial penetration and host-inflammatory response. Cell Microbiol 2006;8:1349–1360.

121 Carmeliet P, Collen D: Genetic analysis of the plasminogen and coagulation system in mice. Haemostasis 1996;26(suppl 4):132–153.

122 Carmeliet P, Collen D: Vascular development and disorders: molecular analysis and pathogenic insights. Kidney Int 1998;53:1519–1549.

123 Degen JL, Drew AF, Palumbo JS, Kombrinck KW, Bezerra JA, Danton MJ, Holmbäck K, Suh TT: Genetic manipulation of fibrinogen and fibrinolysis in mice. Ann N Y Acad Sci 2001;936:276–290.

124 Ploplis VA, French EL, Carmeliet P, Collen D, Plow EF: Plasminogen deficiency differentially affects recruitment of inflammatory cell populations in mice. Blood 1998;91:2005–2009.

125 Candela M, Bergmann S, Vici M, Vitali B, Turroni S, Eikmanns BJ, Hammerschmidt S, Brigidi P: Binding of human plasminogen to *Bifidobacterium*. J Bacteriol 2007;189:5929–5936.

126 Hurmalainen V, Edelman S, Antikainen J, Baumann M, Lähteenmäki K, Korhonen TK: Extracellular proteins of *Lactobacillus crispatus* enhance activation of human plasminogen. Microbiology 2007;153:1112–1122.

127 Bergmann S, Hammerschmidt S: Fibrinolysis and host response in bacterial infections. Thromb Haemost 2007;98:512–520.

Prof. Dr. rer. nat. Sven Hammerschmidt
Inst. für Genetik und funktionelle Genomforschung, Abt. Genetik der Mikroorganismen
Ernst-Moritz-Arndt-Universität Greifswald
Friedrich-Ludwig-Jahn-Str. 15a, 17487 Greifswald, Germany
Tel. +49 3834 86-4160, Fax -4172
E-Mail hammerschmidt@mvp.uni-greifswald.de

Scharf RE (ed): Progress and Challenges in Transfusion Medicine, Hemostasis and Hemotherapy.
Freiburg i.Br., Karger, 2008, pp 89–112

Selective Immune Apheresis Technologies – Where Do We Stand?

Wolfgang Ramlow[a] · Heinrich Prophet[a] · Jörg Emmrich[b]

[a]Apheresis Center, Rostock,
[b]Department of Gastroenterology, University of Rostock, Germany

Key Words

Blood component removal · Immunoadsorption · Autoimmune diseases · Dilated cardiomyopathy · Ulcerative colitis · Transplantation · Pemphigus

Summary

Due to inadequate scientific evidence there are almost no established guidelines for the application of immune apheresis therapy in a specific disease condition. Relatively high costs and the requirement for specially trained staff and special technical equipment are the major reasons that apheresis therapy usually is not considered until life-threatening conditions or end-stage disease have developed. In this complex situation, standardization of treatment and scientific evaluation is extremely difficult to manage. The preparation and conduct of well-designed randomized controlled trials evaluating the clinical effectiveness of immune apheresis therefore requires a close interdisciplinary collaboration of clinicians, researchers and industry. On this background, this review describes the current status and future trends of selective immune apheresis therapy in autoimmune diseases and immune-mediated clinical conditions in which antibodies antagonize special treatment options such as transplantation or coagulation factor substitution. In order to transfer persuasive clinical experience of apheresis experts into scientific evidence and general acceptance of this treatment modality, a more sophisticated patient selection and a harmonization of study protocols on an international perspective, together with prospective data collection by national and international registries, are the main future tasks of the apheresis community.

©2008 S. Karger GmbH, Freiburg i.Br.

Introduction

Because of their high potential to remove immune-relevant cells or proteins, selective immunoadsorption technologies (SIAT) have been increasingly considered as a useful adjunct to immunosuppressive drug therapy in case of contraindication, intolerance or inadequate disease control by drugs alone. Regardless of a superior theoretical background, SIAT are still less frequently used than non-selective apheresis technologies. A longer history and a better local accessibility have generated more clinical experience and scientific evidence for plasma exchange treatment in many diseases.

Nonetheless, during the last decade there has been emerging evidence for a beneficial effect of SIAT treatment in indications such as idiopathic dilated cardiomyopathy (IDCM), solid organ transplantation, blistering skin diseases, ulcerative colitis (UC), and hemophilia with coagulation factor inhibitors. Randomized controlled trials are already under way or in preparation for IDCM, UC and autoimmune blistering skin diseases. In other special fields of application such as solid organ transplantation (human leukocyte antigen (HLA) presensitization, humoral allograft rejection, blood group incompatibility) or inhibitor-mediated bleeding in hemophiliacs, local acceptance could be achieved by several groups based on the superior cost effectiveness of SIAT treatment in comparison to other treatment alternatives.

Definition

In common use, apheresis technologies are rather categorized by the nature of targets or by clinical indications than by technological features. In this perspective, all apheresis technologies aiming at the removal or modulation of immune factors/cells are subsumed under the term immune apheresis, regardless of the physicochemical nature of their interactions with the biological components.

Selective Immunoadsorption Technologies

SIAT do allow selective or even specific removal of relevant target(s) while leaving essential components widely unaffected. In contrast to plasma exchange, there is no need for protein replacement with the potential risk of transferring infectious agents. SIAT can be differentiated by
- the setting in which the adsorber module is being used (plasmaperfusion vs. hemoperfusion),
- the level of selectivity of the adsorption process,
- the nature of the adsorption process (e.g. hydrophobic interactions, antigen-antibody interactions),
- the number of adsorber columns used during one procedure (single-column immunoadsorption (IA) system = SC-IA vs. double-column IA system = DC-IA),
- the reusability of the adsorber devices (single use vs. re-use systems).

Table 1 provides an overview of the main features of SIAT.

Table 1. Overview on major SIAT

Product	Company	Matrix	Ligand	Reusability	Technical setting
Adacolumn®	Jimro / Otsuka	cellulose diacetate	–	no	hemoperfusion
Cellsorba®	Asahi Kasei / Diamed	nonwoven polyester fabric	–	no	hemoperfusion
Globaffin®	Fresenius	sepharose	synthetic peptide	yes	plasmaperfusion
Glycosorb®	Glycorex	sepharose	carbohydrate epitope	not approved	plasmaperfusion
Ig-Therasorb™	Miltenyi	sepharose	polyclonal sheep anti-human Ig	yes	plasmaperfusion
Immunosorba®	Fresenius	sepharose	protein A	yes	plasmaperfusion
Immusorba®	Asahi Kasei / Diamed	polyvinyl alcohol gel	hydrophobic amino acids (PH, TR)	no	plasmaperfusion
Prosorba®	Fresenius	silica gel	protein A	no	plasmaperfusion
Selesorb®	Kaneka	cellulose	dextrane sulfate	not approved	plasmaperfusion

Plasmaperfusion Devices

Because of their inadequate biocompatibility, adsorber devices preferentially have been developed for the use in plasma in order to prevent interactions between blood cells and foreign surfaces. The typical devices used as disposable single columns in a plasmaperfusion setting are Glycosorb® (Glycorex AB Transplantation, Sweden), Immusorba-PH/-TR® (Asahi-Kasei Medical, Japan), and Prosorba® (Fresenius Medical Care, Germany). Due to saturation of single-column systems, the reduction rates for immune factors (antibodies, immune complexes) during one session usually are limited to a maximum of 30–50%.

To increase the elimination capacity, regenerative double-column systems have been introduced that allow adsorption and regeneration during the apheresis procedure in an alternate fashion. By this technology, DC-IA systems can realize reduction rates for immunoglobulins of up to 75–90% during one single session when utilizing about 2.5 times the patient's plasma volume. Because of the regeneration techniques, the adsorbers have to be used in a plasmaperfusion setting. The typical adsorber devices of this group are Ig-Therasorb™ (Miltenyi Biotec, Germany), Ig-Adsopak® (Pocard, Russia), Immunosorba® (Fresenius, Medical Care Germany), and Globaffin® (Fresenius Medical Care, Germany). All adsorbers are approved for re-use in the same patient. In some countries, re-use of medical products is not permitted.

Therefore, these systems are not available in Japan, for example. For the same reason, the Japanese Selesorb® system (Kaneka Corporation, Japan), which is indicated for removal of anti-DNA antibodies in systemic lupus erythematosus (SLE) patients, is not approved for re-use.

Hemoperfusion Devices

Currently, two hemoperfusion systems are available for the treatment of autoimmune diseases. Adacolumn® (Jimro / Otsuka Pharmaceutical, Japan) is an extracorporeal adsorptive cytapheresis device using cellulose diacetate beads, which preferentially adsorb granulocytes, monocytes/macrophages but only small numbers of lymphocytes. The Cellsorba® (Asahi-Kasei Medical, Japan) cytapheresis system consists of a column filled with nonwoven polyester fabric and captures lymphocytes, granulocytes, monocytes/macrophages and platelets to a much higher extent than the Adacolumn system [1, 2]. Both systems are easy to handle and a standard treatment schedule consist of 5–10 apheresis sessions during the first 5–10 weeks, usually performed in a weekly interval. The required blood flow is between 30–50 ml/min that usually can be achieved easily using peripheral venous access. Treatment time is only 1–2 h, which is very convenient for the patients.

Suggested Mode(s) of Action of Selective Immunoadsorption Technologies

The traditional aim of apheresis therapy is the depletion of relevant pathogenic factors and/or cells. This strategy usually requires the prior identification of one or more target(s) playing a key role in initiation or perpetuation of the specific disease or medical condition. Other than in low-density lipoprotein (LDL) apheresis where LDL cholesterol is a clearly defined target, the situation in autoimmune diseases is more complex.

T cells for many years have been considered as the major players in the orchestra of immunological interactions, but the introduction of new laboratory technologies has unveiled a more substantial role of the humoral immune system in the development of an autoimmune attack than originally thought [3, 4]. In certain autoimmune diseases, the elimination of (auto)antibodies has been shown to be beneficial [5–14]. Table 2 provides an overview on relevant antibodies known for their significant role in certain immune-mediated disorders.

On the other hand, the selective removal of granulocytes, monocytes or even platelets by use of adsorptive techniques has been shown to be beneficial as well [1, 15–24]. The observation that antibody depletion as well as cellular removal can induce clinical improvement in the same diseases requires a careful reconsideration on how immune apheresis works [20, 25–34]. Because of the transient nature of the depletion of

Table 2. Key antibodies in specific immune-mediated conditions

(Auto)antibodies (AAB)	Disease / Condition
Acetylcholine receptor antibodies AAB	myasthenia gravis
Coagulation factor inhibitor(s)	hemophilia
Desmoglein 1/3 AAB	pemphigus / pemphigoid
Glomerular basement membrane AAB	Goodpasture's syndrome
$\beta1$-Adrenergic receptor AAB	idiopathic dilated cardiomyopathy
HLA antibodies	HLA-presensitized transplant recipients antibody-mediated allograft rejection
Blood group antibodies	ABO-incompatible transplant recipients

suggested pathogens, long-lasting beneficial effects after SIAT therapy can only be explained by induction of modulatory effects. Therefore, the impact on one or more key mechanisms of the immune response might be the crucial step to induce long-term modulation. The principle of neutralizing/inhibiting one key player or key process of the inflammatory cascade works very effectively in anti-cytokine drug treatment in several autoimmune diseases.

Major Indications of Selective Immunoadsorption Technologies

Rheumatoid Arthritis

Rheumatoid arthritis (RA) is a systemic disease that predominantly affects peripheral joints in a typical symmetric manner. The persistent inflammatory synovitis leads to progressive destruction and deformation. Today, there is sufficient evidence that this chronic inflammatory process results from a dysregulation of the immune network, involving both humoral and cellular mechanisms.

Despite of the complex pathophysiology of RA, apheresis therapy was intensely evaluated during the early 80s of the last century, probably due to the high prevalence of the disease. From today's viewpoint, all these studies were inadequately designed to investigate apheresis therapy in the specific subgroup of drug-refractory RA patients.

Several groups reported on the successful application of IA in drug-refractory RA patients in uncontrolled trials utilizing various SC-IA systems [35–42]. Moreover, Kashiwagi et al. [43] conducted a randomized controlled trial in RA patients investigating safety and effectiveness of the Adacolumn system by utilizing two different apheresis regimens (4 weekly treatments vs. 4 × 2 weekly treatments). Clinical improvement developed in about 50% of the 143 patients who had been eligible for final evaluation, without showing any significant difference between the two groups.

Two randomized double-blind, sham-controlled trials finally provided evidence for the clinical benefit of SC-IA treatment in drug-refractory RA patients. Both studies were published in 1999 [29, 32].

Based on two promising pilot trials with the Prosorba column in RA patients [35, 41], a double-blind, sham-controlled multicenter trial had been initiated involving 12 rheumatologic centers throughout the USA. In this study, drug-refractory RA patients were randomly assigned to receive either 12 weekly treatments with Prosorba or sham apheresis. Final evaluations were performed at weeks 19 and 20. The study was terminated early by an independent data safety monitoring board due to successful outcome after 91 patients had completed the protocol. The overall response rate (according to 20% improvement criteria of the American College of Rheumatology = ACR20) was 31.9% in 47 patients of the active treatment arm versus 11.4% in the 44 patients of the group receiving sham apheresis [32]. Based on these results, the Prosorba column was finally approved and reimbursed in the USA and later in Germany. Today, this product is not marketed any more for this indication, probably due to the relatively high incidence of vasculitis-like side effects [44–46] and a continuously growing competition on the RA market arising from anti-cytokine drug treatment.

Hidaka et al. [29] evaluated the clinical efficacy of the Cellsorba system for drug-refractory RA patients in a randomized double-blind, sham-controlled multicenter trial with a suggested 3:1 randomization ratio. Finally, 25 patients received active treatment, whereas 7 patients in the control group received sham apheresis. The patients received one apheresis (or sham) per week for 3 weeks. Medication remained unchanged in both groups through the study period. According to established ACR20 criteria, 79.2% of the patients in the active group responded to the apheresis treatment. None of the patients in the control group showed an improvement. Based on these results and additional data from uncontrolled studies [28, 47], the Cellsorba system was approved by the Japanese Ministry of Health and Welfare for the treatment of drug-refractory RA patients. Until now, more than 1500 patients have already been treated with this system in Japan [48].

Ulcerative Colitis

UC is a chronic inflammatory bowel disease (IBD) that primarily affects the colorectal mucosa. Treatment options include the application of anti-inflammatory and immunosuppressive drugs with a wide variety of known side effects, in particular in long-term use. Surgical intervention is needed in severe cases with fulminant disease refractory to medical therapy or to prevent the development of colorectal cancer.

Today, there is sufficient evidence that UC arises from a complex inflammatory process involving genetic, environmental, microbiological, and immunoregulatory factors.

The rationale for the cytapheresis treatment in UC is based on the observation that the inflammation of the mucosal wall is amplified by the influx of neutrophils and monocytes, which interact with lymphocytes in further enhancing the inflammatory response [49].

In two major prospective randomized controlled multicenter trials in Japan, the safety and effectiveness of adsorptive cytapheresis (Adacolumn, Cellsorba) in UC was originally evaluated in comparison to patients with high-dose steroid treatment by Shimoyama, Sawada and coworkers [50–52]. All patients in both groups received standard medication with 5-aminosalicylic acid as baseline therapy. Clinical activity and endoscopic indexes showed better improvements in the cytapheresis than in the steroid group. These two studies, conducted in agreement with the Japanese Ministry of Health and Welfare, led to approval and reimbursement of Adacolumn and Cellsorba cytapheresis treatment in UC patients in Japan.

Although large-scale sham-controlled trials are still missing, there is emerging evidence for the beneficial effect of adsorptive cytapheresis. It has been shown by many trials that the remission rate is about 50–70% in average, depending on the clinical phase of the disease, concomitant medication and apheresis treatment schedule. It is obvious that in an earlier disease state or even in naive patients the response rates are the highest. Hanai et al. [49] and Suzuki et al. [53] reported response rates of 85 and 88%, respectively, when treating steroid-naive patients with active UC with Adacolumn cytapheresis. On the other hand, Sawada et al. [23] could demonstrate that Cellsorba therapy is effective even in severe cases. In 4/6 patients with toxic megacolon, colectomy could be prevented by cytapheresis treatment.

Several groups [1, 50, 54–56] reported long-term remission up to 1 year in about 50–80% of patients with steroid-dependent or steroid-refractory UC at study entry.

Until now, more than 10,000 UC patients have already been treated with the two systems in Japan [48].

Idiopathic Dilated Cardiomyopathy

IDCM is the most common cause of heart transplantation worldwide. The hallmark of IDCM is the non-ischemic dilation of the cardiac ventricles leading to progressive cardiac insufficiency. Regular drug treatment consists of β-blockers plus angiotensin-converting enzyme (ACE) inhibitors or angiotensin receptor blocking agents. In advanced stages, left ventricular assist devices and finally heart transplantation are the only therapeutic options.

The etiology of the disease still remains unclear, but there has been emerging evidence for a strong contribution of autoantibodies against cardiac structures (vs. myosin, β1-adrenergic receptor, muscarinic cholinergic receptor, ADP and ATP carrier proteins) to the maintenance and the progression of the disease [3, 57–62]. For autoantbodies directed towards the β1-adrenergic receptor, meanwhile even the fulfillment of the classical Witebsky critera for autoimmunity has been demonstrated [59–61].

Several studies have demonstrated the clinical benefit of SIAT in IDCM patients. In 1996, Wallukat et al. [63] firstly described positive short-term hemodynamic effects in 7 IDCM patients treated with the Ig-Therasorb DC-IA system. The original therapeutic strategy consisted in elimination of autoantibodies directed against the β1-adrenergic receptor. In consideration of missing specific IA technologies, the aggressive removal of all immunoglobulins was intended, suggesting a parallel elimination of anticardiac antibodies. Therefore 5 apheresis sessions were performed for 5 consecutive days, followed by intravenous immunoglobulin (ivIg) substitution at the end of the apheresis cycle. Originally, ivIg was given only for prophylactic reasons, but it cannot be excluded that even minor doses of ivIg cause modulatory effects when administered in patients whose immunoglobulin levels had been extremely lowered before.

In 2000, two Berlin groups published results of two controlled trials. Muller et al. [64] used the same treatment regimen as described above in 17 patients in a case-controlled trial comparing the clinical outcome of an apheresis group to 17 matched controls receiving standard medication only. Although only treated for 5 days by apheresis, the patients developed a long-term clinical response as demonstrated by an improvement in cardiac function and a shift to lower New York Heart Association (NYHA) grades in the treatment group. In addition, the autoantibody titers against β1-adrenergic receptor remained low for 1 year without additional apheresis sessions.

Felix et al. [65] used a slightly different apheresis protocol (3 sessions with Ig-Therasorb for 3 consecutive days followed by 2 sessions every month for 3 months plus ivIg) in a controlled trial. 18 patients with IDCM (NYHA III-IY; left ventricular ejection fraction <30%) were randomly assigned either to the apheresis group (n = 9) or a control group without apheresis. All patients were kept on stable drug medication throughout the 3-month study period. Hemodynamic parameters and clinical symptoms improved remarkably in the apheresis group in contrast to the controls.

In particular, the group of Felix and Staudt has substantially contributed not only to the development of standardized protocols for the apheresis treatment in IDCM patients but also to gaining new insights into the mode of action of DC-IA in IDCM patients. They were able to demonstrate a cardiodepressant effect of antibodies eliminated from IDCM patients by DC-IA treatment on rat cardiomyocytes [8]. Another important contribution by the group was the observation that an effective removal of antibodies belonging to the IgG$_3$ subclass is essential to achieve the expected clinical benefit [6, 66]. This finding led to a modification of the apheresis protocol towards an intensified treatment when using the Immunosorba DC-IA.

The successful application of DC-IA in IDCM has been reported also by other groups, supporting these positive results [67, 68]. In long-term follow-ups, not only a sustained clinical benefit in this special group of patients could be demonstrated but also an excellent cost effectiveness [69, 70].

ABO-Incompatible Solid Organ Transplantation

Blood group incompatibility for many years was considered a major contraindication for solid organ transplantation in living donor kidney transplantation as well as in emergency cadaveric donor transplantation. Strategies to overcome the restrictions in the recruitment of suitable donor organs have been preferentially developed by Japanese groups due to the fact that cadaveric organ transplantation could not be performed for legal restrictions until a transplantation law was settled in Japan in 1997.

Tanabe [71] recently summarized the Japanese experience of ABO-incompatible kidney transplantation. Between 1989 and 2005, a total of 851 ABO-incompatible kidney transplantations were performed in 82 institutions throughout Japan, demonstrating 1-, 3-, 5-, and 10-year graft survival rates of 89, 85, 79, and 61%, respectively. In Japan, plasma exchange and double membrane filtration have been widely used in combination with standard immunosuppression and splenectomy for many years. Graft survival has increasingly improved after the introduction of tacrolimus and mycophenolate mofetil. Since 2005, splenectomy in most protocols was replaced by the usage of rituximab. With these new protocols, in the most recent years graft survival has almost reached the results of blood group-compatible donor transplantation now [71, 72].

In 2001, a Swedish group introduced a new protocol for ABO-incompatible kidney transplantation in their center, consisting of antigen-specific IA in addition to a standard triple drug immunosuppression plus rituximab [11, 73]. The new adsorber columns (Glycosorb A/B) utilize trisaccharide carbohydrate epitopes on a sepharose matrix to specifically adsorb blood group antibodies [74]. Two different columns are available, one with antigenic properties of the A blood group and one with antigenic properties of the B blood group. Meanwhile, many European groups have also successfully implemented the original Swedish protocol [75–78]. Last year, Tyden et al. [11] published a 3-center-pooled analysis on 60 consecutive ABO-incompatible living donor kidney transplantations. Graft survival at a mean follow-up of 17.5 months was excellent with 97%, equalizing the results of 274 living donor ABO-compatible transplantations (95% at a mean follow-up of 21.1 months).

While initially patients with high antibody titers were excluded, now the Freiburg group has reported on successful transplantation even in this subgroup of patients by using a more intensive apheresis treatment protocol (increase of the plasma volume treated during single sessions) [77, 79]. Another important observation has been made by this group, suggesting that preemptive apheresis treatments post transplantation might not be necessary in all patients [80, 81].

Successful transplantation of cadaveric organs across the ABO barrier utilizing antigen-specific IA or selective DC-IA in addition to standard immunosuppression has already been reported for lung, liver and heart transplants in case reports or small case series, too [82–86].

The potential of DC-IA for high-capacity elimination of HLA alloantibodies makes this treatment an excellent choice to enable successful cadaveric kidney transplantation in highly sensitized recipients, as well as to treat antibody-mediated kidney allograft rejection that often causes severe graft dysfunction. By far, the most clinical experience in these two indications has been collected by the Vienna group of Derfler and Böhmig [13, 14, 87–89]. Although the numbers of patients evaluated in uncontrolled clinical trials is still limited, the results are quite remarkable. A randomized controlled two-center trial evaluating the effectiveness of DC-IA in acute C4d-positive kidney allograft rejection was terminated early after the first interim analysis of the first 10 patients because of the high rate of graft losses in the non-apheresis group (4/5 versus 1/5 in the apheresis group) [14]. Many reports of other groups support the Vienna observations for a beneficial effect of peri-transplant IA treatment in presensitized kidney transplant recipients as well as in acute humoral allograft rejection, not only for kidney transplants but also for other solid organs [90–111].

Coagulation Factor Inhibitors

Coagulation factor-neutralizing inhibitors can be detected in hemophiliac patients with genetic background, but also in patients originally not having shown any signs of hemophilia before. In hemophiliac patients, antibodies develop in reaction to substitution of missing coagulation factors. In hemophilia A inhibitors develop in about 10–35% of patients whereas in hemophilia B inhibitors can be detected in about 3–5% of patients [112]. The spontaneous development of inhibitors in primarily unaffected patients is a very rare disorder with an estimated incidence rate of 0.2–1.0 annual cases per million population. Various immunosuppressive regimens have been tried without convincing results. A meta-analysis in patients with acquired hemophilia revealed a high mortality rate of 42% in patients in whom the inhibitor could not be eliminated [113]. The overall mortality rate in this analysis of 245 patients was 16%, whereby not only bleeding but also complications of cytotoxic drug therapy contributed substantially to this rate. The inhibitors usually belong to the IgG fraction of immunoglobulins and therefore can be easily eliminated by all re-usable DC-IA techniques.

Nilsson firstly described the successful application of protein A DC-IA in a patient with hemophilia B and inhibiting antibodies directed towards coagulation factor IX in 1981 [114]. Later, the so-called Malmö protocol was developed, consisting of coagulation factor replacement, immunosuppressive drugs and protein A DC-IA. Freiburghaus summarized 15 years experience of successful application of this protocol to 10 patients in 1998 [115]. Jansen et al. from the Vienna group reported on their experience with the Ig-Therasorb system in 11 patients, showing complete remission in 7 and partial remission in 1 patient [116].

A German group [117] adapted the original Malmö and Bonn protocols to the modified Bonn-Malmö protocol (MBMP) in 1996. In 2005, Zeitler et al. reported on the successful application of this protocol in 35 acquired hemophilia patients with high titers and critical bleeding [5]. The data were updated for 45 patients in 2006, confirming the original results. Using the MBMP, bleeding could be controlled immediately. Inhibitor levels decreased within a median of 3 days to undetectable levels, and long-term follow-up (mean 48 months) showed an overall response for complete remission in 91% of patients (97% without cancer patients) [118].

Although randomized controlled trials are missing, the use of DC-IA is highly recommended in these special subgroups of patients, not only because of the dramatic response to apheresis therapy but also because of superior cost effectiveness in comparison to alternative treatment options.

Autoimmune Bullous Diseases

Pemphigus and pemphigoid belong to a group of autoimmune bullous diseases of the skin and mucous membranes. Without adequate treatment, the blisters develop progressively and spread out over the body, causing debilitating disease or even fatal outcome. The standard therapy consists of corticosteroids and immunosuppressants, preferentially azathioprine, mycophenolate mofetil, cyclophosphamide and methotrexate. In patients with inadequate response, ivIg and eventually rituximab might be used.

In pemphigus, pemphigoid as well as epidermolysis bullosa acquisita there is clear evidence for a pathogenic role of autoantibodies directed towards skin structures such as desmogleins, collagen, laminin, and annexin [9, 10]. In particular, titers of antibodies directed towards desmogleins correlate with disease activity [119].

After plasma exchange treatments had revealed conflicting clinical results, the successful application of IA was reported for 2 pemphigoid patients in 1997 and 1 year later for 1 patient with paraneoplastic pemphigus [120, 121]. Several groups thereafter demonstrated impressive clinical responses using various DC-IA systems for aggressive lowering of autoantibodies as an adjunctive treatment in autoimmune bullous disease, mainly pemphigus [122–127]. Clinical improvement utilizing the Immusorba-TR column was also reported, but the effect was not as pronounced, probably due to less effective antibody elimination [128–130].

A consensus conference was held in 2005 in Hamburg, Germany, in order to develop guidelines for the use of immune apheresis treatment in bullous diseases. The recommendations of the expert panel consisting of dermatologists and apheresis experts were published by Zillikens et al. in a review article [10]. Briefly, the IA therapy is recommended for severe or drug-refractory cases, in addition to basic immunosuppressive drug medication consisting of corticosteroids and azathioprine or mycophenolate mofetil. Other combinations using cyclophosphamide or rituximab are possible. 3–4 treatments on consecutive days with DC-IA should be performed during the induction phase, followed by weekly single DC-IA treatments or repetition of the 3–4-day induction cycle in 4-week intervals, depending on disease activity during the maintenance phase.

In cases with contraindication to immunosuppressants, IA treatment should be considered as well.

SC-IA treatment is recommended by the expert panel only for selected cases.

Other Indications

In many other immune-mediated disorders (table 3) there is a rationale for the application of SIAT [16, 20, 30, 31, 33, 34, 42, 55, 131–214]. But until now, randomized controlled trials with adequate numbers of patients proving the effectiveness of SIAT therapy in a required scientific manner are still missing. For this reason, the use of SIAT outside clinical trials can only be recommended in emergency situations like myasthenic crisis, bleeding disorders, loss of visual acuity or other critical organ involvement, such as in Goodpasture's syndrome or rapidly progressive glomerulonephritis or severe central nervous involvement in SLE or other autoimmune vasculitidies.

In addition, SIAT might be considered as a preferred treatment option in situations where immunosuppressive drug treatment is contraindicated, as in pregnancy or the lactation period.

Recommendations for the Clinical Application of Selective Immunoadsorption Technologies

Intensive treatment regimens using repeated DC-IA treatments can induce rapid clinical improvement in line with aggressive elimination of (auto)antibodies and immune complexes. Due to the complexity and the initial financial burden of DC-IA systems, their application should be preferentially considered in critical organ involvement and life-threatening disease conditions as well as in circumstances in which other treatment alternatives exceed the costs of apheresis therapy.

In other immune-mediated conditions that presumably require only a few treatments, non-selective technologies or single-column systems might be considered as first choice.

Adsorptive cytapheresis systems should be preferentially considered in cases with mild to moderate disease activity allowing a delayed onset of clinical response. Because of the simple design and superior safety profile, an application in earlier disease stages should be encouraged in the future.

Table 3. Other immune-mediated disorders with suggested indication for SIAT

Immune-mediated disease / condition	Literature
Autoimmune vasculitidies / SLE	[20, 30, 31, 33, 34, 131–149]
Crohn's disease	[16, 55, 150–159]
Myasthenia gravis	[42, 160–177]
Guillain-Barré syndrome	[172, 178–183]
Chronic inflammatory demyelinating polyneuropathy	[184, 185]
Multiple sclerosis	[186–188]
Idiopathic thrombocytopenic purpura	[189–195]
Thrombotic thrombocytopenic purpura	[191, 196, 197]
Hemolytic-uremic syndrome	[198, 199]
Psoriasis	[200–203]
ABO-incompatible allogeneic hematopoietic stem cell transplantation with isoagglutinin persistence	[204, 205]
Endocrine ophthalmopathy	[206]
(Recurrent) focal segmental glomerulosclerosis	[207–214]

Approval and Reimbursement

SIAT, which mostly has been developed and introduced in Japan and Europe, still waits for adequate acceptance outside the apheresis community due to poor scientific evidence arising from inadequately planned and performed clinical trials during the last 30 years. In most circumstances, studies covered only patients in end-stage diseases who already demonstrated a very complex medical condition at study entry. In almost all controlled clinical trials, the apheresis therapy was used as an adjunct to combined drug treatment for only a relatively short period of time. These protocols did not clearly allow discriminating between the various treatment alternatives applied. For this reason, clear recommendations for the use of SIAT are still missing.

In addition, national differences concerning regulatory affairs and reimbursement guidelines have impeded the progress of apheresis therapy in a substantial way during the past by enforcing the industry to meet rather local requirements than internationally accepted standards. Under today's economic pressure, the apheresis community is facing the situation that valid scientific data will not be sufficient for the future establishment of the apheresis therapy without clearly demonstrating cost effectiveness.

Conclusions and Future Directions

Innovative strategies on a global perspective are needed for the future to convince the scientific and medical community that apheresis therapy might be a beneficial and cost-effective alternative even in earlier stages of the disease, in which more sophisticated patient selection and harmonization of study protocols could be achieved.

The scientific apheresis societies should enhance their activities in establishing national and international registries for prospective data collection on apheresis therapy as well as in international harmonization of study protocols.

Disclosure of Conflict of Interests

The authors state that they have no conflict of interests.

References

1 Emmrich J, Petermann S, Nowak D, Beutner I, Brock P, Klingel R, Mausfeld-Lafdhiya P, Liebe S, Ramlow W: Leukocytapheresis (LCAP) in the management of chronic active ulcerative colitis – results of a randomized pilot trial. Dig Dis Sci 2007;52:2044–2053.

2 Pineda AA: Developments in the apheresis procedure for the treatment of inflammatory bowel disease. Inflamm Bowel Dis 2006;12(suppl 1):S10–14.

3 Tozzoli R: Review: The diagnostic role of autoantibodies in the prediction of organ-specific autoimmune diseases. Clin Chem Lab Med 2008;46:577–587.

4 Buse C, Altmann F, Amann B, Hauck SM, Poulsen Nautrup C, Ueffing M, Stangassinger M, Deeg CA: Discovering novel targets for autoantibodies in dilated cardiomyopathy. Electrophoresis 2008;29:1325–1332.

5 Zeitler H, Ulrich-Merzenich G, Hess L, Konsek E, Unkrig C, Walger P, Vetter H, Brackmann HH: Treatment of acquired hemophilia by the Bonn-Malmo protocol: Documentation of an in vivo immunomodulating concept. Blood 2005;105:2287–2293.

6 Staudt A, Dorr M, Staudt Y, Bohm M, Probst M, Empen K, Plotz S, Maschke HE, Hummel A, Baumann G, Felix SB: Role of immunoglobulin G3 subclass in dilated cardiomyopathy: Results from protein A immunoadsorption. Am Heart J 2005;150:729–736.

7 Mobini R, Staudt A, Felix SB, Baumann G, Wallukat G, Deinum J, Svensson H, Hjalmarson A, Fu M: Hemodynamic improvement and removal of autoantibodies against beta1-adrenergic receptor by immunoadsorption therapy in dilated cardiomyopathy. J Autoimmun 2003;20:345–350.

8 Felix SB, Staudt A, Landsberger M, Grosse Y, Stangl V, Spielhagen T, Wallukat G, Wernecke KD, Baumann G, Stangl K: Removal of cardiodepressant antibodies in dilated cardiomyopathy by immunoadsorption. J Am Coll Cardiol 2002;39:646–652.

9 Shimanovich I, Nitschke M, Rose C, Grabbe J, Zillikens D: Treatment of severe pemphigus with protein A immunoadsorption, rituximab and intravenous immunoglobulins. Br J Dermatol 2008;158:382–388.

10 Zillikens D, Derfler K, Eming R, Fierlbeck G, Goebeler M, Hertl M, Hofmann SC, Karlhofer F, Kautz O, Nitschke M, Opitz A, Quist S, Rose C, Schanz S, Schmidt E, Shimanovich I, Michael M, Ziller F: Recommendations for the use of immunoapheresis in the treatment of autoimmune bullous diseases. J Dtsch Dermatol Ges 2007;5:881–887.

11 Tyden G, Donauer J, Wadstrom J, Kumlien G, Wilpert J, Nilsson T, Genberg H, Pisarski P, Tufveson G: Implementation of a protocol for ABO-incompatible kidney transplantation – a three-center experience with 60 consecutive transplantations. Transplantation 2007;83:1153–1155.

12 Tyden G, Kumlien G, Efvergren M: Present techniques for antibody removal. Transplantation 2007;84:S27–29.

13 Bohmig GA, Regele H, Exner M, Derhartunian V, Kletzmayr J, Saemann MD, Horl WH, Druml W, Watschinger B: C4d-positive acute humoral renal allograft rejection: Effective treatment by immunoadsorption. J Am Soc Nephrol 2001;12:2482–2489.

14 Bohmig GA, Wahrmann M, Regele H, Exner M, Robl B, Derfler K, Soliman T, Bauer P, Mullner M, Druml W: Immunoadsorption in severe C4d-positive acute kidney allograft rejection: A randomized controlled trial. Am J Transplant 2007;7:117–121.

15 Waitz G, Petermann S, Liebe S, Emmrich J, Ramlow W: Reduction of dendritic cells by granulocyte and monocyte adsorption apheresis in patients with ulcerative colitis. Dig Dis Sci 2008, DOI: 10.1007/s10620-007-0168-8.

16 Fukunaga K, Miwa H, Matsumoto T: Role of leukocytapheresis in the management of inflammatory bowel disease. Trop Gastroenterol 2007;28:11–15.

17 Yamamoto T, Umegae S, Matsumoto K: Safety and clinical efficacy of granulocyte and monocyte adsorptive apheresis therapy for ulcerative colitis. World J Gastroenterol 2006;12:520–525.

18 Yamamoto T, Saniabadi AR, Umegae S, Matsumoto K: Impact of selective leukocytapheresis on mucosal inflammation and ulcerative colitis: Cytokine profiles and endoscopic findings. Inflamm Bowel Dis 2006;12:719–726.

19 Suzuki Y, Yoshimura N, Fukuda K, Shirai K, Saito Y, Saniabadi AR: A retrospective search for predictors of clinical response to selective granulocyte and monocyte apheresis in patients with ulcerative colitis. Dig Dis Sci 2006;51:2031–2038.

20 Soerensen H, Schneidewind-Mueller JM, Lange D, Kashiwagi N, Franz M, Yokoyama T, Ramlow W: Pilot clinical study of Adacolumn cytapheresis in patients with systemic lupus erythematosus. Rheumatol Int 2006;26:409–415.

21 Hanai H: Positions of selective leukocytapheresis in the medical therapy of ulcerative colitis. World J Gastroenterol 2006;12:7568–7577.

22 Fukunaga K, Fukuda Y, Yokoyama Y, Ohnishi K, Kusaka T, Kosaka T, Hida N, Ohda Y, Miwa H, Matsumoto T: Activated platelets as a possible early marker to predict clinical efficacy of leukocytapheresis in severe ulcerative colitis patients. J Gastroenterol 2006;41:524–532.

23 Sawada K, Egashira A, Ohnishi K, Fukunaga K, Kusaka T, Shimoyama T: Leukocytapheresis (LCAP) for management of fulminant ulcerative colitis with toxic megacolon. Dig Dis Sci 2005;50:767–773.

24 Andoh A, Tsujikawa T, Inatomi O, Deguchi Y, Sasaki M, Obata H, Mitsuyama K, Fujiyama Y: Leukocytapheresis therapy modulates circulating T cell subsets in patients with ulcerative colitis. Ther Apher Dial 2005;9:270–276.

25 Hasegawa M, Ohashi A, Kabutan N, Hiramatsu S, Kato M, Murakami K, Tomita M, Nabeshima K, Hiki Y, Sugiyama S: Cytapheresis for the treatment of myeloperoxidase antineutrophil cytoplasmic autoantibody-associated vasculitis: A pilot study of 21 patients. Ther Apher Dial 2006;10:412–418.

26 Sanmarti R, Marsal S, Valverde J, Casado E, Lafuente R, Kashiwagi N, Rodriguez-Cros JR, Erra A, Reina D, Gratacos J: Adsorptive granulocyte/monocyte apheresis for the treatment of refractory rheumatoid arthritis: An open pilot multicentre trial. Rheumatology 2005;44:1140–1144.

27 Hidaka T, Suzuki K: Leukocytapheresis for rheumatic disease. Ther Apher Dial 2003;7:161–164.

28 Ueki Y, Yamasaki S, Kanamoto Y, Kawazu T, Yano M, Matsumoto K, Miyake S, Tominaga Y, Iwamoto U, Suemitsu J, Matsuno Y, Sizume Y, Takenaka Y, Eguchi K: Evaluation of filtration leucocytapheresis for use in the treatment of patients with rheumatoid arthritis. Rheumatology 2000;39:165–171.

29 Hidaka T, Suzuki K, Matsuki Y, Takamizawa-Matsumoto M, Kataharada K, Ishizuka T, Kawakami M, Nakamura H: Filtration leukocytapheresis therapy in rheumatoid arthritis: A randomized, double-blind, placebo-controlled trial. Arthritis Rheum 1999;42:431–437.

30 Braun N, Erley C, Klein R, Kotter I, Saal J, Risler T: Immunoadsorption onto protein A induces remission in severe systemic lupus erythematosus. Nephrol Dial Transplant 2000;15:1367–1372.

31 Braun N, Junger M, Klein R, Gutenberger S, Guagnin M, Risler T: Dextran sulfate (Selesorb) plasma apheresis improves vascular changes in systemic lupus erythematosus. Ther Apher 2002;6:471–477.

32 Felson DT, LaValley MP, Baldassare AR, Block JA, Caldwell JR, Cannon GW, Deal C, Evans S, Fleischmann R, Gendreau RM, Harris ER, Matteson EL, Roth SH, Schumacher HR, Weisman MH, Furst DE: The Prosorba column for treatment of refractory rheumatoid arthritis: A randomized, double-blind, sham-controlled trial. Arthritis Rheum 1999;42:2153–2159.

33 Stummvoll GH, Aringer M, Smolen JS, Schmaldienst S, Jimenez-Boj E, Horl WH, Graninger WB, Derfler K: IgG immunoadsorption reduces systemic lupus erythematosus activity and proteinuria: A long term observational study. Ann Rheum Dis 2005;64:1015–1021.

34 Suzuki K: The role of immunoadsorption using dextran-sulfate cellulose columns in the treatment of systemic lupus erythematosus. Ther Apher 2000;4:239–243.

35 Caldwell J, Gendreau RM, Furst D, Wiesenhutter C, Quagliata F, Spindler J, Bertram J: A pilot study using a staph protein A column (Prosorba) to treat refractory rheumatoid arthritis. J Rheumatol 1999;26:1657–1662.

36 Fujimori J, Yoshino S, Koiwa M, Hirai H, Shiga H, Hayama N, Iino Y: Improvement in rheumatoid arthritis following application of an extracorporeal granulotrap column, G-1. Rheumatol Int 1996;15:175–180.

37 Lazarus HM, Cohen SB, Clegg DO, Menitove JE, Sorin SB, Hinkle S, Markenson JA, Saal S, Goodnough LT, Fleischmann RM: Selective in vivo removal of rheumatoid factor by an extracorporeal treatment device in rheumatoid arthritis patients. Transfusion 1991;31:122–128.

38 Nagashima M, Yoshino S, Tanaka H, Yoshida N, Kashiwagi N, Saniabadi AR: Granulocyte and monocyte apheresis suppresses symptoms of rheumatoid arthritis: A pilot study. Rheumatol Int 1998;18:113–118.

39 Ohara M, Saniabadi AR, Kokuma S, Hirata I, Adachi M, Agishi T, Kasukawa R: Granulocytapheresis in the treatment of patients with rheumatoid arthritis. Artif Organs 1997;21:989–994.

40 Takahashi K, Yoshinoya S, Yoshizawa H, Miyamoto T: Extracorporeal hydrophobic amino acid adsorbent therapy in rheumatoid arthritis. Clin Rheumatol 1987;6:553–563.

41 Wiesenhutter CW, Irish BL, Bertram JH: Treatment of patients with refractory rheumatoid arthritis with extracorporeal protein A immunoadsorption columns: A pilot trial. J Rheumatol 1994;21:804–812.

42 Yamazaki Z, Idezuki Y, Inoue N, Yoshizawa H, Yamawaki N, Inagaki K, Tsuda N: Extracorporeal immunoadsorption with IM-PH or IM-TR column. Biomater Artif Cells Artif Organs 1989;17:117–124.

43 Kashiwagi N, Hirata I, Kasukawa R: A role for granulocyte and monocyte apheresis in the treatment of rheumatoid arthritis. Ther Apher 1998;2:134–141.

44 Scroggie D, Harris MD, Abel M, Sakai L, Arroyo R: Vasculitis following treatment of rheumatoid arthritis with extracorporeal staphylococcal protein A immunoadsorption column (Prosorba). J Clin Rheumatol 2001;7:238–241.

45 Deodhar A, Allen E, Daoud K, Wahba I: Vasculitis secondary to staphylococcal protein A immunoadsorption (Prosorba column) treatment in rheumatoid arthritis. Semin Arthritis Rheum 2002;32:3–9.

46 Iglesias J, D'Agati VD, Levine JS: Acute glomerulonephritis occurring during immunoadsorption with staphylococcal protein A column (Prosorba). Nephrol Dial Transplant 2004;19:3155–3159.

47 Ueki Y, Eguchi K: [Leukocytapheresis for therapy of rheumatoid arthritis]. Nippon Rinsho 2005;63(suppl 1):649–652.

48 Watanabe M, Kubota D, Nagahori M, Kanai T: Treatment of inflammatory immunologic disease. 1. Leukocytapheresis for inflammatory immunologic disease (tentative). Intern Med 2007;46:1305–1306.

49 Hanai H, Iida T, Yamada M, Sato Y, Takeuchi K, Tanaka T, Kondo K, Kikuyama M, Maruyama Y, Iwaoka Y, Nakamura A, Hirayama K, Saniabadi AR, Watanabe F: Effects of Adacolumn selective leukocytapheresis on plasma cytokines during active disease in patients with active ulcerative colitis. World J Gastroenterol 2006;12:3393–3399.

50 Sawada K, Muto T, Shimoyama T, Satomi M, Sawada T, Nagawa H, Hiwatashi N, Asakura H, Hibi T: Multicenter randomized controlled trial for the treatment of ulcerative colitis with a leukocytapheresis column. Curr Pharm Des 2003;9:307–321.

51 Shimoyama T, Sawada K, Hiwatashi N, Sawada T, Matsueda K, Munakata A, Asakura H, Tanaka T, Kasukawa R, Kimura K, Suzuki Y, Nagamachi Y, Muto T, Nagawa H, Iizuka B, Baba S, Nasu M, Kataoka T, Kashiwagi N, Saniabadi AR: Safety and efficacy of granulocyte and monocyte adsorption apheresis in patients with active ulcerative colitis: A multicenter study. J Clin Apher 2001;16:1–9.

52 Shimoyama T, Sawada Y, Onishi K, Egashira A, Kaneda M, Hida N, Fukunaga K, Tomita T, Satomi M: [Leukocyte adsorption and removal for the treatment of ulcerative colitis]. Nihon Naika Gakkai zasshi 1999;88:724–730.

53 Suzuki Y, Yoshimura N, Saniabadi AR, Saito Y: Selective granulocyte and monocyte adsorptive apheresis as a first-line treatment for steroid naive patients with active ulcerative colitis: A prospective uncontrolled study. Dig Dis Sci 2004;49:565–571.

54 Ricart E, Esteve M, Andreu M, Casellas F, Monfort D, Sans M, Oudovenko N, Lafuente R, Panes J: Evaluation of 5 versus 10 granulocyteapheresis sessions in steroid-dependent ulcerative colitis: A pilot, prospective, multicenter, randomized study. World J Gastroenterol 2007;13:2193–2197.

55 Ljung T, Thomsen OO, Vatn M, Karlen P, Karlsen LN, Tysk C, Nilsson SU, Kilander A, Gillberg R, Grip O, Lindgren S, Befrits R, Lofberg R: Granulocyte, monocyte/macrophage apheresis for inflammatory bowel disease: The first 100 patients treated in Scandinavia. Scand J Gastroenterol 2007;42:221–227.

56 Hanai H, Watanabe F, Yamada M, Sato Y, Takeuchi K, Iida T, Tozawa K, Tanaka T, Maruyama Y, Matsushita I, Iwaoka Y, Kikuch K, Saniabadi AR: Adsorptive granulocyte and monocyte apheresis versus prednisolone in patients with corticosteroid-dependent moderately severe ulcerative colitis. Digestion 2004;70:36–44.

57 Tozzoli R: Recent advances in diagnostic technologies and their impact in autoimmune diseases. Autoimmun Rev 2007;6:334–340.

58 Takahashi R, Asai T, Murakami H, Murakami R, Tsuzuki M, Numaguchi Y, Matsui H, Murohara T, Okumura K: Pressure overload-induced cardiomyopathy in heterozygous carrier mice of carnitine transporter gene mutation. Hypertension 2007;50:497–502.

59 Jahns R, Boivin V, Hein L, Triebel S, Angermann CE, Ertl G, Lohse MJ: Direct evidence for a beta 1-adrenergic receptor-directed autoimmune attack as a cause of idiopathic dilated cardiomyopathy. J Clin Invest 2004;113:1419–1429.

60 Chen J, Larsson L, Haugen E, Fedorkova O, Angwald E, Waagstein F, Fu M: Effects of autoantibodies removed by immunoadsorption from patients with dilated cardiomyopathy on neonatal rat cardiomyocytes. Eur J Heart Fail 2006;8:460–467.

61 Buvall L, Tang MS, Isic A, Andersson B, Fu M: Antibodies against the beta1-adrenergic receptor induce progressive development of cardiomyopathy. J Mol Cell Cardiol 2007;42:1001–1007.

62 Caforio AL, Tona F, Bottaro S, Vinci A, Dequal G, Daliento L, Thiene G, Iliceto S: Clinical implications of anti-heart autoantibodies in myocarditis and dilated cardiomyopathy. Autoimmunity 2008;41:35–45.

63 Wallukat G, Reinke P, Dorffel WV, Luther HP, Bestvater K, Felix SB, Baumann G: Removal of autoantibodies in dilated cardiomyopathy by immunoadsorption. Int J Cardiol 1996;54:191–195.

64 Muller J, Wallukat G, Dandel M, Bieda H, Brandes K, Spiegelsberger S, Nissen E, Kunze R, Hetzer R: Immunoglobulin adsorption in patients with idiopathic dilated cardiomyopathy. Circulation 2000;101:385–391.

65 Felix SB, Staudt A, Dorffel WV, Stangl V, Merkel K, Pohl M, Docke WD, Morgera S, Neumayer HH, Wernecke KD, Wallukat G, Stangl K, Baumann G: Hemodynamic effects of immunoadsorption and subsequent immunoglobulin substitution in dilated cardiomyopathy: Three-month results from a randomized study. J Am Coll Cardiol 2000;35:1590–1598.

66 Staudt A, Bohm M, Knebel F, Grosse Y, Bischoff C, Hummel A, Dahm JB, Borges A, Jochmann N, Wernecke KD, Wallukat G, Baumann G, Felix SB: Potential role of autoantibodies belonging to the immunoglobulin G-3 subclass in cardiac dysfunction among patients with dilated cardiomyopathy. Circulation 2002;106:2448–2453.

67 Burgstaler EA, Cooper LT, Winters JL: Treatment of chronic dilated cardiomyopathy with immunoadsorption using the staphylococcal A-agarose column: A comparison of immunoglobulin reduction using two different techniques. J Clin Apher 2007;22:224–232.

68 Cooper LT, Belohlavek M, Korinek J, Yoshifuku S, Sengupta PP, Burgstaler EA, Winters JL: A pilot study to assess the use of protein A immunoadsorption for chronic dilated cardiomyopathy. J Clin Apher 2007;22:210–214.

69 Dorffel WV, Wallukat G, Dorffel Y, Felix SB, Baumann G: Immunoadsorption in idiopathic dilated cardiomyopathy, a 3-year follow-up. Int J Cardiol 2004;97:529–534.

70 Knebel F, Bohm M, Staudt A, Borges AC, Tepper M, Jochmann N, Wernicke KD, Felix S, Baumann G: Reduction of morbidity by immunoadsorption therapy in patients with dilated cardiomyopathy. Int J Cardiol 2004;97:517–520.

71 Tanabe K: Japanese experience of ABO-incompatible living kidney transplantation. Transplantation 2007;84:S4–7.

72 Takahashi K, Saito K: Present status of ABO-incompatible kidney transplantation in Japan. Xenotransplantation 2006;13:118–122.

73 Tyden G, Kumlien G, Fehrman I: Successful ABO-incompatible kidney transplantations without splenectomy using antigen-specific immunoadsorption and rituximab. Transplantation 2003;76:730–731.

74 Rydberg L, Bengtsson A, Samuelsson O, Nilsson K, Breimer ME: In vitro assessment of a new ABO immunosorbent with synthetic carbohydrates attached to sepharose. Transpl Int 2005;17:666–672.

75 Tyden G: The European experience. Transplantation 2007;84:S2–3.

76 Norden G, Briggs D, Cockwell P, Lipkin G, Mjornstedt L, Molne J, Ready A, Rydberg L, Samuelsson O, Svalander CT, Breimer ME: ABO-incompatible live donor renal transplantation using blood group A/B carbohydrate antigen immunoadsorption and anti-CD20 antibody treatment. Xenotransplantation 2006;13:148–153.

77 Donauer J, Wilpert J, Geyer M, Schwertfeger E, Kirste G, Drognitz O, Walz G, Pisarski P: ABO-incompatible kidney transplantation using antigen-specific immunoadsorption and rituximab: A single center experience. Xenotransplantation 2006;13:108–110.

78 Beimler J, Zeier M: ABO-incompatible transplantation – a safe way to perform renal transplantation? Nephrol Dial Transplant 2007;22:25–27.

79 Wilpert J, Geyer M, Teschner S, Schaefer T, Pisarski P, Schulz-Huotari C, Gropp A, Wisniewski U, Goebel H, Gerke P, Walz G, Donauer J: ABO-incompatible kidney transplantation – proposal of an intensified apheresis strategy for patients with high initial isoagglutinine titers. J Clin Apher 2007;22:314–322.

80 Wilpert J, Geyer M, Pisarski P, Drognitz O, Schulz-Huotari C, Gropp A, Goebel H, Gerke P, Teschner S, Walz G, Donauer J: On-demand strategy as an alternative to conventionally scheduled post-transplant immunoadsorptions after ABO-incompatible kidney transplantation. Nephrol Dial Transplant 2007;22:3048–3051.

81 Geyer M, Donauer J, Pisarski P, Drognitz O, Schulz-Huotari C, Wisniewski U, Gropp A, Gobel H, Gerke P, Teschner S, Walz G, Wilpert J: Preemptive postoperative antigen-specific immunoadsorption in ABO-incompatible kidney transplantation: Necessary or not? Transplantation 2007;84:S40–43.

82 Pierson RN, 3rd, Loyd JE, Goodwin A, Majors D, Dummer JS, Mohacsi P, Wheeler A, Bovin N, Miller GG, Olson S, Johnson J, Rieben R, Azimzadeh A: Successful management of an ABO-mismatched lung allograft using antigen-specific immunoadsorption, complement inhibition, and immunomodulatory therapy. Transplantation 2002;74:79–84.

83 Banner NR, Rose ML, Cummins D, de Silva M, Pottle A, Lyster H, Doyle P, Carby M, Khaghani A: Management of an ABO-incompatible lung transplant. Am J Transplant 2004;4:1192–1196.

84 Bucin D, Johansson S, Malm T, Jogi P, Johansson J, Westrin P, Lindberg LO, Olsson AK, Gelberg J, Peres V, Harling S, Bennhagen R, Kornhall B, Ekmehag B, Kurkus J, Otto G: Heart transplantation across the antibodies against HLA and ABO. Transpl Int 2006;19:239–244.

85 Troisi R, Noens L, Montalti R, Ricciardi S, Philippe J, Praet M, Conoscitore P, Centra M, de Hemptinne B: ABO-mismatch adult living donor liver transplantation using antigen-specific immunoadsorption and quadruple immunosuppression without splenectomy. Liver Transpl 2006;12:1412–1417.

86 Boberg KM, Foss A, Midtvedt K, Schrumpf E: ABO-incompatible deceased donor liver transplantation with the use of antigen-specific immunoadsorption and anti-CD20 monoclonal antibody. Clin Transplant 2006;20:265–268.

87 Bohmig GA, Regele H, Saemann MD, Exner M, Druml W, Kovarik J, Horl WH, Zlabinger GJ, Watschinger B: Role of humoral immune reactions as target for antirejection therapy in recipients of a spousal-donor kidney graft. Am J Kidney Dis 2000;35:667–673.

88 Lorenz M, Regele H, Schillinger M, Kletzmayr J, Haidbauer B, Derfler K, Druml W, Bohmig GA: Peritransplant immunoadsorption: A strategy enabling transplantation in highly sensitized crossmatch-positive cadaveric kidney allograft recipients. Transplantation 2005;79:696–701.

89 Haas M, Bohmig GA, Leko-Mohr Z, Exner M, Regele H, Derfler K, Horl WH, Druml W: Peri-operative immunoadsorption in sensitized renal transplant recipients. Nephrol Dial Transplant 2002;17:1503–1508.

90 Schneidewind J, Gliesche T, Sehland D, Ramlow W, Wolfsdorff B, Bast R, Wegener S, Decker S, Schmidt R: [Protein A immunoadsorption as a new apheresis procedure for elimination of HLA antibodies]. Beitr Infusionsther Transfusionsmed 1994;32:360–365.

91 Braun N, Wernet D, Schnaidt M, Bevan DJ, Viebahn R, Risler T: Successful treatment of accelerated vascular rejection in a highly immunised renal transplant recipient with immunoadsorption and 15-deoxyspergualin. Transpl Int 2004;17:384–386.

92 Mastrangelo F, Pretagostini R, Berloco P, Poli L, Cinti P, Patruno P, Alfonso L, Pompei L, Carboni F, Rizzelli S, Alfani D, Cortesini R: Immunoadsorption with protein A in humoral acute rejection of kidney transplants: Multicenter experience. Transplant Proc 1995;27:892–895.

93 Persson NH, Bucin D, Ekberg H, Kallen R, Omnell Persson M, Simanaitis M, Sterner G, Swedenborg P: Immunoadsorption in acute vascular rejection after renal transplantation. Transplant Proc 1995;27:3466.

94 Reisaeter AV, Leivestad T, Albrechtsen D, Holdaas H, Hartmann A, Sodal G, Flatmark A, Fauchald P: Pretransplant plasma exchange or immunoadsorption facilitates renal transplantation in immunized patients. Transplantation 1995;60:242–248.

95 Higgins RM, Bevan DJ, Carey BS, Lea CK, Fallon M, Buhler R, Vaughan RW, O'Donnell PJ, Snowden SA, Bewick M, Hendry BM: Prevention of hyperacute rejection by removal of antibodies to HLA immediately before renal transplantation. Lancet 1996;348:1208–1211.

96 Higgins RM, Bevan DJ, Vaughan RW, Phillips AO, Snowden S, Bewick M, Scoble JE, Hendry BM: 5-year follow-up of patients successfully transplanted after immunoadsorption to remove anti-HLA antibodies. Nephron 1996;74:53–57.

97 Hickstein H, Korten G, Bast R, Barz D, Templin R, Schneidewind JM, Kittner C, Nizze H, Schmidt R: Protein A immunoadsorption (IA) in renal transplantation patients with vascular rejection. Transfus Sci 1998;19(suppl):53–57.

98 Hickstein H, Korten G, Bast R, Barz D, Nizze H, Schmidt R: Immunoadsorption of sensitized kidney transplant candidates immediately prior to surgery. Clin Transplant 2002;16:97–101.

99 Tschernia A, LeLeiko NS, Grima K, Whittset C, Molnar K, Spencer RW, Sloves MF, Gondolesi G, Kaufman SS, Fishbein TM: Anti-HLA antibody removal by extracorporeal immunoadsorption in two hyperimmunized pediatric patients awaiting hepatointestinal transplantation. Transplant Proc 2002;34:900–901.

100 Appel JZ, 3rd, Hartwig MG, Davis RD, Reinsmoen NL: Utility of peritransplant and rescue intravenous immunoglobulin and extracorporeal immunoadsorption in lung transplant recipients sensitized to HLA antigens. Hum Immunol 2005;66:378–386.

101 Ji SM, Liu ZH, Chen JS, Sha GZ, Ji DX, Li LS: Rescue therapy by immunoadsorption in combination with tacrolimus and mycophenolate mofetil for C4d-positive acute humoral renal allograft rejection. Transplant Proc 2006;38:3459–3463.

102 Palmer A, Taube D, Welsh K, Brynger H, Delin K, Gjorstrup P, Konar J, Soderstrom T: Extracorporeal immunoadsorption of anti-HLA antibodies: Preliminary clinical experience. Transplant Proc 1987;19:3750–3751.

103 Brocard JF, Farahmand H, Fassi S, Plaisant B, Fries E, Cantarovich M, Bismuth A, Lambert T, Hiesse C, Lantz O, Fries D, Charpenter B: Attempt at depletion of anti-HLA antibodies in sensitized patients awaiting transplantation using extracorporeal immunoadsorption, polyclonal IgG, and immunosuppressive drugs. Transplant Proc 1989;21:733–734.

104 Palmer A, Taube D, Welsh K, Bewick M, Gjorstrup P, Thick M: Removal of anti-HLA antibodies by extracorporeal immunoadsorption to enable renal transplantation. Lancet 1989;1:10–12.

105 Hakim RM, Milford E, Himmelfarb J, Wingard R, Lazarus JM, Watt RM: Extracorporeal removal of anti-HLA antibodies in transplant candidates. Am J Kidney Dis 1990;16:423–431.

106 Wingard RL: Immunoadsorption: A novel treatment for sensitized kidney transplant candidates. ANNA J 1990;17:288–294,328.

107 Alarabi AA, Wikstrom B, Backman U, Danielson BG, Tufvesson G, Sjoberg O: Pretransplantation immunoadsorption therapy in patients immunized with human lymphocyte antigen: Effect of treatment and three years' clinical follow-up of grafts. Artif Organs 1993;17:702–707.

108 Olivari MT, May CB, Johnson NA, Ring WS, Stephens MK: Treatment of acute vascular rejection with immunoadsorption. Circulation 1994;90: II70–73.

109 Kriaa F, Laurian Y, Hiesse C, Tchernia G, Charpentier B: Five years' experience at one centre with protein A immunoadsorption in patients with deleterious allo/autoantibodies (anti-HLA antibodies, autoimmune bleeding disorders) and post-transplant patients relapsing with focal glomerular sclerosis. Nephrol Dial Transplant 1995;10(suppl 6):108–110.

110 Kaczmarek I, Deutsch MA, Sadoni S, Brenner P, Schmauss D, Daebritz SH, Weiss M, Meiser BM, Reichart B: Successful management of antibody-mediated cardiac allograft rejection with combined immunoadsorption and anti-CD20 monoclonal antibody treatment: Case report and literature review. J Heart Lung Transplant 2007;26:511–515.

111 Koller H, Steurer W, Mark W, Margreiter R, Lhotta K, Mayer G, Rosenkranz AR: Clearance of C4d deposition after successful treatment of acute humoral rejection in follow-up biopsies: A report of three cases. Transpl Int 2004;17:177–181.

112 Freedman J, Garvey MB: Immunoadsorption of factor VIII inhibitors. Curr Opin Hematol 2004;11:327–333.

113 Delgado J, Jimenez-Yuste V, Hernandez-Navarro F, Villar A: Acquired haemophilia: Review and meta-analysis focused on therapy and prognostic factors. Br J Haematol 2003;121:21–35.

114 Nilsson IM, Jonsson S, Sundqvist SB, Ahlberg A, Bergentz SE: A procedure for removing high titer antibodies by extracorporeal protein-A-sepharose adsorption in hemophilia: Substitution therapy and surgery in a patient with hemophilia B and antibodies. Blood 1981;58:38–44.

115 Freiburghaus C, Berntorp E, Ekman M, Gunnarsson M, Kjellberg BM, Nilsson IM: Immunoadsorption for removal of inhibitors: Update on treatments in Malmo-Lund between 1980 and 1995. Haemophilia 1998;4:16–20.

116 Jansen M, Schmaldienst S, Banyai S, Quehenberger P, Pabinger I, Derfler K, Horl WH, Knobl P: Treatment of coagulation inhibitors with extracorporeal immunoadsorption (Ig-Therasorb). Br J Haematol 2001;112:91–97.

117 Brackmann HH, Oldenburg J, Schwaab R: Immune tolerance for the treatment of factor VIII inhibitors – twenty years ,Bonn protocol'. Vox Sang 1996;70(suppl 1):30–35.

118 Zeitler H, Ulrich-Merzenich G, Walger P, Dusing R, Vetter H, Brackmann HH: [The modified Bonn Malmo protocol (MBMP) in the treatment of acquired haemophilia A]. Dtsch Med Wochenschr 2006;131:141–147.

119 Eming R, Hertl M: Immunoadsorption in pemphigus. Autoimmunity 2006;39:609–616.

120 Schoen H, Foedinger D, Derfler K, Amann G, Rappersberger K, Stingl G, Volc-Platzer B: Immunoapheresis in paraneoplastic pemphigus. Arch Dermatol 1998;134:706–710.

121 Ino N, Kamata N, Matsuura C, Shinkai H, Odaka M: Immunoadsorption for the treatment of bullous pemphigoid. Ther Apher 1997;1:372–376.

122 Wohrl S, Geusau A, Karlhofer F, Derfler K, Stingl G, Zillikens D: Pemphigoid gestationis: Treatment with immunoapheresis. J Dtsch Dermatol Ges 2003;1:126–130.

123 Schmidt E, Klinker E, Opitz A, Herzog S, Sitaru C, Goebeler M, Mansouri Taleghoni B, Brocker EB, Zillikens D: Protein A immunoadsorption: A novel and effective adjuvant treatment of severe pemphigus. Br J Dermatol 2003;148:1222–1229.

124 Frost N, Messer G, Fierlbeck G, Risler T, Lytton SD: Treatment of pemphigus vulgaris with protein A immunoadsorption: Case report of long-term history showing favorable outcome. Ann N Y Acad Sci 2005;1051:591–596.

125 Eming R, Rech J, Barth S, Kalden JR, Schuler G, Harrer T, Hertl M: Prolonged clinical remission of patients with severe pemphigus upon rapid removal of desmoglein-reactive autoantibodies by immunoadsorption. Dermatology 2006;212:177–187.

126 Shimanovich I, Herzog S, Schmidt E, Opitz A, Klinker E, Brocker EB, Goebeler M, Zillikens D: Improved protocol for treatment of pemphigus vulgaris with protein A immunoadsorption. Clin Exp Dermatol 2006;31:768–774.

127 Niedermeier A, Eming R, Pfutze M, Neumann CR, Happel C, Reich K, Hertl M: Clinical response of severe mechanobullous epidermolysis bullosa acquisita to combined treatment with immunoadsorption and rituximab (anti-CD20 monoclonal antibodies). Arch Dermatol 2007;143:192–198.

128 Herrero-Gonzalez JE, Sitaru C, Klinker E, Brocker EB, Zillikens D: Successful adjuvant treatment of severe bullous pemphigoid by tryptophan immunoadsorption. Clin Exp Dermatol 2005;30:519–522.

129 Luftl M, Stauber A, Mainka A, Klingel R, Schuler G, Hertl M: Successful removal of pathogenic autoantibodies in pemphigus by immunoadsorption with a tryptophan-linked polyvinylalcohol adsorber. Br J Dermatol 2003;149:598–605.

130 Ogata K, Yasuda K, Matsushita M, Kodama H: Successful treatment of adolescent pemphigus vulgaris by immunoadsorption method. J Dermatol 1999;26:236–239.

131 Laczika K, Knapp S, Derfler K, Soleiman A, Horl WH, Druml W: Immunoadsorption in Goodpasture's syndrome. Am J Kidney Dis 2000;36:392–395.

132 Graninger M, Schmaldienst S, Derfler K, Graninger WB: Immunoadsorption therapy (Therasorb) in patients with severe lupus erythematosus. Acta Med Austriaca 2002;29:26–29.

133 Stummvoll GH, Aringer M, Jansen M, Smolen JS, Derfler K, Graninger WB: Immunoadsorption (IAS) as a rescue therapy in SLE: Considerations on safety and efficacy. Wien Klin Wochenschr 2004;116:716–724.

134 Stegmayr BG, Almroth G, Berlin G, Fehrman I, Kurkus J, Norda R, Olander R, Sterner G, Thysell H, Wikstrom B, Wiren JE: Plasma exchange or immunoadsorption in patients with rapidly progressive crescentic glomerulonephritis. A Swedish multicenter study. Int J Artif Organs 1999;22:81–87.

135 Suzuki K, Hara M, Harigai M, Ishizuka T, Hirose T, Matsuki Y, Kawaguchi Y, Kitani A, Kawagoe M, Nakamura H: Continuous removal of anti-DNA antibody, using a new extracorporeal immunoadsorption system, in patients with systemic lupus erythematosus. Arthritis Rheum 1991;34:1546–1552.

136 Suzuki K, Matsuki Y, Hidaka T, Ishizuka T, Kawakami M, Takata S, Kutsuki H, Nakamura H: Anti-DNA antibody kinetics following selective removal by adsorption using dextran sulphate cellulose columns in patients with systemic lupus erythematosus. J Clin Apher 1996;11:16–22.

137 Gaubitz M, Seidel M, Kummer S, Schotte H, Perniok A, Domschke W, Schneider M: Prospective randomized trial of two different immunoadsorbers in severe systemic lupus erythematosus. J Autoimmun 1998;11:495–501.

138 Funauchi M, Ikoma S, Imada A, Kanamaru A: Combination of immunoadsorption therapy and high-dose methylprednisolone in patients with lupus nephritis; possible indications in patients with early stage. J Clin Lab Immunol 1997;49:47–57.

139 Matsuki Y, Suzuki K, Kawakami M, Ishizuka T, Kawaguchi Y, Hidaka T, Nakamura H: High-avidity anti-DNA antibody removal from the serum of systemic lupus erythematosus patients by adsorption using dextran sulfate cellulose columns. J Clin Apher 1996;11:30–35.

140 Suzuki K, Hara M, Ishizuka T, Hirose T, Harigai M, Kitani K, Kawagoe M, Nakamura H: Continuous anti-dsDNA antibody apheresis in systemic lupus erythematosus. Lancet 1990;336:753–754.

141 Hu W, Liu Z, Ji D, Xie H, Gong D, Li L: Staphylococcal protein A immunoadsorption for Goodpasture's syndrome in four chinese patients. J Nephrol 2006;19:312–317.

142 Hasegawa M, Kawamura N, Kasugai M, Koide S, Murase M, Asano S, Toba T, Kushimoto H, Murakami K, Tomita M, Shikano M, Sugiyama S: Cytapheresis for the treatment of myeloperoxidase antineutrophil cytoplasmic antibody-associated vasculitis: Report of five cases. Ther Apher 2002;6:443–449.

143 Hasegawa M, Kawamura N, Murase M, Koide S, Kushimoto H, Murakami K, Tomita M, Hiki Y, Shikano M, Sugiyama S: Efficacy of granulocytapheresis and leukocytapheresis for the treatment of microscopic polyangiitis. Ther Apher Dial 2004;8:212–216.

144 Hasegawa M, Watanabe A, Takahashi H, Takahashi K, Kasugai M, Kawamura N, Kushimoto H, Murakami K, Tomita M, Nabeshima K, Oohashi A, Kondou F, Ooshima H, Hiki Y, Sugiyama S: Treatment with cytapheresis for antineutrophil cytoplasmic antibody-associated renal vasculitis and its effect on anti-inflammatory factors. Ther Apher Dial 2005;9:297–302.

145 Yamagata K, Hirayama K, Mase K, Yamaguchi N, Kobayashi M, Takahashi H, Koyama A: Apheresis for MPO-ANCA-associated RPGN-indications and efficacy: Lessons learned from Japan nationwide survey of RPGN. J Clin Apher 2005;20:244–251.

146 Hotta O, Ishida A, Kimura T, Taguma Y: Improvements in treatment strategies for patients with antineutrophil cytoplasmic antibody-associated rapidly progressive glomerulonephritis. Ther Apher Dial 2006;10:390–395.

147 Matic G, Michelsen A, Hofmann D, Winkler R, Tiess M, Schneidewind JM, Muller W, Ramlow W: Three cases of C-ANCA-positive vasculitis treated with immunoadsorption: Possible benefit in early treatment. Ther Apher 2001;5:68–72.

148 Palmer A, Cairns T, Dische F, Gluck G, Gjorstrup P, Parsons V, Welsh K, Taube D: Treatment of rapidly progressive glomerulonephritis by extracorporeal immunoadsorption, prednisolone and cyclophosphamide. Nephrol Dial Transplant 1991;6:536–542.

149 Harscher S, Rummler S, Oelzner P, Mentzel HJ, Brodhun M, Witte OW, Terborg C, Isenmann S: [Selective immunoadsorption in neurologic complications of systemic lupus erythematosus]. Nervenarzt 2007;78:441–444.

150 Sawada K, Ohnishi K, Kosaka T, Fukui S, Yamamura M, Amano K, Satomi M, Shimoyama T: Leukocytapheresis therapy with leukocyte removal filter for inflammatory bowel disease. J Gastroenterol 1995;30(suppl 8):124–127.

151 Rembacken BJ, Newbould HE, Richards SJ, Misbah SA, Dixon ME, Chalmers DM, Axon AT: Granulocyte apheresis in inflammatory bowel disease: Possible mechanisms of effect. Ther Apher 1998;2:93–96.

152 Kosaka T, Sawada K, Ohnishi K, Egashira A, Yamamura M, Tanida N, Satomi M, Shimoyama T: Effect of leukocytapheresis therapy using a leukocyte removal filter in Crohn's disease. Intern Med 1999;38:102–111.

153 Sawada K, Ohnishi K, Egashira A, Kaneda M, Yano T, Ohkusu K, Chikano S, Kosaka T, Nagase K, Fukunaga K, Okui M, Fukuda Y, Tamura K, Satomi M, Shimoyama T, Nishigami T: [Induction of long-term remission for the first onset of severe enterocolitis Crohn's disease treated by leukocytapheresis alone]. Nippon Shokakibyo Gakkai zasshi 1999;96:1386–1391.

154 Kohgo Y, Ashida T, Maemoto A, Ayabe T: Leukocytapheresis for treatment of IBD. J Gastroenterol 2003;38(suppl 15):51–54.

155 Matsui T, Nishimura T, Matake H, Ohta T, Sakurai T, Yao T: Granulocytapheresis for Crohn's disease: A report on seven refractory patients. Am J Gastroenterol 2003;98:511–512.

156 Domenech E, Hinojosa J, Esteve-Comas M, Gomollon F, Herrera JM, Bastida G, Obrador A, Ruiz R, Saro C, Gassull MA: Granulocyteaphaeresis in steroid-dependent inflammatory bowel disease: A prospective, open, pilot study. Aliment Pharmacol Ther 2004;20:1347–1352.

157 Fukuda Y, Matsui T, Suzuki Y, Kanke K, Matsumoto T, Takazoe M, Matsumoto T, Motoya S, Honma T, Sawada K, Yao T, Shimoyama T, Hibi T: Adsorptive granulocyte and monocyte apheresis for refractory Crohn's disease: An open multicenter prospective study. J Gastroenterol 2004;39:1158–1164.

158 Kusaka T, Fukunaga K, Ohnishi K, Kosaka T, Tomita T, Yokoyama Y, Sawada K, Fukuda Y, Miwa H, Matsumoto T: Adsorptive monocyte-granulocytapheresis (M-GCAP) for refractory Crohn's disease. J Clin Apher 2004;19:168–173.

159 Giampaolo B, Giuseppe P, Michele B, Alessandro M, Fabrizio S, Alfonso C: Treatment of active steroid-refractory inflammatory bowel diseases with granulocytapheresis: Our experience with a prospective study. World J Gastroenterol 2006;12:2201–2204.

160 Sato T, Ishigaki Y, Komiya T, Tsuda H: Therapeutic immunoadsorption of acetylcholine receptor antibodies in myasthenia gravis. Ann N Y Acad Sci 1988;540:554–556.

161 Somnier FE, Langvad E: Plasma exchange with selective immunoadsorption of anti-acetylcholine receptor antibodies. J Neuroimmunol 1989;22:123–127.

162 Hosokawa S, Oyamaguchi A: Safety, stability, and effectiveness of immunoadsorption under membrane plasmapheresis treatment for myasthenia gravis. ASAIO Trans 1990;36:M207–208.

163 Yamamoto Y, Sameshima T, Akaike T: Selective removal of anti-acetylcholine receptor antibodies and IgG in vitro with an immunoadsorbent containing immobilized sulfathiazole. Artif Organs 1990;14:334–341.

164 Ichikawa M, Koh CS, Hata Y, Tohyama M, Tsuno T, Komiyama A: Immunoadsorption plasmapheresis for severe generalised myasthenia gravis. Arch Dis Child 1993;69:236–238.

165 Antozzi C, Berta E, Confalonieri P, Zuffi M, Cornelio F, Mantegazza R: Protein-A immunoadsorption in immunosuppression-resistant myasthenia gravis. Lancet 1994;343:124.

166 Shibuya N, Sato T, Osame M, Takegami T, Doi S, Kawanami S: Immunoadsorption therapy for myasthenia gravis. J Neurol Neurosurg Psychiatry 1994;57:578–581.

167 Grob D, Simpson D, Mitsumoto H, Hoch B, Mokhtarian F, Bender A, Greenberg M, Koo A, Nakayama S: Treatment of myasthenia gravis by immunoadsorption of plasma. Neurology 1995;45:338–344.

168 Yamawaki T, Suzuki N: Can immunoadsorption plasmapheresis be used as the first choice therapy for neuroimmunological disorders? Ther Apher 1997;1:348–352.

169 Yoshida M, Tamura Y, Yamada Y, Yamawaki N, Yamashita Y: Immusorba TR and immusorba PH: Basics of design and features of functions. Ther Apher 1998;2:185–192.

170 Benny WB, Sutton DM, Oger J, Bril V, McAteer MJ, Rock G: Clinical evaluation of a staphylococcal protein A immunoadsorption system in the treatment of myasthenia gravis patients. Transfusion 1999;39:682–687.

171 Yeh JH, Chiu HC: [Immunoadsorption therapy for myasthenia gravis: Study on the adsorption capacity of an immunoadsorption column]. J Microbiol Immunol Infect 1999;32:121–125.

172 Haupt WF, Rosenow F, van der Ven C, Birkmann C: Immunoadsorption in Guillain-Barré syndrome and myasthenia gravis. Ther Apher 2000;4:195–197.

173 Schneidewind JM, Zettl UK, Winkler RE, Ramlow W, Tiess M, Michelsen A, Hebestreit G, Prophet H, Patow W, Benecke R: The outcome in myasthenia gravis patients – an eight-year follow-up after finishing immunoabsorption therapy. Transfus Apher Sci 2001;24:95–98.

174 Haas M, Mayr N, Zeitlhofer J, Goldammer A, Derfler K: Long-term treatment of myasthenia gravis with immunoadsorption. J Clin Apher 2002;17:84–87.

175 Splendiani G, Cipriani S, Passalacqua S, Sturniolo A, Costanzi S, Fulignati P, Staffolani E, Casciani CU: Plasmaperfusion on tryptophan columns can improve the clinical outcome of patients affected with myasthenia gravis. Artif Cells Blood Substit Immobil Biotechnol 2003;31:69–79.

176 Ishizeki J, Nishikawa K, Kunimoto F, Goto F: Postoperative myasthenic crisis successfully treated with immunoadsorption therapy. J Anesth 2005;19:320–322.

177 Zeitler H, Ulrich-Merzenich G, Hoffmann L, Kornblum C, Schmidt S, Vetter H, Walger P: Long-term effects of a multimodal approach including immunoadsorption for the treatment of myasthenic crisis. Artif Organs 2006;30:597–605.

178 Haupt WF, Rosenow F, van der Ven C, Borberg H, Pawlik G: Sequential treatment of Guillain-Barré syndrome with extracorporeal elimination and intravenous immunoglobulin. Ther Apher 1997;1:55–57.

179 Dittrich E, Schmaldienst S, Derfler K: [Plasma exchange and immunoadsorption]. Wien Klin Wochenschr 2007;119:39–53;quiz 54.

180 Seta T, Nagayama H, Katsura K, Hamamoto M, Araki T, Yokochi M, Utsumi K, Katayama Y: Factors influencing outcome in Guillain-Barré syndrome: Comparison of plasma adsorption against other treatments. Clin Neurol Neurosurg 2005;107:491–496.

181 Okamiya S, Ogino M, Ogino Y, Irie S, Kanazawa N, Saito T, Sakai F: Tryptophan-immobilized column-based immunoadsorption as the choice method for plasmapheresis in Guillain-Barré syndrome. Ther Apher Dial 2004;8:248–253.

182 Takei H, Komaba Y, Araki T, Iino Y, Katayama Y: Plasma immunoadsorption therapy for Guillain-Barré syndrome: Critical day for initiation. J Nippon Med Sch 2002;69:557–563.

183 Diener HC, Haupt WF, Kloss TM, Rosenow F, Philipp T, Koeppen S, Vietorisz A: A preliminary, randomized, multicenter study comparing intravenous immunoglobulin, plasma exchange, and immune adsorption in Guillain-Barré syndrome. Eur Neurol 2001;46:107–109.

184 Ullrich H, Mansouri-Taleghani B, Lackner KJ, Schalke B, Bogdahn U, Schmitz G: Chronic inflammatory demyelinating polyradiculoneuropathy: Superiority of protein A immunoadsorption over plasma exchange treatment. Transfus Sci 1998;19(suppl):33–38.

185 Zinman LH, Sutton D, Ng E, Nwe P, Ngo M, Bril V: A pilot study to compare the use of the excorim staphylococcal protein immunoadsorption system and ivIg in chronic inflammatory demyelinating polyneuropathy. Transfus Apher Sci 2005;33:317–324.

186 Schmitt E, Behm E, Buddenhagen F, Ernst B, Hitzschke B, Kracht M, Korten G, Kundt G, Meyer-Rienecker H, Osten B: Immunoadsorption (IA) versus plasma exchange (PE) in multiple sclerosis – first results of a double blind controlled trial. Prog Clin Biol Res 1990;337:289–292.

187 Schneidewind JM, Winkler R, Ramlow W, Tiess M, Hertel U, Sehland D: Immunoadsorption – a new therapeutic possibility for multiple sclerosis? Transfus Sci 1998;19(suppl):59–63.

188 Moldenhauer A, Haas J, Wascher C, Derfuss T, Hoffmann KT, Kiesewetter H, Salama A: Immunoadsorption patients with multiple sclerosis: An open-label pilot study. Eur J Clin Invest 2005;35:523–530.

189 Muroi K, Sasaki R, Miura Y: The effect of immunoadsorption therapy by a protein A column on patients with thrombocytopenia. Semin Hematol 1989;26:10–14.

190 Snyder HW, Jr., Cochran SK, Balint JP, Jr., Bertram JH, Mittelman A, Guthrie TH, Jr., Jones FR: Experience with protein A-immunoadsorption in treatment-resistant adult immune thrombocytopenic purpura. Blood 1992;79:2237–2245.

191 Snyder HW, Jr., Seawell BW, Cochran SK, Balint JP, Jr., Jones FR: Specificity of antibody responses affected by extracorporeal immunoadsorption of plasma over columns of protein A silica. J Clin Apher 1992;7:110–118.

192 Balint JP, Cochran SK, Jones FR: Modulation of idiotypic and antiidiotypic immunoglobulin g responses in an immune thrombocytopenic purpura patient as a consequence of extracorporeal protein A immunoadsorption. Artif Organs 1995;19:496–499.

193 Cahill MR, Macey MG, Cavenagh JD, Newland AC: Protein A immunoadsorption in chronic refractory ITP reverses increased platelet activation but fails to achieve sustained clinical benefit. Br J Haematol 1998;100:358–364.

194 Fabrizio F, Luzzatto G, Ramon R, Randi ML, De Silvestro G, Girolami A: Treatment of refractory ITP with extracorporeal immunoadsorption over a protein-A sepharose column: A report of two cases. Haematologica 2000;85:889–890.

195 Quintini G, Barbera V, Dieli M, Marino C, Mariani G: Prolonged response of chronic immune thrombocytopenic purpura (ITP) to extracorporeal immunoadsorption. Int J Artif Organs 2000;23:407–408.

196 Mittelman A, Puccio C, Ahmed T, Arlin Z, Wuest D, Ciavarella D, Seawell BW, Snyder HW, Jr.: Response of refractory thrombotic thrombocytopenic purpura to extracorporeal immunoadsorption. N Engl J Med 1992;326:711–712.

197 Knobl P, Haas M, Laczika K, Varadi K, Turecek PL: Immunoadsorption for the treatment of a patient with severe thrombotic thrombocytopenic purpura resistant to plasma exchange: Kinetics of an inhibitor of ADAMTS13. J Thromb Haemost 2003;1:187–189.

198 D'Souza RJ, Kwan JT, Hendry BM, Fallon M, Cunningham D: Successful outcome of treating hemolytic uremic syndrome associated with cancer chemotherapy with immunoadsorption. Clin Nephrol 1997;47:58–59.

199 Mistry B, Kimmel PL, Hetzel PC, Phillips TM, Braden GL: The role of circulating immune complexes and biocompatibility of staphylococcal protein A immunoadsorption in mitomycin c-induced hemolytic uremic syndrome. Am J Kidney Dis 2004;44:e50–58.

200 Kanekura T, Yoshii N, Yonezawa T, Kawabata H, Saruwatari H, Kanzaki T: Treatment of pustular psoriasis with granulocyte and monocyte adsorption apheresis. J Am Acad Dermatol 2003;49:329–332.

201 Kanekura T, Kawabata H, Maruyama I, Kanzaki T: Treatment of psoriatic arthritis with granulocyte and monocyte adsorption apheresis. J Am Acad Dermatol 2004;50:242–246.

202 Liumbruno GM, Centoni PE, Molfettini P, Ceretelli S, Ceccarini M, Bachini L, Pomponi A, Bagnoni G, Vitolo M, Eberle O, Biondi A, Sodini ML: Lymphocytapheresis in the treatment of psoriasis vulgaris. J Clin Apher 2006;21:158–164.

203 Seishima M, Mizutani Y, Shibuya Y, Nagasawa C, Aoki T: Efficacy of granulocyte and monocyte adsorption apheresis for pustular psoriasis. Ther Apher Dial 2008;12:13–18.

204 Rabitsch W, Knobl P, Greinix H, Prinz E, Kalhs P, Horl WH, Derfler K: Removal of persisting isohaemagglutinins with Ig-Therasorb immunoadsorption after major ABO-incompatible non-myeloablative allogeneic haematopoietic stem cell transplantation. Nephrol Dial Transplant 2003;18:2405–2408.

205 Rabitsch W, Knobl P, Prinz E, Keil F, Greinix H, Kalhs P, Worel N, Jansen M, Horl WH, Derfler K: Prolonged red cell aplasia after major ABO-incompatible allogeneic hematopoietic stem cell transplantation: Removal of persisting isohemagglutinins with Ig-Therasorb immunoadsorption. Bone Marrow Transplant 2003;32:1015–1019.

206 Prophet H, Matic GB, Winkler RE, Tiess M, Schneidewind JM, Hebestreit G, Michelsen A, Ramlow W: Two cases of refractory endocrine ophthalmopathy successfully treated with extracorporeal immunoadsorption. Ther Apher 2001;5:142–146.

207 Dantal J, Testa A, Bigot E, Soulillou JP: Disappearance of proteinuria after immunoadsorption in a patient with focal glomerulosclerosis. Lancet 1990;336:190.

208 Dantal J, Testa A, Bigot E, Soulillou JP: Effects of plasma-protein A immunoadsorption on idiopathic nephrotic syndrome recurring after renal transplantation. Ann Med Interne 1992;143(suppl 1):48–51.

209 Dantal J, Godfrin Y, Koll R, Perretto S, Naulet J, Bouhours JF, Soulillou JP: Antihuman immunoglobulin affinity immunoadsorption strongly decreases proteinuria in patients with relapsing nephrotic syndrome. J Am Soc Nephrol 1998;9:1709–1715.

210 Esnault VL, Besnier D, Testa A, Coville P, Simon P, Subra JF, Audrain MA: Effect of protein A immunoadsorption in nephrotic syndrome of various etiologies. J Am Soc Nephrol 1999;10:2014–2017.

211 Moriconi L, Passalacqua S, Pretagostini R, Battaglia G, Russo G, De Palo T, Rindi P, Puccini R, Batini V, Carraro M, Faccini L, Artero M, Zennaro C, Cristofani R: Apheresis in primary focal segmental glomerulosclerosis of native and transplanted kidneys: A therapeutic protocol. J Nephrol 2000;13:347–351.

212 Ponikvar R, Bren A, Kandus A, Buturovic Ponik-var J: Treatment of recurrence of focal segmental glomerular sclerosis after kidney transplantation with plasma exchange and immunoadsorption. Transplant Proc 2001;33:3365–3367.

213 Kuhn C, Kuhn A, Markau S, Kastner U, Osten B: Effect of immunoadsorption on refractory idiopathic focal and segmental glomerulosclerosis. J Clin Apher 2006;21:266–270.

214 Meyer TN, Thaiss F, Stahl RA: Immunoadsorb-tion and rituximab therapy in a second living-related kidney transplant patient with recurrent focal segmental glomerulosclerosis. Transpl Int 2007;20:1066–1071.

Dr. Wolfgang Ramlow
Apheresis Center
Nobelstr. 53
18059 Rostock, Germany
Tel. +49 381 4050 223, Fax -257
E-Mail ramlow@apherese.de

Immunomodulation and Therapeutic Apheresis

Scharf RE (ed): Progress and Challenges in Transfusion Medicine, Hemostasis and Hemotherapy.
Freiburg i.Br., Karger, 2008, pp 113–122

Cytapheresis as a Nonpharmacological Therapy for Inflammatory Bowel Disease

Takayuki Matsumoto · Ken Fukunaga · Koji Kamikozuru ·
Katsutoshi Tozawa · Yoko Yokoyama · Takeshi Kusaka · Kunio Onishi ·
Hiroto Miwa · Shiro Nakamura

Division of Lower G-I Disease, Hyogo College of Medicine, Nishinomiya, Japan

Key Words

Inflammatory bowel disease · Ulcerative colitis · Cytapheresis · Nonpharmacological therapy · Regulatory T cell

Summary

Inflammatory bowel disease (IBD), including ulcerative colitis (UC) and Crohn's disease (CD), is a chronic recurrent disease with unknown etiology; however, recent studies suggest that impaired immune responses to intestinal tissue and/or intestinal flora play important roles in the pathogenesis of IBD. For patients with IBD, 5-aminosalycilates are often used in case of mild disease and corticosteroids are mainly used for moderate to severe disease. However, we often encounter patients who are resistant to or dependent on conventional therapy, which is likely to lead to future problems concerning the quality of life due to adverse effects of the drugs used, especially the corticosteroids. Extracorporeal leukocyte removal therapy (cytapheresis) is one of the adjunctive therapies for IBD patients refractory to steroids, through suppression of the impaired immune response by removing activated leukocytes from the circulating blood system, especially granulocytes and lymphocytes. The present paper reviews the latest evidences in order to propose the current status of cytapheresis in the therapeutic strategy for IBD, especially for UC and CD. Although there are a few randomized controlled trials, clinical experience so far suggests that cytapheresis has superior efficiency as a nonpharmacological immunomodulative therapy for steroid-resistant moderate to severe UC. Moreover, cytapheresis is characterized by higher safety compared with other conventional medications for severe UC.   ©2008 S. Karger GmbH, Freiburg i.Br.

Introduction

Ulcerative colitis (UC) and Crohn's disease (CD) are chronic intestinal inflammatory diseases of yet unknown origin and are called idiopathic inflammatory bowel diseases (IBD). They may lead to an impairment of the quality of life through long-lasting symptoms such as diarrhea, bloody stool and abdominal pain [1]. In Japan, the number of UC and CD cases has increased ten times compared to that in the 1980s. The etiology of IBD has not been proven; however, an autoimmune disturbance is thought to play an important role in this incurable disease.

So far, systemic administration of corticosteroids has been widely used as the standard therapy for moderately to severe UC, which often results in dose-dependent adverse effects such as moon face, infections, diabetic disease and osteoporosis. For patients with steroid-resistant or steroid-dependent types of disease, immunomodulators such as cyclosporine and tacrolimus for severe disease, or 6-mercaptopurine and azathiopurin for mild to moderate disease, have been widely used.

Cytapheresis, which removes leukocyte from the peripheral blood, has been reported as an adjunctive therapy for steroid-resistant UC in 1995 [2]. The primary aim of cytapheresis is to suppress and reduce the impaired immune responses in the diseased intestine by removing circulating over-activated leukocytes, especially granulocytes, which have been identified as characteristic leukocytes in the diseased tissue and as the cause of crypt abscesses, using a specially designed device. The currently available cytapheresis techniques for active IBD patients are filtration leukocytapheresis (LCA), adsorption granulocyte/monocyte apheresis (GMA), and centrifugal lymphocytapheresis (CLA). GMA and LCA have been approved by the national health insurance policy for active UC patients since 2000 and 2001, respectively, in Japan. They have been widely used as nonpharmacological and nonsurgical therapeutic options for intractable UC patients. On the other hand, although GMA has been on the final stage for getting the government approval, cytapheresis has not been approved for CD by the health insurance system in Japan.

However, there have been a few data showing which types of patients are more likely to respond to the therapy or what are the true mechanisms of action of cytapheresis in IBD.

Cytapheresis Techniques Currently Available for Patients with Active Inflammatory Bowel Disease

Filtration Leukocytapheresis

LCA is carried out using a Cellsorba EX™ (Asahi Kasei Kuraray Medical Co., Ltd., Tokyo, Japan) column which is filled with a polyester unwoven filter. This filter is designed to remove almost 100% of the granulocytes and monocytes and 64% of the lymphocytes [3]. Furthermore, approximately 35% of the platelets can be trapped on the filter from the processed peripheral blood [3]. LCA is usually performed weekly using a Cellsorba EX™ set on a simple one-way hemofiltration circuit [2–4]. In case the patient is in severe active condition, two sessions are allowed in the first week of the treatment, followed by consecutive weekly sessions [4]. A roller pump drains the patient's peripheral blood from an antecubital vein at a constant flow rate of 30–50 ml/min. The optimal amount of the anti-coagulant Nafamostat mesilate (Torii Pharmacol. Co., Ltd., Tokyo, Japan) or heparin was mixed with saline and was added to the patient's drained peripheral whole blood as anti-coagulant before infusion into the column. Although the use of Nafamostat is sometimes associated with allergic adverse effects, the half-life of the drug is short enough to prevent bleeding accompanied with ulcerative lesions in UC. When analyzing anti-Nafamostat IgE antibodies in UC patients who developed allergic reactions to Nafamostat, the anti-Nafamostat IgE was present in 12% of the symptomatic patients, whose adverse effects were possibly induced by Nafamostat [5]. However, 43% of the patients did not show anti-Nafamostat IgE, in spite of the fact that their adverse effects were also caused by Nafamostat.

Adsorption Granulocyte/Monocyte Apheresis

GMA is carried out with the Adacolumn (JIMRO Co. Ltd., Takasaki, Japan), which is filled with cellulose acetate beads. The beads are designed to adsorb about 65% of the granulocytes, 55% of the monocytes/macrophages and a smaller fraction of the lymphocytes from peripheral blood. One of the mechanisms how leukocytes adsorb to the beads is through the so-called Fcγ receptor and complement receptors [6–8]. The circuit diagram for GMA is almost the same as that for LCA. The duration of one GMA session was 60 min, at 30 ml/min, with the optimal amount of Nafamostat mesilate or heparin as anti-coagulant. As GMA does not remove platelets, this method is preferably used in patients with moderate to severe bleeding.

Centrifugal Lymphocytapheresis

CLA is performed using a centrifugal cell separator (Component Correction System: CCS, Haemonetics Japan, Tokyo, Japan). Peripheral whole blood drained from a patient is collected into a polycarbonate disposable bowl. The CCS makes the 125-ml bowl spin to generate a centrifugal force, and the refined lymphocyte-rich layer (buffy coat) is then selectively removed. After the lymphocyte removal, the separated blood is returned to the patient through the same catheter. CLA processes approximately 2,400 ml of the patient's whole blood. In LCA for patients with UC, a relatively heavy layer of the leukocytes is removed to increase the efficacy.

Cytapheresis for Patients with Ulcerative Colitis

Lymphocytapheresis for Patients with Ulcerative Colitis

LCA and GMA have been widely used in Japan as effective therapeutic options for active UC patients who do not respond well to the conventional treatments; however, our current level of knowledge of LCA is still fragmental. Although the mechanisms underlying the therapeutic efficacy have not been fully elucidated, immune modulations induced during LCA have been reported previously, especially from the point of view of cytokine production and immune regulation. It has been shown that LCA enhances the ability of the peripheral lymphocytes to produce interleukin (IL)-4, an anti-inflammatory cytokine [9]. Furthermore, LCA showed an ability to decrease IL-6 release (a pro-inflammatory cytokine) from peripheral blood lymphocytes. This modification is accompanied with a concomitant increase in IL-10 production. This modification to lymphocyte function in producing inflammatory and anti-inflammatory cytokines can induce the inhibition of IL-1 on the protein level and the mRNA expression level during the cytapheresis procedure [10].

On the other hand, approximately 35% of the peripheral blood platelets are removed by LCA, which adhere to the surface of the polyester filter of the Cellsorba EX™ column [4]. Recently, it has been reported that circulating platelets are important cells not only in hemostasis but also in a variety of inflammatory responses [11]. An increase of peripheral platelet counts has often been recognized as a common feature during the chronic active phase of IBD [12]. As it has been reported previously that the high platelet number correlates well with disease severity [13], we hypothesized that this significant platelet removal achieved during LCA might have an active role in down-regulating the severe immunological reactions in UC patients with an acute flare. We have proven that activated platelets may be used to predict the clinical efficacy of LCA in severe UC patients [14].

Sawada et al. reported a multicenter randomized controlled trial of LCA for active UC patients [3]. In this study, moderate to severe UC patients who were resistant to conventional steroid therapy of at least 30 mg/day were randomized into either an LCA group (add LCA) or a high-dose steroid group (prednisolone 60 mg/day). The LCA group showed a significantly higher efficacy rate compared with the conventional high-dose corticosteroid group (h-PSL) (LCA vs. h-PSL = 74.1 vs. 31.8%, $p < 0.05$). However, there were no significant differences between LCA and h-PSL in the clinical efficiency. A major advantage of LCA was its safety profile which showed that no serious adverse side effect was observed in the LCA group, while a substantial number of patients in the h-PSL group showed severe adverse effects such as infection.

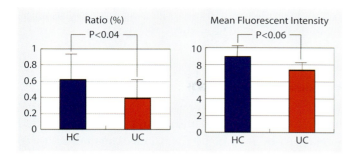

Fig. 1. Percentages of CD25high+CD4+ lymphocytes (regulatory T cells); UC vs. healthy control [33].

Granulocyte/Monocyte Apheresis for Patients with Ulcerative Colitis

Several studies [15–19] showed remission induction rates of GMA in patients with UC. As stated above, GMA uses cellulose acetate beads that adhere to granulocytes through Fc receptors. Cellular contact to the beads may produce other immunological effects on other types of cells such as lymphocytes. We have demonstrated that in the first session of GMA, the proportion of regulatory T cells in the peripheral blood of patients with UC increases, which may suppress the impaired immune responses in UC. In patients with active IBD, peripheral blood granulocytes and monocytes/macrophages are elevated, show activation behavior and increased survival time [20–25]. As these leukocytes are major sources of inflammatory cytokines [26, 27], they may contribute to the exacerbation and perpetuation of IBD [28, 29]. Furthermore, the level of neutrophil infiltration into the mucosal tissue in patients with active IBD is related to the severity of intestinal inflammation and clinical relapse [30–32].

We showed that peripheral regulatory T cells (CD25highCD4+ T cells), which were suppressed in active UC compared to the healthy control, were significantly increased after a single GMA session (fig. 1) [33]. The impaired activity and/or proportion of regulatory T cells results in an over-activation of immune responses including polyclonal antibody production, and leads to autoimmunity-mediated tissue destruction. The increase in CD25high+CD4+ regulatory T cells after GMA should contribute to improved immune function of the patient. The rise could reflect depletion of non-CD25high+CD4+ T cells by the GMA procedure. The changes in regulatory T cells in the intestinal mucosa, however, have not been clarified yet. Likewise, several other investigators have reported favorable immunological observations associated with GMA [34, 35]. Andoh et al. reported a significant decrease of IL-1β- and TNF-α-induced IL-8 and IL-6 release from peripheral leukocytes following GMA [35]. Collectively, GMA may correct a part of the impaired immune responses through regulatory T cells and cytokine production from lymphocytes in the peripheral blood. The mechanisms how the changes in the peripheral blood immune cells cause changes in the intestinal immune cells should be further examined. A multicenter trial of GMA for active UC patients [36] showed that GMA had a significant efficiency for relapsing UC patients compared with the conventional h-PSL therapy (GMA vs. h-PSL = 54.8

vs. 39.5%, p < 0.05), and GMA had a significantly lower ratio of adverse events compared with that of h-PSL (GMA vs. h-PSL = 89.9 vs. 58.9%, p < 0.001).

Cytapheresis for Patients with Crohn's Disease

The efficacy of cytapheresis for active CD has been examined and we have conducted a multicenter open label study on GMA in Japan for active CD patients refractory to enteral nutrition with more than 1200 kcal/day of elemental diet [37]. Prior to this multicenter study, we reported the efficacy of cytapheresis in active CD as a preliminary clinical trial [38]. According to these two studies, adsorptive cytapheresis therapy (GMA) showed preferable effects in active CD patients with colonic disease evaluated by clinical activity. Fukuda et al. [7] reported that significant improvements in CD activity index (CDAI), International Organization for the Study of IBD (IOIBD) and IBD questionnaire (IBDQ) scores were observed at week 7 of GMA therapy. The CDAI, IOIBD, and IBDQ scores before GMA were 275.6, 3.4, and 152, respectively. The corresponding values of CDAI after GMA were 214.8 ± 89.2 (p = 0.0005), 2.54 (p = 0.0224), and 165 (p = 0.0327), respectively. Currently, GMA for CD is considered as an optional medical therapy. Although LCA has previously been reported to have superior efficiency for active CD patients [39], there are no sufficient data eligible for getting approval from the government.

Cytapheresis for Inflammatory Bowel Disease in the Western World

In the USA, Hanauer [29] (The University of Chicago) and Mayer et al. (Mount Sinai School of Medicine) have conducted a pilot study of LCA for active UC patients refractory to steroids and 5-aminosalychric acid. However, their treatment schedule and column were different from those of the Japanese trial. Their regimen was designed to perform LCA twice a week for 3 weeks (total 6 sessions), and the column (Cellsorba FX) used in the study was modified to be usable with acid-citrate dextrose sodium (ACD) instead of Nafamostat mesilate or heparin as anti-coagulant. GMA has also been evaluated for moderate to severe active UC patients in the USA with a multicenter double-blind randomized sham-controlled trial.

Cellsorba FX™ had the CE mark and has been approved as medical device in Europe. The column used in Europe is modified to be used with ACD as in the USA. A clinical trial has been started for active UC refractory to conventional medication therapy in Germany.

Future Development in Cytapheresis for the Management of Inflammatory Bowel Diseases

The factors that may influence the clinical effectiveness of LCA and GMA include blood flow speed, proceeding time, and proceeding frequency. Basically, a slower flow speed increases the leukocyte removal rate of the column. However, Cellsorba, the column used in LCA, may cause a coagulation problem in the column under 20 ml/min of slow flow speed conditions since the platelets in the column cause foamy thromboses. On the other hand, Adacolumn, the column used in GMA, adsorbs granulocytes, monocytes/macrophages and a smaller fraction of the lymphocytes from the patients' peripheral whole blood on the cellulose acetate beads filling the device. As peripheral blood leukocytes bear an Fcγ receptor and complement receptors [8, 40], and the column is not likely to adhere to platelets, GMA is suitable for processing under slow flow speed conditions. We then focused on the platelet removal performances of LCA and GMA as a possible factor to understand their therapeutic mechanisms. GMA may be better if the patient is in a severe inflammatory condition and/or dehydrated status because of hyper blood viscosity. Conversely, LCA can be primarily used for patients with severe inflammatory condition of the colonic mucosa, such as grade 4 in Matts' classification [41] which is often seen in intractable patients.

The clinical response to cytapheresis is usually seen at week 5 by the clinical and the endoscopic indices. During this period, there could be serious deteriorations together with a debilitating impact on the quality of life for patients who become nonresponders. Since the established evidences suggest that both functional suppression of the circulating leukocytes and the quantitative removal of activated leukocytes contribute to the efficacy of this nonpharmacological therapy, it has been hypothesized that there might be an inverse proportion between proceeding frequency and immunological effect of cytapheresis. A recent unpublished randomized controlled study comparing intensive and once-a-week regimens showed that intensive treatment, which consists of 2 apheresis sessions in a week for 5 consecutive weeks, results in a higher remission rate both by clinical and endoscopic criteria and shorter duration before getting a clinical response.

However, for steroid-resistant severe UC, intravenous infusion therapy of cyclosporine has been widely accepted as an adjunct therapy [42]; a large proportion of the patients may need surgery in several years. Clinical experience so far suggests that cytapheresis has superior efficiency as a nonpharmacological immunomodulative therapy for steroid-resistant UC patients before colectomy [1–4].

Conclusions and Future Directions

Cytapheresis is an effective nonpharmacological therapy for steroid-resistant moderate to severe UC. We have to clarify which types of the patients are good candidates for cytapheresis and what are the most reliable parameters in predicting responders for cytapheresis in UC in the near future. Clinical efficacy and indication based on the mode of action for patients with steroid-naive UC should be determined to improve the patients' quality of life.

Disclosure of Conflict of Interests

Takayuki Matsumoto has research grants from Asahi-Kasei Kuraray Medical Co., Ltd., JIMRO (Japan Immunoresearch Laboratories Co., Ltd.), Eisai Co., Ltd., Tanabe-Mitsubishi Pharmaceuticals, Otsuka Pharmaceuticals, Nisshin-Kyorin Pharmaceuticals and Asteras Pharmaceutical Co, Ltd.

References

1   Hibi T, Ogata H: Novel pathophysiological concepts of inflammatory bowel disease. J Gastroenterol 2006;41:10–16.
2   Sawada K, Ohnishi K, Fukui S, Yamamura M, Amano K, Satomi M, Shimoyama T: Leukocytapheresis therapy, performed with leukocyte removal filter, for inflammatory bowel disease. J Gastroenterol 1995;30:322–329.
3   Sawada K, Muto T, Shimoyama T, Satomi M, Sawada T, Nagawa H, Hiwatashi N, Asakura H, Hibi T: Multicenter randomized controlled trial for the treatment of ulcerative colitis with a leukocytapheresis column. Curr Pharm Des 2003;9:307–321.
4   Shibata H, Kuriyama T, Yamawaki N: Cellsorba. Ther Apher Dial 2003;7:44–47.
5   Nagase K, Fukunaga K, Ohnishi K, Kusaka T, Matoba Y, Sawada K: Detection of specific IgE antibodies to Nafamostat mesilate as an indication of possible adverse effects of leukocytapheresis using Nafamostat mesilate as anticoagulant. Ther Apher Dial 2004;8:45–51.
6   Saniabadi AR, Hanai H, Suzuki Y, Ohmori T, Sawada K, Yoshimura N, Saito Y, Takeda Y, Umemura K, Kondo K, Ikeda Y, Fukunaga K, Nakashima M, Beretta A, Bjarnason I, Lofberg R: Adacolumn for selective leukocytapheresis as a non-pharmacological treatment for patients with disorders of the immune system: an adjunct or an alternative to drug therapy? J Clin Apher 2005;20:171–184.
7   Hiraishi K, Takeda Y, Shiobara N, Shibusawa H, Jimma F, Kashiwagi N, Saniabadi AR, Adachi M: Studies on the mechanisms of leukocyte adhesion to cellulose acetate beads: an in vitro model to assess the efficacy of cellulose acetate carrier-based granulocyte and monocyte adsorptive apheresis. Ther Apher Dial 2003;7:334–340.
8   D'Arrigo C, Candal-Couto JJ, Greer M, Veale DJ, Woof JM: Human neutrophil Fc receptor-mediated adhesion under flow: a hallow fiber model of intravascular arrest. Clin Exp Immunol 1993;100:173–179.
9   Noguchi M, Hiwatashi N, Hayakawa T, Toyota T: Leukocyte removal filter-passed lymphocytes produce large amounts of interleukin-4 in immunotherapy for inflammatory bowel disease: Role of bystander suppression. Ther Apher 1998;2:109–114.
10 Hanai H, Iida T, Takeuchi K, Tanaka T, Kondo K, Kikuyama M, Maruyama Y, Iwaoka Y, Nakamura A, Hirayama K, Saniabadi AR, Watanabe F: Decrease of reactive-oxygen-producing granulocytes and release of IL-10 into the peripheral blood following leukocytapheresis in patients with active ulcerative colitis. World J Gastroenterol 2005;11:3085–3090.
11 Danese S, Motte C, Fiocchi C: Platelets in inflammatory bowel disease: clinical, pathogenic, and therapeutic implications. Am J Gastroenterol 2004;99:938–945.
12 Talstad I, Rootwelt K, Gjone E: Thrombocytosis in ulcerative colitis and Crohn's disease. Scand J Gastroenterol 1973;8:135–138.
13 Harries AD, Fitzsimons E, Fifield R, Dew MJ, Rhoades J: Platelet count: A simple measure of activity in Crohn's disease. Br Med J 1983;286:1476.
14 Fukunaga K, Fukuda Y, Yokoyama Y, Ohnishi K, Kusaka T, Kosaka T, Hida N, Ohda Y, Miwa H, Matsumoto T: Activated platelet as a possible early marker to predict clinical efficacy of leukocytapheresis in severe ulcerative colitis patients. J Gastroenterol 2006;41:524–532.
15 Kanke K, Nakano M, Hiraishi H, Terano A: Clinical evaluation of granulocyte/monocyte apheresis therapy for active ulcerative colitis. Dig Liv Dis 2004;36:512–518.

16 Naganuma M, Funakoshi S, Sakuraba A, Takagi H, Inoue N, Ogata H, Iwao Y, Ishi H, Hibi T: Granulocytapheresis is useful as an alternative therapy in patients with steroid-refractory or -dependent ulcerative colitis. Inflamm Bowel Dis 2004;10:251–257.

17 Yamamoto T, Umegae S, Kitagawa T, Yasuda Y, Yamada Y, Takahashi D, Mukumoto M, Nishimura N, Yasue K, Matsumoto K: Granulocyte and monocyte adsorptive apheresis in the treatment of active distal ulcerative colitis: a prospective, pilot study. Aliment Pharmacol Ther 2004;20:783–792.

18 Domenech E, Hinojosa J, Esteve-Comas M, Gomollón F, Herrera JM, Bastida G, Obrador A, Ruiz R, Saro C, Gassull MA; Spanish Group for the Study of Crohn's Disease and Ulcerative Colitis (GETECCU): Granulocytapheresis in steroid-dependent inflammatory bowel disease: a prospective, open, pilot study. Aliment Pharmacol Ther 2004;20:1347–1352.

19 Suzuki Y, Yoshimura N, Saito Y, Saniabadi AR: A retrospective search for predictors of clinical response to selective granulocyte and monocyte apheresis in patients with ulcerative colitis. Dig Dis Sci 2006;51:2031–2038.

20 Saniabadi AR, Hanai H, Takeuchi K, Umemura K, Nakashima M, Adachi T, Shima C, Bjarnason I, Lofberg R: Adacolumn, an adsorptive carrier based granulocyte and monocyte apheresis device for the treatment of inflammatory and refractory diseases associated with leukocytes. Ther Apher Dial 2003;7:48–59.

21 Hanai H, Watanabe F, Takeuchi K, Iida T, Yamada M, Iwaoka Y, Saniabadi A, Matsushita I, Sato Y, Tozawa K, Arai H, Furuta T, Sugimoto K, Bjarnason I: Leukocyte adsorptive apheresis for the treatment of active ulcerative colitis: a prospective uncontrolled pilot study. Clin Gastroenterol Hepatol 2003;1:28–35.

22 McCarthy DA, Rampton DS, Liu Y-C: Peripheral blood neutrophils in inflammatory bowel disease: morphological evidence of in vivo activation in active disease. Clin Exp Immunol 1991;86:489–493.

23 Rugtveit J, Brandtzaeg P, Halstensen TS, Fausa O, Scott H: Increased macrophage subsets in inflammatory bowel disease: apparent recruitment from peripheral blood monocytes. Gut 1994;35:669–674.

24 Meuret G, Bitzi A, Hammer B: Macrophage turnover in Crohn's disease and ulcerative colitis. Gastroenterology 1978;74:501–503.

25 Brannigan AE, O'Connell PR, Hurley H: Neutrophil apoptosis is delayed in patients with inflammatory bowel disease. Shock 2000;13:361–366.

26 Cassatella MA: The production of cytokines by polymorph nuclear neutrophils. Immunol Today 1995;16:21–26.

27 Nikolaus S, Bauditz J, Gionchetti P: Increased secretion of pro-inflammatory cytokines by circulating polymorph nuclear neutrophils and regulation by interleukin-10 during intestinal inflammation. Gut 1998;42:470–476.

28 Mahida YR: The key role of macrophages in the immunopathogenesis of inflammatory bowel disease. Inflamm Bowel Dis 2000;6:21–33.

29 Hanauer SB: Inflammatory bowel disease: Epidemiology, pathogenesis, and therapeutic opportunities. Inflamm Bowel Dis 2006;12:S3–S9.

30 Allison MC, Dhillon AP, Lewis WG, Pounder RE (eds): Inflammatory Bowel Disease. London, Mosby, 1998, pp 15–95.

31 Tibble JA, Sigthorsson G, Bridger D, Fagerhol MK, Bjarnason I: Surrogate markers of intestinal inflammation are predictive of relapse in patients with inflammatory bowel disease. Gastroenterology 2000;119:15–22.

32 Limburg P, David M, Ahlquist A, Sandborn WJ: Faecal calprotectin levels predict colorectal inflammation among patients with chronic diarrhoea referred for colonoscopy. Am J Gastroenterol 2000;95:2831–2837.

33 Yokoyama Y, Fukunaga K, Fukuda Y, Tozawa K, Kamikozuru K, Ohnishi K, Kusaka T, Kosaka T, Hida N, Ohda Y, Miwa H, Matsumoto T: Demonstration of low CD25high+CD4+ and high CD28–CD4+ T-cell subsets in patients with ulcerative colitis: modified by selective leucocytapheresis. Dig Dis Sci 2007;52:2725–2731.

34 Kashiwagi N, Sugimura K, Koiwai H, Saniabadi A: Immunomodulatory effects of granulocyte and monocyte adsorption apheresis as a treatment for patients with ulcerative colitis. Dig Dis Sci 2002;6:1334–1341.

35 Andoh A, Tsujikawa T, Inatomi O, Deguchi Y, Hata K, Kitoh K, Sasaki M, Mitsuyama K, Fujiyama Y: Suppression of inflammatory cytokines secretion by granulocyte/monocytes adsorptive apheresis in active ulcerative colitis. Ther Apher Dial 2005;2:123–127.

36 Shimoyama T, Sawada K, Hiwatashi N, Sawada T, Matsueda K, Munakata A, Asakura H, Tanaka T, Kasukawa R, Kimura K, Suzuki Y, Nagamachi Y, Muto T, Nagawa H, Iizuka B, Baba S, Nasu M, Kataoka T, Kashiwagi N, Saniabadi AR: Safety and efficacy of granulocytes and monocyte adsorption apheresis in patients with active ulcerative colitis: a multicenter study. J Clin Apher 2001;16:1–9.

37 Fukuda Y, Matsui T, Suzuki Y, Matsumoto T, Takazoe M, Matsumoto T, Motoya S, Honma T, Sawada K, Yao T, Shimoyama T, Hibi T: Adsorptive granulocyte and monocyte apheresis for refractory Crohn's disease: an open multicenter prospective study. J Gastroenterol 2004;39:1158–1164.

38 Kusaka T, Fukunaga K, Ohnishi K, Kosaka T, Tomita T, Yokoyama Y, Sawada K, Fukuda Y, Miwa H, Matsumoto T: Adsorptive monocyte-granulocytapheresis (M-GCAP) for refractory Crohn's disease. J Clin Apher 2004;19:168–173.

39 Kosaka T, Sawada K, Ohnishi K, Egashira A, Yamamura M, Tanida N, Satomi M, Shimoyama T: Effect of leukocytapheresis therapy using a leukocyte removal filter in Crohn's disease. Intern Med 1999;38:102–111.

40 Hiraishi K, Takeda Y, Shiobara N: Studies on the mechanisms of leukocyte adhesion to cellulose acetate beads: an in vitro model to assess the efficacy of cellulose acetate carrier-based granulocyte and monocyte adsorptive apheresis. Ther Apher Dial 2003;7:334–340.

41 Matts SGF: The value of rectal biopsy in the diagnosis of ulcerative colitis. Q J Med 1961;120:393–407.

42 Fukunaga K, Fukuda Y, Sawada K, Hori K, Matoba Y, Sagayama K, Ohnishi K, Fukui S, Shimoyama T: Poorly controlled ulcerative colitis treated by colectomy during remission induced by extracorporeal leukocyte removal therapy. J Gastroenterol 2003;38:684–689.

Professor Takayuki Matsumoto, M.D., Ph.D.
Division of Lower G-I Disease, Department of Internal Medicine
Hyogo College of Medicine
Mukogawa-cho, Nishinomiya, Japan 663–8131
Tel. +81 798 456660, Fax 456661
E-Mail matsut@hyo-med.ac.jp

Immunomodulation and Therapeutic Apheresis

Scharf RE (ed): Progress and Challenges in Transfusion Medicine, Hemostasis and Hemotherapy.
Freiburg i.Br., Karger, 2008, pp 123–131

Immunoadsorption in Dilated Cardiomyopathy

Alexander Staudt · Stephan B. Felix

Department of Internal Medicine B, University of Greifswald, Germany

Key Words

Immunoadsorption · Heart failure · Dilated cardiomyopathy

Summary

Disturbances of the humoral immune system have been described in patients with dilated cardiomyopathy (DCM). Various circulating cardiac antibodies have been detected among DCM patients. Circulating antibodies are extractable by immunoadsorption. Recent studies have shown that removal of antibodies by immunoadsorption induces improvement of cardiac function in DCM. Furthermore, it decreases myocardial inflammation. Antibodies belonging to the IgG-3 subclass play an important role in cardiac dysfunction of patients suffering from DCM. The removal of negative inotropic antibodies which induce their functional effects via Fc_γ receptor IIa may play an important role in the effects of immunoadsorption. Therapy by immunoadsorption may offer a new therapeutic option for patients with severe heart failure due to DCM.   ©2008 S. Karger GmbH, Freiburg i.Br.

Introduction

Dilated cardiomyopathy (DCM) is a myocardial disease characterized by progressive depression of myocardial contractile function, and by ventricular dilatation in the absence of abnormal loading conditions or ischemic heart disease sufficient to cause global myocardial contractile dysfunction. The current accepted therapeutic approach for therapy of heart failure takes the form of administration, for example, of angiotensin-converting enzyme inhibitors and angiotensin-1 antagonists, β-blockers, as well as spironolactone. Now as before, however, the prognosis of DCM is not promising, despite therapeutic intervention in this way [1]. A number of innovative therapeutic options have accordingly been examined to enhance the clinical outcome for DCM patients.

Disturbances of the Humoral Immune System in Dilated Cardiomyopathy

Patients with myocarditis and DCM demonstrate abnormalities of the humoral immune system. In addition, the presence of various autoantibodies has been confirmed in DCM patients, including antibodies against mitochondrial proteins, contractile proteins, cardiac-β_1 receptors, and muscarinergic receptors [2–6]. In the case of particular antibodies, in vitro evidence has suggested a negative influence on cardiac performance [2, 7]. A DCM model, created by Matsui et al., is based on immunization of rabbits with peptides that match the sequence of the second extracellular loop of either β_1 adrenoceptors or M2-muscarinic receptors [8]. In the sera of immunized animals, Matsui et al. have discovered high titers of anti-peptide antibodies. Both groups of immunized rabbits studied by these authors exhibited morphological heart alterations similar to those established in human DCM. In addition, Jahns et al. employed an animal model to confirm that antibodies against the β_1 receptor itself are capable of inducing DCM [9]. Publications in recent time have disclosed that mice showing deficiencies in the programmed death (PD)-1 receptor develop DCM [10]. Deficiencies in the immunoregulatory PD-1 receptor result in creation of autoantibodies against cardiac troponin which, in turn, account for the cardiac dysfunction in these animals [11]. In addition, troponin antibodies induce severe inflammation in myocardial tissue [12]. In DCM patients, the detection of antibodies against myosin is associated with a deterioration of left ventricular function [13].

Cardiac autoantibodies play an active role in pathogenesis of DCM, by virtue of triggering the disease process or by aggravating myocardial contractile malfunction after it has developed. Under the hypothesis that cardiac autoantibodies actually play a functional role in DCM, one would expect that their elimination could improve the hemodynamics of DCM patients. Immunoadsorption (IA) makes it possible to extract cardiac antibodies.

Clinical Effects of Immunoadsorption

We executed a preliminary, primary uncontrolled pilot study to investigate the short-term hemodynamic effects of IA in patients with severe heart failure resulting from DCM [14]. Extraction of immunoglobulin (Ig) from the plasma of these patients resulted in a significant increase in cardiac index (CI), in conjunction at the same time with a reduction in systemic vascular resistance (SVR). These results imply that elimination of antibodies may enhance hemodynamics among DCM patients.

We conducted an additional randomized study to investigate the hemodynamic influence of IA in patients with DCM (New York Heart Association (NYHA) III–IV, left ventricular ejection fraction (LVEF) < 30%, CI < 2.5 l/min/m²) who had previously been on a stable regimen of oral medication for treatment of heart failure [15]. We continued oral medication throughout 3 months in the control group. In

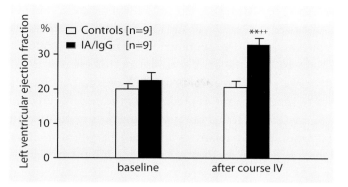

Fig. 1. Changes in LVEF in the IA/IgG group (filled bars) and in the control group (controls, open bars) [15]. **p < 0.01 significantly different from baseline; ++p < 0.01 significantly different from controls.

the treatment group, first we administered medication in one single IA session daily, throughout 3 consecutive days. This was followed by repetition of IA at 1-month intervals, for a total of 3 further courses, until month 3. Following each course, we substituted IgG to reduce infection risk and to block rebound of antibody production in B cells following IgG depletion. In the control group, we determined no alteration in hemodynamics or LVEF during the 3 months. Among the treatment groups, on the other hand, CI and stroke volume index (SVI) rose significantly (30%), accompanied by a concomitant parallel reduction in SVR. The enhancement recorded in CI, SVI, and SVR continued in the following 3 months. LVEF likewise appreciably rose within the treatment group, which indicates that IA followed by IgG substitution enhances cardiovascular function in DCM patients [15] (fig. 1). A case-controlled study conducted by other authors performed IA in 1 course of 5 consecutive days, without subsequent IgG substitution [16]. That study did not repeat IA during follow-up. LVEF increased significantly in contrast to the control group without IA therapy over 1 year. In the case of other autoimmune diseases, repetition of IA or plasmapheresis is, as a rule, conducted at periodic intervals. As part of a recent randomized study, we compared the results of IA repeated at monthly intervals with 1 IA course carried out over 5 days. One interesting result was that both groups experienced comparable hemodynamic benefits over 6 months [17].

Mechanisms of Immunoadsorption in Dilated Cardiomyopathy

In one of our experimental studies, we studied the potential mechanisms of advantageous acute hemodynamic effects brought about by IA, by investigating the effects of the eliminated antibodies in isolated rat cardiomyocytes [18]. We employed confocal laser scanning microscopy to analyze the effects of DCM antibodies on cell contraction and on Ca^{2+}-dependent fluorescence in isolated field-stimulated rat cardiomyocytes. The antibodies that we obtained from the blood of healthy donors (controls) had no effect on Ca^{2+} transients or on cardiomyocyte cell shortening. In contrast, the antibodies from DCM patients obtained during the initial regeneration cycle of the first IA session immediately elicited a decrease in Ca^{2+} transients and cell shortening that was a function of concentration. The acute hemodynamic enhancement determined in patients correlated well with the cardiodepressant influence of DCM antibodies on isolated cardiomyocytes [18]. Detection of cardiodepressant antibodies in plasma of DCM patients prior to IA could serve as predictor of the possible efficacy of this therapeutic approach. We therefore carried out a subsequent investigation to study systematically, for the first time, and in a relatively large patient cohort whether detection of the cardiodepressant effects of antibodies as determined in patients' plasma prior to IA can successfully predict acute, long-term hemodynamic enhancement during IA [19]. Since, moreover, IA successfully removes cardiac autoantibodies from plasma, a technique of this type enables assessment of the role played by the humoral immune system in cardiac dysfunction among DCM patients. Our investigation revealed that, in the majority of DCM patients, it is possible to detect functionally active autoantibodies. Interestingly, we determined that IA elicits advantageous effects in this subgroup of DCM patients alone. The presence of cardiodepressant antibodies accordingly serves as predictor of acute and long-lasting hemodynamic benefits during IA. The results of our investigation indicate that the humoral immune system, with production of circulating antibodies, can play a significant role in cardiac dysfunction for the majority of DCM patients [19].

In a following study, we investigated the mechanisms of the functional effects induced by the DCM antibodies on cardiomyocytes. The data of this study suggests that DCM IgGs, while binding to their respective cardiac epitopes via their Fab parts, induce their negative inotropic effects via their Fc part by binding to the newly detected Fc_γ receptor IIa on cardiomyocytes (fig. 2). In this study, for the first time Fc_γ receptors IIa were detected on human and rat cardiomyocytes (fig. 3). Fc_γ receptors IIa can induce an activating signal via their cytoplasmic domains, thereby possibly triggering the negative inotropic effect [20].

In hematopoietic cells, activation of Fc_γ receptor IIa induces an increase of intracellular calcium levels via tyrosine kinase pathways [21]. Inhibition of the cardiosuppressant effects of DCM antibodies by the tyrosin kinase inhibitor 4-amino-5-(4-chlorophenyl)-7-(t-butyl)pyrazolo[3,4-d]pyrimidine (PP2) provides further evidence of an important role of Fc_γ receptors IIa in DCM. The proposed model of Fc_γ receptor-dependent activation of cardiomyocytes by DCM autoantibodies provides an explanation of why antibodies directed against different antigens on cardiomyocytes can induce the same functional effects. However, we can merely speculate about the potential role of the interaction between antibodies and the Fc_γ receptor on the pathogenesis of DCM. This study has parallel implications with respect to another severe immune-mediated disorder in cardiovascular medicine: heparin-induced thrombocytopenia [22]. In heparin-induced thrombocytopenia, antibodies are generated against the self protein, platelet factor 4, when platelet factor 4 forms multimolecular complexes with heparin [23]. This results in immune complexes that activate platelets

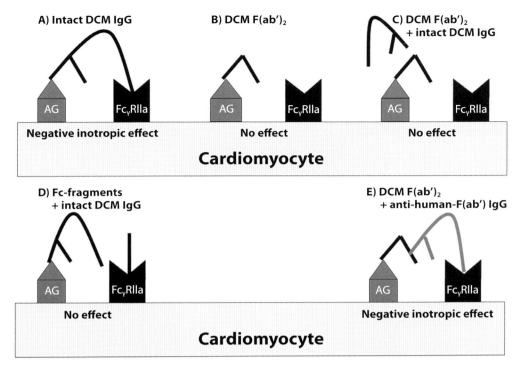

Fig. 2. Intact IgG of DCM patients induced negative inotropic effects by binding via their Fab part to the antigenic epitope on cardiomyocytes and then via their Fc part to the Fc$_\gamma$ receptor IIa (Fc$_\gamma$R) (A). The F(ab')$_2$ fragments of these antibodies inhibited the effect of intact DCM IgG (B), as did Fc fragments of normal IgG (C). Reconstitution of Fc parts by sequential incubation of cardiomyocytes with DCM F(ab')$_2$ fragments and goat anti-human F(ab) IgG induced a negative inotropic effect (D) comparable to findings for intact DCM IgG [20]. AG = antigen.

by cross-linking their Fc$_\gamma$ receptors IIa. Intravascular activation of platelets results in enhanced thrombin generation and can lead to catastrophic thromboembolic complications [24].

It is feasible that IA not merely enhances hemodynamics but likewise influences myocardial inflammation in patients with DCM. We accordingly conducted a randomized study to investigate the immunohistological changes induced by IA therapy and subsequent IgG substitution. This study was performed in four courses, at 1-month intervals, in patients with DCM, and in comparison with controls without immunomodulatory therapy [25]. We conducted immunohistological analysis by performing right ventricular biopsies obtained from all patients: at baseline and after 3 months. Among control patients, the number of lymphocytes (CD3, CD4, and CD8) and of leucocyte common antigen (LCA)-positive cells in the myocardium maintained stability throughout 3 months. We moreover determined no alteration in expression of human leukocyte antigen (HLA) class II. In contrast, IA therapy and subsequent IgG substitution effected an appreciable reduction in lymphocytes and

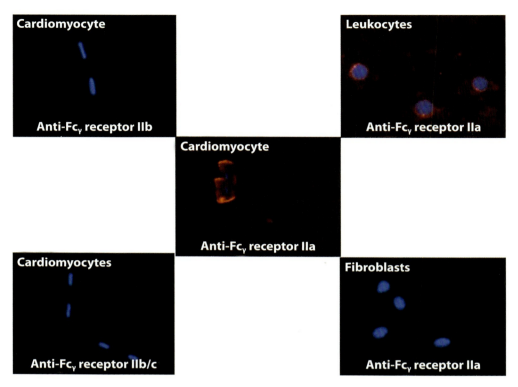

Fig. 3. Immunofluorescent staining of isolated rat cardiomyocytes with a rhodamine-conjugated bovine anti-goat secondary antibody after pre-incubation with polyclonal goat primary antibodies against Fc_γ receptor IIa, Fc_γ receptor IIb, or Fc_γ receptor IIb/c. Immunofluorescence of fibroblasts and rat leukocytes with a rhodamine-conjugated bovine anti-goat secondary antibody after pre-incubation with polyclonal goat primary antibodies against Fc_γ receptor IIa served as negative and positive control subjects, respectively (counterstaining with 4',6-diamidino-2-phenylindole, dilactate (DAPI); representative figures of n = 6 experiments for each antibody) [20].

LCA-positive cells in the myocardium within the follow-up period: a finding paralleled by a significant reduction in HLA class II antigen expression [25] (fig. 4).

Immunological differences prevail throughout the IgG subclasses: Complement activation, for example, is most successful with IgG-3. Long-term IgG-mediated complement activation in myocardial tissue may play a role in promoting development of DCM. The significance of the action of IgG-3 autoantibodies in cardiac dysfunction in DCM patients has not yet been elucidated. A recent study that employed protein A and anti-IgG columns for IA has suggested that antibodies belonging to IgG-3 could exert a pathogenic influence in DCM [26]. Protein A binds with high affinity to the Fc part of human IgG-1, -2, and -4, and the affinity of protein A to IgG-3 is about 10 times less pronounced than to the other subclasses. The less effective removal of IgG-3 by protein A could consequently exhibit hemodynamic effects unlike those observed for anti-IgG adsorption – which effectively eliminates total IgG, including sub-

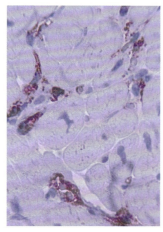

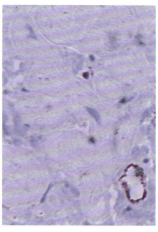

HLA-class II antigen
before IA/IgG therapy

HLA-class II antigen
post IA/IgG therapy

Fig. 4. Changes in HLA class II antigen expression of the same patient before and after 3 months of therapy with IA and subsequent IgG substitution (magnification × 400) [25].

class IgG-3. Unlike work with IA that employs anti-IgG columns, we determined no change of left ventricular function throughout follow-up in DCM patients receiving protein A IA with ineffective reduction in IgG-3 [26]. This investigation indicates that antibodies belonging to IgG-3 could play a key role in cardiac dysfunction in DCM patients. A following study has disclosed that protein A IA – with administration of an enhanced therapy regime for IgG-3 removal – effects hemodynamic enhancement in DCM patients [27]. These results verify the possible importance for DCM of autoantibodies belonging to IgG-3.

Conclusions and Future Directions

The findings from the studies cited above suggest that activation of the humoral immune system, with production of cardiac autoantibodies, could play a functional role in the cardiac dysfunction of DCM patients. Influencing the humoral immune system through IA could therefore offer a hopeful treatment approach in DCM for intervention in this autoimmune process. A large-scale multicenter study would, however, be required to elucidate the effects of IA on the morbidity and mortality of DCM patients.

Disclosure of Conflict of Interests

Various studies were supported by grants from the German Research Foundation (DFG) and by Fresenius Medical Care.

References

1 Roger VL, Weston SA, Redfield MM, Hellermann-Homan JP, Killian J, Yawn BP, Jacobsen SJ: Trends in heart failure incidence and survival in a community-based population. JAMA 2004;292:344–350.

2 Schulze K, Becker BF, Schauer R, Schultheiss HP: Antibodies to ADP-ATP carrier – an autoantigen in myocarditis and dilated cardiomyopathy – impair cardiac function. Circulation 1990;81:959–969.

3 Caforio AL, Grazzini M, Mann JM, Keeling PJ, Bottazzo GF, McKenna WJ, Schiaffino S: Identification of alpha- and beta-cardiac myosin heavy chain isoforms as major autoantigens in dilated cardiomyopathy. Circulation 1992;5:1734–1742.

4 Limas CJ, Goldenberg IF, Limas C: Autoantibodies against beta-adrenoceptors in human idiopathic dilated cardiomyopathy. Circ Res 1989;64:97–103.

5 Magnusson Y, Wallukat G, Waagstein F, Hjalmarson A, Hoebeke J: Autoimmunity in idiopathic dilated cardiomyopathy. Characterization of antibodies against the beta 1-adrenoceptor with positive chronotropic effect. Circulation 1994;89:2760–2767.

6 Fu LX, Magnusson Y, Bergh CH, Liljeqvist JA, Waagstein F, Hjalmarson A, Hoebeke J: Localization of a functional autoimmune epitope on the muscarinic acetylcholine receptor-2 in patients with idiopathic dilated cardiomyopathy. J Clin Invest 1993;91:1964–1968.

7 Schultheiss HP, Kuhl U, Janda I, Melzner B, Ulrich G, Morad M: Antibody-mediated enhancement of calcium permeability in cardiac myocytes. J Exp Med 1988;168:2102–2119.

8 Matsui S, Fu MLX, Katsuda S, Hayase M, Yamaguchi N, Teraoka K, Kurihara T, Takekoshi N, Murakami E, Hoebeke J, Hjalmarson A: Peptides derived from cardiovascular G-protein-coupled receptors induce morphological cardiomyopathic changes in immunized rabbits. J Mol Cell Cardiol 1997;29:641–655.

9 Jahns R, Boivin V, Hein L, Triebel S, Angermann CE, Ertl G, Lohse MJ: Direct evidence for a beta 1-adrenergic receptor-directed autoimmune attack as a cause of idiopathic dilated cardiomyopathy. J Clin Invest 2004;113:1419–1429.

10 Nishimura H, Okazaki T, Tanaka Y, Nakatani K, Hara M, Matsumori A, Sasayama S, Mizoguchi A, Hiai H, Minato N, Honjo T: Autoimmune dilated cardiomyopathy in PD-1 receptor-deficient mice. Science 2001;291:319–322.

11 Okazaki T, Tanaka Y, Nishio R, Mtsuiye T, Mizoguchi A, Wang J, Ishida M, Hiai H, Matsumori A, Minato N, Honjo T: Autoantibodies against troponin-I are responsible for dilated cardiomyopathy in PD-1 deficient mice. Nat Med 2003;9:1477–1483.

12 Göser S, Andrassy M, Buss SJ, Leuschner F, Volz CH, Ottl R, Zittrich S, Blaudeck N, Hardt SE, Pfitzer G, Rose NR, Katus HA, Kaya Z: Cardiac troponin I but not cardiac troponin T induces severe autoimmune inflammation in the myocardium. Circulation 2006;114:1693–1702.

13 Caforio AL, Mahon NG, Baig MK, Tona F, Murphy RT, Elliot PM, McKenna WJ: Prospective familial assessment in dilated cardiomyopathy: Cardiac autoantibodies predict disease development in asymptomatic relatives. Circulation 2007;115:76–83.

14 Dorffel WV, Felix SB, Wallukat G, Brehme S, Bestvater K, Hofmann T, Kleber FX, Baumann G, Reinke P: Short-term hemodynamic effects of immunoadsorption in dilated cardiomyopathy. Circulation 1997;95:1994–1997.

15 Felix SB, Staudt A, Dorffel WV, Stangl V, Merkel K, Pohl M, Döcke WD, Morgera S, Neumayer HH, Wernecke KD, Wallukat G, Stangl K, Baumann G: Hemodynamic effects of immunoadsorption and subsequent immunoglobulin substitution in dilated cardiomyopathy: three-month results from a randomized study. J Am Coll Cardiol 2000;35:1590–1598.

16 Muller J, Wallukat G, Dandel M, Bieda H, Brandes K, Spiegelsberger S, Nissen E, Kunze R, Hetzer R: Immunoglobulin adsorption in patients with idiopathic dilated cardiomyopathy. Circulation 2000;101:385–391.

17 Staudt A, Hummel A, Ruppert J, Dorr M, Trimpert C, Birkenmeier K, Krieg T, Staudt Y, Felix SB: Immunoadsorption in dilated cardiomyopathy: 6-month results from a randomized study. Am Heart J 2006;152:712.e1–6.

18 Felix SB, Staudt A, Landsberger M, Grosse Y, Stangl V, Spielhagen T, Wallukat G, Wernecke KD, Baumann G, Stangl K: Removal of cardiodepressant antibodies in dilated cardiomyopathy by immunoadsorption. J Am Coll Cardiol 2002;39:646–652.

19 Staudt A, Staudt Y, Dörr M, Böhm M, Knebel F, Hummel A, Wunderle L, Tiburcy M, Wernecke KD, Baumann G, Felix SB: Potential role of humoral immunity in cardiac dysfunction of patients suffering from dilated cardiomyopathy. J Am Coll Cardiol 2004;44:829–836.

20 Staudt A, Eichler P, Trimpert C, Felix SB, Greinacher A: Fc_γ receptors IIa on cardiomyocytes and their potential functional relevance in dilated cardiomyopathy. J Am Coll Cardiol 2007;49,1684–1692.

21 Shen Z, Lin CT, Unkeless JC: Correlations among tyrosine phosphorylation of Shc, p72syk, PLC-gamma 1, and $[Ca^{2+}]_i$ flux in Fc gamma RIIA signaling. J Immunol 1994;152:3017–3023.

22 Warkentin TE, Greinacher A: Heparin-induced thrombocytopenia: recognition, treatment, and prevention: the Seventh ACCP Conference on Antithrombotic and Thrombolytic Therapy. Chest 2004;126:311S–37S.

23 Greinacher A, Potzsch B, Amiral J, Dummel V, Eichner A, Mueller-Eckhardt C: Heparin-associated thrombocytopenia: isolation of the antibody and characterization of a multimolecular PF4-heparin complex as the major antigen. Thromb Haemost 1994;71:247–251.

24 Greinacher A, Eichler P, Lubenow N, Kwasny H, Luz M: Heparin-induced thrombocytopenia with thromboembolic complications: meta-analysis of 2 prospective trials to assess the value of parenteral treatment with lepirudin and its therapeutic aPTT range. Blood 2000;96:846–851.

25 Staudt A, Schaper F, Stangl V, Plagemann A, Bohm M, Merkel K, Wallukat G, Wernecke KD, Stangl K, Baumann G, Felix SB: Immunohistological changes in dilated cardiomyopathy induced by immunoadsorption therapy and subsequent immunoglobulin substitution. Circulation 2001;103:2681–2686.

26 Staudt A, Böhm M, Knebel F, Grosse Y, Bischoff C, Hummel A, Dahm JB, Borges A, Jochmann N, Wernecke KD, Wallukat G, Baumann G, Felix SB: Potential role of autoantibodies belonging to the immunoglobulin G-3 subclass in cardiac dysfunction among patients suffering from dilated cardiomyopathy. Circulation 2002;106:2448–2453.

27 Staudt A, Dörr M, Staudt Y, Böhm M, Probst M, Empen K, Plötz S, Maschke HE, Hummel A, Baumann G, Felix SB: Role of immunoglobulin G-3 subclass in dilated cardiomyopathy – results from protein-A immunoadsorption. Am Heart J 2005;150:729–736.

Alexander Staudt, M.D.
Klinik für Innere Medizin B, Medizinische Fakultät
Ernst-Moritz-Arndt-Universität
Loefflerstr. 23a, 17487 Greifswald, Germany
Tel. +49 3834 86-7322, Fax -5609
E-Mail staudt@uni-greifswald.de

Scharf RE (ed): Progress and Challenges in Transfusion Medicine, Hemostasis and Hemotherapy.
Freiburg i.Br., Karger, 2008, pp 132–150

Therapeutic Use of Circulating Peripheral Blood Stem Cells

Rainer Haas · Ingmar Bruns · Guido Kobbe · Ralf Kronenwett

Clinic for Hematology, Oncology and Clinical Immunology, Heinrich Heine University Düsseldorf, Germany

Key Words

CD34+ cells mobilization · Autologous and allogeneic blood stem cell transplantation · Granulocyte colony-stimulating factor (G-CSF) · Very late antigen-4 (VLA-4) · Integrin antagonists · Chemokine receptors

Summary

Hematopoietic stem cells from peripheral blood or bone marrow are characterized by the surface expression of the CD34 antigen. They are commonly used for autologous or allogeneic transplantation following high-dose therapy in patients with malignant diseases of the lymphohematopoietic system. The availability of hematopoietic growth factors such as granulocyte colony-stimulating factor (G-CSF) was an essential prerequisite for the mobilization of CD34+ cells. The molecular processes effective in the context of blood stem cell mobilization are only partially deciphered. It is a complex process with a crosstalk between hematopoietic growth factors, cytokines, and adhesion molecules. In this review, the role of these various cellular and matrix components involved in mobilization and homing of CD34+ cells will be addressed. We will also describe factors influencing the cytokine-induced mobilization in patients and healthy donors. The review closes with an overview of new classes of mobilizing drugs such as monoclonal antibodies or small molecules targeting adhesion molecules.   ©2008 S. Karger GmbH, Freiburg i.Br.

Introduction

High-dose therapy followed by the transplantation of autologous or allogeneic CD34+ peripheral blood stem cells (PBSC) provides a potentially curative treatment for patients with hematological malignancies. In principle, there are different methods in order to mobilize hematopoietic stem and progenitor cells into the peripheral blood (PB). At the time being, the preferred modality is the administration of hematopoietic growth factors (HGF) such as granulocyte colony-stimulating growth factor (G-CSF), which can be given during either steady-state hematopoiesis or following different kinds of disease-related cytotoxic chemotherapy. In this setting, G-CSF enforces the rebound of circulating progenitor cells during the period of hematological recovery

[1, 2]. The mechanisms underlying the process of PBSC mobilization are only partially unravelled. It is a complex process characterized by enhanced proliferation of early hematopoietic stem and progenitor cells, which ultimately migrate through the endothelial barrier within the bone marrow (BM) to enter the blood stream. Adhesive forces are effective between the CD34[+] hematopoietic stem cells (HSC) and progenitors with mesenchymal cells and matrix components of the BM environment. Trafficking of stem cells not only occurs because of cytokine-supported BM recovery following cytotoxic chemotherapy, but constantly during normal steady-state hematopoiesis. Thus, small amounts of CD34[+] cells are always circulating in the PB permitting a continuous migration and exchange of HSC between BM and other organs such as liver or spleen. In the following, we will give an overview of the role of HGF and adhesion molecules for mobilization and homing of CD34[+] cells. In this context, we will also address new modalities of stem cell mobilization such as the targeting of integrins with monoclonal antibodies or the interference with chemokine receptors by small molecules. Ultimately, the use of blood-derived HSC for autologous and allogeneic transplantation will be addressed.

Role of Adhesion Molecules for Mobilization and Homing of CD34[+] Cells

Adhesive interactions between HSC and components of the BM microenvironment are pivotal for migration, circulation, and proliferation of hematopoietic stem and progenitor cells [3–5]. In part, the receptors and ligands involved are members of the β1 and β2 integrin, selectin, and superimmunoglobulin families. These molecules were first described and functionally evaluated in mature leukocytes mostly in the context of inflammation [6–11] (fig. 1). Some of the corresponding ligands are found on endothelial cells or accessory marrow cells. The binding partners may also represent compounds of the extracellular matrix of the BM microenvironment. These interactions are of particular relevance within the BM niche, a specialized location for the lifelong maintenance of the most primitive hematopoietic stem cell population. The BM contains stromal cells that support hematopoiesis including the production of cytokines, such as c-Kit ligand, that stimulate stem cells and progenitors. Cytokines, including interleukins, thrombopoietin (TPO), and erythropoietin (EPO), also influence progenitor function and survival. The examination of *Drosophila* testes and ovarian stem cells provided the basis for concepts of functional niches in other tissues and species [12]. For instance, in the testis, an apical hub cell is found which binds the ligand Upd. The latter one activates the JAK-STAT (Janus kinases, JAKs; signal transducers and activators of transcription, STATs) signaling pathway in neighboring germ cells to regulate their self-renewal. Along this line of reasoning, the concept of the niche within adult BM has emerged. An essential finding was made by Calvi et al. [13] and Zhang et al. [14] demonstrating that mutant mice with a disrupted bone morphogenetic protein (BMP) pathway develop increased numbers of osteoblasts and

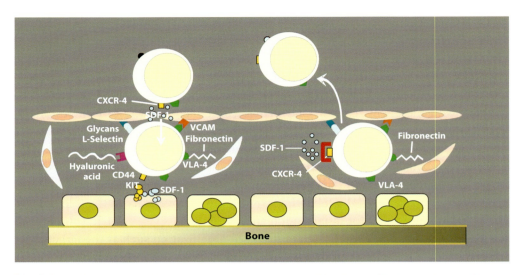

Fig. 1. Role of adhesion molecules and their ligands for mobilization of CD34+ hematopoietic stem cells. SDF-1 = Stromal-derived factor-1; VCAM = vascular cell adhesion molecule; VLA-4 = very late antigen-4.

HSC. These observations imply that osteoblasts apparently represent central components of the BM niche for HSC. Based on findings made by intravital microscopy, HSC are found in the periosteal region of calverium marrow [15], while transplanted GFP-marked or LacZ-marked HSC preferentially lodge close to osteoblasts. Other factors and stroma components such as ligands for Notch receptors and N-cadherin are provided by osteoblasts. Still, their role and contribution to adult hematopoiesis awaits further elucidation. The relevance of N-cadherin as the partner for interactions with osteoblasts [14] and the significance of osteoblasts for HSC adhesion are still not clear [16]. In particular, the concept of the osteoblastic niche has to be reconciled with recent findings placing HSC near vascular cells. Within this model, the chemokine CXCL12 (stromal-derived factor-1, SDF-1) stipulates the migration of HSC to the vascular cells now called the vascular niche [17]. In the light of these findings, one would assume that HSC reside in different sites within the marrow cavity, whereby their functional state and cellular fate might depend on their localization. Some of these seemingly conflicting findings could lose their functional relevance in case that osteoblastic and vascular niche are connected and not entirely separated from each other. It is also conceivable that HSC are truly sitting in distinct subregions, which may be associated with different activities or subset composition. The understanding of the cellular processes within the niche is of greatest interest, particularly in the light of blood stem cell transplantation. For instance, recent results of animal studies suggest that antibody-mediated irradiation of HSC from the recipient facilitates admission to the niche and engraftment of the donor-derived HSC [18].

In the following, we will highlight some of the receptors and ligands of the BM microenvironment, which play a role in migration and homing of HSC. For instance, L-selectin (CD62L) recognizes carbohydrate residues on endothelial cells and mediates the initial attachment of leukocytes to endothelial cells. It is highly expressed on circulating CD34+ stem and progenitor cells, implying an essential role for homing of stem cells following transplantation [19]. The ß1 integrins very late antigen-4 (VLA-4, CD29/CD49d) and VLA-5 (CD29/CD49e) are important candidates permitting adhesion of hematopoietic progenitor cells to components of the BM stroma. In particular, the VLA-4-mediated interaction between HSC and BM stroma is of functional relevance for hematopoiesis as well as for mobilization and homing of CD34+ cells [4, 20–22]. We observed that circulating CD34+ cells express VLA-4 at a lower level in comparison to CD34+ cells in the BM. The release of CD34+ cells and their migratory capacity is apparently related to the presence and expression level of VLA-4 [4, 19, 23–26]. This is in line with the finding that systemic treatment of primates and mice with monoclonal antibodies directed against VLA-4 led to a significant increase of circulating hematopoietic progenitor cells [27–30]. Antibody treatment of mice resulted in engraftment failure of HSC [31]. The adhesive properties of CD34+ cells are not only affected by the expression level but also depend on the functional state of the integrins. Changes of the functional state of integrins are known for other physiological processes such as platelet aggregation [32, 33], cell migration [34], and embryonic development [35]. Looking at the activation state of VLA-4 on CD34+ cells from BM and PB by flow cytometry using a vascular cell adhesion molecule I-immunoglobulin (VCAM-I/IgG) fusion protein as soluble ligand [26], we observed a significantly reduced functional state of the VLA-4 receptor on circulating CD34+ cells from PB during G-CSF-enhanced marrow recovery in comparison to CD34+ cells from steady-state BM. The number of circulating CD34+ cells during marrow recovery was inversely related to the activation state and not to the expression level of VLA-4. This finding implies that the functional state of VLA-4 is altered in circulating CD34+ cells. The mechanisms mediating the inactivation of VLA-4 on circulating CD34+ cells are not clear. On the other hand, we observed that Mg^{2+} ions or contact with endothelial cells led to an activation of the VLA-4 receptor. We therefore concluded that changes in the Mg^{2+} concentration close to the VLA-4 receptor change its activity on CD34+ cells located along the endothelial cells. Besides VLA-4, the ß2 integrin leukocyte function-associated molecule-1 (LFA-1, CD18/CD11a) is also involved in interactions between CD34+ hematopoietic progenitor cells and BM stroma. The ligands of LFA-1 are the members of the superimmunoglobulin family intercellular adhesion molecule (ICAM)-1 and ICAM-2. On circulating CD34+ cells, LFA-1 had a lower expression level in comparison to BM [19]. Functionally, the adhesion to and migration through an endothelial cell layer could be inhibited using LFA-1-directed blocking monoclonal antibodies [19, 36]. There is also a relevant interaction between cell adhesion and signal transduction pathways stimulated by cytokines [37]. Along this line, stem cell factor (SCF), granulocyte-macrophage colony-stimulating factor

(GM-CSF), or interleukin-3 (IL-3) are capable of transiently enhancing the adhesiveness of CD34$^+$ cells via activation of the integrins VLA-4 and VLA-5 [38, 39]. The resulting contact between HSC and stroma is associated with a stronger proliferative effect, i.e., a positive feedback loop is triggered [40]. The need for integrin activation via adhesion could explain why circulating CD34$^+$ cells lacking contact to BM stroma are mainly quiescent cells in the G_0/G_1 phase of the cell cycle.

Other adhesion molecules relevant in the context of mobilization and homing are the platelet endothelial cell adhesion molecule-1 (PECAM-1) and CD44. The latter one is a highly glycosylated surface molecule with at least 10 isoforms resulting from differences in glycosylation and alternative splicing. It is strongly expressed on CD34$^+$ hematopoietic stem and progenitor cells. The ligands of CD44, hyaluronic acid and fibronectin, are components of the stromal microenvironment. Monoclonal antibodies directed against CD44 lower the adhesion of CD34$^+$ cells to BM stroma, induce the mobilization of progenitor cells in mice, and prevent hematopoiesis in long-term BM cultures [41–45].

Beside growth factors and adhesion molecules, the alpha chemokine CXCL12/ SDF-1 plays a relevant role in blood stem cell migration [46]. The cellular receptor of SDF-1 is CXCR-4, which functions as coreceptor for T-cell-tropic HIV-1 strains [47]. CXCR-4 is expressed in CD34$^+$ cells dependent on the degree of differentiation. The subset of CD34$^+$/CD38^{low} and CD34$^+$/human leukocyte antigen (HLA)-DR^{low} cells, representing a population of more immature progenitor cells, stains brightly positive for CXCR-4, whereas a lower level of CXCR-4 expression was observed in the population of CD34$^+$/CD38^{bright} and CD34$^+$/HLA-DR^{bright} cells [48, 49]. SDF-1 acts as chemoattractant for HSC [46, 50, 51].

Role of Cytokines in the Mobilization of Peripheral Blood Stem Cells

Currently, HGF are used for the mobilization of PBSC. The two prototype growth factors in question are G-CSF and GM-CSF, which primarily mediate the differentiation of myeloid progenitors into mature granulocytes and monocytes, respectively. Small quantities of the receptor for G-CSF and GM-CSF are found on the more primitive progenitor cells, while an increasing receptor density is noted during myeloid or myelomonocytic differentiation [52–54]. Interestingly, the G-CSF receptor is also expressed on stromal cells of the BM. This could be of relevance for our understanding of the mobilization process as it could be shown in a mouse model that the expression of the G-CSF receptor on CD34$^+$ cells is not required for their ability to circulate upon exposure to G-CSF. This finding implies that G-CSF may not affect the primitive hematopoietic progenitor cell directly, but via receptors on cells of the BM stroma [55]. Most recently, it could be shown that adrenalin mediates downregulation of CXCL12 via β2-adrenergic receptors on osteoblasts, which results in an increased release of stem cells [56].

As GM-CSF was made available for clinical use somehow earlier than G-CSF, our first studies addressing the mobilizing ability of HGF were carried out using GM-CSF. In a group of 11 patients with different types of hematological malignancies and a history of extensive previous cytotoxic chemotherapy, we observed an approximately 18-fold increase of circulating colony-forming units granulocyte-macrophage (CFU-GM) in comparison to baseline values. Of note, these patients received the cytokine during steady-state hematopoiesis. An even 5-fold greater enhancement was observed when GM-CSF was administered following cytotoxic chemotherapy to increase the natural rebound of circulating CD34$^+$ cells during hematopoietic recovery [57]. Looking at the groundbreaking studies performed with G-CSF, a dose-dependent increase of CFU-GM was found when G-CSF was given during steady-state hematopoiesis for four days [1]. The greatest increase of CFU-GM was 100-fold more in comparison to baseline level. In principle, these findings were confirmed by several other groups in patients with hematological malignancies, a variety of solid tumors such as breast cancer or healthy volunteers [58–63]. Looking at the mobilizing capacity of G-CSF in comparison to GM-CSF, no significant difference became apparent between these two growth factors [64, 65]. In our first study, there was an 8.5-fold increase of CFU-GM in the PB over baseline when GM-CSF was administered as continuous intravenous infusion (250 µg/m^2/day). The patients included into this phase I/II study were extensively pretreated and not eligible for BM harvesting because of radiotherapy to the sites of BM harvesting [66]. The relatively moderate mobilization effect induced by GM-CSF was presumably a consequence of the great amount of previous cytotoxic chemo- and radiotherapy. As noted earlier, in the following studies PBSC mobilization was performed in the context of a cytotoxic chemotherapy. This kind of PBSC mobilization is generally associated with a lower likelihood of harvesting malignant cells, particularly if the malignancy proved to be chemosensitive [2, 67–69]. The advantage of a chemotherapy-based PBSC mobilization is best reflected by the data of a study with an intraindividual comparison. In that setting we observed a 7-fold greater yield of CD34$^+$ cells per leukapheresis after G-CSF-supported chemotherapy compared with steady-state administration of G-CSF at a dose of 5 µg/kg/day [70]. We assume that a greater endogenous G-CSF serum level is effective in the period of chemotherapy-induced neutropenia and therefore less exogenous G-CSF might be required [71, 72]. The situation is different during steady-state hematopoiesis when greater amounts of myeloid precursor cells and mature neutrophils are present to bind G-CSF via high-affinity receptors, ultimately leading to a reduction of bioavailable G-CSF [73]. Thus, since during steady-state hematopoiesis the cellularity of the BM and the number of neutrophils with binding sites for G-CSF are greater than post-chemotherapy, a greater amount of G-CSF is necessary to ensure saturation of the expressed receptors.

Despite the vast amount of data available, there is still no generally accepted recommendation as far as dose and schedule for the administration of G-CSF or GM-CSF are concerned. During steady-state mobilization in normal donors for allogeneic

PBSC transplantation, significantly higher peak levels of circulating CD34$^+$ cells were noted when the daily dose of G-CSF (filgrastim) was 10 µg instead of 3 or 5 µg/kg [74]. The same finding was made when the dose of glycosylated G-CSF (lenograstim) was enhanced from 3, 5, and 7.5 to 10 µg/kg/day in healthy volunteers [75]. The picture is quite different in case of G-CSF administration following cytotoxic chemotherapy. Under those circumstances, no relationship was found between the dose of G-CSF and the peak level of circulating CD34$^+$ cells [76]. Even an increase of the G-CSF dose to 23 µg/kg was not more effective in comparison with a dose of 2.8 µg/kg. As an explanation for this phenomenon, we favor the idea that endogenous serum concentrations of G-CSF post-chemotherapy are sufficiently high to reach a saturation level as soon as the relatively low dose of 2.8 µg/kg is given.

We and other groups looked for differences between CD34$^+$ cells from BM and PB during G-CSF-enhanced marrow recovery and found a 3.7-fold greater peak concentration of CD34$^+$ cells in the PB during G-CSF-supported recovery in comparison with BM samples from steady-state hematopoiesis [77]. Independent of the method of mobilization, the vast majority of circulating CD34$^+$ cells is in the G_0/G_1 phase of the cell cycle suggesting that contact with the BM stroma is a prerequisite for proliferation of hematopoietic progenitor cells [78]. PB during G-CSF treatment contains a greater proportion of more primitive CD34$^+$ cells as indicated by functional assays enumerating the long-term culture-initiating cells and pre-CFU-GM [79]. These data could be confirmed by immunophenotypical findings demonstrating that a greater proportion of mobilized PBSC expressed the early stem cell-associated antigen Thy-1 in comparison with BM [77]. These data provide a strong line of arguments for the use of blood-derived progenitor cells rather than BM for autologous or allogeneic transplantation, since early hematopoietic progenitor cells are particularly relevant for long-term hematopoiesis following high-dose or even myeloablative conditioning therapy. It should be also noted that mobilized CD34$^+$ cells differ from BM CD34$^+$ cells also with regard to their lower expression of c-Kit and CD45RA [77, 80]. The composition of PBSC also depends on whether G-CSF is given during steady-state hematopoiesis or following cytotoxic chemotherapy [70]. In a study including patients with acute leukemia, Hodgkin's disease, non-Hodgkin's lymphoma, or multiple myeloma, the amount of CD34$^+$ cells collected post-chemotherapy was 5.7-fold greater in comparison with PBSC harvest obtained during steady state. In particular, the mean proportion of more primitive CD34$^+$ progenitors lacking HLA-DR or CD38 expression was smaller in patients with PBSC collection following G-CSF-supported chemotherapy than during steady-state mobilization. Still, considering the greater number of CD34$^+$ cells mobilized in total, the absolute amount of CD34$^+$/HLA-DR$^-$ cells was still 2.3-fold greater post-chemotherapy. On the other hand, the proportion of lineage-committed CD34$^+$/CD33$^+$ cells was significantly enhanced post-chemotherapy in comparison with steady-state mobilization. These data are in line with findings of another group showing that CD34$^+$ cells mobilized following G-CSF during steady state contained a greater proportion of CD38$^-$ cells than CD34$^+$ cells mobilized by other regimens [81].

Similarly, adhesion molecules are also differentially expressed on CD34+ cells from PB and BM. We examined this aspect on a molecular level. For that purpose we assessed in 18 volunteers the gene expressions of 1,185 genes in highly enriched BM CD34+ (BM-CD34+) or G-CSF-mobilized PB CD34+ (PB-CD34+) cells by means of cDNA array technology to identify molecular causes underlying the functional differences between circulating and sedentary hematopoietic stem and progenitor cells. In total, 65 genes were significantly differentially expressed. Greater cell cycle and DNA synthesis activity of BM-CD34+ cells than of PB-CD34+ cells were reflected by the 2- to 5-fold higher expression of 9 genes involved in cell cycle progression, 11 genes regulating DNA synthesis, and cell cycle-initiating transcription factor E2F-1. Conversely, 9 other transcription factors, including the differentiation-blocking GATA2 and N-myc, were expressed 2–3 times higher in PB-CD34+ cells than in BM-CD34+ cells. Expression of 5 apoptosis-driving genes was also 2–3 times greater in PB-CD34+ cells, reflecting a higher apoptotic activity. These data molecularly confirmed and explained the finding that CD34+ cells residing in the BM cycle more rapidly, whereas circulating CD34+ cells consist of a higher number of quiescent stem and progenitor cells [82].

Irrespective of the growth factor used and the particular mode of application there is always a wide variation in the mobilization efficacy between normal volunteers as well as among patients [83]. As far as normal volunteers are concerned, there is an inverse correlation between age and yield of CD34+ cells collected following G-CSF administration [62]. Individual factors or characteristics associated with PBSC mobilization in patients are essentially the dose of cytotoxic chemotherapy administered for mobilization, the underlying disease, and the cumulative amount of previous cytotoxic treatment as well as previous radiotherapy. For instance, administration of 7 g/m^2 cyclophosphamide in comparison with 4 g/m^2 resulted in significantly greater peak levels of CD34+ cells in PB of patients with multiple myeloma [84]. In a retrospective study including 61 patients with lymphoma, we looked for patient-associated factors that may influence the yield of CD34+ cells following G-CSF-supported cytotoxic chemotherapy [68]. We found that previous cytotoxic chemotherapy and irradiation adversely affected the yield of CD34+ cells. As a consequence, we proposed to harvest PBSC as early as possible during the course of the disease to ensure a yield sufficient to support high-dose therapy. With regard to diagnosis, we found that patients with Hodgkin's disease had a significantly smaller collection efficacy in comparison to those with non-Hodgkin's lymphoma. Nevertheless, since the patients with Hodgkin's disease had been irradiated, diagnosis could not be evaluated as an independent variable. On the other hand, patients' characteristics without association to the collection efficacy were age, sex, and disease status. At this point, we would like to stress the view that the observations made in normal donors still argue for an age-associated decrease of the stem and progenitor cell pool. BM involvement at the time of PBSC collection was also not associated with the yield of CD34+ cells.

Following the experience made with G-CSF and GM-CSF, other cytokines such as IL-3, IL-8, IL-11, SCF, flt-3 ligand, or macrophage inflammatory protein-1α (MIP-

1α) were considered potential new candidates for the mobilization of CD34+ cells [85–92]. The ability of these cytokines to increase the number of circulating PBSC when given as single agents was either not superior to that of G-CSF or associated with relevant side effects. For instance, the use of SCF, which also acts on mast cells, was associated with a variety of serious side effects attributable to mast cell degranu-lation. The spectrum of toxicity encountered encompassed edema of the glottis and severe hypotension as observed in an anaphylactic shock. Without being associated with undue toxicity, the sequential administration of IL-3 and GM-CSF in patients with high-grade non-Hodgkin's lymphoma following second-line cytotoxic chemo-therapy had a similar mobilization efficacy when compared with a historical control group of patients who had received G-CSF [87].

Still, progress has been made by a chemical modification of G-CSF, i.e., the pegyla-tion of filgrastim. Different from the original compound, pegfilgrastim is character-ized by a significantly longer half-life because of a substantially reduced renal elimi-nation [93]. In two studies including patients with different types of hematological malignancies, we could demonstrate safety and efficacy of this new drug in mobiliz-ing a sufficient number of CD34+ cells required for at least one autologous transplan-tation. Following induction therapy and 4 g/m^2 cyclophosphamide, a single dose of 12 mg polyethyleneglycol-conjugated G-CSF (pegfilgrastim; n = 12) or daily doses of unconjugated G-CSF (8.5 µg/kg/day; n = 12) were administered to myeloma patients. Pegfilgrastim was associated with an earlier leukocyte recovery (12 vs 14 days) and PB CD34+ cell peak (12 vs 15 days). The PB CD34+ cell peak was lower in the pegfilgras-tim group (78 vs 111/µl). Following high-dose melphalan (200 mg/m^2) and autograft-ing, leukocyte and platelet reconstitution was similar in both groups and stable blood counts were observed 100 days post transplant. Thus, a single dose of pegfilgrastim after chemotherapy is capable of mobilizing a sufficient number of CD34+ cells for successful autografting with early engraftment and sustained hematological reconsti-tution in patients with myeloma [94]. In a subsequent study, the use of pegfilgrastim was examined at two dose levels for peripheral blood progenitor cells (PBPC) mobi-lization in patients with stage II or III multiple myeloma. Four days after cytotoxic therapy with cyclophosphamide (4 g/m^2), a single dose of either 6 mg pegfilgrastim (n = 15) or 12 mg pegfilgrastim (n = 15) or daily doses of 8 µg/kg unconjugated G-CSF (n = 15) were administered. The number of circulating CD34+ cells was determined during white blood cell (WBC) recovery, and PBPC harvesting was performed by large-volume apheresis. Pegfilgrastim was equally potent at 6 and 12 mg with regard to mobilization and yield of CD34+ cells. No dose dependence was observed because CD34+ cell concentration peaks were 131 and 85/µl, respectively, and CD34+ cell yield was 10.2 × 10^6 and 7.4 × 10^6/kg of body weight, respectively. Pegfilgrastim in either dose was associated with a more rapid WBC recovery (p = 0.03) and an earlier per-formance of the first apheresis procedure (p < 0.05) in comparison to unconjugated G-CSF. There was no difference regarding CD34+ cell maximum and yield. We there-fore concluded that a single dose of 6 mg pegfilgrastim is equally potent as 12 mg for

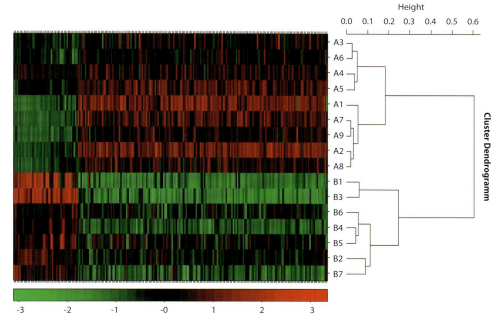

Fig. 2. Hierarchical cluster analysis of Peg-G-CSF- and G-CSF-mobilized CD34$^+$ cell samples on the basis of the differentially expressed genes. The left branch of the dendrogram shows the G-CSF-mobilized samples, and the right branch shows the Peg-G-CSF-mobilized samples. Hierarchical cluster analysis was performed by the hclust function of the 'R' software using an average linkage clustering algorithm. G-CSF = Granulocyte colony-stimulating factor; Peg-G-CSF = pegylated G-CSF.

mobilization and harvest of PBPC in patients with multiple myeloma. Because no dose dependence was seen at these dose levels, this might be also true for even smaller doses. In 3 of 6 patients with insufficient mobilization in response to pegfilgrastim, the additional administration of filgrastim as boost resulted in an adequate increase of CD34$^+$ cells for harvesting. At this point, it is not clear which kind of combinations and schedules might be beneficial particularly in patients with a reduced hematopoietic reserve [95]. In the context of pegfilgrastim, it was interesting to note that the pegfilgrastim-exposed CD34$^+$ cells had a subset composition different from that of filgrastim-mobilized CD34$^+$ cells, i.e., a greater proportion of more primitive CD34$^+$ cells as characterized by the lack of CD38 expression. The different subset composition was accompanied by a significantly different gene expression profile reflecting the preponderance of a more immature CD34$^+$ cell subset on the level of the transcriptome (fig. 2). For instance, the CD34$^+$ cells mobilized by pegylated G-CSF had higher expression levels of genes indicative of early hematopoiesis, including HOXA9, MEIS1, and GATA3. We found lower expression of genes characteristic of erythroid and later stages of myeloid differentiation and a lower functional burst-forming units erythroid (BFU-E)/CFU-GM ratio. Consistently, greater numbers of HSC and common myeloid progenitors and fewer megakaryocyte-erythrocyte progenitors were found in the pegylated-G-CSF-mobilized CD34$^+$ cells. Additionally, sorted pegylated-G-CSF-mobilized HSC displayed higher expression of HOXA9 in comparison to G-CSF-mobilized HSC. In line with the gene expression data, CD34$^+$ cells mobilized by pegylated G-CSF as well as sorted HSC showed a significantly greater cell cycle activity. Thus, stimulation with pegylated G-CSF or G-CSF results in different expression of key regulatory genes and different functional properties of mobilized HSC as well as their progeny, a finding that might be relevant for the application of these cells in blood stem cell transplantation [96].

Fruehauf et al. made a similar observation using the small molecule AMD3100 that is a new CXCR4 antagonist [97]. It induces a rapid release of hematopoietic progenitors from the BM to the PB. They conducted a clinical study where patients with multiple myeloma and non-Hodgkin's lymphoma were treated with AMD3100 (A) to increase the number of PBPC when given a mobilization regimen of G-CSF (G). Because experimental data suggest that A+G-mobilized PBPC are functionally different from G-mobilized PBPC, they performed an intraindividual comparison of the gene expression profile of CD34$^+$ cells in the two different settings. PB CD34$^+$ cells of 3 patients (3 G, 3 A+G samples) were isolated by immunomagnetic followed by flow cytometric sorting. The authors observed a pattern of unanimously higher (81) or lower (29) expressed genes in the A+G-mobilized vs G-mobilized CD34$^+$ PBPC. Genes were grouped according to gene function. Only increased expression was found in the categories antiapoptosis, cell cycle, replication/DNA repair, cell motility, and oxygen transport. Decreased expression occurred in the proapoptosis gene group. CXCR4 receptor gene expression itself was significantly 1.5-fold higher in the A+G vs G group. Apparently, A+G-mobilized CD34$^+$ PBPC express significantly higher amounts of genes that potentially promote superior engraftment after myeloablative therapy than G-mobilized CD34$^+$ PBPC.

Anti-α4- or anti-β2-integrin monoclonal antibodies have already been used for stem cell mobilization in primates [27]. Anti-α4 treatment resulted in a significant increase of circulating hematopoietic progenitor cells with peak levels which were 200-fold over baseline levels within 24 h after injection. In contrast, anti-β2 antibodies had no mobilizing effect. Similar observations were made in mice [28, 29]. The combination of anti-α4 antibodies with either G-CSF or SCF treatment led to a 5- to 8-fold greater mobilization efficacy in comparison with anti-α4 or cytokine treatment alone [28]. These findings indicate a synergistic effect of both mobilizing modalities. Recently, Papayannopoulou et al. showed that peripheralization of progenitor cells using anti-α4 antibodies requires a functional c-Kit/c-Kit ligand pathway [30]. In addition, the increase of hematopoietic progenitors in the blood was associated with a downregulation of c-Kit expression on the cells, suggesting an integrin/cytokine crosstalk during mobilization. In another study, hematopoietic progenitor cells could be mobilized in mice using CD44-directed monoclonal antibodies [98]. Most recently, the group of Papayannopoulou and our group observed in patients with multiple sclerosis who received a treatment with the humanized recombinant antibody natalizumab an increased number of circulating CD34$^+$ cells when compared intraindividually to baseline levels before therapy or in comparison with other patients who received different kinds of treatment [99, 100]. The increased number of CD34$^+$ cells may result from a facilitated release of CD34$^+$ cells from the VCAM-expressing endothelial niche or by a prolonged circulation because of impaired homing due to the lack of VLA-4 mediated transendothelial migration. In animal models, the BM repopulating ability of VLA-4 exposed hematopoietic progenitor cells could be demonstrated [101]. Thus, this antibody provides a new alternative for PBSC mobilization potentially alone or in combination with G-CSF.

Transplantation of Mobilized Peripheral Blood Stem Cells

The ability of PBSC to restore hematopoiesis fully following myeloablative high-dose conditioning was demonstrated by several groups in 1986 [102–105]. Since cytokines were not available at that time, PBSC were either collected during steady-state hematopoiesis without any mobilization aid or following cytotoxic chemotherapy. Transplantation of cytokine-mobilized PBSC and successful hematological reconstitution following marrow ablation were first reported in 1989 [58]. Subsequent studies confirmed unequivocally that cytokine-mobilized PBSC without or following cytotoxic chemotherapy can be used for autografting [2, 66, 67, 69, 106–108]. In these studies, it became apparent that the time needed for hematological recovery and hospitalization was significantly shorter in patients who were autografted using PBSC when compared with BM grafting. At the beginning of PBSC autografting, the number of mononuclear cells or clonogenic progenitors served as surrogate parameter for the characterization of the PBSC grafts. With the introduction of immunofluorescence analyses using directly labeled anti-CD34 antibodies a standardized characterization of PBSC could be developed. Based on this kind of assessment, a minimum number of CD34$^+$ cells emerged as threshold value required for rapid and sustained engraftment. This minimum quantity of CD34$^+$ cells needed for transplantation is generally accepted to lie between 2.5 and 5.0×10^6/kg body weight [2, 108, 109]. In the context of these analyses, a relationship was found between the number of CD34$^+$ cells transplanted and the time required for hematological reconstitution. Not surprisingly, patients who received a greater number of CD34$^+$ cells/kg needed shorter recovery times than patients grafted with a smaller number of CD34$^+$ progenitor cells [2, 110–112].

Following the successful experience made with PBSC in the context of autografting, this source of hematopoietic stem and progenitor cells also serves for allogeneic transplantation [62, 113–115]. Rapid and complete engraftment was obtained with recovery times which were apparently shorter than following allogeneic BM transplantation. There is no doubt that long-term engraftment of donor cells is achieved following allogeneic PBSC transplantation, as cytogenetic and molecular biological examinations have shown. Still, the issue regarding the risk of acute and chronic graft-versus-host disease as well as the induction of a graft-versus-leukemia reaction awaits further clarification.

Conclusions and Future Directions

Hematopoietic growth factors G-CSF or GM-CSF are currently the prototype drugs used for the mobilization of PBSC. A sufficient harvest of HSC including the most primitive ones with a high potential for self-renewal is an essential prerequisite for their successful use for transplantation following high-dose therapy or even myeloablative conditioning regimens. The introduction of other cytokines such as SCF, IL-11, IL-8, or flt-3 ligand was not superior to the 'classical' mobilization factors administered so far. Now, we are witnessing the beginning of a new era with an array of new compounds. This includes the long-lasting pegfilgrastim permitting PBSC mobilization by a single injection as well as the CXCR4 antagonist AMD3100 or the anti-VLA-4 monoclonal antibody natalizumab. The latter two agents are directly interfering with the crosstalk between HGF and adhesion molecules. The inhibition of receptor-ligand interactions may provide a synergistic treatment modality to improve cytokine-based PBSC mobilization.

Disclosure of Conflict of Interests

The authors state that they have no conflict of interest.

References

1 Dührsen U, Villeval JL, Boyd J, Kannourakis G, Morstyn G, Metcalf D: Effects of recombinant human granulocyte colony-stimulating factor on hematopoietic progenitor cells in cancer patients. Blood 1988;72:2074–2081.
2 Hohaus S, Goldschmidt H, Ehrhardt R, Haas R: Successful autografting following myeloablative conditioning therapy with blood stem cells mobilized by chemotherapy plus rhG-CSF. Exp Hematol 1993;21:508–514.
3 Verfaillie C, Hurley R, Bhatia R, McCarthy JB: Role of bone marrow matrix in normal and abnormal hematopoiesis. Crit Rev Oncol Hematol 1994;16:201–224.
4 Prosper F, Stroncek D, McCarthy JB, Verfaillie CM: Mobilization and homing of peripheral blood progenitors is related to reversible downregulation of alpha4 beta1 integrin expression and function. J Clin Invest 1998;101:2456–2467.
5 Whetton AD, Graham GJ: Homing and mobilization in the stem cell niche. Trends Cell Biol 1999;9:233–238.
6 Soligo D, Schiró R, Luksch R, Manara G, Quirici N, Parravicini C, Lambertenghi Deliliers G: Expression of integrins in human bone marrow. Br J Haematol 1990;76:323–332.
7 Verfaillie CM, McCarthy JB, McGlave PB: Differentiation of primitive human multipotent hematopoietic progenitors into single lineage clonogenic progenitors is accompanied by alteration in their interaction with fibronectin. J Exp Med 1991;174:693–703.
8 Simmons PJ, Masinovsky B, Longenecker BM, Berenson R, Torok-Storb B, Gallatin WM: Vascular cell adhesion molecule-1 expressed by bone marrow stromal cells mediates the binding of hematopoietic progenitor cells. Blood 1992;80:388–395.

9   Teixido J, Hemler ME, Greenberger JS, Anklesaria P: Role of beta 1 and beta 2 integrins in the adhesion of human CD34hi stem cells to bone marrow stroma. J Clin Invest 1992;90:358–367.

10 Liesveld JL, Winslow JM, Frediani KE, Ryan DH, Abboud CN: Expression of integrins and examination of their adhesive function in normal and leukemic hematopoietic cells. Blood 1993;81:112–121.

11 Kinashi T, Springer TA: Adhesion molecules in hematopoietic cells. Blood Cells 1994;20:25–44.

12 Decotto E, Spradling AC: The Drosophila ovarian and testis stem cell niches: similar somatic stem cells and signals. Dev Cell 2005;9:501–510.

13 Calvi LM, Adams GB, Weibrecht KW, Weber JM, Olson DP, Knight MC, Martin RP, Schipani E, Divieti P, Bringhurst FR, Milner LA, Kronenberg HM, Scadden DT: Osteoblastic cells regulate the haematopoietic stem cell niche. Nature 2003;425:841–846.

14 Zhang J, Niu C, Ye L, Huang H, He X, Tong WG, Ross J, Haug J, Johnson T, Feng JQ, Harris S, Wiedemann LM, Mishina Y, Li L: Identification of the haematopoietic stem cell niche and control of the niche size. Nature 2003;425:836–841.

15 Sipkins DA, Wei X, Wu JW, Runnels JM, Côté D, Means TK, Luster AD, Scadden DT, Lin CP: In vivo imaging of specialized bone marrow endothelial microdomains for tumour engraftment. Nature 2005;435:969–973.

16 Kiel MJ, Radice GL, Morrison SJ: Lack of evidence that hematopoietic stem cells depend on N-cadherin-mediated adhesion to osteoblasts for their maintenance. Cell Stem Cell 2007;1:204–217.

17 Kiel MJ, Morrison SJ: Maintaining hematopoietic stem cells in the vascular niche. Immunity 2006;25:862–864.

18 Czechowicz A, Kraft D, Weissman IL, Bhattacharya D: Efficient transplantation via antibody-based clearance of hematopoietic stem cell niches. Science 2007;318:1296–1299.

19 Möhle R, Murea S, Kirsch M, Haas R: Differential expression of L-selectin, VLA-4, and LFA-1 on CD34+ progenitor cells from bone marrow and peripheral blood during G-CSF-enhanced recovery. Exp Hematol 1995;23:1535–1542.

20 Miyake K, Weissman IL, Greenberger JS, Kincade PW: Evidence for a role of the integrin VLA-4 in lympho-hemopoiesis. J Exp Med 1991;173:599–607.

21 Yanai N, Sekine C, Yagita H, Obinata M: Roles for integrin very late activation antigen-4 in stroma-dependent erythropoiesis. Blood 1994;83:2844–2850.

22 Hamamura K, Matsuda H, Takeuchi Y, Habu S, Yagita H, Okumura K: A critical role of VLA-4 in erythropoiesis in vivo. Blood 1996;87:2513–2517.

23 Leavesley DI, Oliver JM, Swart BW, Berndt MC, Haylock DN, Simmons PJ: Signals from platelet/endothelial cell adhesion molecule enhance the adhesive activity of the very late antigen-4 integrin of human CD34+ hemopoietic progenitor cells. J Immunol 1994;153:4673–4683.

24 Yamaguchi M, Ikebuchi K, Hirayama F, Sato N, Mogi Y, Ohkawara J, Yoshikawa Y, Sawada K, Koike T, Sekiguchi S: Different adhesive characteristics and VLA-4 expression of CD34(+) progenitors in G0/G1 versus S+G2/M phases of the cell cycle. Blood 1998;92:842–848.

25 Bellucci R, De Propris MS, Buccisano F, Lisci A, Leone G, Tabilio A, de Fabritiis P: Modulation of VLA-4 and L-selectin expression on normal CD34+ cells during mobilization with G-CSF. Bone Marrow Transplant 1999;23:1–8.

26 Lichterfeld M, Martin S, Burkly L, Haas R, Kronenwett R: Mobilization of CD34+ haematopoietic stem cells is associated with a functional inactivation of the integrin very late antigen 4. Br J Haematol 2000;110:71–81.

27 Papayannopoulou T, Nakamoto B: Peripheralization of hemopoietic progenitors in primates treated with anti-VLA4 integrin. Proc Natl Acad Sci U S A 1993;90:9374–9378.

28 Craddock CF, Nakamoto B, Andrews RG, Priestley GV, Papayannopoulou T: Antibodies to VLA4 integrin mobilize long-term repopulating cells and augment cytokine-induced mobilization in primates and mice. Blood 1997;90:4779–4788.

29 Vermeulen M, LePesteur F, Gagnerault MC, Mary JY, Sainteny F, Lepault F: Role of adhesion molecules in the homing and mobilization of murine hematopoietic stem and progenitor cells. Blood 1998;92:894–900.

30 Papayannopoulou T, Priestley GV, Nakamoto B: Anti-VLA4/VCAM-1-induced mobilization requires cooperative signaling through the kit/mkit ligand pathway. Blood 1998;91:2231–2239.

31 Papayannopoulou T, Craddock C, Nakamoto B, Priestley GV, Wolf NS: The VLA4/VCAM-1 adhesion pathway defines contrasting mechanisms of lodgement of transplanted murine hemopoietic progenitors between bone marrow and spleen. Proc Natl Acad Sci U S A 1995;92:9647–9651.

32 Faull RJ, Ginsberg MH: Dynamic regulation of integrins. Stem Cells 1995;13:38–46.

33 Shattil SJ, Kashiwagi H, Pampori N: Integrin signaling: the platelet paradigm. Blood 1998;91:2645–2657.

34 Huttenlocher A, Ginsberg MH, Horwitz AF: Modulation of cell migration by integrin-mediated cytoskeletal linkages and ligand-binding affinity. J Cell Biol 1996;134:1551–1562.

35 Martin-Bermudo MD, Dunin-Borkowski OM, Brown NH: Modulation of integrin activity is vital for morphogenesis. J Cell Biol 1998;141:1073–1081.

36 Möhle R, Moore MA, Nachman RL, Rafii S: Transendothelial migration of CD34+ and mature hematopoietic cells: an in vitro study using a human bone marrow endothelial cell line. Blood 1997;89:72–80.

37 Hughes PE, Pfaff M: Integrin affinity modulation. Trends Cell Biol 1998;8:359–364.

38 Kovach NL, Lin N, Yednock T, Harlan JM, Broudy VC: Stem cell factor modulates avidity of alpha 4 beta 1 and alpha 5 beta 1 integrins expressed on hematopoietic cell lines. Blood 1995;85:159–167.

39 Levesque JP, Leavesley DI, Niutta S, Vadas M, Simmons PJ: Cytokines increase human hemopoietic cell adhesiveness by activation of very late antigen (VLA)-4 and VLA-5 integrins. J Exp Med 1995;181:1805–1815.

40 Schofield KP, Humphries MJ, de Wynter E, Testa N, Gallagher JT: The effect of alpha4 beta1-integrin binding sequences of fibronectin on growth of cells from human hematopoietic progenitors. Blood 1998; 91:3230–3238.

41 Miyake K, Medina KL, Hayashi S, Ono S, Hamaoka T, Kincade PW: Monoclonal antibodies to Pgp-1/CD44 block lympho-hemopoiesis in long-term bone marrow cultures. J Exp Med 1990;171:477–488.

42 Khaldoyanidi S, Denzel A, Zöller M: Requirement for CD44 in proliferation and homing of hematopoietic precursor cells. J Leukoc Biol 1996;60:579–592.

43 Khaldoyanidi S, Schnabel D, Föhr N, Zöller M: Functional activity of CD44 isoforms in haemopoiesis of the rat. Br J Haematol 1997;96:31–45.

44 Oostendorp RA, Spitzer E, Brandl M, Eaves CJ, Dörmer P: Evidence for differences in the mechanisms by which antibodies against CD44 promote adhesion of erythroid and granulopoietic progenitors to marrow stromal cells. Br J Haematol 1998;101:436–445.

45 Rösel M, Khaldoyanidi S, Zawadzki V, Zöller M: Involvement of CD44 variant isoform v10 in progenitor cell adhesion and maturation. Exp Hematol 1999;27:698–711.

46 Aiuti A, Webb IJ, Bleul C, Springer T, Gutierrez-Ramos JC: The chemokine SDF-1 is a chemoattractant for human CD34+ hematopoietic progenitor cells and provides a new mechanism to explain the mobilization of CD34+ progenitors to peripheral blood. J Exp Med 1997;185:111–120.

47 Bleul CC, Farzan M, Choe H, Parolin C, Clark-Lewis I, Sodroski J, Springer TA: The lymphocyte chemoattractant SDF-1 is a ligand for LESTR/fusin and blocks HIV-1 entry. Nature 1996;382:829–833.

48 Deichmann M, Kronenwett R, Haas R: Expression of the human immunodeficiency virus type-1 coreceptors CXCR-4 (fusin, LESTR) and CKR-5 in CD34+ hematopoietic progenitor cells. Blood 1997;89:3522–3528.

49 Viardot A, Kronenwett R, Deichmann M, Haas R: The human immunodeficiency virus (HIV)-type 1 coreceptor CXCR-4 (fusin) is preferentially expressed on the more immature CD34+ hematopoietic stem cells. Ann Hematol 1998;77:193–197.

50 Möhle R, Bautz F, Rafii S, Moore MA, Brugger W, Kanz L: The chemokine receptor CXCR-4 is expressed on CD34+ hematopoietic progenitors and leukemic cells and mediates transendothelial migration induced by stromal cell-derived factor-1. Blood 1998;91:4523–4530.]

51 Voermans C, Gerritsen WR, von dem Borne AE, van der Schoot CE: Increased migration of cord blood-derived CD34+ cells, as compared to bone marrow and mobilized peripheral blood CD34+ cells across uncoated or fibronectin-coated filters. Exp Hematol 1999;27:1806–1814.

52 Wognum AW, de Jong MO, Wagemaker G: Differential expression of receptors for hemopoietic growth factors on subsets of CD34+ hemopoietic cells. Leuk Lymphoma 1996;24:11–25.

53 Shinjo K, Takeshita A, Ohnishi K, Ohno R: Granulocyte colony-stimulating factor receptor at various differentiation stages of normal and leukemic hematopoietic cells. Leuk Lymphoma 1997;25:37–46.

54 Lund-Johansen F, Houck D, Hoffman R, Davis K, Olweus J: Primitive human hematopoietic progenitor cells express receptors for granulocyte-macrophage colony-stimulating factor. Exp Hematol 1999;27:762–772.

55 Liu F, Poursine-Laurent J, Link DC: Expression of the G-CSF receptor on hematopoietic progenitor cells is not required for their mobilization by G-CSF. Blood 2000;95:3025–3031.

56 Katayama Y, Battista M, Kao WM, Hidalgo A, Peired AJ, Thomas SA, Frenette PS: Signals from the sympathetic nervous system regulate hematopoietic stem cell egress from bone marrow. Cell 2006;124:407–421.

57 Socinski MA, Cannistra SA, Elias A, Antman KH, Schnipper L, Griffin JD: Granulocyte-macrophage colony stimulating factor expands the circulating haemopoietic progenitor cell compartment in man. Lancet 1988;1:1194–1198.

58 Gianni AM, Siena S, Bregni M, Tarella C, Stern AC, Pileri A, Bonadonna G: Granulocyte-macrophage colony-stimulating factor to harvest circulating haemopoietic stem cells for autotransplantation. Lancet 1989;2:580–585.

Haas/Bruns/Kobbe/Kronenwett

59 Shimazaki C, Oku N, Ashihara E, Okawa K, Goto H, Inaba T, Ito K, Fujita N, Tsuji H, Murakami S, Haruyama H, Nishio A, Nakagawa M: Collection of peripheral blood stem cells mobilized by high-dose Ara-C plus VP-16 or aclarubicin followed by recombinant human granulocyte-colony stimulating factor. Bone Marrow Transplant 1992;10:341–346.

60 Teshima T, Harada M, Takamatsu Y, Makino K, Taniguchi S, Inaba S, Kondo S, Tanaka T, Akashi K, Minamishima I et al: Cytotoxic drug and cytotoxic drug/G-CSF mobilization of peripheral blood stem cells and their use for autografting. Bone Marrow Transplant 1992;10:215–220.

61 Matsunaga T, Sakamaki S, Kohgo Y, Ohi S, Hirayama Y, Niitsu Y: Recombinant human granulocyte colony-stimulating factor can mobilize sufficient amounts of peripheral blood stem cells in healthy volunteers for allogeneic transplantation. Bone Marrow Transplant 1993;11:103–108.

62 Dreger P, Haferlach T, Eckstein V, Jacobs S, Suttorp M, Löffler H, Müller-Ruchholtz W, Schmitz N: G-CSF-mobilized peripheral blood progenitor cells for allogeneic transplantation: safety, kinetics of mobilization, and composition of the graft. Br J Haematol 1994;87:609–613.

63 Venturini M, Del Mastro L, Melioli G, Balleari E, Garrone O, Pasquetti E, Bason C, Ghio R, Bruzzi P, Rosso R: Release of peripheral blood progenitor cells during standard dose cyclophosphamide, epidoxorubicin, 5-fluorouracil regimen plus granulocyte colony stimulating factor for breast cancer therapy. Cancer 1994;74:2300–2306.

64 Winter JN, Lazarus HM, Rademaker A, Villa M, Mangan C, Tallman M, Jahnke L, Gordon L, Newman S, Byrd K, Cooper BW, Horvath N, Crum E, Stadtmauer EA, Conklin E, Bauman A, Martin J, Goolsby C, Gerson SL, Bender J, O'Gorman M: Phase I/II study of combined granulocyte colony-stimulating factor and granulocyte-macrophage colony-stimulating factor administration for the mobilization of hematopoietic progenitor cells. J Clin Oncol 1996;14:277–286.

65 Hohaus S, Martin H, Wassmann B, Egerer G, Haus U, Färber L, Burger KJ, Goldschmidt H, Hoelzer D, Haas R: Recombinant human granulocyte and granulocyte-macrophage colony-stimulating factor (G-CSF and GM-CSF) administered following cytotoxic chemotherapy have a similar ability to mobilize peripheral blood stem cells. Bone Marrow Transplant 1998;22:625–630.

66 Haas R, Ho AD, Bredthauer U, Cayeux S, Egerer G, Knauf W, Hunstein W: Successful autologous transplantation of blood stem cells mobilized with recombinant human granulocyte-macrophage colony-stimulating factor. Exp Hematol 1990;18:94–98.

67 Haas R, Hohaus S, Egerer G, Ehrhardt R, Witt B, Hunstein W: Recombinant human granulocyte-macrophage colony-stimulating factor (rhGM-CSF) subsequent to chemotherapy improves collection of blood stem cells for autografting in patients not eligible for bone marrow harvest. Bone Marrow Transplant 1992;9:459–465.

68 Haas R, Moos M, Karcher A, Möhle R, Witt B, Goldschmidt H, Frühauf S, Flentje M, Wannenmacher M, Hunstein W: Sequential high-dose therapy with peripheral-blood progenitor-cell support in low-grade non-Hodgkin's lymphoma. J Clin Oncol 1994;12:1685–1692.

69 Haas R, Schmid H, Hahn U, Hohaus S, Goldschmidt H, Murea S, Kaufmann M, Wannenmacher M, Wallwiener D, Bastert G, Hunstein W: Tandem high-dose therapy with ifosfamide, epirubicin, carboplatin and peripheral blood stem cell support is an effective adjuvant treatment for high-risk breast cancer. Eur J Cancer 1997;33:372–378.

70 Möhle R, Pförsich M, Frühauf S, Witt B, Krämer A, Haas R: Filgrastim post-chemotherapy mobilizes more CD34+ cells with a different antigenic profile compared with use during steady-state hematopoiesis. Bone Marrow Transplant 1994;14:827–832.

71 Haas R, Gericke G, Witt B, Cayeux S, Hunstein W: Increased serum levels of granulocyte colony-stimulation factor after autologous bone marrow or blood stem cell transplantation. Exp Hematol 1993;21:109–113.

72 Cairo MS, Suen Y, Sender L, Gillan ER, Ho W, Plunkett JM, van de Ven C: Circulating granulocyte colony-stimulating factor (G-CSF) levels after allogeneic and autologous bone marrow transplantation: endogenous G-CSF production correlates with myeloid engraftment. Blood 1992;79:1869–1873.

73 Layton JE, Hockman H, Sheridan WP, Morstyn G: Evidence for a novel in vivo control mechanism of granulopoiesis: mature cell-related control of a regulatory growth factor. Blood 1989;74:1303–1307.

74 Grigg AP, Roberts AW, Raunow H, Houghton S, Layton JE, Boyd AW, McGrath KM, Maher D: Optimizing dose and scheduling of filgrastim (granulocyte colony stimulating factor) for mobilization and collection of peripheral blood progenitor cells in normal volunteers. Blood 1995;86:4437–4445.

75 Hoglund M, Smedmyr B, Simonsson B, Tötterman T, Bengtsson M: Dose-dependent mobilisation of haematopoietic progenitor cells in healthy volunteers receiving glycosylated rHuG-CSF. Bone Marrow Transplant 1996;18:19–27.

76 Martin-Murea S, Voso MT, Hohaus S, Pförsich M, Fruehauf S, Goldschmidt H, Hegenbart U, Haas R: The dose of granulocyte colony-stimulating factor administered following cytotoxic chemotherapy is not related to the rebound level of circulating CD34+ haematopoietic progenitor cells during marrow recovery. Br J Haematol 1998;101:582–585.

77 Haas R, Möhle R, Pförsich M, Fruehauf S, Witt B, Goldschmidt H, Hunstein W: Blood-derived autografts collected during granulocyte colony-stimulating factor-enhanced recovery are enriched with early Thy-1+ hematopoietic progenitor cells. Blood 1995;85:1936–1943.

78 Roberts AW, Metcalf D: Noncycling state of peripheral blood progenitor cells mobilized by granulocyte colony-stimulating factor and other cytokines. Blood 1995;86:1600–1605.

79 Tarella C, Benedetti G, Caracciolo D, Castellino C, Cherasco C, Bondesan P, Omedé P, Ruggieri D, Gianni AM, Pileri A: Both early and committed haemopoietic progenitors are more frequent in peripheral blood than in bone marrow during mobilization induced by high-dose chemotherapy + G-CSF. Br J Haematol 1995;91:535–543.

80 Dercksen MW, Rodenhuis S, Dirkson MK, Schaasberg WP, Baars JW, van der Wall E, Slaper-Cortenbach IC, Pinedo HM, Von dem Borne AE, van der Schoot CE: Subsets of CD34+ cells and rapid hematopoietic recovery after peripheral-blood stem-cell transplantation. J Clin Oncol 1995;13:1922–1932.

81 To LB, Haylock DN, Dowse T, Simmons PJ, Trimboli S, Ashman LK, Juttner CA: A comparative study of the phenotype and proliferative capacity of peripheral blood (PB) CD34+ cells mobilized by four different protocols and those of steady-phase PB and bone marrow CD34+ cells. Blood 1994;84:2930–2939.

82 Steidl U, Kronenwett R, Rohr UP, Fenk R, Kliszewski S, Maercker C, Neubert P, Aivado M, Koch J, Modlich O, Bojar H, Gattermann N, Haas R: Gene expression profiling identifies significant differences between the molecular phenotypes of bone marrow-derived and circulating human CD34+ hematopoietic stem cells. Blood 2002;99:2037–2044.

83 Roberts AW, DeLuca E, Begley CG, Basser R, Grigg AP, Metcalf D: Broad inter-individual variations in circulating progenitor cell numbers induced by granulocyte colony-stimulating factor therapy. Stem Cells 1995;13:512–516.

84 Goldschmidt H, Hegenbart U, Haas R, Hunstein W: Mobilization of peripheral blood progenitor cells with high-dose cyclophosphamide (4 or 7 g/m²) and granulocyte colony-stimulating factor in patients with multiple myeloma. Bone Marrow Transplant 1996;17:691–697.

85 Andrews RG, Bartelmez SH, Knitter GH, Myerson D, Bernstein ID, Appelbaum FR, Zsebo KM: A c-kit ligand, recombinant human stem cell factor, mediates reversible expansion of multiple CD34+ colony-forming cell types in blood and marrow of baboons. Blood 1992;80:920–927.

86 Brugger W, Bross K, Frisch J, Dern P, Weber B, Mertelsmann R, Kanz L: Mobilization of peripheral blood progenitor cells by sequential administration of interleukin-3 and granulocyte-macrophage colony-stimulating factor following polychemotherapy with etoposide, ifosfamide, and cisplatin. Blood 1992;79:1193–1200.

87 Haas R, Ehrhardt R, Witt B, Goldschmidt H, Hohaus S, Pförsich M, Ehrlich H, Färber L, Hunstein W: Autografting with peripheral blood stem cells mobilized by sequential interleukin-3/granulocyte-macrophage colony-stimulating factor following high-dose chemotherapy in non-Hodgkin's lymphoma. Bone Marrow Transplant 1993;12:643–649.

88 Lemoli RM, Fogli M, Fortuna A, Motta MR, Rizzi S, Benini C, Tura S: Interleukin-11 stimulates the proliferation of human hematopoietic CD34+ and CD34+CD33-DR- cells and synergizes with stem cell factor, interleukin-3, and granulocyte-macrophage colony-stimulating factor. Exp Hematol 1993;21:1668–1672.

89 Jacobsen SE, Okkenhaug C, Myklebust J, Veiby OP, Lyman SD: The FLT3 ligand potently and directly stimulates the growth and expansion of primitive murine bone marrow progenitor cells in vitro: synergistic interactions with interleukin (IL) 11, IL-12, and other hematopoietic growth factors. J Exp Med 1995;181:1357–1363.

90 Mauch P, Lamont C, Neben TY, Quinto C, Goldman SJ, Witsell A: Hematopoietic stem cells in the blood after stem cell factor and interleukin-11 administration: evidence for different mechanisms of mobilization. Blood 1995;86:4674–4680.

91 Laterveer L, Lindley IJ, Heemskerk DP, Camps JA, Pauwels EK, Willemze R, Fibbe WE: Rapid mobilization of hematopoietic progenitor cells in rhesus monkeys by a single intravenous injection of interleukin-8. Blood 1996;87:781–788.

92 Hunter MG, Bawden L, Brotherton D, Craig S, Cribbes S, Czaplewski LG, Dexter TM, Drummond AH, Gearing AH, Heyworth CM, Lord BI, McCourt M, Varley PG, Wood LM, Edwards RM, Lewis PJ: BB-10010: an active variant of human macrophage inflammatory protein-1 alpha with improved pharmaceutical properties. Blood 1995;86:4400–4408.

93 Curran MP, Goa KL: Pegfilgrastim. Drugs 2002;62:1207–1213.

94 Steidl U, Fenk R, Bruns I, Neumann F, Kondakci M, Hoyer B, Gräf T, Rohr UP, Bork S, Kronenwett R, Haas R, Kobbe G: Successful transplantation of peripheral blood stem cells mobilized by chemotherapy and a single dose of pegylated G-CSF in patients with multiple myeloma. Bone Marrow Transplant 2005;35:33–36.

95 Bruns I, Steidl U, Kronenwett R, Fenk R, Graef T, Rohr UP, Neumann F, Fischer J, Scheid C, Hübel K, Haas R, Kobbe G: A single dose of 6 or 12 mg of pegfilgrastim for peripheral blood progenitor cell mobilization results in similar yields of CD34+ progenitors in patients with multiple myeloma. Transfusion 2006;46:180–185.

96 Bruns I, Steidl U, Fischer JC, Czibere A, Kobbe G, Raschke S, Singh R, Fenk R, Rosskopf M, Pechtel S, von Haeseler A, Wernet P, Tenen DG, Haas R, Kronenwett R: Pegylated granulocyte colony-stimulating factor mobilizes CD34+ cells with different stem and progenitor subsets and distinct functional properties in comparison with unconjugated granulocyte colony-stimulating factor. Haematologica 2008;93:347–355.

97 Fruehauf S, Seeger T, Maier P, Li L, Weinhardt S, Laufs S, Wagner W, Eckstein V, Bridger G, Calandra G, Wenz F, Zeller WJ, Goldschmidt H, Ho AD: The CXCR4 antagonist AMD3100 releases a subset of G-CSF-primed peripheral blood progenitor cells with specific gene expression characteristics. Exp Hematol 2006;34:1052–1059.

98 Zöller M: CD44v10 in hematopoiesis and stem cell mobilization. Leuk Lymphoma 2000;38:463–480.

99 Bonig H, Wundes A, Chang KH, Lucas S, Papayannopoulou T: Increased numbers of circulating hematopoietic stem/progenitor cells are chronically maintained in patients treated with the CD49d blocking antibody natalizumab. Blood 2008;111:3439–3441.

100 Zohren F, Toutzaris D, Klärner V, Hartung HP, Kieseier B, Haas R: The monoclonal anti-VLA-4 antibody natalizumab mobilizes CD34+ hematopoietic progenitor cells in humans. Blood 2008;111:3893–3895.

101 Christ O, Kronenwett R, Haas R, Zöller M: Combining G-CSF with a blockade of adhesion strongly improves the reconstitutive capacity of mobilized hematopoietic progenitor cells. Exp Hematol 2001;29:380–390.

102 Reiffers J, Bernard P, David B, Vezon G, Sarrat A, Marit G, Moulinier J, Broustet A: Successful autologous transplantation with peripheral blood hemopoietic cells in a patient with acute leukemia. Exp Hematol 1986;14:312–315.

103 Kessinger A, Armitage JO, Landmark JD, Weisenburger DD: Reconstitution of human hematopoietic function with autologous cryopreserved circulating stem cells. Exp Hematol 1986;14:192–196.

104 To LB, Dyson PG, Juttner CA: Cell-dose effect in circulating stem-cell autografting. Lancet 1986;2:404–405.

105 Körbling M, Dörken B, Ho AD, Pezzutto A, Hunstein W, Fliedner TM: Autologous transplantation of blood-derived hemopoietic stem cells after myeloablative therapy in a patient with Burkitt's lymphoma. Blood 1986;67:529–532.

106 Sheridan WP, Begley CG, Juttner CA, Szer J, To LB, Maher D, McGrath KM, Morstyn G, Fox RM: Effect of peripheral-blood progenitor cells mobilised by filgrastim (G-CSF) on platelet recovery after high-dose chemotherapy. Lancet 1992;339:640–644.

107 Elias AD, Ayash L, Anderson KC, Hunt M, Wheeler C, Schwartz G, Tepler I, Mazanet R, Lynch C, Pap S, Pelaez J, Reich E, Critchlow J, Demetri G, Bibbo J, Schnipper L: Mobilization of peripheral blood progenitor cells by chemotherapy and granulocyte-macrophage colony-stimulating factor for hematologic support after high-dose intensification for breast cancer. Blood 1992;79:3036–3044.

108 Haas R, Möhle R, Frühauf S, Goldschmidt H, Witt B, Flentje M, Wannenmacher M, Hunstein W: Patient characteristics associated with successful mobilizing and autografting of peripheral blood progenitor cells in malignant lymphoma. Blood 1994;83:3787–3794.

109 Reiffers J, Faberes C, Boiron JM, Marit G, Foures C, Ferrer AM, Cony-Makhoul P, Puntous M, Bernard P, Vezon G, Broustet A: Peripheral blood progenitor cell transplantation in 118 patients with hematological malignancies: analysis of factors affecting the rate of engraftment. J Hematother 1994;3:185–191.

110 Bensinger WI, Longin K, Appelbaum F, Rowley S, Weaver C, Lilleby K, Gooley T, Lynch M, Higano T, Klarnet J, Chauncey T, Storb R, Buckner CD: Peripheral blood stem cells (PBSCs) collected after recombinant granulocyte colony stimulating factor (rhG-CSF): an analysis of factors correlating with the tempo of engraftment after transplantation. Br J Haematol 1994;87:825–831.

111 Weaver CH, Hazelton B, Birch R, Palmer P, Allen C, Schwartzberg L, West W: An analysis of engraftment kinetics as a function of the CD34 content of peripheral blood progenitor cell collections in 692 patients after the administration of myeloablative chemotherapy. Blood 1995;86:3961–3969.

112 Ketterer N, Salles G, Raba M, Espinouse D, Sonet A, Tremisi P, Dumontet C, Moullet I, Eljaafari-Corbin A, Neidhardt-Berard EM, Bouafia F, Coiffier B: High CD34$^{(+)}$ cell counts decrease hematologic toxicity of autologous peripheral blood progenitor cell transplantation. Blood 1998;91:3148–3155.

113 Bensinger WI, Weaver CH, Appelbaum FR, Rowley S, Demirer T, Sanders J, Storb R, Buckner CD: Transplantation of allogeneic peripheral blood stem cells mobilized by recombinant human granulocyte colony-stimulating factor. Blood 1995;85:1655–1658.

114 Körbling M, Przepiorka D, Huh YO, Engel H, van Besien K, Giralt S, Andersson B, Kleine HD, Seong D, Deisseroth AB, Andreef M, Champlin R: Allogeneic blood stem cell transplantation for refractory leukemia and lymphoma: potential advantage of blood over marrow allografts. Blood 1995;85:1659–1665.

115 Schmitz N, Dreger P, Suttorp M, Rohwedder EB, Haferlach T, Löffler H, Hunter A, Russell NH: Primary transplantation of allogeneic peripheral blood progenitor cells mobilized by filgrastim (granulocyte colony-stimulating factor). Blood 1995;85:1666–1672.

Prof. Dr. med. Rainer Haas
Klinik für Hämatologie, Onkologie und Klinische Immunologie
Heinrich-Heine-Universität Düsseldorf
Moorenstr. 5, 40225 Düsseldorf, Germany
Tel. +49 211 811-7760, Fax -8853
E-Mail haas@med.uni-duesseldorf.de

Scharf RE (ed): Progress and Challenges in Transfusion Medicine, Hemostasis and Hemotherapy.
Freiburg i.Br., Karger, 2008, pp 151–161

Cultured Red Blood Cells: A New Advance in Stem Cell Engineering

Luc Douay

INSERM, UMR_S 893 and Pierre and Marie Curie University Paris, France

Key Words

Red blood cells · In vitro expansion · Transfusion · Hematopoietic stem cells · Hemoglobin substitute

Summary

For several years, researchers have been trying to find a substitute for red blood cells (RBC). The development of chemical or natural molecules to replace hemoglobin has nevertheless proved difficult, and artificial blood is still unattainable. We have described a methodology permitting the massive ex vivo production of mature human RBC which have all the characteristics of native adult RBC from hematopoietic stem cells (HSC) of diverse origins: blood, bone marrow, or cord blood. This protocol allows both the massive expansion of HSC/progenitors and their complete differentiation to the stage of perfectly functional mature RBC. The levels of amplification obtained (10^5–2×10^5) are compatible with an eventual transfusion application. In this report, we discuss the state of the art of this new concept and evoke the obstacles that need to be overcome to pass from the laboratory model to clinical practice. This concept of cultured RBC opens up potentially considerable therapeutic perspectives in the field of blood transfusion.
©2008 S. Karger GmbH, Freiburg i.Br.

Introduction

Since blood supplies are regularly insufficient to meet demands and certain rare blood groups are lacking, we need to dispose of complementary sources of blood components. For several years, researchers have been trying to find a substitute for red blood cells (RBC). The development of chemical or natural molecules to replace hemoglobin has nevertheless proved difficult, and artificial blood is still unattainable.

Thus, instead of replacing what nature has made, why not try to copy her? Today, we have sufficient knowledge of the biology of blood stem cells, which are present in adult bone marrow, to produce human RBC in the laboratory. In this report, we describe how mature, functional RBC can be obtained from hematopoietic stem cells (HSC) of diverse origins. We have many reasons to think that within a few years it will be possible to produce enough cells to be able to transfuse cultured RBC to patients.

Replace or Copy Nature?

Alternative solutions will become indispensable: either the design of artificial substitutes capable of transporting oxygen, which will replace the blood, or the production of human RBC in culture, which will reproduce natural blood. Blood substitutes have already been developed. On injection into the circulation, they recreate the fundamental function of the red blood cell, oxygen transport. Chemists have focused especially on two types of artificial blood: chemically modified or genetically produced hemoglobin and chemical substances of the perfluorocarbon family.

Hemoglobin substitutes are obtained in this case from three possible sources: blood donations, samples from animals, and production by genetically modified organisms. However, free hemoglobin is toxic: in the circulation, it disintegrates rapidly, and its degradation products induce lesions. To be useful, the hemoglobin has to be encapsulated or chemically modified, which leads in all cases to less efficient oxygen transport as compared to red cells [1–3].

Oxygen transporters are synthetic fluids composed of perfluorocarbons, molecules containing atoms of carbon, hydrogen, and fluorine, which are capable of dissolving large quantities of oxygen. These liquids are not toxic as they are soluble in neither water nor blood. On the other hand, they are used as emulsions in order to be able to disperse in the circulation and, thus, are unstable and have to be eliminated rapidly by the organism. In clinical trials, patients transfused with these substitutes experienced notable side effects. Thus, it is extremely difficult to create an artificial liquid which transports oxygen like natural hemoglobin does, and no substitute has to date been widely used in clinical practice. The hope of producing human RBC by laboratory techniques is therefore a feasible alternative [4, 5].

Hematopoietic Stem Cells: The Source of Red Blood Cells

The HSC which produce the different components of blood are found in the bone marrow. In the 1980s, it became possible to mobilize them and make them enter the blood stream; thus, they could be collected more simply [6]. In 1993, Lu et al. [7] demonstrated the presence of large quantities of these cells in umbilical cord blood.

Consequently, if we dispose of cells capable of generating RBC, it remains to master their transformation. Over the last decade, researchers have been attempting to improve bone marrow grafts by increasing the number of HSC in the grafts, a method called ex vivo expansion [8]. While working on this concept, the idea came to mind to control the proliferation of these stem cells and to force them to differentiate specifically to the erythroid line. The red blood cell has, however, an essential particularity: it is the only cell of the organism which has no nucleus and nevertheless lives for 120 days. At the end of its maturation in the bone marrow, the erythroid cell expels its nucleus by mechanisms still poorly elucidated to become a red blood cell.

Hence, the production of RBC from stem cells in the laboratory must satisfy two conditions: one must obtain complete maturation of the erythroid cells to mature, enucleated, and functional RBC and one must produce a quantity of RBC comparable to that contained in a standard concentrate transfused to a patient (2×10^{12} cells).

The HSC, which constitute 0.01–0.05% of the marrow cells, differentiate according to a well-defined hierarchy and in close contact with the medullar microenvironment [9]. They become myeloid stem cells and then progenitors, which will give rise to the different constituents of blood: RBC, granulocytes, and platelets. The cells of the medullar environment, known as stromal cells, are very numerous and include notably adipocytes, macrophages, and fibroblasts lying on an extracellular matrix [10]. These cells play a key role in the differentiation of the stem cells. They secrete soluble factors regulating activatory and inhibitory cytokines and facilitate interactions between stem cells, which is determinant in the regulation of hematopoiesis. The difficulty resides in constraining a hematopoietic stem cell to commit itself exclusively to the erythroid line and mature into a red blood cell. Since the stem cells are multipotential, i.e. have the capacity to give rise to any blood cell, one has to determine the environmental characteristics responsible for their differentiation into RBC. Attempts were unsuccessful for several years: experiments in the laboratory produced either mature RBC in very small quantities or large quantities of immature RBC still containing a nucleus.

In vitro Generation of Mature and Functional Red Blood Cells

One of the major characteristics of the human red blood cell is that it is the only cell which has a long life span (120 days) despite the absence of a nucleus. Researchers suppose to know the mechanisms of nucleus expulsion which, however, have not been formally established due to a lack of experimental conditions permitting the massive ex vivo production of RBC. Such conditions must in fact satisfy three requirements: (i) the massive amplification of primitive HSC, (ii) the controlled induction of exclusive differentiation to the erythroid line, and (iii) the completion of terminal maturation to the stage of enucleated cells.

We initially described [11] a protocol for the expansion of HSC derived from cord blood (CB) in a well-defined medium and without stroma, based on the sequential addition of growth factors. Starting from CD34+ cells, this protocol allows the massive production (amplification up to 200,000 times) of 99% erythroid precursors containing fetal hemoglobin (HbF). Contrary to their behavior under these ex vivo conditions in the presence of growth factors alone, such progenitors/precursors, when injected into nonobese diabetic/severely compromised immunodeficient (NOD/SCID) mice, are capable of continuing to proliferate in vivo and of differentiating within 4 days to the terminal stage of enucleated cells producing adult hemoglobin (HbA), which points to a major role of the microenvironment in terminal erythroid differentiation.

In vitro Generation of Red Blood Cells
On the basis of these data, we then modified our protocol to obtain the expansion and differentiation of CD34+ cells derived from blood, bone marrow, or CB in three steps [12]: (i) first, in a liquid medium, involving cell proliferation and induction of erythroid differentiation in the presence of stem cell factor (SCF), interleukin-3 (IL-3), and erythropoietin (EPO); (ii) second, based on a model reconstitution of the microenvironment (murine stromal cell line MS-5), in the presence of EPO alone; (iii) third, in the presence of the stromal cells alone, without any growth factors. This cell culture system in a well-defined medium without serum reproduces ex vivo the microenvironment existing in vivo [13] (fig. 1, 2).

Using this protocol, we obtain by day 15 a plateau of the mean amplification of CD34+ cells of 16,000 fold (up to 25,000) for cells derived from bone marrow or peripheral blood, of 29,000 fold (up to 34,000) for cells obtained by leukapheresis after mobilization with granulocyte colony-stimulating factor (G-CSF), and of 140,000 fold (up to 280,000) for cells derived from CB.

A commitment to the erythroid lineage is morphologically evident by day 8 (95% erythroblasts). The subsequent terminal differentiation is rapid as the percentage of enucleated cells is only 1–5% on day 11, but 65–80% by day 15. At this stage, 98% of the cells are reticulocytes with a mean cell volume (MCV) of 130 fl, a mean corpuscular hemoglobin concentration (MCHC) of 18%, and a mean cell hemoglobin (MCH) of 23 pg.

Differentiation of the reticulocytes into mature RBC continues from day 15 to day 18, as shown by the continued disappearance of nuclei and the progressive loss of transferrin receptor CD71 expression and of staining with laser dye styryl (LDS). At this stage, 90–100% of the cells are enucleated. These erythrocytes display characteristics close to those of native RBC, namely an MCV of 113 fl, an MCH of 33 pg, and an MCHC of 29%. The cell yield on day 18 with respect to day 15 is 77% with a mean reticulocyte content of 18%. This complete differentiation of vastly expanded precursors into a pure erythroid lineage is due to the targeted proliferative induction of erythroid progenitors (erythroid burst-forming units, BFU-E and erythroid colony-forming units, CFU-E) and occurs at the expense of granulomacrophagic progenitors (granulomacrophagic colony-forming units, CFU-GM). All progenitors subsequently disappear between days 8 and 11.

Interestingly, the total cell expansion achieved during the first step in the presence of growth factors alone is directly related to the duration of culture. When the culture is prolonged for 3 additional days, the level of expansion increases dramatically to

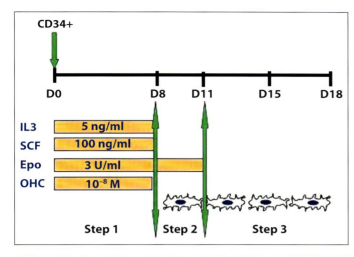

Fig. 1. Overall protocol for the expansion and differentiation of CD34+ cells derived from blood, bone marrow, or cord blood. D0 = Day 0; IL3 = interleukin-3; SCF = stem cell factor; Epo = erythropoietin; OHC = hydrocortisone.

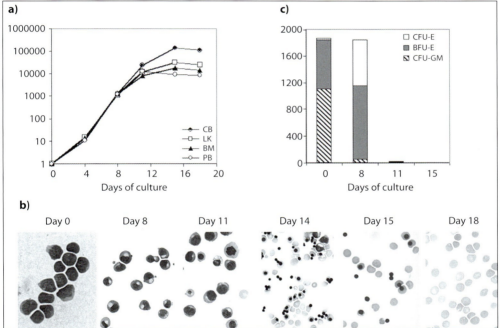

Fig. 2. Amplification of erythroid cells. **a** Human CD34+ cells from cord blood (CB), bone marrow (BM), peripheral blood (PB), or leukapheresis (LK) were cultured in a liquid medium on a layer of stromal cells of murine origin (MS-5) according to a three-phase protocol. Total numbers of viable nonadherent cells were determined at different times. **b** Photographs of the cells on days 0, 8, 11, 14, 15, and 18 of culture after May-Grünwald-Giemsa staining. **c** Progenitor cell counts in semisolid cultures. Results are mean values (per 10^4 seeded cells) for erythroid progenitors (erythroid colony-forming units, CFU-E and erythroid burst-forming units, BFU-E) and granulomacrophagic progenitors (granulomacrophagic colony-forming units, CFU-GM) in experiments using cells from CB cultures. At various time points, aliquots of nonadherent cells were grown in methylcellulose in the presence of stem cell factor (SCF), granulomacrophagic colony-stimulating factor (GM-CSF), granulocyte colony-stimulating factor (G-CSF), interleukin-3 (IL-3), and erythropoietin (EPO) for progenitor evaluation.

reach 2×10^6, 1.20×10^5, or 1×10^5 fold for CB, peripheral blood/leukapheresis, or bone marrow products respectively, with preservation of the terminal differentiation after steps 2 and 3 (70–91% enucleated cells).

The reticulocytes and RBC generated ex vivo have a glucose-6-phosphate dehydrogenase (G6PD) content of 42 U/g Hb and a pyruvate kinase (PK) level of 83 U/g Hb, in keeping with the nature of a young homogeneous red cell population. This indicates that they should be capable of reducing glutathione and maintaining ATP levels, thereby ensuring normal levels of 2,3-diphosphoglycerate (2,3-DPG), a compound which decreases the affinity of Hb for its ligand. The deformability of these reticulocytes and RBC, as evaluated by ektacytometry, is comparable to that of native erythrocytes.

The functionality of Hb in cultured RBC (cRBC) may be assessed by ligand binding kinetics after flash photolysis. The bimolecular kinetics after photodissociation of CO provides a sensitive test for Hb function. On varying the energy of the photolysis pulse, two phases are observed, which correspond to the two Hb conformations (R and T states). The kinetics is thus biphasic, reflecting the two allosteric forms. Like native Hb, cRBC Hb is able to fix and release oxygen.

Oxygen equilibrium measurements confirm the observed affinity and cooperativity. The log P50 value is 1.2 for cRBC Hb as compared to 1.3 for control RBC Hb, and the Hill coefficients are identical (N50 of 2.28 vs. 2.29). The kinetic and equilibrium data thus indicate ligand-binding properties in very close agreement with control values. Methemoglobin (Met-Hb) is not detected, which shows that cRBC are enzymatically capable of reversing Hb oxidation.

In vivo Fate of Cultured Human Red Blood Cells

After intraperitoneal infusion into NOD/SCID mice, carboxyfluorescein diacetate succinimidylester (CFSE)-labeled cRBC and reticulocytes obtained by leukapheresis persist in the circulation to the same extent as native RBC: CFSE+ cells are detected for 3 days in both groups of animals. In vivo, the infused reticulocytes fully mature into RBC, as shown by the appearance of CFSE+/LDS– cells: 36% and 63% on days 1 and 2, respectively. Over 90% of the CFSE+ cells are mature RBC by day 3.

At this stage of development of the model, it has thus been established that it is possible to produce functional human RBC by culture of HSC.

Prerequisites for Clinical Development

In the course of the protocol development, we have identified a number of parameters critical for the achievement of the two fundamental requirements: massive amplification of the erythroid compartment and total enucleation of the precursors. Our observations made under different culture conditions lead us to retain the following major elements for the conception of standardizable conditions for RBC production:

– Maintenance of the microenvironment, which may originate from diverse sources (bone marrow, human or murine stromal cell lines, autologous or allogeneic human mesenchymal cells), throughout culture prevents apoptosis. In cultures without serum, growth factors alone cannot replace the microenvironment.
– EPO can be removed at the end of culture to induce enucleation. This observation contradicts the dogma whereby EPO would be a terminal maturation factor.

We think it should be possible to dispense with the cellular microenvironment while conserving its antiapoptotic effect and the signal inducing nucleus expulsion observed in cocultures and to establish culture conditions permitting cell survival in the presence of a specific microenvironment. Analysis of these experiments should allow us to deduce the parameters involved in the overall process – adhesion protein(s), growth factor(s), antiapoptotic factor(s) – in order to replace the cellular microenvironment.

A New Labile Blood Product: Cultured RBC

Considering on the one hand the levels of cell amplification obtained (2×10^5–2×10^6 fold for apheresis and CB with 90–100% maturation) and on the other hand a mean quantity of 2–8×10^6 CD34+ cells/kg in an apheresis donation or 2–5×10^6 CD34+ cells in a CB unit, it is the equivalent of 2–6 RBC concentrates which theoretically can be produced by this procedure. As for the use of embryonic stem cells, it would allow the preparation of an almost unlimited quantity of red cell concentrates.

This type of product is of course better suited for clinical use than the precedent because, first, it permits perfect control of the dosage of the transfusion and, second, it may be considered a 'pure' RBC concentrate, in any case free of the usual contaminants such as leukocytes, platelets, and plasma.

Prospective Indications

Without pretending to replace 'classical' transfusion, these products could at least find indications in the context of 'impossible' transfusion situations. Such situations are encountered in the two circumstances of rare erythrocyte phenotypes and antierythrocyte polyimmunization. Moreover, certain patients dependent on blood transfusion from a very early age, like those suffering from hemoglobinopathies and notably thalassemia, could also benefit from these products. Finally, one can further evoke the case of transfusion in intensive care.

A rare phenotype is characterized by the absence of an antigen of high frequency on RBC. Such individuals can develop antibodies against these antigens either spontaneously or after initial allogeneic stimulation during pregnancy or transfusion.

Any person with a rare phenotype must receive concentrates of identical rare RBC. These RBC concentrates are stored frozen in a small number of Blood Banks of Rare Phenotypes. However, depending on the frequency, the reserves are not always sufficient to satisfy the demand.

In our experience of blood transfusion in France, this is notably the case for rare specificities found solely in the Afro-Antillean populations, such as certain rare phenotypes of the Rhesus (Rh) system. The problem is magnified because repeated transfusions can be necessary among these populations, notably in patients with sickle cell disease.

One could therefore propose for these patients the constitution of stocks of rare blood obtained either from adult donors of the same rare phenotype or from CB units conserved within the framework of a bank of CB of rare phenotype. Generally, when an individual having a rare phenotype is identified, a family study is performed to determine among other things the possibility of finding among the relatives other individuals carrying the same particularity who would be susceptible to give blood. It would thus be entirely feasible to extend this study to a search for persons susceptible to give HSC from the blood or placenta.

Situations of polyimmunization constitute a second application. The case of a subject immunized against a large number of antigens resembles that of a rare blood group insofar as the blood units compatible with all the antibodies produced are few. In this situation, it would be unrealistic to look for donors presenting an antigen combination compatible with the patient and to ask them to give HSC. Conversely, one could envisage producing RBC from the patient's own CD34+ cells, as the patient is the best potential 'donor' in this case.

The idea of transfusing patients suffering from thalassemia with RBC having a prolonged life span is an old one. Earlier studies, which made use of the fact that young RBC have a lower density than mature or senescent RBC, collected apheresis products that had a half-life (measured by ^{51}Cr labeling) of 44 days as compared with 28 days for conventional RBC concentrates [14]. However, this technique proved to be disappointing in routine practice [15] and was thus abandoned.

The ex vivo preparation of RBC would enable us to transfuse a cell population homogeneous in age whose life span should be close to 120 days, as compared with the mean half-life of 28 days of RBC collected from a donor, due to the simultaneous presence of RBC of variable age [16]. This would reduce the number of transfusions and alleviate the inevitable iron overload, a major complication in multitransfused subjects, particularly in thalassemic patients.

One may bet that cultured RBC might have impact on the adverse effects linked to conventional transfusion. Indeed, the suspension of cultured RBC is free of leukocytes, which is of interest in that it improves the storage of the cells at 4 °C due to the absence of cytokines released by senescent leukocytes and diminishes the residual risk of anti-HLA alloimmunization, at least equally as well as deleukocytation procedures [17].

Similarly, the use of RBC prepared in culture should lead to a reduction of the risks linked to the presence of plasma and notably the risk of transfusion-related acute lung injury (TRALI), whatever the mechanism of this complication of classical blood transfusion [18, 19].

Another important potential application of cultured RBC might be the management of sickle cell disease. The ex vivo synthesis of HbF by cells derived from CB is related to the culture conditions, since the erythroblast progenitors/precursors obtained after 10 days of culture in the absence of a microenvironment give rise in vivo, after transfusion into NOD/SCID mice, to mature RBC containing 96% functional HbA with complete modulation of HbF (ratio γA:γG of 35:65) [11]. This model is thus a new tool to investigate the cellular and molecular mechanisms of the Hb switch.

Stimulation ex vivo of the expression of HbF in subjects with drepanocytosis could represent an interesting therapeutic approach. This activation of HbF should diminish the polymerization of sickle hemoglobin (HbS). One could thus propose an autologous transfusion product modified ex vivo so as to specifically amplify the synthesis of HbF.

This culture system also offers a new approach to the search for 'universal' RBC, i.e. red cells lacking membrane expression of certain antigens of the two principal blood group systems, A and B of the ABO system and antigen D (RH1) of the Rh system. Here, it is no longer a question of trying to eliminate the surface antigens once they have formed, but a matter of preventing their synthesis before the RBC reach maturity. The blood group antigens ABO and RH, which are not expressed on HSC, are already present on erythroblast precursors.

Two approaches may be envisaged: (i) inhibition of gene expression in CD34+ human HSC through the use of interfering RNA (siRNA); (ii) biochemical intracellular inhibition of the glycosyltransferases specific for the antigens A and B.

Whatever the method, this inhibition has to be initiated at the stage of CD34+ HSC and continued to that of RBC. The techniques of this approach can avoid the side effects inherent to the procedures of stripping [20] or masking [21] currently being tested.

Conclusions and Future Directions

Even if the advent of artificial blood has been heralded for a long time, authentic blood substitutes have yet to become available. Is this a sign that, as far as labile blood products are concerned, it is not easy to replace nature? The concept of cultured RBC shows that it is at least possible to imitate her. The technical conditions for their industrial development still have to be created, and the clinical and economic interest in this new labile blood product has to be proven. A concentrate of homogeneous RBC has a long life span, is free of platelets, leukocytes and plasma, has an improved storage capacity, a selected phenotype, and is constantly available. Finally, the development of this new blood product will be conditioned by the establishment of its therapeutic efficacy and safety, like it is the case for any new therapeutic product.

Human embryonic stem cells (huESC), which have an unlimited proliferative potential, could become in the next few years an alternative and attractive source for cell engineering. Some groups have already reported a 20% commitment of huESC to CD34+ hematopoietic cells. Hence, in vitro differentiation of ESC to the erythroid line could eventually permit the massive production of RBC.

This new concept of cultured RBC provides an innovative tool to elucidate the physiopathological mechanisms of erythropoiesis and opens up potentially considerable therapeutic perspectives, notably in the field of blood transfusion [22]. The hopes engendered by this new approach to cell therapy should become concrete reality in the relatively near future, given the right conditions of research and development.

Disclosure of Conflict of Interests

The author states that he has no conflict of interest.

References

1 Buehler PW, Alayash AI: Toxicities of hemoglobin solutions: in search of in-vitro and in-vivo model systems. Transfusion 2004;44:1516–1530.
2 Sharma AC, Gulati A: Yohimbine modulates diaspirin crosslinked hemoglobin-induced systemic hemodynamics and regional circulatory effects. Crit Care Med 1995;23:874–884.
3 Remy B, Deby-Dupont G, D'Ans V, Ernest P, Lamy M: Substituts des globules rouges: émulsions de fluorocarbures et solutions d'hémoglobine. [Red cell substitutes: perfluorocarbon emulsions and hemoglobin solutions.] Ann Fr Anesth Reanim 1999;18:211–224.
4 Kerins DM: Role of the perfluorocarbon fluosol-DA in coronary angioplasty. Am J Med Sci 1994;307:218–221.
5 Krafft MP, Chittofrati A, Riess JG: Emulsions and microemulsions with a fluorocarbon phase. Curr Opin Colloid Interface Sci 2003;8:251–258.
6 Firat H, Douay L: Ex vivo expansion of mobilized peripheral blood stem cells. Baillieres Best Pract Res Clin Haematol 1999;12:99–115.
7 Lu L, Xiao M, Shen PN, Grigsby S, Broxmeyer ME: Enrichment, characterization, and responsiveness of single primitive CD34 human umbilical cord blood hematopoietic progenitors with high proliferative and replating potential. Blood 1993;81:41–48.

8 Douay L: Experimental culture conditions are critical for ex vivo expansion of hematopoietic cells. J Hematother Stem Cell Res 2001;10:341–346.
9 Ogawa M: Differentiation and proliferation of hematopoietic stem cells. Blood 1993;81:2844–2853.
10 Friedenstein AJ, Deriglasova UF, Kulagina NN, Panasuk AF, Rudakowa SF, Luriá EA, Ruadkow IA: Precursors for fibroblasts in different populations of hematopoietic cells as detected by the in vitro colony assay method. Exp Hematol 1974;2:83–92.
11 Neildez-Nguyen TM, Wajcman H, Marden MC, Bensidhoum M, Moncollin V, Giarratana MC, Kobari L, Thierry D, Douay L: Human erythroid cells produced ex vivo at large scale differentiate into red blood cells in vivo. Nat Biotechnol 2002;20:467–472.
12 Giarratana MC, Kobari L, Lapillonne H, Chalmers D, Kiger L, Cynober T, Marden MC, Wajcman H, Douay L: Ex vivo generation of fully mature human red blood cells from hematopoietic stem cells. Nat Biotechnol 2005;23:69–74.
13 Lichtman MA: The ultrastructure of the hemopoietic environment of the marrow: a review. Exp Hematol 1981;9:391–410.
14 Propper RD, Button LN, Nathan DG: New approaches to the transfusion management of thalassemia. Blood 1980;55:55–60.

15 Marcus RE, Wonke B, Bantock HM, Thomas MJ, Parry ES, Taite H, Huehns ER: A prospective trial of young red cells in 48 patients with transfusion-dependent thalassaemia. Br J Haematol 1985;60:153–159.

16 Mollison PL: Methods of determining the post-transfusion survival of stored red cells. Transfusion 1984;24:93–96.

17 Andreu G, Morel P, Forestier F, Debeir J, Rebibo D, Janvier G, Hervé P: Hemovigilance network in France: organization and analysis of immediate transfusion incident reports from 1994 to 1998. Transfusion 2002;42:1356–1364.

18 Kopko PM, Popovsky MA, MacKenzie MR, Paglieroni TG, Muto KN, Holland PV: HLA class II antibodies in transfusion-related acute lung injury. Transfusion 2001;41:1244–1248.

19 Silliman CC, Thurman GW, Ambruso DR: Stored blood components contain agents that prime the neutrophil NADPH oxidase through the platelet-activating-factor receptor. Vox Sang 1992;63:133–136.

20 Kruskall MS, AuBuchon JP, Anthony KY, Herschel L, Pickard C, Biehl R, Horowitz M, Brambilla DJ, Popovsky MA: Transfusion to blood group A and 0 patients of group B RBCs that have been enzymatically converted to group 0. Transfusion 2000;40:1290–1298.

21 Nacharaju P, Boctor FN, Manjula BN, Acharya SA: Surface decoration of red blood cells with maleimidophenyl-polyethylene glycol facilitated by thiolation with iminothiolane: an approach to mask A, B, and D antigens to generate universal red blood cells. Transfusion 2005;45:374–383.

22 Douay L, Andreu G: Ex vivo production of human red blood cells from hematopoietic stem cells: what is the future in transfusion? Transfus Med Rev 2007;21:91–100.

Prof. Luc Douay, M.D.
Inserm Unit UMR_S 893
27, rue de Chaligny
75571 Paris Cedex 12, France
Tel. +33 1 44 73-6222, Fax -6333
E-Mail luc.douay@trs.aphp.fr

Stem Cells and Blood Cell Engineering

Scharf RE (ed): Progress and Challenges in Transfusion Medicine, Hemostasis and Hemotherapy.
Freiburg i.Br., Karger, 2008, pp 162–177

From Hematopoietic Stem Cells to Megakaryocytes and Platelets

Rémi Favier[a, b, c] · William Vainchenker[a, b, d] · Hana Raslova[a, b, d]

[a]INSERM U790,
[b]Institute Gustave Roussy, Villejuif,
[c]Hematological Laboratory, Hospital Armand Trousseau, Paris,
[d]University Paris XI, U790, Villejuif, France

Key Words

Megakaryocyte · Platelet · Proplatelet · Thrombopoietin · Endomitosis · Transcription factors

Summary

Platelets are enucleated blood cells, which participate in many different biological functions such as hemostatic plug, wound repair, innate immunity, metastatic tumor cell dissemination, or viral reservoir. They are produced by fragmentation of the cytoplasm of bone marrow megakaryocytes (MK) through a dynamic process, called proplatelet formation. MK themselves are generated through different biological and cellular steps that include the commitment of hematopoietic stem cells towards MK progenitors, the proliferation of MK progenitors, their polyploidization and terminal maturation. Each human adult produces every day an average of 10^{11} platelets to maintain the platelet pool. The level of platelet production may vary under various exogenous or endogenous stimuli, implicating that megakaryocytopoiesis and platelet production are finely regulated by cellular and molecular mechanisms. This review focuses on the recent insights into megakaryocytopoiesis and platelet production. Numerous platelet disorders are now explained by molecular abnormalities in the activity of some transcription factors or in signaling molecules, like thrombopoietin and its receptor Mpl. These studies have also contributed to a better understanding of the molecular and humoral regulation of megakaryocytopoiesis. The recent development of MPL agonists provides a new and valuable therapeutic option for the management of some thrombocytopenias.
©2008 S. Karger GmbH, Freiburg i.Br.

Introduction

In clinical and transfusion medicine, the importance of megakaryocytopoiesis and thrombopoiesis is attested by the morbidity and mortality from bleeding due to moderate to severe thrombocytopenia. Thrombocytopenia is commonly encountered in numerous pathologies such as immune thrombocytopenia, myelodysplastic syndromes, and chemotherapy-induced thrombocytopenia. The magnitude of this problem can be gauged by considering that in the United States approximately 4 million platelet units are transfused yearly in order to reduce the risk of bleeding. Platelet transfusion therapy is expensive, and it is well known that adverse effects may occur such as immune and cytokine-mediated febrile reactions, refractory state to platelet transfusion, acute pulmonary injury, and graft-versus-host disease. During the last 30 years, many steps have been achieved that have greatly contributed to a better understanding of megakaryocytopoiesis and thrombopoiesis. These include the establishment of clonal assays in culture for megakaryocyte (MK) progenitor cells, the crucial isolation of thrombopoietin (TPO) allowing MK culture in liquid serum-free medium, the development of monoclonal antibodies against platelet glycoproteins used as markers in studies of MK differentiation, the identification of specific transcription factors driving megakaryocytic determination, methods to generate genetically modified MK and platelets using mutant mouse models and cell lines, and in vitro visualization of platelet formation by biphotonic microscopy. This review highlights data that address the cellular and molecular pathways regulating the development of MK and the generation of platelets.

The Cellular Origin of Megakaryocytes and Platelets

Hematopoietic Stem Cells

Sustained production of all hematopoietic lineages, which comprise cells with a relatively short life (including MK and platelets), is supplied by the differentiation from hematopoietic stem cells (HSC). HSC have two important properties: they have the potential to self-renew and to differentiate into various progenitor cells giving rise to all lineages [1, 2]. HSC will first produce a progeny of cells that lose the self-renewal capacity and acquire multipotential properties. Multipotent progenitors (MPP) will then commit to lymphoid or myeloid programs giving rise to common lymphoid (CLP) [3] and common myeloid (CMP) [4] progenitors. Next, CMP will commit to bipotent erythro-megakaryocytic (MEP) and to granulomacrophage (GMP) progenitors. An alternative model suggests that the MEP can directly derive from HSC [5]. MK precursor cells differentiate from MEP progenitors. HSC in bone marrow are largely quiescent, and amplification of the different blood cell compartments occurs from the proliferation of multipotent or bipotent hematopoietic progenitors. In the mouse, HSC and MPP are highly enriched in a Lin$^-$ c-Kit$^+$ Sca-1$^+$ cell population [6]. In this cell population, HSC express the Thy1.1 and CD150 markers, but not CD34 and FLT3, and are characterized by their incapacity to retain vital Hoechst (side population, SP) [7]. MPP do not express the Thy1.1 antigen. In human, HSC are defined by the expression of the CD34, CD133, Thy1, and c-Kit antigens and an absence of CD38 and lineage markers, while MPP are suggested to be CD38$^+$ like other hematopoietic progenitors [8].

Erythro-Megakaryocytic Progenitor

The existence of a common MEP was first suggested by the many common features of erythroid and megakaryocytic cells, like common transcription factors, cell surface molecules, and cytokine receptors. Later on, a bipotent progenitor that gives rise to colonies containing a majority of erythroblasts and a minority of MK was identified [9]. In the mouse, the MEP is characterized by the phenotype Lin⁻ c-Kit⁺ Sca-1⁻ FcγR⁻ CD34⁻ [2] and in human by Lin⁻ CD34⁺CD38⁺IL-3Rα⁻CD45RA⁻ markers [2]. However, the presence of MEP has also been reported in the CD34⁺CD38^low Lin⁻ cell fraction [9].

Megakaryocyte Progenitors

MK progenitor cells, restrictively committed towards the MK lineage, are capable of proliferation, and in vitro they give rise to MK colonies. Hierarchical classification of MK progenitors is essentially based on cell proliferation capacities. Burst-forming unit MK (BFU-MK) are the most primitive MK-committed progenitors with the highest aptitude to proliferate, giving rise to colonies composed of more than 50 cells. Colonies derived from BFU-MK appear after 12 days in the mouse [10] and 21 days in human. Colony-forming unit MK (CFU-MK) have lower capacities of proliferation and give rise to colonies composed of 3–50 cells after 5 days in the mouse [11] and 12 days in human [12]. A third and more mature progenitor has been defined in the mouse that gives rise, in 2–3 days, to colonies composed of a few MK with a high ploidy level [13].

Megakaryocyte Differentiation Stage-Specific Markers

In human, MK progenitors are characterized by the expression of CD34, CD31, and CD133 like other hematopoietic progenitors. The expression of human leukocyte antigen (HLA)-DR permits to differentiate BFU-MK (HLA-DR^low) from CFU-MK (HLA-DR^high). The use of several monoclonal antibodies directed against platelet proteins like the main platelet glycoproteins, GPIIb/IIIa (α2β3 integrin or CD41b) and GPIb complex (GPIbα, GPIbβ, GPIX, and GPV or CD42a, b, c and d) [14] allowed the characterization of the different steps of MK differentiation (fig. 1A). CD41a (GPIIb) or CD41b (GPIIb/IIIa complex) appears relatively specific of the MK lineage, especially in the adult, but can also be expressed on mast cells [15]. CD41 is present on a small fraction of marrow CD34⁺ cells (about 3%), and these CD34⁺CD41⁺ cells are enriched in MK progenitors. CD41 expression precedes the detection of other major platelet proteins including CD42. However, CD42 is present on a fraction of CD34⁺CD41⁺ cells [16]. Thus, CD34⁺CD41⁺CD42⁻ cells correspond to true CFU-

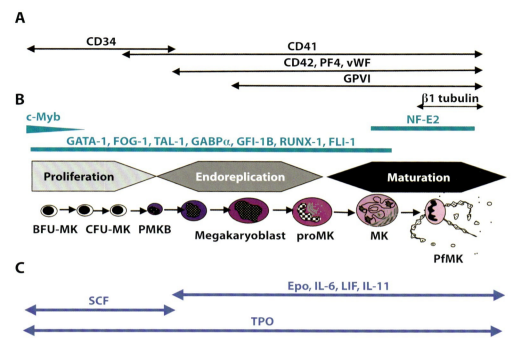

Fig. 1. Megakaryocytic differentiation. **A** Expression of differentiation markers along the human megakaryocytic differentiation. **B** Transcription factors involved in the development of the mega-karyocytic lineage. **C** Effects of cytokines along the human megakaryocytic differentiation. MK = Megakaryocyte; BFU-MK = burst-forming unit MK; CFU-MK = colony-forming unit MK; PMKB = promegakaryoblast; PfMK = proplatelet-forming MK; SCF = stem cell factor; Epo = erythropoietin; IL-6 = interleukin-6; LIF = leukemia-inducing factor; TPO = thrombopoietin. Adapted from Cramer and Vainchenker [71].

MK, whereas CD34⁺CD41⁺CD42⁺ cells give rise in vitro to single MK or to clusters of less than 4 MK. The CD42 antigen is a late MK marker associated with a significant increase in the expression of several membrane receptors like Mpl (TPO receptor), GPVI (collagen receptor), α2β1 integrin (collagen receptor), CD36 (thrombospon-din receptor), as well as α-granule proteins such as PF4 or vWF. The increase in the expression of platelet proteins is accompanied by a disappearance of the CD34 anti-gen during the endomitotic process.

Megakaryocyte and the Endomitotic Process

Committed MK progenitors first proliferate by a mitotic process. Thereafter, when the synthesis of platelet-specific proteins has begun, mitosis switches to endomitosis. MK endomitosis is an incomplete multipolar mitosis characterized by an absence of both nuclear (karyokinesis) and cytoplasmic (cytokinesis) division giving rise to a polyploid MK, which contains a unique multilobulated nucleus. MK are one of the rare cells that become polyploid during their normal differentiation in the absence of any hematopoietic stress. MK undergo several cycles of endoreplication leading to a modal ploidy number of 16N (from 4N to 128N) in human and mouse. The principal role of polyploidization is to increase the MK size, particularly the cytoplasm volume, which may increase even more strikingly than the ploidy level. As platelets arise from MK cytoplasm fragmentation, ploidization is an efficient manner to amplify the MK mass and thus platelet production. It has been suggested that only MK with a ploidy over 4N are capable of forming proplatelets. However, MK with a low ploidy (2N and 4N microMK) are able to shed platelets in culture. After the end of DNA replication, MK undergo terminal differentiation. Protein synthesis that leads to granule biogenesis is markedly increased along with the development of demarcation membranes required for platelet release [17, 18]. Several studies performed on MK either isolated from bone marrow or grown in culture have shown that endomitosis corresponds to an incomplete mitosis with a failure in cytokinesis. Like a mitosis, an endomitosis begins with a duplication of the centrosomes, followed by the development of a mitotic spindle, a prophase with chromatin condensation, a rupture of the nuclear envelope, a chromosome alignment on the equatorial plate during metaphase, and finally a sister chromatids separation in anaphase. The formation of a midzone, a network of antiparallel microtubules between the separating chromosomes, characterizes the metaphase to anaphase transition. The midzone is required for the maintenance of the overall spindle architecture, for spindle elongation, and cleavage furrow positioning. In polyploid MK, the spindle is multipolar with a number of poles corresponding to the ploidy level. However, the spindle remains short and does not elongate like in a normal mitosis. Nevertheless, an accurate midzone structure develops like during a normal mitosis with the presence of proteins necessary to regulate midzone formation and cytokinesis [19]. Recently, using real-time confocal videomicroscopy, we could demonstrate that endomitosis resembles the process called 'retro-cytokinesis' [Chang et al., unpublished data]. Telophase and the formation of a cleavage furrow are present at the 2N to 4N transition, however, mitosis did not proceed further with a reversal of cytokinesis characterized by a backward movement of the two 'potential' daughter cells, which leads to a unique cell with a single nucleus. At the end of endomitosis, MK thus contain a single nucleus with a single nuclear membrane. Each nuclear lobe corresponds to each pole of the multipolar spindle, and their number is a direct reflection of the ploidy.

The polyploidization process includes a succession of G1, S, G2 phases followed by a mitotic phase which is incomplete [20, 21]. After the M phase, MK reenter into G1 to initiate a subsequent cell cycle in order to duplicate their DNA. None of the molecular mechanisms linked to this phase of cell cycle, which were suggested to be at the origin of the endomitotic process, is really involved in MK polyploidization. No defect in cyclin B1 expression and activity was detected [21]. The presence and the correct localization of the main chromosomal passenger proteins such as survivin and aurora B [22, Chang et al., unpublished data] suggest that cytokinesis failure is not related to a defect in the central spindle. Rather, the absence of nonmuscle myosin IIA accumulation at furrowing sites implies that defects may occur in the contractile ring since contractile forces are related to the actin/myosin II complex [23, Chang et al., unpublished data]. Cell cycle exit and accumulation in a quiescent G0/G1 state depend on either the absence of mitogenic stimuli (loss of cyclin D-dependent activity) or the inhibition of CDK4/6. Different inhibitors of members of the INK4 and CIP/KIP families were investigated to explain the arrest of polyploidization because MK exit the cell cycle at different ploidy levels (from 2N to 128N). While p21^{CIP1} and p27^{KIP1} did not seem to be directly responsible for this process, we recently reported that p19^{INK4D} could directly regulate the endomitotic cell cycle arrest [24].

The main goal of MK ploidization is to facilitate the increase in cell size and thus proplatelet formation without losing the energy required for karyo- and cytokinesis. Polyploidization may be a way to markedly increase protein synthesis and to modify gene expression. Indeed, polyploidization is associated with a functional gene amplification without epigenetic silencing [25] and may modify gene expression in a differentiation-related manner [26].

Megakaryocyte and Platelet Shedding

The end of MK maturation is characterized by the formation of pseudopodial proplatelet extension, which will fragment into the platelets. This fragmentation does not occur inside the marrow but in blood circulation. In the bone marrow, MK are located in the extravascular space applied to the subendothelium region in close contact with endothelial cells. At the time of platelet release, long cytoplasm pseudopods invaginate, penetrate the endothelial lining cells, and enter into the marrow sinusoids. It has also been demonstrated that entire or fragmented MK can traverse the marrow-blood barrier and enter the circulation with terminal platelet maturation taking place in blood vessels [27]. This entire process has recently been filmed in vivo in mice [28].

Both the stroma and the extracellular matrix (ECM) play an important role in proplatelet formation. It has been shown that in the marrow microenvironment, fibrillar collagen type I prevents proplatelet formation [29]. On the other hand, during MK migration towards the endothelium and through the blood barrier, MK interact with other compounds of the ECM such as fibrinogen, which may induce or increase proplatelet formation. Immature MK express CXCR4 and respond to its ligand SDF-1 in order to be retained in the marrow. Then, the CXCR4 signaling pathway in response to SDF-1 is partly inactivated in mature MK and platelets. This may permit mature MK to migrate through the endothelial cell barrier and liberate platelets in the circulation [30].

The mechanism of platelet shedding requires the formation of long cytoplasm pseudopod extensions (proplatelet formation) [31]. Three main actors are involved in platelet shedding: the demarcation membrane system (DMS), microtubules, and actin filaments. DMS elaborates a network of MK membrane channels composed of flattened cisternae and tubules that serve as a membrane reservoir for platelet formation. Before proplatelet formation, DMS associates with both microtubules and actin filaments [32]. The assembling of tubulin molecules into linear filaments forms microtubules. While their polymerization is necessary to support the enlarging of proplatelet mass, the sliding of overlapping microtubules acts as a primary motor for proplatelet elongation [32]. During proplatelet elongation, microtubule bundles align in the proplatelet shafts and, at the free end of the extension, they form a loop and reenter the shaft [31]. Platelets are probably generated only at the free end of the proplatelet extension, but not at the swellings along the extensions. Microtubules also serve for the transport of mitochondria, granules, and other vesicular organelles into platelets [33]. The actin-myosin complex is not necessary for the extension of proplatelets, but is needed for proplatelet bending and branching, which leads to the amplification of platelet production [34].

Regulation of Megakaryocytopoiesis

The Molecular Regulation of Megakaryocytopoiesis

Three major transcription factor families are involved in the regulation of megakaryocytopoiesis (fig. 1B), and their implication has been confirmed by the presence of abnormalities in the study of hereditary thrombocytopenias.

GATA
Sequence analyses of MK-specific gene promoters, such as GPIIb, PF4, GPIba, β-TG, GPIX, or GPV, have revealed the presence of a consensus binding sequence (WGA-TAR) for transcription factors of the GATA family, also found in erythroid-specific genes [35, 36]. In some patients with the Bernard-Soulier syndrome, a mutation of the GATA-binding site was found within the GPIb promoter. Two GATA proteins are expressed during erythro-megakaryocytic differentiation. GATA-2 is mainly involved in the proliferation of multipotent progenitors. The knockout of GATA-1 leads to a lethal anemia in the embryo [37] and the knockout of GATA-1 directed in the MK lineage induces a profound macrothrombocytopenia with an excess of small immature MK in the marrow [38]. One of the most important cofactors of GATA-1 is FOG-1 (friend of GATA), which was identified by a yeast double-hybrid approach [39]. The knockout of FOG-1 gives a phenotype similar to that of GATA-1 in the erythroid lineage; in contrast, the phenotype is more profound in the MK lineage with a total absence of progenitors. This suggests that FOG-1 may associate with another partner, such a GATA-2, during the early stage of the MK differentiation. The significance of GATA-1/FOG-1 association has been underlined in human X-linked

congenital thrombocytopenia characterized by macroplatelets and a moderate dys-erythropoiesis. Four distinct GATA-1 mutation types have been detected in X-linked disorders: 1) mutation impairing FOG-1 binding; 2) mutation impairing binding to a GATC motif; 3) mutation affecting the N finger of GATA-1 but disrupting neither FOG-1 nor DNA binding; 4) hereditary mutation generating a truncated form of GATA-1 (GATA-1s) [40]. It should be noted that the severity of anemia and throm-bocytopenia depends on the mutation type mentioned above. In addition, acquired mutations in exon 2 of GATA-1 which generate a short GATA-1 variant (GATA-1s) lacking the N-terminal have been detected in transient myeloproliferative diseases and acute megakaryoblastic leukemia (AML-M7) associated with Down syndrome [41].

RUNX

Recently, it has been shown that the transcription factor AML-1 (RUNX-1), a DNA-binding subunit of the core-binding factor (CBF) transcription complex, may coop-erate with GATA-1 [42, 43]. RUNX sites consisting of TGT/cGGT motifs have been found in several megakaryocytic promoters [43], and both RUNX-1 and CBFβ are highly expressed during megakaryocytic but not erythroid differentiation [43, 44]. Germline heterozygous missense mutations, frameshift mutations, nonsense muta-tions, and a point nucleotide deletion in a single allele of the RUNX-1 gene were de-tected in cases of familial platelet disorder with predisposition to acute myelogenous leukemia (FPD/AML) [45]. All result in a lack of DNA binding. Two mechanisms for FPD/AML induction were proposed that depend on the mutation type: one is linked to a haploinsufficiency and the second to a negative dominant function [46]. In the first, mutated RUNX-1 has lost its capacity to interact with CBFβ; in the second, the RUNX-1/CBFβ interaction is conserved. The predisposition to develop AML seems to be related to the role of RUNX-1 in HSC homeostasis that may be increased when mutant RUNX-1 displays a dominant negative function. The knockout of RUNX-1 in mice shows that it is essential for the establishment of definitive hematopoiesis [47]; an inducible knockout of both RUNX-1 and CBFβ causes a profound disruption of megakaryocytopoiesis [48–50].

ETS

The most studied ETS transcription factor in MK differentiation is FLI-1. In humans, FLI-1 is localized in the 11q23.3 chromosome region deleted in the Paris-Trousseau thrombocytopenia. This disease is characterized by a marked thrombocytopenia with an excess of small immature MK in bone marrow undergoing apoptosis [51]. It has been shown that overexpression of FLI-1 in CD34$^+$ cells of patients partially restores the dysmegakaryocytopoiesis linked to this syndrome [52]. FLI-1 cooper-ates with GATA-1 and FOG-1 to transcriptionally activate the expression of late MK genes such as GPIX, GPIba, and PF4 [53]. Another ETS transcription factor, GABPα, seems to regulate the expression of genes such as GPIIb or c-mpl expressed earlier during MK differentiation [54]. EKLF transcription factor has recently been demonstrated to act as an antagonist of FLI-1. While FLI-1 is involved in the commitment of MEP towards the MK lineage, EKLF plays the same role in the commitment to the erythroid lineage [55]. The inducible knockout of TEL-1, an ETS transcription factor, leads to a dramatic decrease in platelet counts [56]. Recently, it has been shown that ETS-1 expression increases during MK maturation and that its overexpression promotes MK differentiation and enhances the upregulation of GATA-2 and MK-specific genes [57].

Other transcription factors that are necessary for megakaryocytopoiesis include TAL-1, NF-E2, GFI-1B, and c-MYB. Deletion of the bHLH transcription factor TAL-1 (SCL) in adult mice leads to a loss of early progenitors of MK and erythroid lineages [58]. Recent data indicate that TAL-1 plays a major role in platelet production during stress thrombopoiesis by regulating directly NF-E2 transcriptional activity [59]. An active NF-E2 transcription factor is formed by a heterodimerization of p45^{NF-E2} (basic leucine zipper protein) with proteins of the Maf family. The knockout of p45^{NF-E2} is lethal at birth. Mice display a profound thrombocytopenia, an increase in the number of MK presenting a marked defect in both the development of demarcation membranes and the distribution of a-granules [60]. The double knockout of two NF-E2 partners, MafG and MafK, generates mice with the same degree of thrombocytopenia as p45^{NF-E2} knockout mice [61]. Three target genes of p45^{NF-E2}, β1-tubulin, 3β-HSD, and Rab27b, are involved in proplatelet formation. The knockout of GFI-1b is lethal during embryogenesis due to a profound anemia and thrombocytopenia. Fetal liver progenitors from GFI-1b knockout mice give rise to small MK colonies with a decreased level of GPIIb, c-mpl, and NF-E2 compared to wild-type cells [62]. A recent study suggests that c-Myb acts as a negative regulator for the commitment of MPP towards the MK lineage [63].

It should be noted that MK differentiation from HSC via MEP to platelets does not depend at any stage on one single transcription factor, but results from a cooperation of a network of multiple transcription factors belonging to different families.

The Humoral Regulation of Megakaryocytopoiesis

Studies on the regulation of megakaryocytopoiesis have been dominated by two concepts (fig. 1C): (i) a humoral regulation by a late differentiation factor, called TPO [64], which would be the equivalent of erythropoietin for the MK lineage; (ii) a sequential dual regulation corresponding to different developmental stages, one early in differentiation by proliferative factors called MK colony-stimulating factor (MK-CSF), the second late in differentiation by differentiation factors also called potentiators or synergistic factors [65]. The identification of TPO, the humoral factor regulating platelet production, has demonstrated that TPO acts both in early and late stages of megakaryocytopoiesis.

Historical Perspectives

The existence of a factor in the plasma of animals or patients with severe thrombocytopenia which could increase platelet number and size as well as MK number, size, and ploidy was proposed more than 40 years ago. In analogy to the model of erythropoietin (EPO), this factor was termed thrombopoietin or TPO. Thereafter, it was noted that the plasma from aplastic mammals could stimulate the in vitro proliferation of MK progenitor cells. This proliferative activity was referred to as MK-CSF and was thought to be different from TPO. The isolation of several recombinant cytokines and analyses of their in vitro effects led to the concept that megakaryocytopoiesis was regulated at two levels by early factors acting on the proliferation of committed MK progenitor cells (interleukin-3, IL-3; granulomacrophagic colony-stimulating factor, GM-CSF; stem cell factor, SCF) and by TPO-like factors stimulating the later stages of MK maturation (IL-6; IL-11; leukemia-inducing factor, LIF; EPO). However, none of these cytokines is specific for the MK lineage. The breakthrough in the isolation and cloning of the TPO gene stems is the demonstration that the murine myeloproliferative leukemia virus contains a truncated form (v-mpl oncogene) of an orphan cytokine receptor [66].

The c-mpl Proto-Oncogene, a Receptor for Thrombopoietin

Early studies demonstrate that the c-mpl proto-oncogene product (Mpl) plays a key role in megakaryocytopoiesis. In human, c-mpl mRNA is expressed in bone marrow and fetal liver tissues, but its expression is restricted to CD34$^+$ cells, MK, platelets, and endothelial cells [67]. c-mpl knockout mice exhibit a dramatic reduction (85%) in platelet count and a profound decrease in the number of MK in the marrow without alteration of the number of red blood cells or leukocytes [68]. Together, these observations indicated that Mpl could be activated by a regulator acting predominantly on thrombopoiesis. The use of an Mpl-soluble receptor fused to an immunoglobulin Fc fragment or coupled to affinity matrices permits to isolate and clone its ligand, TPO [69].

Structure of the Mpl Ligand/Thrombopoietin

The human TPO cDNA contains an open reading frame of 1,059 nucleotides, which predicts a primary translation product of 353 amino acids. The N-terminus is highly hydrophobic and likely functions as a secretory signal. The protein has a two-domain structure. The amino-terminal domain of 153 amino acids is well conserved among species and shares 25% identity (50% similarity) to EPO. Both TPO and EPO have 4 cysteines, of which 3 are conserved. Based on sequence alignment, it is predicted that the 'EPO-like' domain of TPO would adopt a four-alpha-helical structure similar to that proposed for EPO or other cytokines and shown to be involved in receptor interactions. The carboxy-terminal domain of 179 amino acids is less conserved between species and bears no recognizable homology with other known protein sequences. This domain is rich in serine, threonine, and proline residues and contains all potential N-linked glycosylation sites (6 for the human, porcine, canine TPO and 7 for the murine TPO). The 'EPO-like' and the C-terminal domains of TPO are separated by a dibasic Arg-Arg sequence, that is conserved at the same position among the species examined and that could serve as proteolytic site. The mature EPO is also processed from a precursor polypeptide by proteolytic cleavage at an arginine residue located in a similar position. Therefore, TPO might be expressed as a precursor protein, which undergoes proteolysis to generate a mature active ligand. The biological activity of TPO resides in the N-terminal 'EPO-like' domain. Recombinant forms of a truncated human and murine TPO deleted of the carboxy domain are competent for receptor binding, stimulation of proliferation in c-mpl-transfected cells, and proliferation and maturation of MK in vitro. The role of the carboxy domain is not yet clearly established [70].

Site of TPO Production and Regulation

In humans, the liver appears to be the major TPO production site, but TPO mRNA is also detected in kidney and skeletal muscle or, at a low level, in testis, bone marrow fibroblasts, and umbilical endothelial cells. The molecular basis for the regulation of plasma TPO levels is still under investigation. Prior studies demonstrate that serum TPO levels are inversely related to platelet mass [69]. It is usually considered that TPO gene expression is constitutive with TPO serum level being modulated by the number of platelets and MK through a mechanism of uptake and catabolism. However, TPO synthesis might be regulated by the platelet level in marrow stromal cells or by inflammatory cytokines.

The Biological Activity of TPO

In vivo injection of TPO induces a thrombopoietic response considerably greater than the effects seen following administration of other cytokines, such as IL-6, IL-11, or SCF. In vitro, TPO can induce a complete MK differentiation from CD34+ cells leading to polyploidy and fully mature MK capable of shedding platelets. However, a combination of growth factors such as SCF plus IL-6 and IL-3 can have a similar effect as TPO. c-mpl or TPO knockout mice have a marked but nonlethal thrombocytopenia. In addition, in response to 5-fluorouracil (5-FU), these mice exhibit a rebound thrombocytosis. This result clearly suggests that other factors regulate platelet formation. It has been recently suggested that the residual platelet formation is related to fibroblast growth factor-4 (FGF-4) and SDF-1, which allow an interaction between MK and endothelial cells [71].

A surprising result was that TPO also regulates the HSC compartment, as demonstrated with c-mpl or TPO knockout mice. These mice have a decrease in long-term reconstituting cells, which becomes more pronounced with aging. It has been recently reported that TPO regulates both the quiescence of HSC and the amplification of multipotent progenitors [72]. Interestingly, the homozygous losses of function by mutation of c-mpl in humans lead to congenital amegakaryocytic thrombocytopenia, a disease characterized by a very profound thrombocytopenia quickly progressing to a lethal aplastic anemia. Thus, in human, TPO regulates both platelet production and HSC. In addition, TPO acts on dendritic cells and mast cells.

In vivo Generation of Platelets

Advances in the understanding of the TPO structure have enabled the development of the first generation of TPO-like growth factors, i.e., recombinant human TPO and pegylated recombinant human megakaryocyte growth and development factor (PEG-rHuMGDF – the pegylated 'cytokine' domain of TPO). In clinical trials, these agents were effective in promoting a significant increase in platelet counts in different thrombocytopenic disorders. However, these first trials were stopped when neutralizing antibodies cross-reacting with endogenous TPO and causing thrombocytopenia in healthy donors were detected. A second generation of thrombopoietic growth factors, including TPO peptide and nonpeptide mimetics and TPO agonist antibodies, was subsequently developed. Two Mpl agonists, a TPO peptide mimetic (AMG 531), and a nonpeptide mimetic (eltrombopag) are currently in advanced clinical trials. Both resulted in dose-dependent platelet increases in patients with immune thrombocytopenic purpura (ITP) and in patients with thrombopenia due to severe hepatic diseases [73, 74]. The median time from the first dose to peak platelet count was 10 days. Efficacy was highest with a dose equivalent to >1 µg/kg.

Clinical trials are also conducted to test the efficacy and safety of eltrombopag for the treatment of thrombocytopenia in ITP. The efficacy, safety, and tolerability of this agent have been demonstrated in a randomized, controlled trial including more than 100 adults with chronic ITP [75]. Eltrombopag is also used in hepatitis C virus-infected patients.

From these preliminary studies, it appears that these new agents are well tolerated and that the formation of antibodies against TPO is not detected. Increases in marrow reticulin have been demonstrated with some growth factors in some patients, but this phenomenon is reversible. No increased incidence of thrombotic events in patients who achieve high platelet counts was observed. Supplementary data are necessary concerning the effects induced by the long-term use of these drugs, and the clinical use in children must be determined also. Other agents have been developed by several companies and begin to be tested (romiplostim).

Conclusions and Future Directions

In these last years, a lot of progress has been made in the understanding of megakaryocytopoiesis and the mechanisms of platelet production. This knowledge has already permitted to better understand the mechanisms of numerous congenital or acquired disorders of platelet production including megakaryoblastic leukemia and myeloproliferative syndromes. The recent development of new thrombopoietic agents, agonists of the TPO receptor (Mpl), offers novel strategies inducing in vivo generation of platelets in the treatment of thrombocytopenia. In parallel to these encouraging results, several issues remain to be addressed before realizing large-scale ex vivo generation of platelets for a clinical applicability, and serious obstacles need to be overcome before these new methods can be used for clinical platelet transfusion.

Disclosure of Conflict of Interests

The authors state that they have no conflict of interest.

Acknowledgements

We are grateful to F. Wendling for critical reading of the manuscript and helpful suggestions.
Our laboratory is supported by grants from the Institut National de la Santé et de la Recherche Médicale (INSERM), the Ligue Nationale contre le Cancer (LNCC), the Association de Recherche contre le Cancer (ARC), and the Agence Nationale de la Recherche (ANR).

References

1 Till JE, McCulloch EA: A direct measurement of the radiation sensitivity of normal mouse bone marrow cells. Radiat Res 1961;14:213–222.

2 Bryder D, Rossi DJ, Weissman IL: Hematopoietic stem cells: the paradigmatic tissue-specific stem cell. Am J Pathol 2006;169:338–346.

3 Kondo M, Weissman IL, Akashi K: Identification of clonogenic common lymphoid progenitors in mouse bone marrow. Cell 1997;91:661–672.

4 Akashi K, Traver D, Miyamoto T, Weissman IL: A clonogenic common myeloid progenitor that gives rise to all myeloid lineages. Nature 2000;404:193–197.

5 Forsberg EC, Serwold T, Kogan S, Weissman IL, Passegue E: New evidence supporting megakaryocyte-erythrocyte potential of flk2/flt3+ multipotent hematopoietic progenitors. Cell 2006;126:415–426.

6 Osawa M, Nakamura K, Nishi N, Takahasi N, Tokuomoto Y, Inoue H, Nakauchi H: In vivo self-renewal of c-Kit+ Sca-1+ Lin(low/–) hemopoietic stem cells. J Immunol 1996;156:3207–3214.

7 Goodell MA, Brose K, Paradis G, Conner AS, Mulligan RC: Isolation and functional properties of murine hematopoietic stem cells that are replicating in vivo. J Exp Med 1996;183:1797–1806.

8 Manz MG, Miyamoto T, Akashi K, Weissman IL: Prospective isolation of human clonogenic common myeloid progenitors. Proc Natl Acad Sci U S A 2002;99:11872–11877.

9 Debili N, Coulombel L, Croisille L, Katz A, Guichard J, Breton-Gorius J, Vainchenker W: Characterization of a bipotent erythro-megakaryocytic progenitor in human bone marrow. Blood 1996;88:1284–1296.

10 Long MW, Gragowski LL, Heffner CH, Boxer LA: Phorbol diesters stimulate the development of an early murine progenitor cell. The burst-forming unit-megakaryocyte. J Clin Invest 1985;76:431–438.

11 McLeod DL, Shreeve MM, Axelrad AA: Induction of megakaryocyte colonies with platelet formation in vitro. Nature 1976;261:492–494.

12 Vainchenker W, Bouget J, Guichard J, Breton-Gorius J: Megakaryocyte colony formation from human bone marrow precursors. Blood 1979;54:940–947.

13 Chatelain C, De Bast M, Symann M: Identification of a light density murine megakaryocyte progenitor (LD-CFU-M). Blood 1988;72:1187–1192.

14 Vinci G, Tabilio A, Deschamps JF, Van Haeke D, Henri A, Guichard J, Tetteroo P, Lansdorp PM, Hercend T, Vainchenker W, Breton-Gorius J: Immunological study of in vitro maturation of human megakaryocytes. Br J Haematol 1984;56:589–605.

15 Kirshenbaum AS, Akin C, Goff JP, Metcalfe DD: Thrombopoietin alone or in the presence of stem cell factor supports the growth of KIT(CD117)low/MPL(CD110)+ human mast cells from hematopoietic progenitor cells. Exp Hematol 2005;33:413–421.

16 Debili N, Issaad C, Masse JM, Guichard J, Katz A, Breton-Gorius J, Vainchenker W: Expression of CD34 and platelet glycoproteins during human megakaryocytic differentiation. Blood 1992;80:3022–3035.

17 Behnke O: An electron microscope study of the megakaryocyte of the rat bone marrow. I. The development of the demarcation membrane system and the platelet surface coat. J Ultrastruct Res 1968;24:412–433.

18 Cramer EM, Norol F, Guichard J, Breton-Gorius J, Vainchenker W, Masse JM, Debili N: Ultrastructure of platelet formation by human megakaryocytes cultured with the Mpl ligand. Blood 1997;89:2336–2346.

19 Geddis AE, Kaushansky K: Endomitotic megakaryocytes form a midzone in anaphase but have a deficiency in cleavage furrow formation. Cell Cycle 2006;5:538–545.

20 Ravid K, Lu J, Zimmet JM, Jones MR: Road to polyploidy: the megakaryocyte example. J Cell Physiol 2002;190:7–20.

21 Vitrat N, Cohen-Solal K, Pique C, Le Couedic JP, Norol F, Larsen AK, Katz A, Vainchenker W, Debili N: Endomitosis of human megakaryocytes are due to abortive mitosis. Blood 1998;91:3711–3723.

22 Geddis AE, Kaushansky K: Megakaryocytes express functional Aurora-B kinase in endomitosis. Blood 2004;104:1017–1024.

23 Geddis AE, Fox NE, Tkachenko E, Kaushansky K: Endomitotic megakaryocytes that form a bipolar spindle exhibit cleavage furrow ingression followed by furrow regression. Cell Cycle 2007;6:455–460.

24 Gilles L, Guieze R, Bluteau D, Cordette-Lagarde V, Lacout C, Favier R, Larbret F, Debili N, Vainchenker W, Raslova H: p19^INK4D links endomitotic arrest and megakaryocyte maturation and is regulated by AML-1. Blood 2008;111:4081–4091.

25 Raslova H, Roy L, Vourc'h C, Le Couedic JP, Brison O, Metivier D, Feunteun J, Kroemer G, Debili N, Vainchenker W: Megakaryocyte polyploidization is associated with a functional gene amplification. Blood 2003;101:541–544.

26 Raslova H, Kauffmann A, Sekkai D, Ripoche H, Larbret F, Robert T, Le Roux DT, Kroemer G, Debili N, Dessen P, Lazar V, Vainchenker W: Interrelation between polyploidization and megakaryocyte differentiation: a gene profiling approach. Blood 2007;109:3225–3234.

27 Italiano JE Jr, Shivdasani RA: Megakaryocytes and beyond: the birth of platelets. J Thromb Haemost 2003;1:1174–1182.

28 Junt T, Schulze H, Chen Z, Massberg S, Goerge T, Krueger A, Wagner DD, Graf T, Italiano JE Jr, Shivdasani RA, von Andrian UH: Dynamic visualization of thrombopoiesis within bone marrow. Science 2007;317:1767–1770.

29 Sabri S, Jandrot-Perrus M, Bertoglio J, Farndale RW, Mas VM, Debili N, Vainchenker W: Differential regulation of actin stress fiber assembly and proplatelet formation by alpha2beta1 integrin and GPVI in human megakaryocytes. Blood 2004;104:3117–3125.

30 Riviere C, Subra F, Cohen-Solal K, Cordette-Lagarde V, Letestu R, Auclair C, Vainchenker W, Louache F: Phenotypic and functional evidence for the expression of CXCR4 receptor during megakaryocytopoiesis. Blood 1999;93:1511–1523.

31 Italiano JE Jr, Lecine P, Shivdasani RA, Hartwig JH: Blood platelets are assembled principally at the ends of proplatelet processes produced by differentiated megakaryocytes. J Cell Biol 1999;147:1299–1342.

32 Patel SR, Richardson JL, Schulze H, Kahle E, Galjart N, Drabek K, Shivdasani RA, Hartwig JH, Italiano JE Jr: Differential roles of microtubule assembly and sliding in proplatelet formation by megakaryocytes. Blood 2005;106:4076–4085.

33 Richardson JL, Shivdasani RA, Boers C, Hartwig JH, Italiano JE Jr: Mechanisms of organelle transport and capture along proplatelets during platelet production. Blood 2005;106:4066–4075.

34 Schulze H, Korpal M, Hurov J, Kim SW, Zhang J, Cantley LC, Graf T, Shivdasani RA: Characterization of the megakaryocyte demarcation membrane system and its role in thrombopoiesis. Blood 2006;107:3868–3875.

35 Ravid K, Doi T, Beeler DL, Kuter DJ, Rosenberg RD: Transcriptional regulation of the rat platelet factor 4 gene: interaction between an enhancer/silencer domain and the GATA site. Mol Cell Biol 1991;11:6116–6127.

36 Martin F, Prandini MH, Thevenon D, Marguerie G, Uzan G: The transcription factor GATA-1 regulates the promoter activity of the platelet glycoprotein IIb gene. J Biol Chem 1993;268:21606–21612.

37 Pevny L, Simon MC, Robertson E, Klein WH, Tsai SF, D'Agati V, Orkin SH, Costantini F: Erythroid differentiation in chimaeric mice blocked by a targeted mutation in the gene for transcription factor GATA-1. Nature 1991;349:257–261.

38 Shivdasani RA, Fujiwara Y, McDevitt MA, Orkin SH: A lineage-selective knockout establishes the critical role of transcription factor GATA-1 in megakaryocyte growth and platelet development. EMBO J 1997;16:3965–3973.

39 Tsang AP, Visvader JE, Turner CA, Fujiwara Y, Yu C, Weiss MJ, Crossley M, Orkin SH: FOG, a multitype zinc finger protein, acts as a cofactor for transcription factor GATA-1 in erythroid and megakaryocytic differentiation. Cell 1997;90:109–119.

40 Goldfarb AN: Transcriptional control of megakaryocyte development. Oncogene 2007;26:6795–6802.

41 Wechsler J, Greene M, McDevitt MA, Anastasi J, Karp JE, Le Beau MM, Crispino JD: Acquired mutations in GATA1 in the megakaryoblastic leukemia of Down syndrome. Nat Genet 2002;32:148–152.

42 Waltzer L, Ferjoux G, Bataille L, Haenlin M: Cooperation between the GATA and RUNX factors Serpent and Lozenge during Drosophila hematopoiesis. EMBO J 2003;22:6516–6525.

43 Elagib KE, Racke FK, Mogass M, Khetawat R, Delehanty LL, Goldfarb AN: RUNX1 and GATA-1 coexpression and cooperation in megakaryocytic differentiation. Blood 2003;101:4333–4341.

44 Kundu M, Chen A, Anderson S, Kirby M, Xu L, Castilla LH, Bodine D, Liu PP: Role of Cbfb in hematopoiesis and perturbations resulting from expression of the leukemogenic fusion gene Cbfβ-MYH11. Blood 2002;100:2449–2456.

45 Song WJ, Sullivan MG, Legare RD, Hutchings S, Tan X, Kufrin D, Ratajczak J, Resende IC, Haworth C, Hock R, Loh M, Felix C, Roy DC, Busque L, Kurnit D, Willman C, Gewirtz AM, Speck NA, Bushweller JH, Li FP, Gardiner K, Poncz M, Maris JM, Gilliland DG: Haploinsufficiency of CBFA2 causes familial thrombocytopenia with propensity to develop acute myelogenous leukaemia. Nat Genet 1999;23:166–175.

46 Michaud J, Wu F, Osato M, Cottles GM, Yanagida M, Asou N, Shigesada K, Ito Y, Benson KF, Raskind WH, Rossier C, Antonarakis SE, Israels S, McNicol A, Weiss H, Horwitz M, Scott HS: In vitro analyses of known and novel RUNX1/AML1 mutations in dominant familial platelet disorder with predisposition to acute myelogenous leukemia: implications for mechanisms of pathogenesis. Blood 2002;99:1364–1372.

47 Okuda T, van Deursen J, Hiebert SW, Grosveld G, Downing JR: AML1, the target of multiple chromosomal translocations in human leukemia, is essential for normal fetal liver hematopoiesis. Cell 1996;84:321–330.

48 Ichikawa M, Asai T, Saito T, Seo S, Yamazaki I, Yamagata T, Mitani K, Chiba S, Ogawa S, Kurokawa M, Hirai H: AML-1 is required for megakaryocytic maturation and lymphocytic differentiation, but not for maintenance of hematopoietic stem cells in adult hematopoiesis. Nat Med 2004;10:299–304.

49 Sun W, Downing JR: Haploinsufficiency of AML1 results in a decrease in the number of LTR-HSCs while simultaneously inducing an increase in more mature progenitors. Blood 2004;104:3565–3572.

50 Talebian L, Li Z, Guo Y, Gaudet J, Speck ME, Sugiyama D, Kaur P, Pear WS, Maillard I, Speck NA: T-lymphoid, megakaryocyte, and granulocyte development are sensitive to decreases in CBFbeta dosage. Blood 2007;109:11–21.

51 Breton-Gorius J, Favier R, Guichard J, Cherif D, Berger R, Debili N, Vainchenker W, Douay L: A new congenital dysmegakaryopoietic thrombocytopenia (Paris-Trousseau) associated with giant platelet alpha-granules and chromosome 11 deletion at 11q23. Blood 1995;85:1805–1814.

52 Raslova H, Komura E, Le Couedic JP, Larbret F, Debili N, Feunteun J, Danos O, Albagli O, Vainchenker W, Favier R: FLI1 monoallelic expression combined with its hemizygous loss underlies Paris-Trousseau/Jacobsen thrombopenia. J Clin Invest 2004;114:77–84.

53 Wang X, Crispino JD, Letting DL, Nakazawa M, Poncz M, Blobel GA: Control of megakaryocyte-specific gene expression by GATA-1 and FOG-1: role of Ets transcription factors. EMBO J 2002;21:5225–5234.

54 Pang L, Xue HH, Szalai G, Wang X, Wang Y, Watson DK, Leonard WJ, Blobel GA, Poncz M: Maturation stage-specific regulation of megakaryopoiesis by pointed-domain Ets proteins. Blood 2006;108:2198–2206.

55 Starck J, Cohet N, Gonnet C, Sarrazin S, Doubeikovskaia Z, Doubeikovski A, Verger A, Duterque-Coquillaud M, Morle F: Functional cross-antagonism between transcription factors FLI-1 and EKLF. Mol Cell Biol 2003;23:1390–1402.

56 Hock H, Meade E, Medeiros S, Schindler JW, Valk PJ, Fujiwara Y, Orkin SH: Tel/Etv6 is an essential and selective regulator of adult hematopoietic stem cell survival. Genes Dev 2004;18:2336–2341.

57 Lulli V, Romania P, Morsilli O, Gabbianelli M, Pagliuca A, Mazzeo S, Testa U, Peschle C, Marziali G: Overexpression of Ets-1 in human hematopoietic progenitor cells blocks erythroid and promotes megakaryocytic differentiation. Cell Death Differ 2006;13:1064–1074.

58 Hall MA, Curtis DJ, Metcalf D, Elefanty AG, Sourris K, Robb L, Gothert JR, Jane SM, Begley CG: The critical regulator of embryonic hematopoiesis, SCL, is vital in the adult for megakaryopoiesis, erythropoiesis, and lineage choice in CFU-S12. Proc Natl Acad Sci U S A 2003;100:992–997.

59 McCormack MP, Hall MA, Schoenwaelder SM, Zhao Q, Ellis S, Prentice JA, Clarke AJ, Slater NJ, Salmon JM, Jackson SP, Jane SM, Curtis DJ: A critical role for the transcription factor Scl in platelet production during stress thrombopoiesis. Blood 2006;108:2248–2256.

60 Shivdasani RA, Rosenblatt MF, Zucker-Franklin D, Jackson CW, Hunt P, Saris CJ, Orkin SH: Transcription factor NF-E2 is required for platelet formation independent of the actions of thrombopoietin/MGDF in megakaryocyte development. Cell 1995;81:695–704.

61 Onodera K, Shavit JA, Motohashi H, Yamamoto M, Engel JD: Perinatal synthetic lethality and hematopoietic defects in compound mafG:mafK mutant mice. EMBO J 2000;19:1335–1345.

62 Saleque S, Cameron S, Orkin SH: The zinc-finger proto-oncogene Gfi-1b is essential for development of the erythroid and megakaryocytic lineages. Genes Dev 2002;16:301–306.

63 Emambokus N, Vegiopoulos A, Harman B, Jenkinson E, Anderson G, Frampton J: Progression through key stages of haemopoiesis is dependent on distinct threshold levels of c-Myb. EMBO J 2003;22:4478–4488.

64 Kelemen E, Cserhati I, Tanos B: Demonstration and some properties of human thrombopoietin in thrombocythaemic sera. Acta Haematol 1958;20:350–355.

65 Williams N, Eger RR, Jackson HM, Nelson DJ: Two-factor requirement for murine megakaryocyte colony formation. J Cell Physiol 1982;110:101–104.

66 Souyri M, Vigon I, Penciolelli JF, Heard JM, Tambourin P, Wendling F: A putative truncated cytokine receptor gene transduced by the myeloproliferative leukemia virus immortalizes hematopoietic progenitors. Cell 1990;63:1137–1147.

67 Methia N, Louache F, Vainchenker W, Wendling F: Oligodeoxynucleotides antisense to the proto-oncogene c-mpl specifically inhibit in vitro megakaryocytopoiesis. Blood 1993;82:1395–1401.

68 Gurney AL, Carver-Moore K, de Sauvage FJ, Moore MW: Thrombocytopenia in c-mpl-deficient mice. Science 1994;265:1445–1447.

69 Kaushansky K: Historical review: megakaryopoiesis and thrombopoiesis. Blood 2008;111:981–986.

70 Kaushansky K, Drachman JG: The molecular and cellular biology of thrombopoietin: the primary regulator of platelet production. Oncogene 2002;21:3359–3367.

71 Cramer E, Vainchenker W: Platelet production: cellular and molecular regulation; in Colman RW, Hirsh J, Marder VJ, Clowes AW, George JN (eds): Hemostasis and Thrombosis: Basic Principles and Clinical Practice, ed 5. Philadelphia, Lippincott Williams & Wilkins, 2006, pp 443–461.

72 Qian H, Buza-Vidas N, Hyland CD, Jensen CT, Antonchuk J, Mansson R, Thoren LA, Ekblom M, Alexander WS, Jacobsen SE: Critical role of thrombopoietin in maintaining adult quiescent hematopoietic stem cells. Cell Stem Cell 2007;1:671–684.

73 Newland A, Caulier MT, Kappers-Klunne M, Schipperus MR, Lefrere F, Zwaginga JJ, Christal J, Chen CF, Nichol JL: An open-label, unit dose-finding study of AMG 531, a novel thrombopoiesis-stimulating peptibody, in patients with immune thrombocytopenic purpura. Br J Haematol 2006;135:547–553.

74 Bussel JB, Kuter DJ, George JN, McMillan R, Aledort LM, Conklin GT, Lichtin AE, Lyons RM, Nieva J, Wasser JS, Wiznitzer I, Kelly R, Chen CF, Nichol JL: AMG 531, a thrombopoiesis-stimulating protein, for chronic ITP. N Engl J Med 2006;355:1672–1681.

75 Bussel JB, Cheng G, Saleh MN, Psaila B, Kovaleva L, Meddeb B, Kloczko J, Hassani H, Mayer B, Stone NL, Arning M, Provan D, Jenkins JM: Eltrombopag for the treatment of chronic idiopathic thrombocytopenic purpura. N Engl J Med 2007;357:2237–2247.

Hana Raslova, Ph.D.
Institut Gustave Roussy
INSERM U790
39, rue Camille Desmoulins, 94805 Villejuif, France
Tel. +33 1 42 11-4671, Fax -5240
E-Mail hraslova@igr.fr

Molecular Immunohematology

Scharf RE (ed): Progress and Challenges in Transfusion Medicine, Hemostasis and Hemotherapy.
Freiburg i.Br., Karger, 2008, pp 178–188

The Bloodgen Project of the European Union

Neil D. Avent, on behalf of the Bloodgen consortium

Centre for Research in Biomedicine, Faculty of Health and Life Sciences, University of the West of England, Bristol, UK

Key Words

Blood group antigens · Genotyping · Mass scale · Microarray

Summary

Blood group genotyping has existed since the mid 1990s following the definition of the molecular basis of the major clinically significant blood group antigens. Initially at least, the application of molecular genotyping for blood group status was applied to situations where blood was difficult or risky to obtain, most notably in prenatal diagnosis in instances of maternal alloimmunisation to RhD, other Rh antigens, Kell and Duffy, and thus used in the clinical management of haemolytic disease of the foetus and new-born (HDFN). The genotyping assays implemented were low-throughput, and generally not applicable for routine use. For genotyping to be considered a viable replacement for routine blood group serology, the development of high-throughput platforms that are automatable is essential. The Bloodgen project was intended to demonstrate the use of gene chip technology as a prelude to the development of a high-throughput, fully automatable genotyping system that may provide a suitable alternative to serological determination of blood group status. The Bloodgen consortium assisted in the development of the commercial product, BLOODchip, which is capable of genotyping 116 blood group-specific single-nucleotide polymorphisms taken from 9 different blood group systems. A small-scale trial was conducted in order to obtain Conformité Européenne-marking for Rh CcEe, Kell and Duffy diagnostic use, and was successful. Furthermore, genotyping using the BLOODchip platform was shown to be more accurate than the serological typing of the same cohort, which comprised routine blood donors, patients, weak D phenotype individuals and newborns.   ©2008 S. Karger GmbH, Freiburg i.Br.

Introduction

Blood group genotyping has a relatively short history in the field of transfusion medicine, and can be traced to the initial analysis of foetal *RHD* status in cases of maternal alloimmunisation to a paternally inherited RhD antigen during pregnancy. Bennett et al. [1] were first to describe a clinically applicable assay for the clinical management of haemolytic disease of the foetus and newborn (HDFN). Genotyping for blood groups was only possible once the genes responsible for the expression of the relevant antigens were identified, largely by the cDNA cloning of their appropriate transcripts. Blood group antigens on red cell glycophorins were first to be deciphered at the molecular level, glycophorin A which carries the MN antigens in 1986 [2], glycophorin B (Ss antigens) in 1987 [3] and glycophorin C (Gerbich antigens) also in 1986 [4]. The amino acids responsible for MNS antigenicity were, however, defined by protein chemical techniques some years earlier [5–7]. Then the major clinically significant blood group systems were defined: ABO [8, 9] and RH [10, 11] in 1990, KEL in 1991 [12], RhD in 1992 [13], the molecular basis of the Rh CcEe antigens in 1993 [14], and Duffy in the same year [15]. Throughout the remainder of the 1990s the majority of other minor blood group antigens were defined at the molecular level, and these have been reviewed extensively in the literature [16–19].

With the knowledge in place regarding the molecular background of most clinically significant blood group antigens, it then became a theoretical possibility that genotyping could be used for routine blood typing. But in order for this to be a realistic possibility, testing needed to be of much higher throughput than the standard PCR assays used at that time. There have been significant advances in high-throughput genotyping methods, and notably those performed on microarray formats.

With this background in the early 2000s, a consortium of academic units, blood centres and companies with interest in the transfusion medicine market formed the Bloodgen consortium. The consortium bid to the fifth framework programme of the European commission in 2002 and received EUR 2.35 million funding for a 3-year project which ran from 2003 to 2006. The project consortium was named Bloodgen, and included the University of the West of England (co-ordinators), Bristol; Sanquin Foundation, Amsterdam; University of Ulm; University Hospital Lund; CTBT, Barcelona; UHKT, Prague; BITS, Bristol; and Progenika Biopharma AG. Originally, Biotest AG were members, but withdrew half way into the project. For further details concerning the structure of the consortium see www.bloodgen.com and a consortium review published in *Transfusion* which followed a blood group genotyping workshop held at the Food and Drug Administration (FDA) in September 2006 [20].

The Bloodgen Work Programme

Using the standard structures of EC-funded projects, the Bloodgen project work programme involved several overlapping work packages with key deliverables and milestones. These included (1) fabrication of microarrays, (2) parallel development of fluoro-single-sequence primer (SSP) assays for blood groups, (3) standardisation of DNA extraction and multiplex (MPX) PCR development, (4) a small-scale clinical trial using a biobank of assembled genomic DNAs from rare blood group phenotype individuals, (5) a large-scale clinical trial using a prototype BLOODchip. The technical annex of the project included descriptions of how two commercially available blood group genotyping kits would be released onto the market – fluoro-SSP by Biotest AG and BLOODchip by Progenika Biopharma.

The first deliverable of the project included the definition of a list of single-nucleotide polymorphisms (SNPs) and blood group genotypes required to be detected by BLOODchip. This list was based on the clinical significance of the corresponding blood group antigens, with the most important being considered mandatory and those of minor clinical significance considered obligatory. SNPs were selected from the following blood group systems: ABO, RH, MNS, KEL, FY, JK DO, CO, and DI. Within the genetically complex ABO and RH systems, a combination of SNPs was devised so that hybrid genes (a hallmark of some partial D phenotypes) could be defined by 'exon scanning', using probes located in specific exons of the ABO and *RHD* genes. A comprehensive list of RH alleles that can be detected using BLOODchip is described in table 1. Once the SNP list was defined, probes corresponding to each were designed and validated for incorporation onto BLOODchip.

The protocol for BLOODchip entails amplification of the relevant regions of blood group-active genes encoding the polymorphic SNPs using an MPX PCR. This MPX involves primers that have at their 3' ends gene-specific sequences and at their 5' ends common sequences, known as MPX-amplifiable probe hybridisation (MAPH) tags. Uniform amplification within the MPX is then achieved by including MAPH-specific primers within the amplification mix, which includes the MAPH-tagged gene-specific primers. Once MPX PCR products are produced, they are fragmented, then labelled with fluorescent dyes and denatured before application to the array. Reproducible hybridisation is an essential prerequisite for accurate genotyping with BLOODchip, and use of a Ventana hybridisation station ensures that this is achieved. Hybridisation to the various probes corresponding to each allelic SNP permits the scoring of each allele; strong binding to probes is achieved where there is a perfect match, weak binding when mismatched. Bespoke software designed by Progenika has allowed the prediction of homozygosity or heterozygosity for each SNP by using an algorithm that computes the ratio of fluorescent intensity of binding of each labelled PCR product to the allelic probe pair. Thus, BLOODchip scores zygosity for each probe using a process of allele-specific hybridisation.

During the Bloodgen project, a collection of genomic DNAs prepared from individuals with rare blood group phenotypes was assembled by the consortium and held at a biobank at the University of Ulm. This collection included a large collection of Rh variant samples and is probably a unique collection of this type in the world. These samples were then analysed by a prototype of BLOODchip in a small-scale exercise organised by the activities of work package 4 led by the University of Ulm. This exercise permitted optimisation of probe sequences and improvements to be made of the design of the MPX PCRs, which was essential before the final work package of the project (5), the large-scale clinical trial. Work package 5 included an analysis of 1,000 genomic DNA samples, which was sufficient to permit an application for Conformité Européenne (CE)-marking (for Rh CcEe, Kell, Duffy; Kidd,

Table 1. RhD variant alleles detected by BLOODchip. Although there has been some debate recently that all *RHD* alleles should be described as Rh variants, this table has segregated *RHD* alleles into their phenotypic variation: partial D phenotypes, weak D phenotypes, D-elute or very weak D phenotypes and D-negative phenotypes. The probe combinations and BLOODchip software permit the genotypic assignments of a very large number of Rh variants – the major strength of this genotyping platform. LFA = Low frequency antigen associated with various partial D phenotypes

Phenotype	Name	SNP(s)	Comment
Partial D	DII	C1061A	1 proband
Partial D	DIIIa	exon scanning, A455C, C602G, T667G	LFA = DAK
Partial D	DIIIb	exon scanning, A178C, G203A, T307C*; no exon 2	* = C in Dpos Gneg
Partial D	DIIIc	exon scanning, A455C; no exon 3	
Partial D	DIII type IV	exon scanning, A455C, C410T	
Partial D	DIII type V	C410T, A455C, C602G, T667G	
Partial D	DIII type VI	C410T, A455C, C602G, T667G	
Partial D	DIII type VII	exon scanning, C410T, A455C, C602G, T667G	
Partial D	DIVa	exon scanning, G1048C, A455C	LFA = Goa
Partial D	DIVb	exon scanning, A1193T; no exons 7, 8, 9	LFA = Evans (RH37)
Partial D	DIV type III	exon scanning; no exons 6, 7, 8, 9	
Partial D	DIV type IV	exon scanning, G1048C, C1061A	
Partial D	DVa type I	exon scanning, G697C, T667G	LFA = RH23
Partial D	DVa type II	exon scanning; no exon 5	LFA = RH23
Partial D	DVa type III	exon scanning, G697C, T667G, G676C, G712A	LFA = RH23
Partial D	DVa type IV	G697C	LFA = RH23
Partial D	DVa type V	G697A	LFA = RH23
Partial D	DVa type VI	exon scanning, G697C, T667G, G712A	LFA = RH23
Partial D	DVa type VII	exon scanning; no exon 5	LFA = RH23
Partial D	DVa type VIII	exon scanning, G697C, G712A	LFA = RH23
Partial D	DVa type IX	697 G>C, 712 G>A	
Partial D	DVI type I	exon scanning	
Partial D	DVI type II	exon scanning	LFA = BARC (RH52)
Partial D	DVI type III	exon scanning	LFA = BARC (RH52)
Partial D	DVI type IV	exon scanning	LFA = BARC (RH52)
Partial D	DVII	T329C	LFA = Tar
Partial D	DVII type II	T307C, T329C	
Partial D	DBT I and II	exon scanning	LFA = RH32
Partial D	DFR I and II	exon scanning (DFRI = A514T, T509C)	LFA = FPTT (RH50)
Partial D	DHar (RoHar)	exon scanning (CE1–4, D5, CE6–10)	LFA = FPTT (RH50)
Partial D	DCS	G676C, T667G	DCS I and II
Partial D	DNB	G1063A	
Partial D	DOL	T509C, T667G	DOL-2 and DOL-3 also known, LFA = DAK
Partial D	DHMi	C848T	
Partial D	DFW	A497C	
Partial D	DHR	G686A	
Partial D	DIM	G854A	

▶

Phenotype	Name	SNP(s)	Comment
Partial D	DNU	G1057A	
Partial D	DWI	T1073C	
Partial D	DAR	T1025C, C602G, T667G	(same as weak D 4.2)
Partial D	DAR-E	C602G, T667G, T1025C, G697C	
Partial D	DMH	T161C	
Partial D	DFV	T667G	

Partial D genotypes on BLOODchip = 43

Phenotype	Name	SNP(s)	Comment
Weak D	Weak D type 1	T809G	
Weak D	Weak D type 2	G1154C	
Weak D	Weak D type 3	C8G	
Weak D	Weak D type 4.0	C602G, T667G	
Weak D	Weak D type 4.1	G48C, C602G, T667G	
Weak D	Weak D type 5	C446A	
Weak D	Weak D type 7	G1016A	
Weak D	Weak D type 11	G885T	weak D with cDe (Del when CDe)
Weak D	Weak D type 14	T554A, A594T, C602G	
Weak D	Weak D type 15	G845A	
Weak D	Weak D type 17	C340T	
Weak D	Weak D type 29	A178C, G203A, A594T, T667G, T1025C	DAU cluster
Weak D	Weak D type 41	A1193T	
Weak D	Weak D type 51	A594T, C602G	

Weak D alleles detected by BLOODchip = 13 (14 incl. weak D type 4.2)

Phenotype	Name	SNP(s)	Comment
D-elute	Del (K409K)	G1227A	
D-elute	RHD (IVS3+1G>A)	IVS3+1G>A	splice site
D-elute	RHD (Δ exon 9)	exon scanning (minus exon 9)	
D-elute	RHD (L153P)	T458C	
D-elute	RHD (Δ exon 8)	exon scanning (minus exon 8)	
D-elute	RHD (M295I)	G885T	Del when with CDe
D-elute	RHD (785delA)	Del 785A	D-neg or D-elute, Rhesus base
D-elute	RHD (147delA)	Del147A	very likely to be D-neg
D-elute	RHD (X418L)	1252 Ins T	extended C-terminus to RhD
D-elute	RHD (IVS1+G>A)	IVS1+G>A	splice site
D-elute	RHD (IVS3+2T>A)	IVS3+2T>A	splice site (D-neg or D-elute)
D-elute	RHD (Q405X)	C1213T	
D-elute	RHD (X418L)	insT1253	

D-elute alleles typed by BLOODchip = 13

▶

Phenotype	Name	SNP(s)	Comment
D-Neg	RHD deletion	exon scanning (Δ all RHD exons)	predominant in Caucasians
D-Neg	RHD Ψ	T807G, T667G	predominant in Africans
D-Neg	Ccdees (r's)	exon scanning (hybrid exon 3)	common in Africans
D-Neg	RHCE (1–9)RHD(10)	exon scanning, RHD exon 10	common with Cde
D-Neg	RHD (W16X)	G48A	Caucasian
D-Neg	RHD (Q41X)	C121T	
D-Neg	RHD (W90X)	G270A	
D-Neg	RHD (488del4)	488CAGA deleted	called 487 ACAG in original paper
D-Neg	RHD (G212V)	G635T	
D-Neg	RHD (IVS6+1del4)	906instggct IVS6+1del4	
D-Neg	RHD (G314V)	G941T	
D-Neg	RHD (Y330X)	C990G	
D-Neg	RHD (IVS8+1G>A)	IVS8+1G>A	
D-Neg	RHD (711delC)	Del 711C	
D-Neg	RHD (Y269X)	T807A	
D-Neg	RHD (Y311X)	C933A	
D-Neg	RHD (343delC)	Del 343C	not in deliverable 4 (SNP list)
D-Neg	RHD (449delT)	Del 449T	not in deliverable 4 (SNP list)
D-Neg	RHD (785delA)	Del 785A	D-neg or D-elute, Rhesus base
D-Neg	RHD (Y401X)	T1203A	not in deliverable 4
D-Neg	RHD (94insT (FS, 35X))	94Tins	
D-Neg	RHD (361del11nt (FS, 155X))	361Del 11nt	
D-Neg	RHD (IVS4+1 G>T)	IVS4+1G>T	
D-Neg	RHD-CE(2–8)-D	exon scanning	
D-Neg	RHD-CE(2–7)-D	exon scanning	
D-Neg	RHD-CE(3–7)-D	exon scanning	
D-Neg	RHD-CE(4–7)-D	exon scanning	
D-Neg	RHD-CE(3–9)-D	exon scanning	
D-Neg	RHCE (1–3)D(4–10)	exon scanning	
D-Neg	RHCE (1–7)D(8–9)CE(10)	exon scanning	
D-Neg	RHCE (1–5)D(6)CE(7–10)	exon scanning	

RhD-neg haplotypes scored by BLOODchip = 31

MNS, Dombrock, Colton and Diego) as described in the EC legislation for in vitro diagnostics, and the blood directive. The results of work package 5 are illustrated in table 2. CE-marking is also to be sought for *RHD* genotyping after testing of 3,000 samples is concluded. A number of ABO and Rh variants were found in the analysis of the initial 1,000 samples, and these have been described elsewhere (Avent ND, Brit J Haem 2008, submitted). With the Bloodgen project completed in September 2006, studies are ongoing in several Bloodgen participant laboratories to enable the development of new versions of BLOODchip and to complete the CE-marking progress for *RHD* genotyping.

Conclusions and Future Directions

The potential impact of mass-scale genotyping has recently been discussed in some depth and the reader is referred to this review [21], but here I consider three immediate applications of BLOODchip in transfusion medicine.

Target Patient Groups – Multi-Transfused Patients

BLOODchip was designed to be a comprehensive blood group genotyping platform, and for use to genotype for all clinically significant blood group antigens. In multi-transfused patients (for example those suffering from haemoglobinopathies), genotyping represents the best practise for blood group typing, as these individuals will be difficult to type by serology due to the presence of the transfused blood. Such an approach has been published by several workers [22–25] and is a prime initial use of a blood group genotyping platform such as BLOODchip.

Routine Blood Donors (and Patients?)

To be most effective, the added benefit of genotyping and potential reduction of alloimmunisation events must be coupled with an extended typing programme by blood banks. A cohort of comprehensively genotyped regular blood donors may thus serve this purpose. Electronic cross-matching, which has been in practise for over a decade [26, 27], may therefore be extended without any requirement for serological cross-matching. Logistically, however, it will be difficult to achieve full matching of donor and recipient, but an intelligent assessment of the potential clinical implications of mismatched transfusions can be made. The application of blood group genotyping to patients does not at present appear to be a likely area where genotyping will be adopted. Rapid determination of blood groups in emergency situations would not be possible for genotyping at present (although refer to discussion in future directions

Table 2. CE-marking exercise of BLOODchip, Rh CcEe, Kell, Duffy, Kidd, Dombrock, Diego and Colton antigens, versus serological typings, 1000 genomic DNA samples (work package 5)

Blood group antigen (system)	Serological testing	BLOODchip	Comments
Rh C/c (RH)	998/1000	999/1000	
Rh E/e (RH)	997/1000	1000/1000	includes one typographical error
CW+ (RH)	18*	28	*serological confirmation of genotype
CX+ (RH)	0*	2	*serological confirmation of genotype
VS+ (RH)	9*	15	*serological confirmation of genotype
K/k (KEL)	1000/1000	1000/1000	
Kpa/Kpb (KEL)	358/358	357/358	
Jsa/Jsb (KEL)	122/123	123/123	
Jka/Jkb (JK)	596/597	597/597	
Fya/Fyb/Fy(a–b–) (FY)	498/506	506/506	
MN (MNS)	425/455	455/455	
Ss (MNS)	479/483	483/483	
Dia/Dib (DI)		120/120	confirmed by DNA sequencing
Doa/Dob (DO)		120/120	confirmed by DNA sequencing
Coa/Cob (CO)	169/170	170/170	

section). In such situations, complex serology is not performed either, preferring to use O-RhD-negative blood, and perhaps the cross-match test.

Women of Childbearing Age/Pregnant Women?

In several European countries, anti-D serotyping reagents are deliberately selected so that DVI partial D phenotype pregnant women are typed as D negative. This ensures that they receive prophylactic anti-D at the end of the pregnancy, which is important if they are carrying a normal D-positive infant. However, there are a large number of partial D phenotype individuals (some of the known ones are shown in table 1), and if such individuals are pregnant and incorrectly typed as D positive (a possibility), then they are vulnerable to making anti-D if they carry a foetus with a normally expressed, paternally inherited *RHD* gene. As foetal genotyping using non-invasive maternal plasma-based methods is proliferating in Europe [28–35], it appears likely that all D-negative pregnant women will be offered prenatal *RHD* genotyping of their foetuses early in the pregnancy. It makes good practical sense therefore to use the same sample (i.e. maternal leukocyte-extracted DNA) to define the maternal *RHD* genotype simultaneously. Indeed, this process could readily be unified with the recent suggestions for maternal HPA-1a/HPA-1b genotyping as a measure to identify potentially at risk foetuses that may suffer from neonatal alloimmune thrombocytopaenia (NAITP) due to anti-HPA-1a [36].

The relatively small cohort of samples tested using the BLOODchip platform during the Bloodgen project has proven beyond doubt that the accuracy of the genotyping technology is high enough for routine application. Clearly, further validation of BLOODchip, and for that matter any genotyping platform capable of typing for blood group status, is essential. There remain some concerns regarding routine implementation of genotyping for ABO typing, due to the large number of O alleles, and A,B variants that exist. Whilst genotyping for known ABO alleles is not problematic, unclassified alleles certainly remain to be discovered, although the implementation of genotyping platforms worldwide may accelerate their discovery and characterisation. However, what is urgently required is for large blood centres to work with the Bloodgen consortium (perhaps via framework VII funding) to investigate the feasibility of introducing routine genotyping in the blood bank setting.

As genotyping for a variety of inborn errors of metabolism is becoming a reality, a comprehensive approach to genotyping of all individuals at birth remains a possibility. Indeed advances in rapid genome resequencing by pyrolysis-based procedures appear to be progressing rapidly so that there is the distinct possibility that the complete genome sequence of individuals can be performed at low cost, and quickly. With this being a potential eventuality, genotyping for blood groups and, for example, human leukocyte antigen (HLA) status can comparatively simply be included in a 'whole genome screen' that will follow the determination of an individual's complete genome sequence. With such information being processed shortly after birth, this information will be electronically available if that individual becomes a patient or blood donor during adult life. There is no doubt that blood group genotyping will become more mainstream in the armoury of the transfusion medicine specialist within the next decade, rather than the current situation where it is of relatively specialist interest.

Disclosure of Conflict of Interests

Neil Avent is a member of the Scientific Advisory Board of Progenika Biopharma AG.

References

1 Bennett PR, Le Van Kim C, Colin Y, Warwick RM, Cherif-Zahar B, Fisk NM, Cartron JP: Prenatal determination of fetal RhD type by DNA amplification. N Engl J Med 1993;329:607–610.
2 Siebert PD, Fukuda M: Isolation and characterization of human glycophorin A cDNA clones by a synthetic oligonucleotide approach: nucleotide sequence and mRNA structure. Proc Natl Acad Sci U S A 1986;83:1665–1669.
3 Siebert PD, Fukuda M: Molecular cloning of a human glycophorin B cDNA: nucleotide sequence and genomic relationship to glycophorin A. Proc Natl Acad Sci U S A 1987;84:6735–6739.
4 Colin Y, Rahuel C, London J, Romeo PH, d'Auriol L, Galibert F, Cartron JP: Isolation of cDNA clones and complete amino acid sequence of human erythrocyte glycophorin C. J Biol Chem 1986;261:229–233.
5 Wasniowska K, Drzeniek Z, Lisowska E: The amino acids of M and N blood group glycopeptides are different. Biochem Biophys Res Commun 1976;76:385–390.
6 Dahr W, Uhlenbruck G, Janssen E, Schmalisch R: Different N-terminal amino acids in the MN-glycoprotein from MM and NN erythrocytes. Hum Genet 1977;35:335–343.

7   Dahr W, Beyreuther K, Steinbach H, Gielen W, Kruger J: Structure of the Ss blood group antigens, II: a methionine/threonine polymorphism within the N-terminal sequence of the Ss glycoprotein. Hoppe Seylers Z Physiol Chem 1980;361:895–906.

8   Yamamoto F, Clausen H, White T, Marken J, Hakomori S: Molecular genetic basis of the histo-blood group ABO system. Nature 1990;345:229–233.

9   Yamamoto F, Marken J, Tsuji T, White T, Clausen H, Hakomori S: Cloning and characterization of DNA complementary to human UDP-GalNAc: Fuc alpha 1----2Gal alpha 1----3GalNAc transferase (histo-blood group A transferase) mRNA. J Biol Chem 1990;265:1146–1151.

10 Avent ND, Ridgwell K, Tanner MJ, Anstee DJ: cDNA cloning of a 30 kDa erythrocyte membrane protein associated with Rh (Rhesus)-blood-group-antigen expression. Biochem J 1990;271:821–825.

11 Cherif-Zahar B, Bloy C, Le Van Kim C, Blanchard D, Bailly P, Hermand P, Salmon C, Cartron JP, Colin Y: Molecular cloning and protein structure of a human blood group Rh polypeptide. Proc Natl Acad Sci U S A 1990;87:6243–6247.

12 Lee S, Zambas ED, Marsh WL, Redman CM: Molecular cloning and primary structure of Kell blood group protein. Proc Natl Acad Sci U S A 1991;88:6353–6357.

13 Le van Kim C, Mouro I, Cherif-Zahar B, Raynal V, Cherrier C, Cartron JP, Colin Y: Molecular cloning and primary structure of the human blood group RhD polypeptide. Proc Natl Acad Sci U S A 1992;89:10925–10929.

14 Mouro I, Colin Y, Cherif-Zahar B, Cartron JP, Le Van Kim C: Molecular genetic basis of the human Rhesus blood group system. Nat Genet 1993;5:62–65.

15 Chaudhuri A, Polyakova J, Zbrzezna V, Williams K, Gulati S, Pogo AO: Cloning of glycoprotein D cDNA, which encodes the major subunit of the Duffy blood group system and the receptor for the *Plasmodium vivax* malaria parasite. Proc Natl Acad Sci U S A 1993;90:10793–10797.

16 Avent ND: Human erythrocyte antigen expression: its molecular bases. Br J Biomed Sci 1997;54:16–37.

17 Cartron JP, Colin Y: Structural and functional diversity of blood group antigens. Transfus Clin Biol 2001;8:163–199.

18 Daniels G: The molecular genetics of blood group polymorphism. Transpl Immunol 2005;14:143–153.

19 Reid ME, Mohandas N: Red blood cell blood group antigens: structure and function. Semin Hematol 2004;41:93–117.

20 Avent ND, Martinez A, Flegel WA, Olsson ML, Scott ML, Nogues N, Pisacka M, Daniels G, van der Schoot E, Muniz-Diaz E, Madgett TE, Storry JR, Beiboer SH, Maaskant-van Wijk PA, von Zabern I, Jimenez E, Tejedor D, Lopez M, Camacho E, Cheroutre G, Hacker A, Jinoch P, Svobodova I, de Haas M: The BloodGen project: toward mass-scale comprehensive genotyping of blood donors in the European Union and beyond. Transfusion 2007;47(suppl 1):40S–46S.

21 Avent ND: Large scale blood group genotyping. Transfus Clin Biol 2007;14:10–15.

22 Wenk RE, Chiafari PA: DNA typing of recipient blood after massive transfusion. Transfusion 1997;37:1108–1110.

23 Reid ME, Rios M, Powell VI, Charles-Pierre D, Malavade V: DNA from blood samples can be used to genotype patients who have recently received a transfusion. Transfusion 2000;40:48–53.

24 Rozman P, Dovc T, Gassner C: Differentiation of autologous ABO, RHD, RHCE, KEL, JK, and FY blood group genotypes by analysis of peripheral blood samples of patients who have recently received multiple transfusions. Transfusion 2000;40:936–942.

25 Legler TJ, Eber SW, Lakomek M, Lynen R, Maas JH, Pekrun A, Repas-Humpe M, Schroter W, Kohler M: Application of RHD and RHCE genotyping for correct blood group determination in chronically transfused patients. Transfusion 1999;39:852–855.

26 Butch SH, Judd WJ, Steiner EA, Stoe M, Oberman HA: Electronic verification of donor-recipient compatibility: the computer crossmatch. Transfusion 1994;34:105–109.

27 Judd WJ: Requirements for the electronic crossmatch. Vox Sang 1998;74(suppl 2):409–417.

28 Finning KM, Martin PG, Soothill PW, Avent ND: Prediction of fetal D status from maternal plasma: introduction of a new noninvasive fetal RHD genotyping service. Transfusion 2002;42:1079–1085.

29 Finning K, Martin P, Daniels G: A clinical service in the UK to predict fetal Rh (Rhesus) D blood group using free fetal DNA in maternal plasma. Ann N Y Acad Sci 2004;1022:119–123.

30 Daniels G, Finning K, Martin P, Soothill P: Fetal blood group genotyping from DNA from maternal plasma: an important advance in the management and prevention of haemolytic disease of the fetus and newborn. Vox Sang 2004;87:225–232.

31 Legler TJ, Liu Z, Mavrou A, Finning K, Hromadnikova I, Galbiati S, Meaney C, Hulten MA, Crea F, Olsson ML, Maddocks DG, Huang D, Fisher SA, Sprenger-Haussels M, Soussan AA, van der Schoot CE: Workshop report on the extraction of foetal DNA from maternal plasma. Prenat Diagn 2007;27:824–829.

32 Rouillac-Le Sciellour C, Puillandre P, Gillot R, Baulard C, Metral S, Le Van Kim C, Cartron JP, Colin Y, Brossard Y: Large-scale pre-diagnosis study of fetal RHD genotyping by PCR on plasma DNA from RhD-negative pregnant women. Mol Diagn 2004;8:23–31.

33 Van der Schoot CE, Soussan AA, Koelewijn J, Bonsel G, Paget-Christiaens LG, de Haas M: Non-invasive antenatal RHD typing. Transfus Clin Biol 2006;13:53–57.

34 van der Schoot CE: Molecular diagnostics in immunohaematology. Vox Sang 2004;87(suppl 2):189–192.

35 Daniels G, van der Schoot CE, Olsson ML: Report of the First International Workshop on molecular blood group genotyping. Vox Sang 2005;88:136–142.

36 Ahya R, Turner ML, Urbaniak SJ: Fetomaternal alloimmune thrombocytopenia. Transfus Apher Sci 2001;25:139–145.

Prof. Neil Avent
Centre for Research in Biomedicine, Faculty of Health and Life Sciences
University of the West of England, Bristol
Coldharbour Lane, Frenchay, Bristol BS16 6DT, UK
Tel. +44 117 3282-147, Fax -904
E-Mail neil.avent@uwe.ac.uk

Molecular Immunohematology

Scharf RE (ed): Progress and Challenges in Transfusion Medicine, Hemostasis and Hemotherapy.
Freiburg i.Br., Karger, 2008, pp 189–198

Genotyping of Red Blood Cell, Granulocyte and Platelet Antigens: Current Applications in the German-Speaking Countries

Willy A. Flegel[a, b] · Franz F. Wagner[c]

[a]Institute for Transfusion Medicine, University Hospital Ulm,
[b]DRK Blutspendedienst Baden-Württemberg – Hessen, Institute Ulm,
[c]DRK Blutspendedienst NSTOB, Institute Springe, Germany

Key Words

Consensus statement · Genotyping · Blood groups · Granulocytes · Platelets · Immunohematology

Summary

More than 10 years ago molecular methods for blood group, platelet and granulocyte antigen prediction became available, but today they are still less established than HLA genotyping, which has often re-placed HLA serology. The implementation varies considerably among different health care systems, and a wider availability is desirable and feasible for more patients to benefit from such genotyping. A consensus statement for the established clinical indications of genotyping in the German-speaking countries was published in 2000. This summary is based on the recent literature and discussions at the biannual workshops organized by the Working Party Immunohematology/Gene Technology of the German Society for Transfusion Medicine and Immunohematology (DGTI). As a prerequisite for wider use, commercial kits for routine molecular blood group testing have become available. Publications, conference contributions and genotyping workshop participation indicated increasing application and acceptance in Germany, Switzerland and Austria. The benefit for the patients and the cost efficacy was established for many indications: weak D testing in patients and, particularly, pregnant women; blood group genotyping in perinatal care, in transfused patients and in patients with immunohematologic problems; *RHD* genotyping in donors for DEL and D+/– chimera; and *RHD* zygosity testing. We propose an update of the Consensus Statement 2000 to reflect the currently much wider indications for blood group, platelet and granulocyte antigen genotyping.
©2008 S. Karger GmbH, Freiburg i.Br.

Introduction

Already 10 years ago, we considered blood group phenotype prediction by molecular methods, dubbed 'genotyping', as feasible and, for some applications, as superior to standard serologic 'phenotyping' [1]. In 2000, a turning point was reached in these health care systems when the molecular testing was applied routinely for the benefit of the patients [2–6]. At that time, the Working Party Immunohematology/Gene Technology published a consensus statement (table 1) [7]. The specified established indications have today become common practice, and many samples from all over Germany, Switzerland and Austria are sent to reference laboratories.

In the last years an increasing number of customized Conformité Européenne (CE)-labeled test kits have been marketed [8] and in-house test procedures were established [9] that allow the wider adoption of these techniques in a larger number of routine laboratories. Concurrently, the understanding of many molecular details has been refined, which has also facilitated the improvement and implementation of molecular methods in blood group, granulocyte and platelet genotyping.

This summary details the currently established indications for red blood cell (RBC), granulocyte and platelet genotyping. We argue that the Consensus Statement 2000 should be revised and updated. An implementation of the consensus indication in the national and European guidelines would allow a wider adoption of such methods and ensure that a larger number of patients would benefit from genotyping of blood group, platelet and granulocyte antigens.

Advances since 2000

Since the consensus statement of 2000, considerable advances in molecular testing techniques have been achieved: (i) The molecular basis of the antigens and the rare non-expressing alleles have been defined for multiple, particularly Central European, populations [10–14]. As a result, the accuracy of the antigen prediction has been improved [15]. (ii) Multiplex polymerase chain reaction (PCR) methods have been introduced [16, 17]. This multiplexing may be used to increase accuracy (like by testing more polymorphisms for one antigen prediction), to reduce costs (like by the concurrent prediction of several antigens), or both. As a result, molecular testing has now become advantageous in many situations in which both serologic and molecular testing were an option in 2000. (iii) Proficiency testing has been expanded, enhancing and ensuring the quality of antigen prediction on a routine basis [4, 9]. (iv) Considerable knowledge has been accrued on pitfalls of fetal testing from mothers' peripheral plasma and on ways to circumvent these pitfalls [18, 19].

Current Clinical Applications in Which Genotyping Is Superior to Phenotyping

We propose a revision and update of the Consensus Statement 2000 to reflect the currently much wider indications for blood group, platelet and granulocyte genotyping (table 2) [7, 18–44]. In the following paragraph, we summarize clinical situations in

Table 1. German Consensus Statement 2000 on blood group genotyping [6]

Blood group genotyping may be indicated[a] in the following clinical situations
(i)   In fetus from amniotic fluid or trophoblastic cells (chorionic villi)
(ii) In multipl transfused patients, if standard serology fails
(iii) In case of auto- and allo-immunohemolytic anemia, if standard serology fails
(iv) For *weak D types* and other variant *RH* alleles, if serology is inconclusive

[a] Indication (i) was recommended as first choice because less invasive and hazardous sampling procedures are required. Indications (ii) to (iv) were considered very cost efficient if applied prudently [2, 7].

which molecular typing is superior to phenotyping. Genotyping may thus be considered as a supplementary or the preferred method for these clinical applications.

Situations in Which the Cells to Type Are Not Available or Cannot Be Typed for Technical Reasons

Typing of the Fetus from Amniocytes or Chorionic Biopsy

This procedure is considered superior to serologic testing because it is less invasive [7, 18]. It should preferably be applied in any situation in which otherwise serologic typing of fetal material would be performed. Molecular methods for the prediction of the antigens of interest (usually Rhesus antigens or K) have a very high accuracy, and the relationship between molecular basis and phenotype has been studied for many populations. Molecular prediction of the D antigen should include typing for at least two polymorphisms in the central region of the *RHD* gene (exon 4 to exon 7) and testing for relevant D-negative alleles (including at least *RHDψ* if the ethnicity of the parents is unknown). If the phenotype determination is a major predictor of clinical interventions, high-resolution typing, e.g. by DNA chips, may be advantageous.

Typing of the Fetus from Peripheral Blood of the Mother

This procedure is even less invasive and does not imply any harm for the fetus. Recent studies suggest a high accuracy if testing for the allele of interest is combined with testing for the presence of fetal DNA [19, 20]. To insure high-quality results, this procedure should be performed in laboratories with sufficient experience. In addition, high-resolution typing is not yet in use for this application. A major current controversy focuses on whether it is safe and advantageous to withhold prenatal anti-D prophylaxis, given that a D-negative status of the fetus has been assured by typing from the peripheral blood of the mother. The optimal decision will depend on the

Table 2. Proposal for an updated consensus statement on blood group, platelet and granulocyte antigen prediction by genotyping: Clinical situations in which molecular typing is superior to phenotyping and genotyping may be indicated

Cells are not available for typing or cannot be typed for technical reasons

Typing of the fetus	from amniocytes or chorionic biopsy to predict fetus at risk for hemolytic disease of the fetus and newborn (HDFN) [7, 18]
	from peripheral plasma of the mother to avoid exposure to human-derived RhIg and to advise clinical care in the presence of maternal antibodies [19, 20]
Typing after recent transfusion	like in chronically transfused patients [7]
Typing in the presence of a serologic problem	like in auto- and allo-immunohemolytic anemia with positive direct antiglobulin test [7]

Detection of low-copy number and weakly expressed antigens that are known to be missed by serology

Blood donor typing for *RHD*	like DEL and weak D [21–26]
Patient typing for, e.g., *FY*B* or *FY*X*	like in African people with sickle cell disease [27]
	like weak D types in mother to avoid exposure to human-derived RhIg [28–32]
	like phenotype-negative patients who may receive antigen-positive RBC [28–32]

Suitable antisera are unavailable or the serologically obtained information is insufficient for the resolution of the clinical problem

Antigen testing when suitable antisera or sufficient quantities are lacking	like for typing of Do^a and Do^b antigens [33, 34]
Testing for phenotypes that cannot safely be determined by serology	determination of weak D types and of DIII-like phenotypes [35]
	determination of a *DAR* allele combined with rare *RHCE* alleles [36]

Determination of zygosity and quantity of antigen expression

Predictive clinical zygosity testing	testing of a father for *RHD* zygosity if, for instance, the mother carries a clinically relevant alloantibody [37, 38]
Quality control and labeling of serologic reagents like identification panels	homozygosity for *RHD*, *FY*A* and *FY*B*, *DO*A* and *DO*B* [33]
	exalted RBC antigen expression by distinct *RHD* alleles [37]

Replacement of serological testing in high-throughput situations

Screen for donors with rare antigen combinations or rare antigen-negative status	even if testing has to be confirmed by serology [17]
	like 'extended' genotyping for rare antigen combinations [39]
	including null RBC [40–42], platelets [43] and granulocytes [44] that lack distinct antigen systems
Typing of donors for antigens that cannot be determined by serology with sufficient ease	like for typing of Do^a and Do^b antigens [33]
General typing of donors for antigens	if molecular typing is sufficiently safe and less costly than serologic typing [17]

cost and availability of anti-D for prophylaxis, the cost, availability and accuracy of fetal testing from the peripheral blood of the mother, and possible unwanted effects of such a new policy, like missed prophylaxis in women with low compliancy. Although fetal genotyping from maternal plasma seems to be reliable and is strongly advocated in some countries, current guidelines prevent its use in Germany.

Typing after Recent Transfusion and in Chronically Transfused Patients

It has been shown that molecular typing is possible after recent, even massive transfusion, and in chronically transfused patients [7]. Furthermore, it has been shown that 'most probable phenotypes' deduced from the observed phenotype considering mixed field patterns are misleading in a high percentage of cases, especially in chronically transfused patients. While this indication has been known and accepted for years, its use is still hampered by logistic reasons. Long timelines, limited availability and lack of reimbursement for molecular testing need to be considered and overcome. However, while these reasons may be real in the case of urgent blood need for a massively transfused patient, it is likely that for the multiply transfused patient, incorrect and unreliable serologic antigen determinations triggering selection of special, rare units may infringe considerable costs, too. The unnecessary utilization of rare RBC units of limited availability may delay transfusions and increase transfusion costs which may easily outnumber the cost of timely genotyping.

Typing in the Presence of a Serologic Problem

Typing in the presence of a serologic problem, e.g. RBC coated with immunoglobulin, is very similar to typing after recent transfusion [7]. While there is no doubt that molecular typing is possible in these situations, its use is often hampered by long timelines and lack of accessibility of the genotyping. In multiply transfused patients, indirect costs caused by wrong serologic antigen guesses should be considered, and molecular typing is likely advantageous for these patients. Genotyping may also enhance the safety of ABO-matched neonatal transfusion in the absence of a reverse grouping.

Situations in Which Weak Antigens Should Be Detected but May Be Missed by Serology

RHD Testing of Blood Donors

There have been several cases of anti-D immunization caused by D antigens missed in serologic donor typing [21–26, 45]. Based on several studies, it is obvious that (i) weak D, partial D and D-positive/D-negative chimeric donors may be found among historically 'D-negative' donors and pose a moderate anti-D immunization risk to recipients and that (ii) DEL donors are missed even with current routine serologic methods and occur with a relevant frequency in European populations. Their RBC units may eventually cause anti-D immunizations in recipients. Such cases will be prevented by *RHD* testing of blood donors. There are two possible approaches: *RHD* testing could either supplement current testing or replace parts of current testing. Addition of *RHD* PCR to current testing is safe but may have a low cost efficiency. Replacement of some serologic testing, like the indirect antiglobulin test, by *RHD* PCR is probably cost-efficient and considered safe, provided the *RHD* PCR detects all critical *RHD* and *RHCE* alleles expressing D epitopes. A consensus should be established in which the *RHD* screening strategy sufficiently fulfils these criteria. Similar examples can be enumerated for patient testing (table 2) [27–32].

Situations without Suitable Antisera or without Sufficient Resolution of Serology

Testing for Antigens for Which No Suitable Antisera Are Available or Not Available in Sufficient Amounts

Molecular testing is generally preferred if no suitable antisera are available. The most important example is the determination of the Dombrock phenotype [33, 34]. A similar situation may exist for the Yt^a and Yt^b antigens, for which commercial antisera are lacking, are available in only small quantities or are expensive. In addition, serologic testing is difficult and complicated for most platelet and granulocyte antigens, and molecular testing is today the first choice for determining many of these antigens.

Testing for Phenotypes That Cannot Safely Be Determined by Serology

Molecular testing is indicated for the discrimination of phenotypes that cannot be determined with sufficient certainty by serology, if the determination of the correct type has clinical consequences. The most important applications are: *(i) Determination of the weak D type.* The determination of the weak D type is indicated, if there are clinical consequences, like for instance change of transfusion strategy and withholding of anti-D prophylaxis. These approaches may be very cost-efficient because only one genotyping is required for the lifetime of the recipient. Serological techniques cannot discriminate weak D types with possible anti-D immunization risk and some partial D from weak D that may be safely transfused with D-positive blood. Transfusion strategies without genotyping may lead to unnecessarily risky, too conservative treatment strategies and waste of D-negative RBC units. *(ii) Determination of DIII-like phenotypes, DAR, combined rare RHCE alleles in individuals of African ancestry.* DIII-like phenotypes, DAR and combined rare *RHCE* alleles are frequent in individuals of African ancestry and cannot be determined by serology with sufficient safety [35, 36]. Because incompatible transfusion of these phenotypes and antigens may pose a relevant immunization risk for patients with these phenotypes, including multiple immunizations that effectively prevent further transfusions, molecular analysis may be indicated for these patients if chronic or repeated transfusion need is anticipated, like in sickle cell patients, and for partly immunized patients who need further transfusions.

Determination of Zygosity

Predictive Zygosity Testing

Determination of the zygosity allows the prediction of the likelihood of an antigen in a fetus of a current or future pregnancy [37, 38]. For example, if a father is homozygous for alleles expressing the D antigen, all his children will be D positive and further costly measures to determine the fetus's phenotype may be dropped.

Quality Control of Serologic Reagents

For some antigens, like Fy^a and Fy^b, antigen dosing derived from the presence of the antithetical antigen may be misleading, because non-expressed alleles are known to occur with relevant frequencies. Molecular determination of the zygosity of antibody screening and antibody identification panels may obviate this pitfall and is advocated [33, 37].

Replacement of Serologic Testing in High-Throughput Situations

Recently, several high-throughput methods have been developed that allow the prediction of donor phenotypes. These methods differ in the antigens predicted, the accuracy of the prediction, the necessity to confirm the predicted phenotype by serology and in their costs [17, 33, 39–44]. Use of these methods may be indicated to (i) screen for donors with rare antigen combinations or rare phenotypes, even if testing has to be confirmed by serology; (ii) typing of donors for antigens that cannot be determined by serology with sufficient ease; and (iii) general typing of donors for antigens if molecular typing is sufficiently safe and less costly than serologic typing (this situation is possible even for antigens that may be easily determined by serology, because in multiplex testing, the cost of adding another antigen is negligible and molecular typing may be indicated for other reasons).

Conclusions and Future Directions

We propose an update of the Consensus Statement 2000 to account for the advancements in molecular immunohematology, which by now allow much wider indications for blood group, platelet and granulocyte genotyping.

The advent of CE-labeled test kits renders it technically and legally possible, within the specifications of the CE-certification process for in vitro diagnostic devices in the European Union, to replace several blood group serology tasks by genotyping [6]. INSTAND offers a biannual proficiency workshop, 'External Quality Assurance (EQA) scheme blood group molecular genotyping', which besides blood group antigens also covers platelet and neutrophil antigens. The International Society of Blood Transfusion (ISBT) Workshop on Blood Group Molecular Genotyping is offered every other year and recommended the INSTAND workshop for EQA purposes in the intervening year 2007 to the international participants of the ISBT Workshop when ISBT did not offer its own EQA scheme [46].

As the example of antenatal care has shown, genetic blood group typing has led to a better quality of care because potential side effects can be avoided and costs reduced. This is a rare combination and justifies the extra costs involved in optimizing care via the use of genetic diagnostic techniques. As well as improving patient care, these methods can promote the development of new methods, which will also be used for health care outside of the German-speaking countries [1, 35]. Transfusion medicine specialists, with the help of national and European guidelines, have formulated solutions that transformed many practices in immunohematology and have proved beneficial for the patients. Now is the time to implement the recommended strategies by an appropriate adaptation of the clinical guidelines.

Disclosure of Conflict of Interests

The authors are current or former employees of the DRK Blutspendedienst Baden-Württemberg – Hessen. DRK and W.A.F. are holding patents or have patents pending on nucleotide sequences and their use in molecular genetics for weak D, DEL and the Rhesus boxes.

Acknowledgement

The authors thank Thomas H. Müller and Ingeborg von Zabern for their reviewing the manuscript, and the colleagues in the Deutsche Gesellschaft für Transfusionsmedizin und Immunhämatologie (DGTI) and in the Association Suisse de Médecine Transfusionnelle (ASMT/SVTM) whose important contributions were instrumental in devising the proposed genotyping strategies.

References

1 Flegel WA, Wagner FF, Müller TH, Gassner C: Rh phenotype prediction by DNA typing and its application to practice. Transfus Med 1998;8:281–302.

2 Flegel WA, Wagner FF: Molecular biology of partial D and weak D: implications for blood bank practice. Clin Lab 2002;48:53–58.

3 Legler TJ, Lynen R, Maas JH, Pindur G, Kulenkampff D, Suren A, Osmers R, Köhler M: Prediction of fetal Rh D and Rh CcEe phenotype from maternal plasma with real-time polymerase chain reaction. Transfus Apher Sci 2002;27:217–223.

4 Kroll H, Carl B, Santoso S, Bux J, Bein G: Workshop report on the genotyping of blood cell alloantigens. Transfus Med 2001;11:211–219.

5 van der Schoot CE, Tax GH, Rijnders RJ, de Haas M, Christiaens GC: Prenatal typing of Rh and Kell blood group system antigens: the edge of a watershed. Transfus Med Rev 2003;17:31–44.

6 Flegel WA: Blood group genotyping in Germany. Transfusion 2007;47:47S-53S.

7 Legler TJ, Kroll H, Wagner FF, Flegel WA, Hallensleben M: Indikation und Durchführung einer Genotypisierung erythrozytärer Antigene [Indication and method of red cell antigen genotyping]. Infusionsther Transfusionsmed 2000;27:215–216.

8 Prager M: Molecular genetic blood group typing by the use of PCR-SSP technique. Transfusion 2007;47:54S–59S.

9 Daniels G, van der Schoot CE, Olsson ML: Report of the First International Workshop on molecular blood group genotyping. Vox Sang 2005;88:136–142.

10 Wagner FF, Flegel WA: Review: the molecular basis of the Rh blood group phenotypes. Immunohematol 2004;20:23–36.

11 Doescher A, Flegel WA, Petershofen EK, Bauerfeind U, Wagner FF: Weak D type 1.1 exemplifies another complexity in weak D genotyping. Transfusion 2005;45:1568–1573.

12 Körmöczi GF, Förstemann E, Gabriel C, Mayr WR, Schönitzer D, Gassner C: Novel weak D types 31 and 32: adsorption-elution-supported D antigen analysis and comparison to prevalent weak D types. Transfusion 2005;45:1574–1580.

13 Wagner FF, Blaszczyk R, Seltsam A: Nondeletional ABO*O alleles frequently cause blood donor typing problems. Transfusion 2005;45:1331–1334.

14 Seltsam A, das Gupta C, Bade-Doeding C, Blaszyk R: A weak blood group A phenotype caused by a translation-initiator mutation in the ABO gene. Transfusion 2006;46:434–440.

15 Denomme GA, Wagner FF, Fernandes BJ, Li W, Flegel WA: Partial D, weak D types, and novel RHD alleles among 33,864 multiethnic patients: implications for anti-D alloimmunization and prevention. Transfusion 2005;45:1554–1560.

16 Bugert P, McBride S, Smith G, Dugrillon A, Klüter H, Ouwehand WH, Metcalfe P: Microarray-based genotyping for blood groups: comparison of gene array and 5'-nuclease assay techniques with human platelet antigen as a model. Transfusion 2005;45:654–659.

17 Avent ND, Martinez A, Flegel WA, Olsson ML, Scott ML, Nogués N, Písǎcka M, Daniels G, van der Schoot E, Muñiz-Diaz E, Madgett TE, Storry JR, Beiboer SH, Maaskant-van Wijk PA, von Zabern I, Jiménez E, Tejedor D, López M, Camacho E, Cheroutre G, Hacker A, Jinoch P, Svobodova I, de Haas M: The BloodGen project: toward mass scale comprehensive genotyping of blood donors in the European Union and beyond. Transfusion 2007;47:40S–46S.

18 Denomme GA, Fernandes BJ: Fetal blood group genotyping. Transfusion 2007;47:64S–68S.

19 Grootkerk-Tax MG, Soussan AA, de Haas M, Maaskant-van Wijk PA, van der Schoot CE: Evaluation of prenatal RHD typing strategies on cell-free fetal DNA from maternal plasma. Transfusion 2006;46:2142–2148.

20 Minon JM, Gerard C, Senterre JM, Schaaps JP, Foidart JM: Routine fetal RHD genotyping with maternal plasma: a four-year experience in Belgium. Transfusion 2008;48:373–381.

21 Kumpel BM: Are weak D RBCs really immunogenic? [Letter]. Transfusion 2006;46:1061–1062.

22 Gassner C, Doescher A, Drnovsek TD, Rozman P, Eicher NI, Legler TJ, Lukin S, Garritsen H, Kleinrath T, Egger B, Ehling R, Körmöczi GF, Kilga-Nogler S, Schoenitzer D, Petershofen EK: Presence of RHD in serologically D–, C/E+ individuals: a European multicenter study. Transfusion 2005;45:527–538.

23 Wagner T, Körmöczi GF, Buchta C, Vadon M, Lanzer G, Mayr WR, Legler TJ: Anti-D immunization by DEL red blood cells. Transfusion 2005;45:520–526.

24 Lüttringhaus TA, Cho D, Ryang DW, Flegel WA: An easy RHD genotyping strategy for D– East Asian persons applied to Korean blood donors. Transfusion 2006;46:2128–2137.

25 Polin H, Danzer M, Hofer K, Gassner W, Gabriel C: Effective molecular RHD typing strategy for blood donations. Transfusion 2007;47:1350–1355.

26 Nogues N, Tarrago M, Subirana L, Boto N, Salgado M, Ibañez M, Montero R, Fornes G, Muñiz-Diaz E: RHD null alleles in the Spanish population [abstract]. Vox Sang 2007;93:205.

27 Castilho L: The value of DNA analysis for antigens in the Duffy blood group system. Transfusion 2007;47:28S–31S.

28 Flegel WA: Homing in on D antigen immunogenicity. Transfusion 2005;45:466–468.

29 Flegel WA: How I manage donors and patients with a weak D phenotype. Curr Opin Hematol 2006;13:476–483.

30 Flegel WA, Denomme GA, Yazer MH: On the complexity of D antigen typing: a handy decision tree in the age of molecular blood group diagnostics. J Obstet Gynaecol Can 2007;29:746–752.

31 Noizat-Pirenne F, Verdier M, Lejealle A, Mercadier A, Bonin P, Peltier-Pujol F, Fialaire-Legendre A, Tournamille C, Bierling P, Ansart-Pirenne H: Weak D phenotypes and transfusion safety: where do we stand in daily practice? Transfusion 2007;47:1616–1620.

32 Christiansen M, Samuelsen B, Christiansen L, Morbjerg T, Bredahl C, Grunnet N: Correlation between serology and genetics of weak D types in Denmark. Transfusion 2008;48:187–193.

33 Storry JR, Olsson ML, Reid ME: Application of DNA analysis to the quality assurance of reagent red blood cells. Transfusion 2007;47:73S–78S.

34 Hult A, Hellberg A, Wester ES, Olausson P, Storry JR, Olsson ML: Blood group genotype analysis for the quality improvement of reagent test red blood cells. Vox Sang 2005;88:265–270.

35 Flegel WA: Genetik des Rhesus-Blutgruppensystems. Dtsch Ärzteblatt 2007;104:A651–A657.

36 Grootkerk-Tax MG, van Wintershoven JD, Ligthart PC, van Rhenen DJ, van der Schoot CE, Maaskant-van Wijk PA: RHD(T201R, F223V) cluster analysis in five different ethnic groups and serological characterization of a new Ethiopian variant DARE, the DIII type 6 and the RHD (F223V). Transfusion 2006;46:606–615.

37 Yu X, Wagner FF, Witter B, Flegel WA: Outliers in RhD membrane integration are explained by variant RH haplotypes. Transfusion 2006;46:1343–1351.

38 Krog GR, Clausen FB, Dziegiel MH: Quantitation of RHD by real-time polymerase chain reaction for determination of RHD zygosity and RHD mosaicism/chimerism: an evaluation of four quantitative methods. Transfusion 2007;47:715–722.

39 St Louis M, Perreault J, Lemieux R: Extended blood grouping of blood donors with automatable PCR-ELISA genotyping. Transfusion 2003;43:1126–1132.

40 Karpasitou K, Drago F, Crespiatico L, Paccapelo C, Truglio F, Frison S, Scalamogna M, Poli F: Blood group genotyping for Jk(a)/Jk(b), Fy(a)/Fy(b), S/s, K/k, Kp(a)/Kp(b), Js(a)/Js(b), Co(a)/Co(b), and Lu(a)/Lu(b) with microarray beads. Transfusion 2007;48:505–512.

41 Wagner FF, Döscher A, Bittner R, Petershofen EK: Multiplex PCR without DNA purification to screen blood donors for rare phenotypes [abstract]. Transfusion 2005;45:5A.

42 Wagner FF, Döscher A, Bittner R, Petershofen EK: Identifying donors with specific antigen combinations by multiplex PCR and pooled capillary electrophoresis [abstract]. Transfus Med Hemother 2007;34:54.

43 Denomme GA: The structure and function of the molecules that carry human red blood cell and platelet antigens. Transfus Med Rev 2004;18:203–231.

44 Chu CC, Lee HL, Chu TW, Lin M: The use of genotyping to predict the phenotypes of human platelet antigens 1 through 5 and of neutrophil antigens in Taiwan. Transfusion 2001;41:1553–1558.

45 Flegel WA: Will MICA glitter for recipients of kidney transplants? N Engl J Med 2007;357:1337–1339.

46 Daniels G, van der Schoot CE, Olsson ML: Report of the Second International Workshop on molecular blood group genotyping. Vox Sang 2007;93:83–88.

Prof. Dr. med. Willy A. Flegel
Institut für Klinische Transfusionsmedizin und Immungenetik Ulm
Helmholtzstraße 10
89081 Ulm, Germany
Tel. +49 731 150600, Fax -602
E-Mail willy.flegel@uni-ulm.de

Molecular Immunohematology

Scharf RE (ed): Progress and Challenges in Transfusion Medicine, Hemostasis and Hemotherapy.
Freiburg i.Br., Karger, 2008, pp 199–208

Molecular Methods in Immunohematology: Use of the PCR-SSP Technique

Martina Prager

Molecular Genetics Department, BAG Health Care GmbH, Lich, Germany

Key Words

Immunohematology · Molecular methods · Blood group typing · PCR-SSP · Application · Intended use

Summary

Molecular biological methods based on the well-known polymerase chain reaction with sequence-specific priming are established for different applications in laboratory routine. Therefore, it was obvious to implement this easy-to-handle and robust technique in transfusion medicine for enhancing immunohematology typings. Ready-to-use Conformité Européenne-marked test kits allow the examination of weak, unexpected or unclear serologic findings with acceptable costs.   ©2008 S. Karger GmbH, Freiburg i.Br.

Introduction

DNA typing has become possible for many blood group antigens which are mostly defined by single-amino acid polymorphisms. Since about 1993, scientific literature dealing with molecular typing in immunohematology has appeared with increased frequency [1, 2]. In 1998, blood group genotyping, mainly the determination of *RHD* including weak D phenotypes, was introduced at the University Hospital in Ulm to determine anti-D prophylaxis as well as prenatal and postpartum settings [3]. Meanwhile, many other German university medical centers and transfusion centers also apply molecular typing for the examination of different blood group systems. Indications and benefits of the polymerase chain reaction with sequence-specific priming (PCR-SSP) technique in the practice of blood group diagnosis will be depicted in this article.

Intended Use

The molecular determination of blood group antigens by the use of PCR-SSP [4, 5] has to be performed in conjunction with serology. Current assays (e.g. BAGene DNA-SSP kits; BAG Health Care GmbH, Lich, Germany) are available as a supplementary technique to examine weak or discrepant serological findings, but are neither intended to replace serology nor suitable for high throughput. In case of discrepant or unclear genotyping results, transfusion guidelines have to be followed in accordance with serologic results. Final clarification by sequencing analysis is recommended.

Application

A variety of sensitive reagents and well-established easy-to-handle serology techniques allow reliable blood group determination in most cases of donor and patient typing, but there is a need to clarify doubtful findings in order to prevent alloimmunizations or the waste of rare blood units if unnecessary. Since a long time, PCR-SSP test systems have often helped to investigate ambiguous tissue typing results in HLA (human leukocyte antigen) laboratories and, meanwhile, have also been introduced as a useful supplementary technique to examine questionable findings in immunohematology. The SSP method is based on the principle that under stringent conditions oligonucleotide primers only bind when their sequences entirely match the target sequences of the test DNA. Therefore, a successful PCR relies on an exact match at the 3' end of sense and anti-sense primers and is required to obtain amplicons that finally can be visualized by agarose gel electrophoresis. Ready-to-use PCR-SSP typing kits allow the determination of common, rare or weak alleles of the ABO blood group, Rhesus, Kell/Kidd/Duffy and MNS systems as well as alleles of the human platelet antigens (HPA) (fig. 1) [6]. A summary of the different uses of PCR-SSP for molecular blood group typing in clinical practice is described in this article and presented in table 1.

Determination of ABO Blood Groups

The genes for A and B transferase are located on the long arm of chromosome 9 (9q34) [7–9]. They consist of seven exons with a total length of 1065 base pairs. The majority of clinically relevant polymorphisms (base substitutions, deletions, insertions) are located on exons 6 and 7 [10]. Five common alleles are described in the literature: A^1, A^2, B^1, O^1, and O^2, and there are also numerous variants and subgroups. Unusual ABO typing results are a common problem in blood grouping. Rare *ABO* alleles have been shown to encode for the expression of aberrant ABO phenotypes, resulting in weak antigen activity as well as unexpected findings in reverse typing [11]. BAGene ABO-

ABO Genotyping

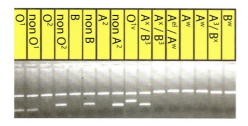

Column labels (left to right): O¹, non O¹, O², non O², B, non B, A², non A², Aᵉˡ/Aʷ, Aʷ, Aˣ/B³, A³/Bˣ, Bʷ, O¹ᵛ, Aˣ

BAGene ABO-TYPE variant genotype $O^{Tv}A^x$

RHD, RHCE Genotyping

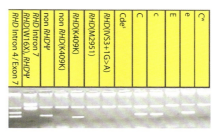

Column labels (left to right): RHD Intron 4 / Exon 7, RHD(W16X), RHDψ, non RHDψ, non RHD(K409K), RHD(K409K), RHD(M295I), RHD(IVS3+1G>A), Cdeˢ, C, c, E, e, Cʷ

BAGene RH-TYPE genotype $RHD(K409K)$ Ccee

Genotyping partial D

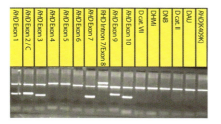

Column labels (left to right): RHD Exon 1, RHD Exon 2 / C, RHD Exon 3, RHD Exon 4, RHD Exon 5, RHD Exon 6, RHD Exon 7, RHD Intron 7/Exon 8, RHD Exon 9, RHD Exon 10, D cat. VII, DHMi, DNB, D cat. II, DAU, RHD(K409K)

BAGene Partial D-TYPE genotype *D cat. VI type II*

Genotyping weak D

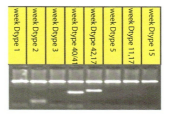

Column labels (left to right): weak Dtype 1, weak Dtype 2, weak Dtype 3, weak Dtype 40/41, weak Dtype 42,17, weak Dtype 5, weak Dtype 11,17, weak Dtype 15

BAGene Weak D-TYPE genotype *weak D type 4.2*

RHD Zygosity

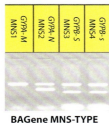

DD   Dd   dd

(columns: Downstream Rhesus Box, Hybrid Rhesus Box)

BAGene D Zygosity-TYPE

Genotyping KEL, JK, FY

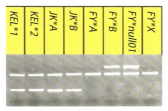

Column labels (left to right): KEL*1, KEL*2, JK*A, JK*B, FY*A, FY*B, FY*null01, FY*X

BAGene KKD-TYPE
genotype *KEL*1/KEL*2; JK*A/JK*B; FY*B/FY*null01*

Genotyping MNS

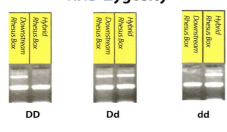

Column labels (left to right): GYPA-M MNS1, GYPA-N MNS2, GYPB-S MNS3, GYPB-s MNS4

BAGene MNS-TYPE
genotype *NSs*

Genotyping HPA

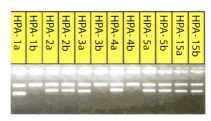

Column labels (left to right): HPA-1a, HPA-1b, HPA-2a, HPA-2b, HPA-3a, HPA-3b, HPA-4a, HPA-4b, HPA-5a, HPA-5b, HPA-15a, HPA-15b

BAGene HPA-TYPE
genotype *HPA-1a/a; 2a/b; 3a/a; 4a/a; 5a/b; 15a/b*

Fig. 1. Examples of gel pictures using PCR-SSP test kits for typing of different blood group loci.

Table 1. Practical applications of PCR-SSP in immunohematology

Genotype multi-transfused recipients
Genotype patients after ABO-incompatible bone marrow transplantation
Determine *RHD* zygosity of partners from alloimmunized D-negative women before pregnancies
Genotype D-negative donors with C or E in order to exclude the presence of the *RHD* gene and thus prevent anti-D alloimmunization of recipients caused by very weak Rh D variants in blood donors
Identify genotype in case of weakly expressed Rh D (e.g. DEL) in donors
Confirm weak D genotypes in recipients in order to avoid unnecessary use of D-negative blood units
Quality control of serological methods
External quality assurance

TYPE variant allows the molecular genetic determination of these 5 main alleles as well as the common O^{lv} allele and the subgroup variants A^3, A^x, A^{el}, A^w, B^3, B^x, B^w (fig. 2) [12–16].

Determination of *RHD/RHCE* Alleles

The two *RH* genes, *RHD* and *RHCE,* are located on the short arm of chromosome 1 (p34.3 to p36.1) [17]. Their 3' ends are oriented to each other and separated by 30,000 base pairs. A further gene (*SMP1*) is located in this section, which encodes for a membrane protein [18, 19]. The *RHD* gene encodes the antigen D; the *RHCE* gene encodes the antigens C, c, E and e. The *RHD* and *RHCE* genes consist of 10 exons with a common size of 69 kilobases. Approximately 18% of Europeans are serologically D-negative. In almost all D-negative Caucasians, the *RHD* gene is completely deleted on both chromosomes [20]. In D-negative individuals from other ethnic groups (Africans, Asians), the seemingly inactive *RHD* associated with a Cde^s haplotype and *RHD*Ψ are found [21–23]. BAGene RH-TYPE allows the molecular genetic determination of standard *RHD/RHCE* alleles [24, 25] as well as the typing of a few *RHD* variants (D cat. VI, D cat. IV type III, Cde^s, *RHD*Ψ, *RHD*(W16X), *RHD-CE*(8–9)-D, *RHD-E*(3–7)-D) and *DEL* (*RHD*(K409K), *RHD*(M295I), *RHD*(IVS3+1G>A)) [26]. The determination of C^w [27] is included as well. *RHD* variants with a higher frequency in Asian than in other ethnic groups (*RHD*(K409K), weak D type 15, 17) [28] can be detected using BAGene *RHD*-TYPE Asia.

Genotyping Partial D and Weak D

Variations of the antigen structure of RhD result either in a partial D or a weak D phenotype. Molecular genetic examinations of these D variants have shown that weak

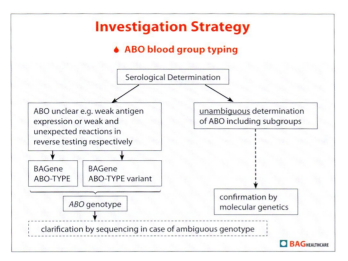

Fig. 2. Clear-cut serological determination of the ABO blood group cannot be achieved with samples of poly-transfused recipients. Weak expression of A and B antigens, either associated with normal or with unexpected reverse typing, also hampers the evaluation of results. This flow chart depicts a strategy using the BAGene ABO-TYPE variant kit which allows resolving most of the unclear serologic findings.

D phenotypes as well as some partial D types are caused by point mutations. In other partial D types, one or several exons of the *RHD* gene are exchanged with the corresponding segments of the *RHCE* gene, thus forming RhD-CE-D fusion proteins. In these fusion proteins, epitopes of the complete RhD protein are missing [29]. Therefore, individuals with partial D types (e.g. with the clinically relevant D category VI [30]) may be immunized by transfusion of erythrocytes expressing the normal RhD protein. According to the literature, amino acid substitutions in partial D phenotypes are localized mainly extracellularly. The substitution of amino acids in weak D is mainly limited to intracellular or transmembrane sections of the RhD protein [31, 32]. BAGene Partial D-TYPE allows the molecular genetic determination of the D categories II, III, IV, V [33, 34], VI, VII [35] as well as partial D *DAU* [36], *DBT* [37], *DFR, DHMi, DHMii, DNB* [38], *DHAR* (Rh33) and *DEL* (*RHD*(K409K)). BAGene Weak D-TYPE allows the molecular genetic determination of the weak D types 1, 2, 3, 4.0/4.1, 4.2, 5, 11, 15 and 17 (fig. 3).

Genotyping *RHD* Zygosity

In the RhD-positive haplotype, the *RHD* gene is flanked by two highly homologous DNA segments, the so-called *Rhesus Boxes*, which are localized 5' (upstream *Rhesus Box*) and 3' (downstream *Rhesus Box*) of the *RHD* gene [39]. In D-negative Caucasians, the *RHD* gene is generally completely deleted on both chromosomes. This results in a hybrid *Rhesus Box* that comprises the 5' end of the upstream *Rhesus Box* and the 3' end of the downstream *Rhesus Box*. BAGene D Zygosity-TYPE allows the determination of the *RHD* zygosity (homozygosity or hemizygosity of D) by the amplification of the downstream *Rhesus Box* (DD), or the hybrid *Rhesus Box* (dd), or by the downstream and the hybrid *Rhesus Box* (Dd), respectively [40].

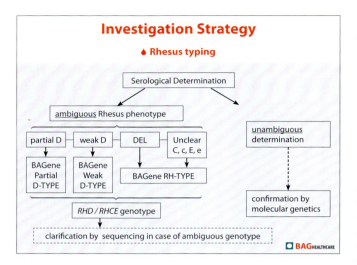

Fig. 3. Unclear Rh phenotypes can be investigated selecting suitable SSP kits depending on specific purposes. This figure shows an approach how to proceed in case of a questionable partial D pre-typed by serology: Quite often, a weak D is hidden behind a partial D. We recommend testing for weak D first. In case that the most common weak D types can be excluded, typing with the Partial D-TYPE kit should follow. An additional kit is available to examine D-negative samples for instance with a big C or big E. The RH-TYPE kit enables to detect D-negative *RHD* alleles, such as *DEL* types, *RHDψ* or *Cde^s*. RhCE antigens can also be cross-checked with this SSP kit.

Genotyping *KEL*, *JK* and *FY*

The significant difference between *KEL1* and *KEL2* (serologic nomenclature K and k – Cellano) is caused by a single base substitution in exon 6 of its gene [41, 42]. The Kidd system is located on chromosome 18 and consists of three different specificities Jk^a, Jk^b, Jk^null. The alleles *JK*A* and *JK*B* of the Kidd system differ in one single nucleotide substitution at position 838 of the *SLC14A1* gene [43].

The *FY* gene is localized on chromosome 1. It consists of the alleles *FY*A*, *FY*B*, *FY*X* and *FY*null01*, which may be represented mutually at the gene locus. Regarding serologic nomenclature, the *FY*A* allele corresponds to the Fy^a antigen and the *FY*B* allele to the Fy^b antigen [44, 45]. The weakly expressed allele *FY*X* (Fy^X) is serologically determined as Fy^{b weak} [46]. In the African population, the phenotype Fy(a–b–) can be observed with a frequency of 68%, whereas in Europeans, Fy(a–b–) is extremely rare (<0,1%). The most frequent cause of a Duffy-negative, i.e. Fy(a–b–), erythrocyte phenotype in black people is a polymorphism in the GATA motif of the Duffy gene (DARC) promoter, disrupting a binding site for the GATA1 erythroid transcription factor. Individuals with this silent allele called *FY*null01* [47, 48] are resistant to Malaria tertiana (*Plasmodium vivax*) due to the lack of an antigen determinant [49]. BAGene KKD-TYPE allows a clear identification of the main Kell, Kidd and Duffy alleles as well as of the immunologically relevant alleles Fy^{b weak} (*Fy*X*) and *FY*null01*. The kit consists of eight different PCR reaction mixes and enables the laboratory to perform the following assays: Kell (K, k), Kidd (Jk^a, Jk^b), and Duffy (Fy^a, Fy^b, Fy^{null}, Fy^X) [50].

Genotyping *MNS*

The antigens M and N were discovered in 1927 by Landsteiner and Levine [51], S and s in 1947 by Walsh und Montgomery [52]. Human glycophorins are the major sialoglycoproteins expressed on the red cell membrane that carry the antigens of the MNS blood group system [53]. Glycophorin A (GPA) has two allelic forms carrying the M or N antigen. Glycophorin B (GPB) also occurs in two allelic forms carrying the antigen S or s. GPA and GPB are encoded by *GYPA* and *GYPB*, respectively, which are members of a gene family on chromosome 4 [54]. The BAGene MNS-TYPE test kit allows the determination of the four main alleles of the MNS system (*M, N, S* and *s*).

Determination of *HPA*

Alloimmunothrombocytopenias such as neonatal alloimmunothrombocytopenia, post-transfusional purpura or refractory condition after thrombocyte transfusions are caused by antibodies directed against HPA which may be formed within the scope of transfusions or pregnancies. A reliable determination of the HPA specificities is necessary for diagnosing and providing suitable blood components for patients with these types of disease [55–60]. The thrombocyte antigens HPA represent a group of polymorphous allelic markers localized on the human thrombocyte glycoproteins GPIIb/IIa, GPIa, GPIbα, and GPIbβ. The polymorphisms are based on point mutations that result in the exchange of individual amino acids [59].

BAGene HPA-TYPE allows the molecular genetic determination of the *HPA* specificities *HPA-1a/b, HPA-2a/b, HPA-3a/b, HPA-4a/b, HPA-5a/b*, and *HPA-15a/b*.

Conclusions and Future Directions

The PCR-SSP technique is helpful to resolve most of the problems caused by discrepant or doubtful serologic results. It is an easy-to-handle and robust method. Questionable cases in donor, recipient and patient typing can be examined with acceptable costs. The current test kits cannot replace serology and are not suitable for high throughput. Results from external studies comparing genotyping for *ABO, RHD* and *RHCE* with serology have been presented in several congresses [61, 62]. Especially genotyping results for *ABO* have to be interpreted with caution in non-white individuals due to the hybrid genes found in these populations and the serious clinical consequences of ABO major incompatible transfusion of red cells. Further studies on different ethnic groups will be presented in the near future.

Disclosure of Conflict of Interests

The author states that she is Director of Molecular Genetics of BAG Health Care GmbH, Lich, Germany.

References

1 Müller TH, Hallensleben M, Schunter F, Blasczyk R: Molekulargenetische Blutgruppendiagnostik. Dt Ärztebl 2001;98:A317–322.
2 Bennett PR, Le Van Kim C, Colin Y, Warwick RM, Chérif-Zahar B, Fisk NM, Cartron JP: Prenatal determination of fetal RhD type by DNA amplification. N Engl J Med 1993;329:607–610.
3 Flegel WA: Blood group genotyping in Germany. Transfusion 2007;47(suppl):47S–53S.
4 Olerup O, Zetterquist H: HLA-DR typing by PCR amplification with sequence-specific primers (PCR-SSP) in 2 hours: an alternative to serological DR typing in clinical practice including donor-recipient matching in cadaveric transplantation. Tissue Antigens 1992;39:225–235.
5 Olerup O, Zetterquist H: DR "low-resolution" PCR-SSP typing – a correlation and an update. Tissue Antigens 1993;1:55–56.
6 Prager M: Molecular genetic blood group typing by the use of PCR-SSP technique. Transfusion 2007;47(suppl):54S–59S.
7 Ferguson-Smith MA, Aitken DA, Turleau C, de Grouchy J: Localisation of the human ABO. Np-1: AK-1 linkage group by regional assignment of AK-1 to 9q34. Hum Genet 1976;34:35–43.
8 Chester MA, Olsson ML: The ABO blood group gene. A locus of considerable genetic diversity. Transfus Med Rev 2001;15:177–200.
9 Yip SP: Sequence variation at the human ABO locus. Ann Hum Genet 2002;66:1–27.
10 Seltsam A, Hallensleben A, Kollmann A, Burkhart J, Blasczyk R: Systematic analysis of the ABO gene diversity within exons 6 and 7 by PCR-screening revealed new ABO alleles. Transfusion 2003;43:428–439.
11 Prager M, Scharberg EA, Wagner FF, Burkhart J, Seltsam A: ABO genotyping for diagnosis of unusual ABO blood groups: A comparative study in German blood donor centers. Transfusion 2007;47(3S): SP305.
12 Yamamoto F, McNeill PD, Yamamoto M, Hakomori S, Harris T, Judd WJ, Davenport RD: Molecular genetic analysis of the ABO blood group system: 1. Weak subgroups: A^3 and B^3 alleles. Vox Sang 1993;64:116–119.
13 Yamamoto F, McNeill PD, Yamamoto M, Hakomori S, Harris T: Molecular genetic analysis of the ABO blood group system: 3. A^x and $B^{(A)}$ alleles. Vox Sang 1993;64:171–174.
14 Olsson ML, Irshaid NM, Hosseini-Maaf B, Hellberg A, Moulds MK, Sareneva H, Chester MA: Genomic analysis of clinical samples with serologic ABO blood grouping discrepancies: Identification of 15 novel A and B subgroup alleles. Blood 2001;98:1585–1593.
15 Seltsam A, Hallensleben M, Kollmann A, Blasczyk R: The nature of diversity and diversification at the ABO locus. Blood 2003;102:3035–3042.
16 Seltsam A, Das Gupta C, Wagner FF, Blasczyk R: Non-deletional ABO*O alleles express weak blood group A phenotypes. Transfusion 2005;45:359–365.
17 Chérif-Zahar B: Localization of the human Rh blood group gene structure to chromosome region 1p34.3–1p36.1 by in situ hybridisation. Hum Genet 1991;86:398–400.
18 Wagner FF, Gassner C, Müller TH, Schönitzer D, Schunter F, Flegel WA: Molecular basis of weak D phenotypes. Blood 1999;93:385–393.
19 Flegel WA, Wagner FF: Molecular genetics of RH. Vox Sang 2000;78(suppl 2):109–115.
20 Blunt T, Daniels G, Carritt B: Serotype switching in a partially deleted RHD gene. Vox Sang 1994;67:397–401.
21 Okada H, Kawano M, Iwamoto S, Tanaka M, Seno T, Okubo Y, Kajii E: The RHD gene is highly detectable in RhD-negative Japanese donors. J Clin Invest 1997;100:373–379.
22 Singleton BK, Green CA, Avent ND, Martin PG, Smart E, Daka A, Narter-Olaga EG, Hawthorne LM, Daniels G: The presence of an RHD pseudogene containing a 37 base pair duplication and a nonsense mutation in Africans with the RhD-negative blood group phenotype. Blood 2000;95:12–18.
23 Wagner FF, Fromajer A, Flegel WA: RHD positive haplotypes in D negative Europeans. BMC Genetics 2001;2:10.
24 Gassner C, Schmarda A, Kilga-Nogler S, Jenny-Feldkircher B, Rainer E, Müller TH, Wagner FF, Flegel WA, Schönitzer D: RHD/CE typing by polymerase chain reaction using sequence-specific primers. Transfusion 1997;37:1020–1026.

25 Flegel WA, Wagner FF, Müller TH, Gassner C: Rh phenotype prediction by DNA typing and its application to practice. Transfus Med 1998;8:281–302.

26 Shao CP, Maas JH, Su YQ, Köhler M, Legler TJ: Molecular background of RhD-positive, D-negative, D_{el} and weak D phenotypes in Chinese. Vox Sang 2002;83:156–161.

27 Mouro I, Colin Y, Sistonen P, Le Pennec PY, Cartron JP, Le Van Kim C: Molecular basis of the RhC^w (Rh8) and RhC^x (Rh9) blood group specificities. Blood 1995;86:1196–1201.

28 Luettringhaus TA, Cho D, Ryang DW, Flegel WA: An easy *RHD* genotyping strategy for D– East Asian persons applied to Korean blood donors. Transfusion 2006;46:2128–2137.

29 Rouillac C, Colin Y, Hughes-Jones NC, Beolet M, D'Ambrosio AM, Cartron JP, Le Van Kim C: Transcript analysis of D category phenotypes predicts hybrid Rh D-CE-D proteins associated with alteration of D epitopes. Blood 1995;85:2937–2944.

30 Wagner FF, Gassner C, Müller TH, Schönitzer D, Schunter F, Flegel WA: Three molecular structures cause Rhesus D category VI phenotypes with distinct immunohematologic features. Blood 1998;91:2157–2168.

31 Legler TJ, Maas JH, Blaschke M, Malekan H, Ohto R, Lynen R, Bustami N, Schwartz DWM, Mayr WR, Köhler M, Panzer S: *RHD* genotyping in weak D phenotypes by multiple polymerase chain reactions. Transfusion 1998;38:434–440.

32 Wagner FF, Frohmajer A, Ladewig B, Eicher NI, Lonicer CB, Muller TH, Siegel MH, Flegel WA: Weak D alleles express distinct phenotypes. Blood 2000;95:2699–2708.

33 Omi T, Takahashi J, Tsudo N, Okuda H, Iwamoto S, Tanaka M, Seno T, Tani Y, Kajii E: The genomic organization of the partial D category DVa: the presence of a new partial D associated with the DVa phenotype. Biochem Biophys Res Commun 1999;254:786–794.

34 Legler TJ, Wiemann V, Ohto H, Matuda I, Obara T, Uchikawa M, Köhler M: D(Va) category phenotype and genotype in Japanese families. Vox Sang 2000;78:194–197.

35 Rouillac C, Le Van Kim C, Beolet M, Cartron JP, Colin Y: Leu110Pro substitution in the RhD polypeptide is responsible for the DVII category blood group phenotype. Am J Hematol 1995;49:87–88.

36 Wagner FF, Ladewig B, Angert KS, Heymann GA, Eicher NI, Flegel WA: The *DAU* allele cluster of the *RHD* gene. Blood 2002;100:306–311.

37 Beckers EAM, Faas BHW, Simsek S, Overbeeke MA, van Rhenen DJ, Wallace M, von dem Borne AE, van der Schoot CE: The genetic basis of a new partial D antigen: D^{DBT}. Br J Haematol 1996;93:720–727.

38 Wagner FF, Eicher NI, Jørgensen JR, Lonicer CB, Flegel WA: DNB: a partial D with anti-D frequent in Central Europe. Blood 2002;100:2253–2256.

39 Wagner FF, Flegel WA: *RHD* gene deletion occurred in the *Rhesus box*. Blood 2000;95:3662–3668.

40 Perco P, Shao CP, Mayr WR, Panzer S, Legler TJ: Testing for the D zygosity with three different methods revealed altered Rhesus boxes and a new weak D type. Transfusion 2003;43:335–339.

41 Lee S, Naime DS, Reid ME, Redman CM: Molecular basis for the high-incidence antigens of the Kell blood group system. Transfusion 1997;37:1117–1122.

42 Lee S, Wu X, Reid M, Zelinski T, Redman C: Molecular basis of the Kell (K1) phenotype. Blood 1995;85:912–916.

43 Lucien N, Sidoux-Walter F, Olives B, Moulds J, Le Pennec PY, Cartron JP, Bailly P: Characterization of the gene encoding the human Kidd blood group/urea transporter protein. Evidence for splice site mutations in Jknull individuals. J Biol Chem 1998;273:12973–12980.

44 Neote K, Mak JY, Kolakowski LFJ, Schall TJ: Functional and biochemical analysis of the cloned Duffy antigen: identity with the red blood cell chemokine receptor. Blood 1994;84:44–52.

45 Tournamille C, Le van Kim C, Gane P, Cartron JP, Colin Y: Molecular basis and PCR-DNA typing of the Fya/Fyb blood group polymorphism. Hum Genet 1995;95:407–410.

46 Tournamille C, Le van Kim C, Gane P, Le Pennec PY, Roubinet F, Babinet J, Cartron JP, Colin Y: Arg89Cys substitution results in very low membrane expression of the Duffy antigen/receptor for chemokines in Fy(x) individuals. Blood 1998;92:2147–2156.

47 Tournamille C, Colin Y, Cartron JP, Le van Kim C: Disruption of a GATA motif in the Duffy gene promoter abolishes erythroid gene expression in Duffy-negative individuals. Nat Genet 1995;10:224–228.

48 Mallinson G, Soo KS, Schall TJ, Pisacka M, Anstee DJ: Mutations in the erythrocyte chemokine receptor (Duffy) gene: the molecular basis of the Fya/Fyb antigens and identification of a deletion in the Duffy gene of an apparently healthy individual with the Fy(a–b–) phenotype. Br J Haematol 1995;90:823–829.

49 Chitnis CE, Chaudhuri A, Horuk R, Pogo AO, Miller LH: The domain on the Duffy blood group antigen for binding *Plasmodium vivax* and *P. knowlesi* malarial parasites to erythrocytes. J Exp Med 1996;184:1531–1536.

50 Rožman P, Dovč T, Gassner C: Differentiation of autologous ABO, RHD, RHCE, KEL, JK, and FY blood group genotypes by analysis of peripheral blood samples of patients who have recently received multiple transfusions. Transfusion 2000;40:936–942.

51 Landsteiner K, Levine P: A new agglutinable factor differentiating individual human bloods. Proc Soc Exp Biol 1927;24:600.

52 Walsh RJ, Montgomery C: A new human isoagglutinin subdividing the MN blood groups. Nature 1947;160:504.

53 Shih MC, Yang LH, Wang NM, Chang JG: Genomic typing of human red cell Miltenberger glycophorins in a Taiwanese population. Transfusion 2000;40:54–61.

54 Storry JR, Reid ME, Fetics S, Huang CH: Mutations in *GYPB* exon 5 drive the S–s–U+^{var} phenotype in persons of African descent: implications for transfusion. Transfusion 2003;43:1738–1747.

55 Ballem PJ, Buskard NA, Decary F, Doubroff P: Posttransfusion purpura secondary to passive transfer of anti-Pl^{A1} by blood transfusion. Br J Hematol 1987;66:113–114.

56 Mueller-Eckhardt C, Kiefel V, Grubert A, Kroll H, Weisheit M, Schmidt S, Mueller-Eckhardt G, Santoso S: 348 cases of suspected neonatal alloimmune thrombocytopenia. Lancet 1989;1:363–366.

57 Panzer S, Kiefel V, Bartram CR, Haas OA, Hinterberger W, Mueller-Eckhardt C, Lechner K: Immune thrombocytopenia more than a year after allogeneic marrow transplantation due to antibodies against donor platelets with anti-Pl^{A1} specificity: evidence for a host derived immune reaction. Br J Hematol 1989;71:259–264.

58 Mueller-Eckhardt C, Kiefel V, Santoso S: Review and update of platelet alloantigen systems. Transfus Med Rev 1990;4:98–109.

59 Santoso S, Kiefel V: Human platelet specific alloantigens: update. Vox Sang 1998;74(suppl):249–253.

60 Lyou JY, Chen YJ, Hu HY, Lin JS, Tzeng CH: PCR with sequence-specific primer-based simultaneous genotyping of human platelet antigen-1 to -13w. Transfusion 2002;42:1089–1095.

61 Legler TJ, Binder E, Smart E, Prager M, Maas JH: RHD and RHCE genotyping in South African blood donors with prepipetted PCR-SSP kits. Transfusion 2004;44(suppl):SP285.

62 Thierbach J, Jung A, Hitzler WE: Retrospective, comparative typing of Rh(D) negative and weak D blood donors with serological and genotyping methods. Transfus Med Hemother 2006;33(suppl 1):49(P6.26).

Martina Prager
Leitung Produktion Molekulargenetik
BAG Health Care GmbH
Amtsgerichtsstraße 1–5, 35423 Lich, Germany
Tel. +49 6404 925222, Fax 92533222
E-Mail prager.martina@bag-healthcare.com

Scharf RE (ed): Progress and Challenges in Transfusion Medicine, Hemostasis and Hemotherapy.
Freiburg i.Br., Karger, 2008, pp 209–218

Fetal Blood Group Genotyping

Axel Seltsam

Institute for Transfusion Medicine, Hannover Medical School, Germany

Key Words

Blood groups · Rhesus · Genotyping · Hemolytic disease of the newborn · Noninvasive fetal genotyping · Maternofetal incompatibility

Summary

Despite the use of anti-D immunoglobulin prophylaxis, RhD alloimmunization still remains the major cause of severe hemolytic disease of the fetus and the newborn. Many of the current methods rely on invasive methods and are associated with an inherent risk of fetal loss. The cloning of blood group genes and the identification of the molecular bases of blood group polymorphisms has made it possible to predict blood group phenotypes from DNA with a reasonable degree of accuracy. This has also opened new possibilities for RhD typing in prenatal diagnostics and pregnancy precaution. Fetal DNA in maternal plasma can be used for noninvasive determination of the RhD status of fetuses carried by RhD-negative pregnant women. Moreover, noninvasive fetal *RHD* typing could be systematically proposed to all RhD-negative pregnant women for a better targeted prenatal follow-up and an increased efficacy of anti-D prophylaxis. Finally, paternal *RHD* zygosity testing offers the opportunity to assess the risk of RhD incompatibility in alloimmunized women.   ©2008 S. Karger GmbH, Freiburg i.Br.

Introduction

Historically, hemolytic disease of the fetus and newborn (HDFN) was a significant cause of fetal and neonatal death (4 to 5 for every 1,000 live births) [1]. HDFN is usually caused by immunoglobulin G (IgG) antibodies to the D blood group antigen of the Rhesus (Rh) system in an RhD-negative mother crossing the placenta and facilitating the immune destruction of RhD-positive fetal red cells. Because the antibody is usually formed in response to immunization by fetal RhD-positive red cells during the delivery of a previous baby, prevention of antibody production by injecting RhD-negative mothers with anti-D immunoglobulin shortly after delivery of each RhD-positive baby has substantially reduced the prevalence of HDFN. Since the introduction of immune prophylaxis to prevent D alloimmunization in the late 1960s, the risk of anti-D alloimmunization has been markedly reduced. In addition, antenatal anti-D prophylaxis was introduced to prevent D immunization during pregnancy. The anti-D immunization rate of RhD-negative pregnant women is now about 0.2–0.5% [2]. Techniques such as OD450 bilirubin estimation of amniotic fluid, noninvasive fetal ultrasound evaluation, and medial cerebral artery flow as a surrogate marker of anemia, all have helped to prevent deaths and allowed for interventions before complications arise. Intrauterine venous blood transfusion and neonatal exchange transfusions can change severe hemolytic disease, complicated by kernicterus and neurologic impairment, into a healthy live birth with little or no long-term health problems.

Serologic typing of red cells for ABO, Rhesus and Kell and alloantibody detection in the blood of pregnant women are routinely performed to identify pregnancies at risk for HDFN, to identify RhD-negative women who need anti-D prophylaxis, and to provide compatible blood for obstetric emergencies. Once an alloantibody is detected in maternal blood and the laboratory parameters such as titer or tests on the biological activity are indicative of possible hemolysis, it is important to know the phenotype of the fetus [3]. Before the molecular bases of the blood group antigens were known, the phenotype had to be determined by serological testing of fetal red cells, which could be obtained by cordocentesis or by chorionic villus sampling [4]. These are invasive and difficult procedures, with some risk for the fetus, and are only available in specialized centers. However, the discovery of circulating cell-free fetal DNA in maternal plasma by Lo and coworkers has opened up new possibilities for noninvasive prenatal diagnosis [5].

Sources of Fetal DNA

Several sources of fetal tissue have been explored for their potential use in blood group genotyping. Blood obtained by cordocentesis was not used routinely because of the risk of transplacental hemorrhage and rise in the antibody titer and fetal demise. An alternative is chorionic villi, which provide sufficient tissue for DNA extraction without a significant risk of a maternal-fetal hemorrhage. But chorionic villus sampling has not gained wide acceptance because of the risk of fetal limb deformities. Amniotic fluid is the most common 'tissue' to use for fetal blood group genotyping. Amniocentesis carries a 0.3% pregnancy loss procedural risk. Transplacental hemorrhage or a rise in the antibody titer occurs in approximately 3% of alloimmunized pregnancies, a risk that is reduced by avoiding puncture of the placenta.

Lo et al. were the first to describe that fetal sex can be determined by Y chromosome-specific polymerase chain reaction (PCR) on cellular DNA isolated from maternal blood samples [6]. The same group and others have shown that it is possible to determine the fetal RhD status with similar methods [7–9]. In particular, fetal erythroblasts that express blood group antigens were enriched from the peripheral maternal blood and used for reverse transcription (RT)-PCR-based *RHD* genotyping strategies [10]. However, none of the applied methodologies for cell enrichment have resulted in tests that meet the accuracy needed for clinical usage. The low sensitivity of these methods might be based on immunological clearance of the erythroblasts owing to ABO incompatibility between mother and child. In addition, the persistence of fetal cells from previous pregnancies can cause false-positive results.

In 1997, the Lo group showed that Y-chromosomal sequences could be amplified from DNA isolated from the plasma from pregnant women carrying male fetuses [5]. The likely resource of fetal DNA is apoptotic villous trophoblasts within the fetal compartment of the placenta. These could be released into the maternal blood via the fetomaternal interface [11]. It has also been demonstrated that microvesicles containing RNA and DNA are shed into the maternal circulation and are rapidly eliminated there with a half-life of about 15 min.

Mostly, RT-PCR techniques with sequence-specific primers and probes have been used to detect the fetal *RHD* status. In contrast to the methods based on fetal cells in the maternal circulation, false positivity due to the persistence of fetal cells from previous pregnancies is excluded when cell-free fetal DNA is used as template [12]. The fact that most of the circulating fetal (<300 bp) DNA fragments are shorter than the maternal DNA molecules should be taken into account when designing fetal genotyping assays [13]. Fetal DNA can be detected in maternal plasma already at the 5th week of gestation and the concentration of fetal DNA increases with gestational age [14]. The finding of *RHD*-positive DNA in the range of 5 to 708 genome equivalents in 160 RhD-negative women pregnant with RhD-positive fetuses reflects the considerable biological variability in the concentration of free fetal DNA [15].

Noninvasive Fetal *RHD* Genotyping in Anti-D Alloimmunized Pregnant Women

Blood group genotyping using free fetal plasma from the maternal circulation is useful to identify fetuses at risk for HDFN because the risks associated with invasive diagnostic procedures can be avoided. Since the discovery of cell-free fetal DNA, many groups have developed robust *RHD* genotyping assays in which several *RHD*-specific nucleotides are present in primers and probes. Fetal *RHD* detection from maternal plasma has reached close to 100% accuracy (table 1) [16]. The technique is sensitive because the maternal Rh genome is often characterized by the deletion of *RHD*, and therefore her plasma DNA will not contain *RHD*-positive genetic material. Because many variant *RHD* alleles exist, multiplex PCR assays should be applied in which several diagnostic regions of the *RHD* gene are amplified in order to limit the rate of false-negative results. False positivity due to the existence of silent *RHD* alleles cannot completely be prevented, but the inclusion of *RHD*-specific PCRs that are negative in the presence of pseudogenes will greatly decrease its incidence. Whereas in Caucasians deletion of the entire *RHD* gene is the most common cause of the RhD-negative phenotype, *RHDψ* and *RHD-CE-D* hybrid genes are the most frequent nonfunctional *RHD* genes in Africans and Asians [17–19]. In white persons, antigen RhD-negative

Group [year]	Number tested	Number correct
Faas [1998]	31	31
Lo [1998]	57	55
Finning [2002]	137	137
Finning [2004]	359	347
Rouillac [2004]	851	842
Van der Schoot [2004]	1257	1249
Gautier [2005]	283	283
Zhou [2005]	98	92
Minon [2007]	545	545
Total accuracy, %		99

Table 1. Diagnostic accuracy of fetal *RHD* genotyping on fetal DNA from maternal plasma

RHD-positive alleles are rare and most frequently associated with hybrid *RHD-CE-D* genes [20]. The original works of Bennett et al. and Wolter et al. suggest that *RHD* typing should include exons 4 to 5 and 10 [21, 22].

For interpretation of typing results, the limitations of the applied genotyping methods have always to be taken into account in order to avoid new risks for the fetus and the pregnant woman that may arise from wrong conclusions. Hence, the genotyping strategy used should include an internal positive control that indicates false-negative results due to low fetal DNA concentration. When *RHD* is not detected, detection of the Y chromosome (male fetus), and other nonmaternal insertions or deletions, and short tandem repeat polymorphic markers are used to confirm the presence of fetal DNA. Figure 1 shows a possible strategy that could be used for fetal *RHD* typing. An accurate medical history is essential when performing this test, as recently demonstrated by the false-positive result observed in a pregnant woman who previously received a male kidney transplant [23]. Recently, detection of the hypermethylated DNA sequence *RASSF41A* has been proposed as universal positive control to detect fetal DNA [24]. This gene is hypermethylated in placental cells, a major source of fetal DNA in the maternal plasma, and hypomethylated in maternal blood cells. However, to date PCR methods based on differential methylation are not sensitive enough for routine application. Thus, according to the guidelines for conventional serologic blood group typing in pregnancy, the results of fetal blood group genotyping should be confirmed by a second testing in anti-D-alloimmunized women.

Since a number of allelic variants and nonfunctional genes are present in humans, in the absence of parallel parental analyses, the interpretation of a genotype can be erroneous. Thus, fetal blood group genotyping as a stand-alone test cannot accurately predict the phenotype of the fetus. In pregnancies at risk for HDFN, it is therefore advisable to evaluate the maternal phenotype and genotype and, if possible, the paternal blood group status along with the fetal blood group. Only then can the fetal phenotype be reliably inferred from the genotype.

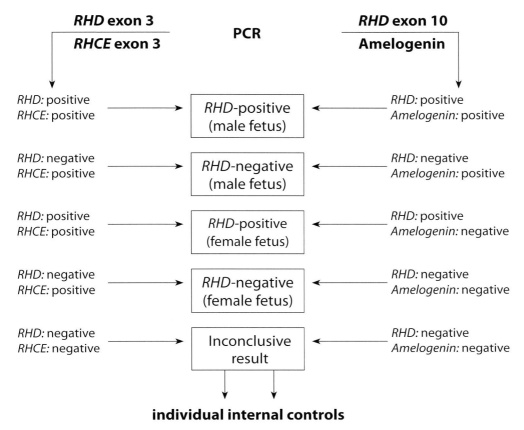

Fig. 1. Example of a strategy for prenatal *RHD* genotyping. The algorithm of a PCR assay is shown in which exons 3 and 10 of the *RHD* gene are amplified. In addition, *RHCE* gene-specific amplification is performed to confirm the presence of DNA in samples from RhD-negative female fetuses. In pregnancies with male fetuses, the detection of the Y chromosome-specific gene *Amelogenin* as an internal positive control confirms the presence of fetal DNA. In the absence of an *Amelogenin*-specific PCR signal, a panel of highly polymorphic markers or short tandem repeats (STRs) can be used as individual internal controls to discriminate fetal from maternal DNA.

Screening for Fetal *RHD* in RhD-Negative Pregnant Women

Fetal blood group genotyping from peripheral maternal blood is a noninvasive method that not only can help to identify RhD incompatibility between mother and child at an early stage of pregnancy but also makes it possible to define the fetal RhD status before administration of the antenatal anti-D prophylaxis (usually at 28 and 34 weeks). The current guidelines do not allow restriction of the antenatal anti-D prophylaxis to only those women at risk for immunization. Because the RhD phenotype of the fetus is not known, about 40% of these RhD-negative women (in a predominantly Caucasian population) carry an RhD-negative fetus and receive this therapy unnecessarily. Administration of this blood-derived product carries a small but real risk of associated blood-borne infection. Furthermore, worldwide supplies of RhD immunoglobulin are limited. A number of studies have shown that fetal *RHD* typing from amniotic fluid or maternal plasma is feasible [16, 25–31]. Automated high-throughput genotyping approaches may reduce the costs below the price of anti-D immunoglobulin. An economic evaluation showed that the implementation of fetal *RHD* typing in the Dutch population is cost effective [16]. The Fetal and Neonatal Evaluation Network (SAFE) is a Network of Excellence established in 2004 under the European Commission Sixth Framework Program with an overriding aim to develop the technology required for robust and cost-effective noninvasive prenatal diagnosis and neonatal screening and to expedite implementation within and beyond the European Community (www.safenoe.org) [32]. SAFE is strongly supporting the application of noninvasive prenatal diagnosis for *RHD* to all RhD-negative pregnant women, who represent in Europe 15–18% of the pregnant population. If such large-scale trials are successful, it could result in significant savings in the use of anti-D immunoglobulin and a reduction in hospital visits for many RhD-negative women. SAFE is evaluating the economic costs and benefits of this strategy, and other partners are investigating strategies for efficient implementation into routine obstetric care.

Paternal Zygosity

Red blood cell alloimmunization in pregnancy must be investigated for its potential risk to the current pregnancy. However, equally important, genetic counseling for future pregnancies requires the determination of the paternal zygosity. If paternity is assured and the father does not express the RBC antigen or is homozygous for the inferred antigen, then the appropriate risk can be assigned. In contrast to all the other common blood group antigens implicated in HDFN, zygosity for RhD cannot be determined serologically. However, since the elucidation of the genomic organization of the *RHD* locus by Flegel and Wagner a few years ago, the *RHD* zygosity can be assigned on the basis of the structure of the Rhesus boxes that flank *RHD* [33]. The upstream and downstream Rhesus boxes share 98.6% identity. In the absence of *RHD* (i.e. deleted *RHD*), a hybrid Rhesus box is present and infers hemizygosity. However, variant Rhesus boxes confounded zygosity assignment and some downstream Rhesus boxes have unacceptable variation for analysis among certain *RHD* alleles [34–36]. At present, there are two assays that can reliably identify the hybrid Rhesus box in certain populations [33, 37]. However, a long-range PCR spanning the whole hybrid Rhesus box and amplifying a 9-kbp fragment when the hybrid Rhesus box is present may not be influenced by the kinds of aberrations and may, although it is technically demanding, prove to be the most reliable assay of choice [36]. The use of real-time quantitative PCR to determine *RHD* dosage complemented by the specific detection of *RHD*ψ is an alternative approach to assign *RHD* zygosity (fig. 2) [37]. Since the

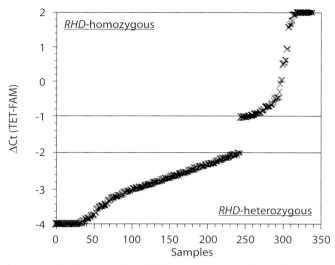

Fig. 2. *RHD* zygosity measured by quantitative real-time PCR in 342 samples. Quantitative real-time PCR was performed with the TaqMan technology and *RHD*-specific primers. Amplification results were reported by cycle threshold (Ct), i.e. the calculated cycle number at which the PCR products crossed a detection threshold. The higher the initial amount of target DNA, the lower the Ct value. It was then determined from the difference between the signals (ΔCt) whether a certain exon was present in homo- or heterozygosity. *RHD*-homozygous individuals showed ΔCt values between +2 and –1, while individuals heterozygous for *RHD* had values between –2 and –4.

RHCE gene is normally present in two copies, it can be used as reference. Thus, an individual is homozygous for *RHD* if the relation of quantity between *RHD* and *RHCE* is 1:1, and heterozygous for *RHD* if the relation of quantity is 1:2.

Fetal Genotyping for Other Blood Groups

After anti-D, the next most common causes of HDFN are anti-c and anti-K, although in both the prevalence of severe disease is much lower than that caused by anti-D [38]. In many cases, HDFN caused by antibodies to c is milder than that caused by anti-D. However, infrequent exceptions have been seen, with perhaps anti-c being more likely than other non-anti-D Rh antibodies to cause severe HDFN [39–41]. The C antigen-specific polymorphisms are defined by a 307C>T single-nucleotide polymorphism and lie in exon 2 of the *RHCE* gene. However, *RHD* and *RHCE*C* are identical in exon 2, which makes *RHCE*C* allelic determination impossible in the background of the Rh-positive haplotype. In contrast, testing for c is more straightforward as cytosine at nucleotide position 307 is unique to *RHCE*c*. Anti-K has also caused severe HDFN, including fatal cases [42]. It has been shown that anti-K may have a greater effect than anti-D in destroying or retarding maturation of erythroid precursor cells [43, 44]. That is, a decrease in red cell production contributes significantly to the anemia as opposed to anti-D HDFN where the anemia is primarily caused by antibody-mediated destruction of red cells. The k/K polymorphism results from a 698C>T nucleotide mutation in exon 6 of the *KEL* gene, allowing for genotyping methods that use restriction enzymes or allele-specific primers [45]. Many other blood group polymorphisms, such as S/s, E/e, Kp^a/Kp^b, Js^a/Js^b, Fy^a/Fy^b, Jk^a/Jk^b, Di^a/Di^b and Co^a/Co^b result from single-nucleotide polymorphisms and have all been involved in HDFN [45]. It would be feasible to develop noninvasive methods for fetal genotyping from maternal blood for all these polymorphisms, but the frequency and severity of HDFN caused by the corresponding antibody specificities is low so that the demand would be also extremely low.

Conclusion and Future Directions

With the many developments both in our understanding of the biology of fetal DNA in maternal plasma and the technological advances in its analysis, it is very likely that maternal plasma DNA analysis will play an increasingly important role in prenatal diagnosis and monitoring. Presently, the lack of a generic positive control for the presence of fetal DNA is a major limitation in fetal blood group genotyping in alloimmunized pregnant women. However, it is to be expected that newer technologies that include the detection of universal fetal DNA markers will overcome this problem.

Indeed, the introduction of fetal blood group genotyping would have a great impact on the management of pregnancies at risk for HDFN or anti-D alloimmunization. Overall, about half of all alloimmunized pregnancies involve a partner who is heterozygous for the target antigen. The identification of an antigen-negative fetus would reduce the number of consultations and, in cases where a hydrops fetalis is present, necessitate the search for another reason for the disorder. Moreover, the anxiety of the parents over the possible outcome of the pregnancy would be diminished with the identification of an antigen-negative fetus. While there is no doubt that fetal blood group genotyping will be beneficial for the management of pregnancies, future studies will have to show its cost effectiveness to improve its acceptance in times of limited resources. Highly automated technologies that include fetal *RHD* typing in mass fetal screening for a variety of inherited conditions hold the promise to allow the widespread utilization of maternal plasma DNA analysis for the noninvasive prenatal diagnosis of blood group mismatches between mother and fetus.

Disclosure of Conflict of Interests

The author states that he has no conflict of interests.

Acknowledgements

The author thanks Dr. Andrea Döscher for providing the figures about fetal *RHD* genotyping.

References

1 Bowman J: The management of hemolytic disease in the fetus and newborn. Semin Perinatol 1997;21:39–44.

2 Huchcroft S, Gunton P, Bowen T: Compliance with postpartum Rh isoimmunization prophylaxis in Alberta. CMAJ 1985;133:871–875.

3 Nicolaides KH, Rodeck CH: Maternal serum anti-D antibody concentration and assessment of Rhesus isoimmunisation. BMJ 1992;304:1155–1156.

4 Gemke RJ, Kanhai HH, Overbeeke MA, Maas CJ, Bennebroek Gravenhorst J, Bernini LF, Engelfriet CP, van't Veer MB: ABO and Rhesus phenotyping of fetal erythrocytes in the first trimester of pregnancy. Br J Haematol 1986;64:689–697.

5 Lo YM, Corbetta N, Chamberlain PF, Rai V, Sargent IL, Redman CW, Wainscoat JS: Presence of fetal DNA in maternal plasma and serum. Lancet 1997;350:485–487.

6 Lo YM, Patel P, Wainscoat JS, Sampietro M, Gillmer MD, Fleming KA: Prenatal sex determination by DNA amplification from maternal peripheral blood. Lancet 1989;2:1363–1365.

7 Hamlington J, Cunningham J, Mason G, Mueller R, Miller D: Prenatal detection of Rhesus D genotype. Lancet 1997;349:540.

8 Lo YM, Noakes L, Bowell PJ, Fleming KA, Wainscoat JS: Detection of fetal RhD sequence from peripheral blood of sensitized RhD-negative pregnant women. Br J Haematol 1994;87:658–660.

9 Sekizawa A, Watanabe A, Kimura T, Saito H, Yanaihara T, Sato T: Prenatal diagnosis of the fetal RhD blood type using a single fetal nucleated erythrocyte from maternal blood. Obstet Gynecol 1996;87:501–505.

10 Cunningham J, Yates Z, Hamlington J, Mason G, Mueller R, Miller D: Non-invasive RNA-based determination of fetal Rhesus D type: a prospective study based on 96 pregnancies. Br J Obstet Gynaecol 1999;106:1023–1028.

11 Poon LL, Lo YM: Circulating fetal DNA in maternal plasma. Clin Chim Acta 2001;313:151–155.

12 Rijnders RJ, Christiaens GC, Soussan AA, van der Schoot CE: Cell-free fetal DNA is not present in plasma of nonpregnant mothers. Clin Chem 2004;50:679–681; author reply 681.

13 Chan KC, Zhang J, Hui AB, Wong N, Lau TK, Leung TN, Lo KW, Huang DW, Lo YM: Size distributions of maternal and fetal DNA in maternal plasma. Clin Chem 2004;50:88–92.

14 Rijnders RJ, Van Der Luijt RB, Peters ED, Goeree JK, Van Der Schoot CE, Ploos Van Amstel JK, Christiaens GC: Earliest gestational age for fetal sexing in cell-free maternal plasma. Prenat Diagn 2003;23:1042–1044.

15 Rijnders RJ, Christiaens GC, Bossers B, van der Smagt JJ, van der Schoot CE, de Haas M: Clinical applications of cell-free fetal DNA from maternal plasma. Obstet Gynecol 2004;103:157–164.

16 Van der Schoot CE, Soussan AA, Koelewijn J, Bonsel G, Paget-Christiaens LG, de Haas M: Non-invasive antenatal RHD typing. Transfus Clin Biol 2006;13:53–57.

17 Colin Y, Cherif-Zahar B, Le Van Kim C, Raynal V, Van Huffel V, Cartron JP: Genetic basis of the RhD-positive and RhD-negative blood group polymorphism as determined by Southern analysis. Blood 1991;78:2747–2752.

18 Singleton BK, Green CA, Avent ND, Martin PG, Smart E, Daka A, Narter-Olaga EG, Hawthorne LM, Daniels G: The presence of an RHD pseudogene containing a 37 base pair duplication and a nonsense mutation in Africans with the RhD-negative blood group phenotype. Blood 2000;95:12–18.

19 Tax MG, van der Schoot CE, van Doorn R, Douglas-Berger L, van Rhenen DJ, Maaskant-van Wijk PA: RHC and RHc genotyping in different ethnic groups. Transfusion 2002;42:634–644.

20 Gassner C, Doescher A, Drnovsek TD, Rozman P, Eicher NI, Legler TJ, Lukin S, Garritsen H, Kleinrath T, Egger B, Ehling R, Kormoczi GF, Kilga-Nogler S, Schoenitzer D, Petershofen EK: Presence of RHD in serologically D–, C/E+ individuals: a European multicenter study. Transfusion 2005;45:527–538.

21 Bennett PR, Warwick R, Letsky E, Fisk NM: Determination of fetal RhD type by DNA amplification from fetal skin following massive fetomaternal haemorrhage and intrauterine fetal death. Br J Obstet Gynaecol 1994;101:636–637.

22 Wolter LC, Hyland CA, Saul A: Rhesus D genotyping using polymerase chain reaction. Blood 1993;82:1682–1683.

23 Minon JM, Senterre JM, Schaaps JP, Foidart JM: An unusual false-positive fetal RHD typing result using DNA derived from maternal plasma from a solid organ transplant recipient. Transfusion 2006;46:1454–1455.

24 Chan KC, Ding C, Gerovassili A, Yeung SW, Chiu RW, Leung TN, Lau TK, Chim SS, Chung GT, Nicolaides KH, Lo YM: Hypermethylated RASSF1A in maternal plasma: A universal fetal DNA marker that improves the reliability of noninvasive prenatal diagnosis. Clin Chem 2006;52:2211–2218.

25 Daniels G, Finning K, Martin P, Soothill P: Fetal blood group genotyping from DNA from maternal plasma: an important advance in the management and prevention of haemolytic disease of the fetus and newborn. Vox Sang 2004;87:225–232.

26 Clausen FB, Krog GR, Rieneck K, Nielsen LK, Lundquist R, Finning K, Dickmeiss E, Hedegaard M, Dziegiel MH: Reliable test for prenatal prediction of fetal RhD type using maternal plasma from RhD negative women. Prenat Diagn 2005;25:1040–1044.

27 van der Schoot CE, Tax GH, Rijnders RJ, de Haas M, Christiaens GC: Prenatal typing of Rh and Kell blood group system antigens: the edge of a watershed. Transfus Med Rev 2003;17:31–44.

28 Brojer E, Zupanska B, Guz K, Orzinska A, Kalinska A: Noninvasive determination of fetal RHD status by examination of cell-free DNA in maternal plasma. Transfusion 2005;45:1473–1480.

29 Finning K, Daniels G, Martin P, Soothill P: Detection of fetal Rhesus D gene in whole blood of women booking for routine antenatal care [Comment on: Eur J Obstet Gynecol Reprod Biol 2003;108:29–32]. Eur J Obstet Gynecol Reprod Biol 2003;110:117; author reply 118.

30 Faas BH, Beuling EA, Christiaens GC, von dem Borne AE, van der Schoot CE: Detection of fetal RHD-specific sequences in maternal plasma. Lancet 1998;352:1196.

31 Legler TJ, Lynen R, Maas JH, Pindur G, Kulenkampff D, Suren A, Osmers R, Kohler M: Prediction of fetal Rh D and Rh CcEe phenotype from maternal plasma with real-time polymerase chain reaction. Transfus Apher Sci 2002;27:217–223.

32 Chitty LS, van der Schoot CE, Hahn S, Avent ND: SAFE – The Special Non-invasive Advances in Fetal and Neonatal Evaluation Network: aims and achievements. Prenat Diagn 2008;28:83–88.

33 Wagner FF, Flegel WA: RHD gene deletion occurred in the Rhesus box. Blood 2000;95:3662–3668.

34 Grootkerk-Tax MG, Maaskant-van Wijk PA, van Drunen J, van der Schoot CE: The highly variable RH locus in nonwhite persons hampers RHD zygosity determination but yields more insight into RH-related evolutionary events. Transfusion 2005;45:327–337.

35 Perco P, Shao CP, Mayr WR, Panzer S, Legler TJ: Testing for the D zygosity with three different methods revealed altered Rhesus boxes and a new weak D type. Transfusion 2003;43:335–339.

36 Wagner FF, Moulds JM, Flegel WA: Genetic mechanisms of Rhesus box variation. Transfusion 2005;45:338–344.

37 Chiu RW, Murphy MF, Fidler C, Zee BC, Wainscoat JS, Lo YM: Determination of RhD zygosity: comparison of a double amplification refractory mutation system approach and a multiplex real-time quantitative PCR approach. Clin Chem 2001;47:667–672.

38 Koelewijn JM, Vrijkotte TG, van der Schoot CE, Bonsel GJ, de Haas M: Effect of screening for red cell antibodies, other than anti-D, to detect hemolytic disease of the fetus and newborn: a population study in The Netherlands. Transfusion 2008;48:941–952.

39 Dudenhausen JW, Pschyrembel W: Praktische Geburtshilfe, ed 19. Opladen, De Gruyter, 2000, pp 99–104, 422–424.

40 Contreras M, Knight RC: Controversies in transfusion medicine. Testing for Du: con. Transfusion 1991;31:270–272.

41 Bowman JM: Treatment options for the fetus with alloimmune hemolytic disease. Transfus Med Rev 1990;4:191–207.

42 Bowman JM, Pollock JM, Manning FA, Harman CR, Menticoglou S: Maternal Kell blood group alloimmunization. Obstet Gynecol 1992;79:239–244.

43 Wagner T, Resch B, Reiterer F, Gassner C, Lanzer G: Pancytopenia due to suppressed hematopoiesis in a case of fatal hemolytic disease of the newborn associated with anti-K supported by molecular K1 typing. J Pediatr Hematol Oncol 2004;26:13–15.

44 Wagner T, Bernaschek G, Geissler K: Inhibition of megakaryopoiesis by Kell-related antibodies. N Engl J Med 2000;343:72.

45 Daniels G: Human blood groups. Oxford, Blackwell, 2002.

Prof. Dr. med. Axel Seltsam
DRK-Blutspendedienst NSTOB
Institut Springe
31830 Springe, Germany
Tel. +49 5041 722-0, Fax -334
E-Mail axel. seltsam@bsd-nstob.de

Scharf RE (ed): Progress and Challenges in Transfusion Medicine, Hemostasis and Hemotherapy.
Freiburg i.Br., Karger, 2008, pp 219–233

Innate Immunity of Platelets: Specific Interactions with Viruses

Claire Flaujac[a, b, c] · Siham Boukour[c] · Elisabeth Cramer Bordé[a, b, c]

[a]Department of Hematology and Immunology, Ambroise Paré Hospital, Boulogne,
[b]Faculty of Medicine Paris-Ile de France-Ouest, University of Versailles,
[c]INSERM U567, Department of Hematology, Cochin Institute, Paris, France

Key Words

Platelets · Megakaryocytes · Viruses · HIV · DC-SIGN receptor · Transfusion

Summary

Thrombocytopenia is a frequent complication of many viral infections (hepatitis C virus, adenoviruses, lentiviruses, etc.), showing that interaction of platelets with viruses is an important pathophysiological phenomenon. Multiple mechanisms are involved depending on the nature of the infecting viruses: immunological platelet destruction, inappropriate platelet activation and consumption, or impaired megakaryopoiesis. Viruses bind platelets through various links, specific receptors and identified ligands. A review of the specific interactions of platelets with other types of viruses and of the different receptors involved in these interactions is presented. We also report on a study, performed in our laboratory, of the reciprocal effects between platelets, megakaryocytes (MKs) and human immunodeficiency virus (HIV)-1, trying to understand the consequences of such interactions. HIV-1 (and replication-deficient HIV-1, insuring optimal biosecurity) were incubated in vitro with human platelets and MKs. HIV-1 internalization was found within two distinct endocytic compartments and occurred preferentially in activated platelets: firstly, endocytic vesicles devoid of platelet secretion contained intact and potentially infectious viruses; secondly, viruses with altered structure were enclosed in the platelet surface-connected canalicular system (SCCS) in contact with platelet secretory products. Similar dual compartments were identified in MKs. Images suggesting that virus internalization by platelets also occurs in vivo were occasionally found of platelets from patients with acquired immune deficiency syndrome (AIDS) and thrombocytopenia. Finally, the pathogen receptor DC-SIGN was identified on platelets and MKs and facilitates HIV-1 internalization within platelets. In conclusion, virus particles can be specifically internalized in platelets and MKs where they can be sheltered, or get into contact with secretory products that lead to their destruction. This occurs in activated platelets (able to interact with macrophages), potentially leading to platelet clearance from the circulation and to the transfer of their viral load into target organs. Moreover, and similarly to platelets, MKs are also potentially colonized by intact infectious viruses, and the relationship between this observation and the occurrence of thrombocytopenia needs to be further examined. Finally, the understanding of the close platelet interaction with viruses emphasizes the importance of pursuing research on pathogen inactivation in platelet concentrates.
©2008 S. Karger GmbH, Freiburg i.Br.

Introduction

The relationship between platelets and infection is well established and thrombocytopenia is a frequent complication during or after bacterial and viral infection. Its responsible mechanism appears to be diverse: increased platelet destruction, due either to the non-specific deposition of immune complexes on platelets or to the presence of specific platelet autoantibodies, and decreased platelet production from megakaryocytes (MKs). In addition, several studies have evidenced direct interactions between platelets, MKs and pathogens: It has been known for a long time that platelets are able to interact with and internalize foreign particles, for example, inert particles like latex beads [1, 2]. However, this was interpreted as passive passage of the particles through the platelet surface-connected canalicular system (SCCS). Some work recently performed in our laboratory using bacteria and viruses, respectively *Staphylococcus aureus* and human immunodeficiency virus (HIV) [3], completed earlier studies [4, 5] showing that platelets were able to interact directly with these microorganisms by engulfing them into specific compartments. Activation and secretory processes by platelets follow engulfment. Alternatively, subcellular compartments were identified where infectious particles were sheltered from platelet attack and secretion. Subsequently, a specific receptor was identified that is able to modulate HIV entry into platelets [6]. Other receptors involved in the interaction of viruses of various types with platelets are reviewed in this chapter. The existence of a direct interaction between platelets and viral particles suggests a role for platelets during infection: either in the protection and defense of the human host against infectious microorganisms or, in contrast, as infection-disseminating agents. Indeed, after injury or disruption of the endothelial surface, one of the first cellular actors to be present in the wound opening is platelets. Therefore platelets very early get into contact with all kinds of foreign invaders, and if specific binding occurs, they may subsequently transport their infectious load, circulating in the body and interacting with other blood and vascular components.

Platelets and Pathogens

It is conceivable that, when platelets interact directly with infectious particles, this event is partly responsible for the thrombocytopenia observed during infection. Several studies performed in vitro on the interaction of platelets with various bacteria showed mutual involvement. Studies performed with *Staphylococcus aureus* indicated that the bacteria are internalized by platelets and induce the platelet release reaction [3]; *Shigella* sp. and *Escherichia coli* endotoxin binds the Toll like receptor 4 expressed by platelets and induces platelet activation, *Streptococci sanguis* induces platelet aggregation, yersiniae get internalized into platelets, borreliae bind and activate platelets in vitro, and interaction with *Helicobacter pylori* is responsible for immune thrombocytopenic purpura.

Flaujac/Boukour/Cramer Bordé

Platelets contain microbicidal substances: Previous studies showed the existence of a bactericidal peptide (platelet microbicidal peptide (PMP)) in the rabbit platelet granules [7] and two components similar to the PMP called thrombocidin in the α-granules of human platelets [8]. α-Granules are the storage place of many chemokines such as neutrophil-activating peptide-2 (NAP2), platelet factor 4, platelet-derived growth factor (PDGF), transforming growth factor β (TGFβ), β-thromboglobulin, and macrophage inflammatory protein-1α (MIP-1α) [9]. These molecules allow the interaction of platelets with other cells, in particular those cells of the immune system that allow acceleration of immunizing responses. Platelets are a significant source of the chemokine RANTES (regulated upon activation normal T cell expressed and secreted) [9–11] which blocks viral infection by its capacity to compete with viral particles by binding their receptors [12, 13]. The virus degradation that we observed within platelets (see below) can be explained by the action of the α-granule content of microbicidal peptides. In another approach, Maurice et al. recently showed a virucidal effect of platelet concentrates in vitro [14]. Three different types of viruses, adenovirus 5, poliovirus 1 and vaccinia virus, were brought into contact with platelet concentrates and the viral titers were significantly decreased [14].

Platelets and HIV

In vitro experiments were performed in our laboratory in order to elucidate the potential interaction of platelets with HIV.

First, the supernatants of peripheral blood monocytic cell (PBMC) cultures were examined by electron microscopy (EM) and immuno-EM to precisely identify the ultrastructure of HIV particles. These were easily identified thanks to their size, regular shape, visible envelope and often eccentric dense core (fig. 1a). Immunogold labeling for the viral core protein p24 confirmed that these little structures were indeed HIV virions (fig 1b).

The ultrastructural examination of platelets incubated for 30 min with the supernatant of a PBMC culture demonstrated that HIVs were internalized by platelets (fig. 2). They were entirely internalized, keeping their ultrastructural integrity, including their envelope; no image of fusion with the platelet plasma membrane could be obtained during this short lapse of time. Immunolabeling for p24 protein confirmed that the internalized particles were indeed HIVs (fig. 3). HIVs were observed in small endocytic vesicles located near the plasma membrane. These images were quite characteristic: viral particles, either isolated or grouped up to four, were tightly enclosed in small vacuoles distinct from the SCCS in that they were frequently located at the platelet periphery and that their content appeared clear, devoid of other content except the viral particles (namely no cellular debris as observed in the PBMC supernatants), indicating a selective uptake of the virions. In addition, several viruses could also be seen in the lumen of the SCCS. At high magnification, lentiviruses located within endocytic vesicles appeared intact, displaying a spherical shape and a well-limited envelope. When located in the SCCS, viral particles appeared swollen and poorly limited, with irregular shape.

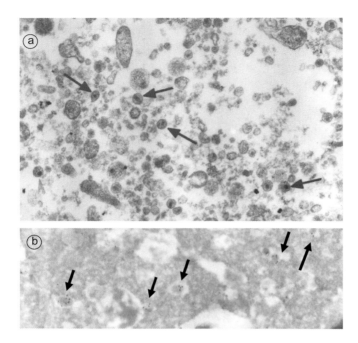

Fig. 1. PBMC supernatant examined by EM (a) and immuno-EM after p24 immunogold labeling (b): HIV particles are indicated by arrows.

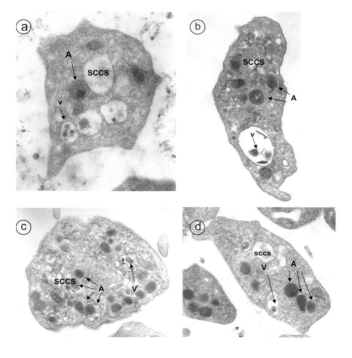

Fig. 2. Platelet incubated with viral suspensions of either modified lentiviruses HIV-e (a) or HIV (b–d): (a) Several well-preserved lentiviruses (v) identified by their size and dense core are observed in a small endocytic vesicle (EV) located near the plasma membrane (PM). The presence of pseudopods (P) indicates that the platelet is activated (m = mitochondria, A = α-granules) (b–d). In the endocytic vesicles, HIVs (v) are intact, displaying spherical shape and well-limited envelopes.

Flaujac/Boukour/Cramer Bordé

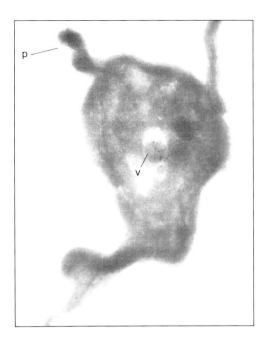

Fig. 3. Platelets incubated with the HIV suspension, immunolabeled for p24 (protein of the viral core): A viral particle (v) has been internalized within a platelet and can be identified thanks to its specific p24 immunolabeling.

Double immunolabeling for p24 protein (protein of the viral core) and fibrinogen (marker of platelet secretion) demonstrated that the intact HIVs enclosed in the endocytic vesicles were sheltered from platelet secretory products whereas, when located in the SCCS, they were in contact with platelet secretion products [6].

We can conclude that:
(1) platelets are able to endocytose HIV virions;
(2) HIVs can be enclosed within platelets, sheltered from host immune system aggression and transported by circulating platelets within the entire human body;
(3) platelets are able to secrete α-granule content and lead to virus destruction.

Moreover, virus/platelet interaction exerts a biological effect on platelets. Indeed, platelets having endocytosed lentiviruses are activated and express P-selectin, the receptor for macrophages, on their membrane. Therefore, they may be cleared from the circulation by macrophages with which they could interact to help HIV killing. Thrombocytopenia complicating HIV infection could in part be the result of this defense mechanism.

DC-SIGN

MKs express the CD4 receptor for HIV [15–17] as well as the co-receptors CXCR1.2.4 and CCR3 [18–20]. Platelets do not express CD4 but only bear the co-receptors

CXCR1.2.4 and CCR3 [18–20]; these are devoted to virus fusion with the plasma membrane and subsequent delivery of the virus genetic material into the host cell.

An alternative receptor-mediated pathway of HIV penetration within host cells was recently described in dendritic cells: DC-SIGN (dendritic cell-specific ICAM-grabbing non-integrin) is a C-type (Ca2+-dependent) lectinic receptor that selectively recognizes high-mannose oligosaccharides [21]. DC-SIGN is expressed on dendritic cells, including those derived from blood monocytes or found in lymphoid tissues and beneath mucosal surfaces [22]. DC-SIGN-expressing cells internalize HIV-1 virions into a trypsin-resistant compartment, and viral infectivity can be retained for several days before transmission to T cells [23, 24]. In downstream DC-SIGN-mediated internalization within dendritic cells, most of the virions are degraded in an acidic compartment [25]. This is a pathogen receptor initially described in dendritic cells. Viral particles are internalized in the endocytic vesicles via DC-SIGN in dendritic cells. After internalization, most of the virions are degraded in an acidic compartment, but some virions escape lysosomal degradation. They are transmitted to permissive CD4+ lymphocytes, whereas another part will gain access to the dendritic cell cytoplasm. Cytosolic viral material may be the source of low levels of productive infection of dendritic cells. The proteasome also degrades cytosolic virions, leading to the MHC class I-restricted presentation of viral epitopes [25]. DC-SIGN binding to intercellular adhesion molecule-3 (ICAM-3) plays an important role in establishing the first contact between dendritic cells and resting T cells [26].

The question could then be raised whether lentivirus particle internalization is a specific function of platelets and MKs. The trafficking of viruses within endocytic vesicles resembles the phenomenon of macropinocytosis described in dendritic cells and mediated by the receptor DC-SIGN. Like in dendritic cells, an intracellular trafficking pathway leading either to lentivirus homing or to lentivirus inactivation was identified in platelets and MKs. The presence and the functionality of the pathogen receptor DC-SIGN was demonstrated on platelets and MKs by various technical approaches.

For this purpose, we used highly sensitive and specific techniques such as flow cytometry, immuno-EM, Western blotting and reverse transcription-polymerase chain reaction (RT-PCR) to show the presence of DC-SIGN in platelets. Flow cytometry revealed that 15% of platelets are DC-SIGN positive, and this proportion is considerable since it is equivalent to the one encountered in dendritic cells. DC-SIGN immunolabeling showed that the protein is mainly localized on the platelet surface (fig. 4). Western blotting revealed and confirmed the presence of DC-SIGN protein in platelets.

Platelets have the capacity to endocytose and store plasma proteins such as fibrinogen [27]. Thus, to rule out the hypothesis that DC-SIGN could be adsorbed on the platelet surface, we studied their precursors, MKs. MKs were obtained from cultured cord blood precursors and cultures were performed without plasma or serum. Under these technical conditions, cultured MKs were found to express DC-SIGN by Western blotting. In addition, MKs were shown to be able to synthesize DC-SIGN since its

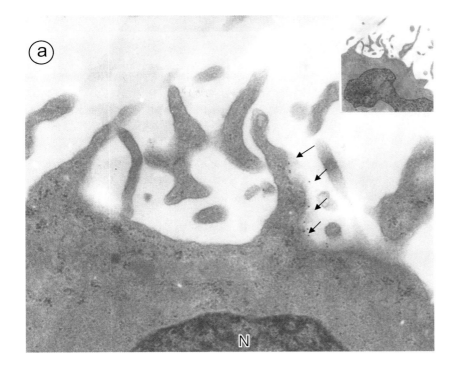

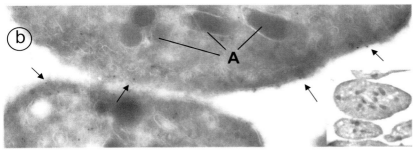

Fig. 4. Dendritic cells and human platelets immunolabeled for DC-SIGN: (a) Gold labeling can be seen on the pseudopod of a dendritic cell (arrows) (N = nucleus) and (b) along the plasma membrane of platelets (arrows) (A = α-granule).

RNA was revealed by RT-PCR. This finding confirmed that the DC-SIGN expression observed on platelets and MKs was specific, since it is the consequence of endogenous synthesis.

To show whether the receptor DC-SIGN is functional in platelets, blocking experiments were performed with specific antibodies. Platelets were brought into contact with the monoclonal anti-DC-SIGN antibody 1B10; then they were incubated with lentivirus suspension. Semi-quantitative estimation of the effect of anti-DC-SIGN antibody on virus internalization was performed: EM examination showed that control platelets consistently internalized HIV-e virions (with HIV envelope), whereas in the

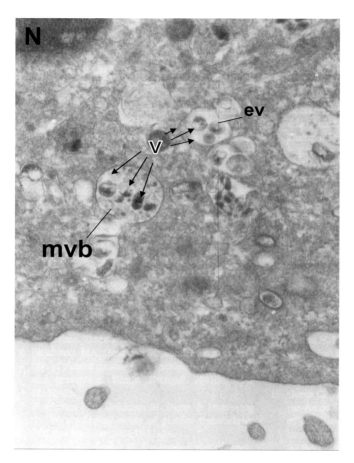

Fig. 5. MKs incubated with lentivirus (HIV-e) suspension: Numerous viruses (v) have been entirely internalized within MKs and are located in small endocytic vesicles (ev) and in multivesicular bodies (mvb). In the endocytic vesicles (ev), the viruses are intact, displaying spherical shape and a well-limited envelope. When located in multivesicular bodies (mvb), the lentiviruses appear swollen and poorly limited, with irregular shape.

presence of anti-DC SIGN antibody virtually no viral internalization was detected but numerous viral particles were found in the extracellular medium.

These findings demonstrated that the DC-SIGN receptor is functional in platelets where it modulates HIV endocytosis.

Finally, platelets also express the C-type lectin-like receptor 2 (CLEC-2), and a combination of DC-SIGN and CLEC-2 inhibitors strongly reduced HIV-1 association with platelets, indicating that these lectins are required for efficient HIV-1 binding to platelets [28].

Modified Lentiviruses

With the experimental model based on the use of intact and live HIV for laboratory purposes being hazardous, in order to continue this study, we have developed an experimental model that confers safety to the experimentator. An experimental model was set up, using non-replicative, genetically modified lentiviruses bearing either the HIV envelope (HIV-e) or vesicular stomatitis virus (VSV) with protein G envelope (VSV-e). Indeed, since the goal of this study was to precisely examine the uptake mechanisms of viral particles, the use of non-replicative lentiviruses was not an obstacle.

Vectors derived from lentiviruses by deletion of the viral coding sequences and of the transcription regulatory sequences of the 3' long terminal repeat (LTR) [29] were used in our study. These two major modifications rendered them replication defective.

We have shown that platelets and Mks are able to internalize the recombinant lentiviruses in the same manner as they internalize HIV, without fusion of their envelope with the cell plasma membrane, since many internalized virus particles displayed a well-preserved envelope (fig. 5).

The ultrastructural examination of platelets incubated with the lentiviral suspension demonstrated that both strains of lentiviruses, HIV and HIV-e, were internalized by platelets (fig. 2c). They were entirely internalized, keeping their ultrastructural integrity, including their envelope; showing endocytosis and not fusion. The primary steps of HIV internalization occur within small endocytic vesicles located near the plasma membrane [3], and modified lentiviruses observed in this compartment indeed exhibited a well-preserved envelope. We concluded that the use of lentiviruses with HIV envelope was a good model for studying platelet interaction with HIV since the capture step is the most important one, with no fusion occurring in these non-nucleated and MK cells.

Platelet Interaction with Other Viruses

Increasing evidence indicates that many viruses can interact with platelets. Indirect binding through to the receptor FcγR2A (CD32) which can bind virus-IgG complexes is commonly admitted. But numerous platelet receptors, such as integrins, have also been implicated in viral particle binding and in cell-pathogen interactions.

Rotavirus contains two outer capsid viral proteins, VP4 (spike protein) and VP7 (major capsid component), both of which are implicated in cell entry. Rotavirus VP4-mediated cell entry involves the α2β1 integrin, whereas VP7 appears to interact with αxβ2 and α4β1 integrins [30, 31]. Since α2β1 is expressed on platelets, one may speculate that rotaviruses interact with platelets.

Adenovirus internalization requires the presence of cell surface integrins that can bind ligands with an arginine-glycine-aspartic acid (RGD) sequence [32] such as the receptor of fibrinogen, α2bβ3, expressed on platelets. The RGD sequence is found in the adenovirus penton base. Other integrins like αvβ3 or αvβ5 may interact with adenoviruses. But despite this interaction, adenoviral vectors (at a wide range of concentrations) do not induce, inhibit or potentiate human platelet aggregation [33]. In contrast, a recent study shows that in a mouse model, after intravenous administration of recombinant adenovirus serotype 5 (usually used as vectors for gene therapy), the viruses rapidly bind to circulating platelets, which causes their activation/aggregation and subsequent entrapment in liver sinusoids and degradation by Kupffer cells [34]. Recently, a specific virus receptor, coxsackie-adenovirus receptor (CAR), has been identified on platelets [35]. Thrombocytopenia following administration of adenoviral gene transfer vectors could originate from platelet activation and accelerated platelet clearance by activation of CAR and/or integrin binding.

Finally, hantaviruses also bind β3 integrins [36], and this binding is likely to be fundamental for virus pathogenesis since β3 integrins are critical adhesive receptors on platelets and endothelial cells [37].

Human platelets also express on their surface the complement (C3d) receptor type II (CR2) [38], which is also a receptor for Epstein Barr virus (EBV). A monoclonal antibody against CR2 (OKB7) blocks the binding of EBV and also inhibits EBV-mediated release of TGFβ [39]. One of the main collagen receptors, glycoprotein VI (GPVI), has been proposed to play a role in viral transport and/or persistence, as hepatitis C virus (HCV) can bind GPVI [40]. Platelets could be a potential transporter of infectious virions to the liver [40].

Megakaryocytes and Viruses

Virus interactions with platelets and MKs have been described for a long time and numerous viruses have been implicated, such as paramyxovirus (Newcastle disease virus) [41], retroviruses (e.g. HIV-1) [5, 6] and herpes viruses (e.g. cytomegalovirus (CMV), human herpesvirus (HHV)-6, HHV-7) [42–44].

HIV

MKs express two HIV receptors: CD4 [15–17] and DC-SIGN. This suggests the existence of two different ways of penetration of viruses in MKs, like in dendritic cells. In dendritic cells, CD4 causes fusion of the viral membrane with the host cell membrane as the mechanism of cell infection, and DC-SIGN causes internalization of lentiviruses in the endocytic vesicles, without fusion of their envelope with the host cell plasma membrane. In MKs, lentiviruses were internalized via endocytic vesicles (fig. 5). In this compartment, lentiviruses appeared intact. Then they accumulated in multivesicular bodies (MVB), where the chemical conditions are poorly compatible with their survival. Indeed, MVB belong to the endosomal system [45–47], and they are considered as late endosomes [48, 49]. In this compartment, the pH is acidic [50] and the detection of acid phosphatase is constantly positive at their level.

Differences in membrane antigen expression between mature MKs and platelets have been highlighted. For example, immature human MKs express the CD4 antigen on their surface, capable of binding HIV-1, but this antigen is not expressed on fully mature MKs and platelets. CD4 expression occurs during hematopoietic differentiation and is an early step in MK maturation [51]. Using this receptor, HIV-1 can infect cells from the MK lineage [15]. In addition, as already mentioned, MKs express the HIV co-receptors CXCR1.2.4 and CCR3 [18–20]. The link between viral particles and MKs is obvious but one can speculate that this binding does not induce particular modification in MKs and/or there is a passive passage of the viral particles through the demarcation membrane. When platelets are incubated with the supernatant of a PBMC culture from HIV-infected patients, HIV is able to penetrate MKs via the demarcation membrane system [5] and HIV mRNA can be detected within MKs. For example, in purified marrow, MKs from HIV-seropositive patients with immune thrombocytopenic purpura, viral transcripts and small amounts of HIV glycoproteins were detected, although heterogeneity among the MKs was observed [52]. Indeed, an in vitro study showed that human MKs are able to internalize the entire HIV particles within endocytic vacuoles and HIV viruses also accumulate in MVB, where they are exposed to the acid phosphatase leading to their destruction [6].

Other Viruses

Nevertheless, viral replication in MKs has been demonstrated for several viruses other than HIV-1 [53–55], HCV [56] and human CMV (HCMV) [42]. These results demonstrate that MKs are susceptible to viral infection and that direct infection of these cells in vivo may contribute to the thrombocytopenia observed in infected patients and/or to virus dissemination.

Moreover, in allogeneic bone marrow transplantation, HCMV is frequently associated with graft failure: This could be due to a direct suppressive effect on thrombopoiesis [42]. Down-regulation of hematopoiesis is probably a protective mechanism of the microenvironment that limits injury to the marrow stem/progenitor cell compartment during the subsequent process of elimination of infected cells, as it has been suggested in dengue virus infection [57]. A study found that HHV-6 viral load was significantly correlated with delayed platelet engraftment and to the number of platelet transfusions required in allogeneic stem cell transplantation [58]. The replication of numerous viruses has been speculated to play a role in delayed engraftment after stem cell transplantation. Some in vitro studies have shown that HHV-6 but not HHV-7 is one of the major causes of thrombopoiesis suppression by a direct effect of HHV-6 on hematopoietic progenitors [43], whereas another in vitro study suggests that HHV-7 impairs the survival/differentiation of megakaryocytic cells [44].

Platelet Transfusion and Viruses

Transfusion of platelet concentrates has been implicated in the transmission of numerous microorganisms. Substantial improvement in the safety of platelet transfusion has been achieved in the last few years [59, 60]. With a combination of serologic determination and nucleic acid testing (NAT) in small pools of samples, the residual risk of contamination with selected viruses has decreased to less than 1:2,000,000 for HIV-1 and HIV-2 and human T lymphotropic virus (HTLV), less than 1:1,000,000 for HCV and less than 1:200,000 for hepatitis B virus (HBV) [61]. Pathogen inactivation with photochemical treatment (as psoralen and derivatives) in platelet concentrates as in other blood products is an innovative approach to blood safety. This approach is clearly important as the interactions between viruses and platelets are not completely understood (surface binding, internalization, etc.). Photochemical treatment could eliminate viruses that are not screened by serologic determination or NAT and emerging viruses whose link with platelets is obviously not yet known.

Conclusions and Future Directions

Platelets have the privilege to circulate within the entire human body where they exert their main role of protection against bleeding. In addition, they are equipped with numerous receptors and proteins that are able to interfere with the inflammatory response. This gives to platelets a major role in non-specific immunity. In the present chapter, we have reviewed the various pathways that platelets use in order to interact with viruses. This interaction is specific, mediated by well-defined functional receptors and leads to mutual alterations of both the platelet host and the viral aggressor. More work needs to be performed to precisely identify the platelet role in viral infections: beneficial and protective or maleficent and pro-infectious. The response might be different depending on the nature of the viral particle involved.

Disclosure of Conflict of Interests

The authors state that they have no conflict of interests.

Acknowledgements

The authors gratefully acknowledge Dr. Tayebeh Youssefian for her collaboration on the HIV study.

References

1 White JG, Clawson CC: Effects of large latex particle uptake of the surface connected canalicular system of blood platelets: a freeze-fracture and cytochemical study. Ultrastruct Pathol 1981;2:277–287.

2 White JG, Clawson CC: Effects of small latex particle uptake on the surface connected canalicular system of blood platelets: a freeze-fracture and cytochemical study. Diagn Histopathol 1982;5:3–10.

3 Youssefian T, Drouin A, Masse JM, Guichard J, Cramer EM: Host defense role of platelets: engulfment of HIV and *Staphylococcus aureus* occurs in a specific subcellular compartment and is enhanced by platelet activation. Blood 2002;99:4021–4029.

4 Zucker-Franklin D: The effect of viral infections on platelets and megakaryocytes. Semin Hematol 1994;31:329–337.

5 Zucker-Franklin D, Seremetis S, Zheng ZY: Internalization of human immunodeficiency virus type I and other retroviruses by megakaryocytes and platelets. Blood 1990;75:1920–1923.

6 Boukour S, Masse JM, Benit L, Dubart-Kupperschmitt A, Cramer EM: Lentivirus degradation and DC-SIGN expression by human platelets and megakaryocytes. J Thromb Haemost 2006;4:426–435.

7 Koo SP, Bayer AS, Sahl HG, Proctor RA, Yeaman MR: Staphylocidal action of thrombin-induced platelet microbicidal protein is not solely dependent on transmembrane potential. Infect Immun 1996;64:1070–1074.

8 Krijgsveld J, Zaat SA, Meeldijk J, van Veelen PA, Fang G, Poolman B, Brandt E, Ehlert JE, Kuijpers AJ, Engbers GH, Feijen J, Dankert J: Thrombocidins, microbicidal proteins from human blood platelets, are C-terminal deletion products of CXC chemokines. J Biol Chem 2000;275:20374–20381.

9 Klinger MH, Wilhelm D, Bubel S, Sticherling M, Schroder JM, Kuhnel W: Immunocytochemical localization of the chemokines RANTES and MIP-1 alpha within human platelets and their release during storage. Int Arch Allergy Immunol 1995;107:541–546.

10 Kameyoshi Y, Dorschner A, Mallet AI, Christophers E, Schroder JM: Cytokine RANTES released by thrombin-stimulated platelets is a potent attractant for human eosinophils. J Exp Med 1992;176:587–592.

11 Bubel S, Wilhelm D, Entelmann M, Kirchner H, Kluter H: Chemokines in stored platelet concentrates. Transfusion 1996;36:445–449.

12 Ferbas J, Giorgi JV, Amini S, Grovit-Ferbas K, Wiley DJ, Detels R, Plaeger S: Antigen-specific production of RANTES, macrophage inflammatory protein (MIP)-1alpha, and MIP-1beta in vitro is a correlate of reduced human immunodeficiency virus burden in vivo. J Infect Dis 2000;182:1247–1250.

13 Stantchev TS, Broder CC: Consistent and significant inhibition of human immunodeficiency virus type 1 envelope-mediated membrane fusion by beta-chemokines (RANTES) in primary human macrophages. J Infect Dis 2000;182:68–78.

14 Maurice A, Marchand-Arvier M, Edert D, Le Faou A, Gondrexon G, Vigneron C: The virucidal effect of platelet concentrates: preliminary study and first conclusions. Platelets 2002;13:219–222.

15 Kouri YH, Borkowsky W, Nardi M, Karpatkin S, Basch RS: Human megakaryocytes have a CD4 molecule capable of binding human immunodeficiency virus-1. Blood 1993;81:2664–2670.

16 Basch RS, Kouri YH, Karpatkin S: Expression of CD4 by human megakaryocytes. Proc Natl Acad Sci U S A 1990;87:8085–8089.

17 Gewirtz AM, Boghosian-Sell L, Catani L, Ratajczak MZ, Shen YM, Schreiber AD: Expression of Fc gamma RII and CD4 receptors by normal human megakaryocytes. Exp Hematol 1992;20:512–516.

18 Kowalska MA, Ratajczak J, Hoxie J, Brass LF, Gewirtz A, Poncz M, Ratajczak MZ: Megakaryocyte precursors, megakaryocytes and platelets express the HIV co-receptor CXCR4 on their surface: determination of response to stromal-derived factor-1 by megakaryocytes and platelets. Br J Haematol 1999;104:220–229.

19 Riviere C, Subra F, Cohen-Solal K, Cordette-Lagarde V, Letestu R, Auclair C, Vainchenker W, Louache F: Phenotypic and functional evidence for the expression of CXCR4 receptor during megakaryocytopoiesis. Blood 1999;93:1511–1523.

20 Lee B, Ratajczak J, Doms RW, Gewirtz AM, Ratajczak MZ: Coreceptor/chemokine receptor expression on human hematopoietic cells: biological implications for human immunodeficiency virus-type 1 infection. Blood 1999;93:1145–1156.

21 Feinberg H, Mitchell DA, Drickamer K, Weis WI: Structural basis for selective recognition of oligosaccharides by DC-SIGN and DC-SIGNR. Science 2001;294:2163–2166.

22 Jameson B, Baribaud F, Pohlmann S, Ghavimi D, Mortari F, Doms RW, Iwasaki A: Expression of DC-SIGN by dendritic cells of intestinal and genital mucosae in humans and rhesus macaques. J Virol 2002;76:1866–1875.

23 Geijtenbeek TB, Kwon DS, Torensma R, van Vliet SJ, van Duijnhoven GC, Middel J, Cornelissen IL, Nottet HS, Kewal-Ramani VN, Littman DR, Figdor CG, van Kooyk Y: DC-SIGN, a dendritic cell-specific HIV-1-binding protein that enhances trans-infection of T cells. Cell 2000;100:587–597.

24 Kwon DS, Gregorio G, Bitton N, Hendrickson WA, Littman DR: DC-SIGN-mediated internalization of HIV is required for trans-enhancement of T cell infection. Immunity 2002;16:135–144.

25 Moris A, Nobile C, Buseyne F, Porrot F, Abastado JP, Schwartz O: DC-SIGN promotes exogenous MHC-I-restricted HIV-1 antigen presentation. Blood 2004;103:2648–2654.

26 Geijtenbeek TB, Torensma R, van Vliet SJ, van Duijnhoven GC, Adema GJ, van Kooyk Y, Figdor CG: Identification of DC-SIGN, a novel dendritic cell-specific ICAM-3 receptor that supports primary immune responses. Cell 2000;100:575–585.

27 Cramer EM, Vainchenker W, Vinci G, Guichard J, Breton-Gorius J: Gray platelet syndrome: immuno-electron microscopic localization of fibrinogen and von Willebrand factor in platelets and megakaryocytes. Blood 1985;66:1309–1316.

28 Chaipan C, Soilleux EJ, Simpson P, Hofmann H, Gramberg T, Marzi A, Geier M, Stewart EA, Eisemann J, Steinkasserer A, Suzuki-Inoue K, Fuller GL, Pearce AC, Watson SP, Hoxie JA, Baribaud F, Pöhlmann S: DC-SIGN and CLEC-2 mediate human immunodeficiency virus type 1 capture by platelets. J Virol 2006;80:8951–8960.

29 Kung SK, An DS, Chen IS: A murine leukemia virus (MuLV) long terminal repeat derived from rhesus macaques in the context of a lentivirus vector and MuLV gag sequence results in high-level gene expression in human T lymphocytes. J Virol 2000;74:3668–36681.

30 Coulson BS, Londrigan SL, Lee DJ: Rotavirus contains integrin ligand sequences and a disintegrin-like domain that are implicated in virus entry into cells. Proc Natl Acad Sci U S A 1997;94:5389–5394.

31 Fleming FE, Graham KL, Taniguchi K, Takada Y, Coulson BS: Rotavirus-neutralizing antibodies inhibit virus binding to integrins alpha 2 beta 1 and alpha 4 beta 1. Arch Virol 2007;152:1087–1101.

32 Zhang Y, Bergelson JM: Adenovirus receptors. J Virol 2005;79:12125–12131.

33 Eggerman TL, Mondoro TH, Lozier JN, Vostal JG: Adenoviral vectors do not induce, inhibit, or potentiate human platelet aggregation. Hum Gene Ther 2002;13:125–128.

34 Stone D, Liu Y, Shayakhmetov D, Li ZY, Ni S, Lieber A: Adenovirus-platelet interaction in blood causes virus sequestration to the reticuloendothelial system of the liver. J Virol 2007;81:4866–4871.

35 Othman M, Labelle A, Mazzetti I, Elbatarny HS, Lillicrap D: Adenovirus-induced thrombocytopenia: the role of von Willebrand factor and P-selectin in mediating accelerated platelet clearance. Blood 2007;109:2832–2839.

36 Gavrilovskaya IN, Shepley M, Shaw R, Ginsberg MH, Mackow ER: Beta3 integrins mediate the cellular entry of hantaviruses that cause respiratory failure. Proc Natl Acad Sci U S A 1998;95:7074–7079.

37 Mackow ER, Gavrilovskaya IN: Cellular receptors and hantavirus pathogenesis. Curr Top Microbiol Immunol 2001;256:91–115.

38 Nunez D, Charriaut-Marlangue C, Barel M, Benveniste J, Frade R: Activation of human platelets through gp140, the C3d/EBV receptor (CR2). Eur J Immunol 1987;17:515–520.

39 Ahmad A, Menezes J: Binding of the Epstein-Barr virus to human platelets causes the release of transforming growth factor-beta. J Immunol 1997;159:3984–3988.

40 Zahn A, Jennings N, Ouwehand WH, Allain JP: Hepatitis C virus interacts with human platelet glycoprotein VI. J Gen Virol 2006;87(Pt 8):2243–2251.

41 Jerushalmy Z, Kaminski E, Kohn A, Devries A: Interaction of Newcastle disease virus with megakaryocytes in cell cultures of guinea pig bone marrow. Proc Soc Exp Biol Med 1963;114:687–690.

42 Crapnell K, Zanjani ED, Chaudhuri A, Ascensao JL, St Jeor S, Maciejewski JP: In vitro infection of megakaryocytes and their precursors by human cytomegalovirus. Blood 2000;95:487–493.

43 Isomura H, Yoshida M, Namba H, Fujiwara N, Ohuchi R, Uno F, Oda M, Seino Y, Yamada M: Suppressive effects of human herpesvirus-6 on thrombopoietin-inducible megakaryocytic colony formation in vitro. J Gen Virol 2000;81(Pt 3):663–673.

44 Gonelli A, Mirandola P, Grill V, Secchiero P, Zauli G: Human herpesvirus 7 infection impairs the survival/differentiation of megakaryocytic cells. Haematologica 2002;87:1223–1225.

45 Geuze HJ: The role of endosomes and lysosomes in MHC class II functioning. Immunol Today 1998;19:282–287.

46 Mellman I: Endocytosis and molecular sorting. Annu Rev Cell Dev Biol 1996;12:575–625.

47 Lindwasser OW, Resh MD: Human immunodeficiency virus type 1 gag contains a dileucine-like motif that regulates association with multivesicular bodies. J Virol 2004;78:6013–6023.

48 Mukherjee S, Ghosh RN, Maxfield FR: Endocytosis. Physiol Rev 1997;77:759–803.

49 Gruenberg J, Maxfield FR: Membrane transport in the endocytic pathway. Curr Opin Cell Biol 1995;7:552–563.

50 Kaiser J, Stockert RJ, Wolkoff AW: Effect of monensin on receptor recycling during continuous endocytosis of asialoorosomucoid. Exp Cell Res 1988;174:472–480.

51 Basch RS, Dolzhanskiy A, Zhang XM, Karpatkin S: The development of human megakaryocytes. II. CD4 expression occurs during haemopoietic differentiation and is an early step in megakaryocyte maturation. Br J Haematol 1996;94:433–442.

52 Louache F, Bettaieb A, Henri A, Oksenhendler E, Farcet JP, Bierling P, Seligmann M, Vainchenker W: Infection of megakaryocytes by human immunodeficiency virus in seropositive patients with immune thrombocytopenic purpura. Blood 1991;78:1697–1705.

53 Sakaguchi M, Sato T, Groopman JE: Human immunodeficiency virus infection of megakaryocytic cells. Blood 1991;77:481–485.

54 Monte D, Groux H, Raharinivo B, Plouvier B, Dewulf J, Clavel T, Grangette C, Torpier G, Auriault C, Capron A: Productive human immunodeficiency virus-1 infection of megakaryocytic cells is enhanced by tumor necrosis factor-alpha. Blood 1992;79:2670–2679.

55 Chelucci C, Federico M, Guerriero R, Mattia G, Casella I, Pelosi E, Testa U, Mariani G, Hassan HJ, Peschle C: Productive human immunodeficiency virus-1 infection of purified megakaryocytic progenitors/precursors and maturing megakaryocytes. Blood 1998;91:1225–1234.

56 Li X, Jeffers LJ, Garon C, Fischer ER, Scheffel J, Moore B, Reddy KR, Demedina M, Schiff ER: Persistence of hepatitis C virus in a human megakaryoblastic leukaemia cell line. J Viral Hepat 1999;6:107–114.

57 La Russa VF, Innis BL: Mechanisms of dengue virus-induced bone marrow suppression. Baillieres Clin Haematol 1995;8:249–270.

58 Ljungman P, Wang FZ, Clark DA, Emery VC, Remberger M, Ringdén O, Linde A: High levels of human herpesvirus 6 DNA in peripheral blood leucocytes are correlated to platelet engraftment and disease in allogeneic stem cell transplant patients. Br J Haematol 2000;111:774–781.

59 Pelletier JP, Transue S, Snyder EL: Pathogen inactivation techniques. Best Pract Res Clin Haematol 2006;19:205–242.

60 Bryant BJ, Klein HG: Pathogen inactivation: the definitive safeguard for the blood supply. Arch Pathol Lab Med 2007;131:719–733.

61 Dodd RY, Notari EP 4th, Stramer SL: Current prevalence and incidence of infectious disease markers and estimated window-period risk in the American Red Cross blood donor population. Transfusion 2002;42:975–979.

Prof. Elisabeth Cramer Bordé, M.D., Ph.D.
Service d'Hématologie et d'Immunologie
Hôpital Ambroise Paré
92100 Boulogne, France
Tel. +33 1 49 09 54-12, Fax -15
E-Mail elisabeth.borde@apr.aphp.fr

Scharf RE (ed): Progress and Challenges in Transfusion Medicine, Hemostasis and Hemotherapy.
Freiburg i.Br., Karger, 2008, pp 234–247

Bacterial Contamination of Platelet Components: Prevalence and Measures to Prevent Transfusion-Transmitted Bacterial Infection

Laurence Corash

Medical Affairs, Cerus Corporation, Concord, CA,
Department of Laboratory Medicine, University of California, San Francisco, CA, USA

Key Words

Bacteria · Transfusion-transmitted sepsis · Platelet components · Pathogen inactivation/reduction

Summary

Bacterial contamination of platelet components represents the most prevalent transfusion-transmitted infectious risk, with the exception of viral epidemics. Transfusion services have grappled with this problem for more than 50 years. It is only within the last 2 decades that the magnitude of the risk and the clinical outcomes associated with bacterial contamination of platelet components have been fully appreciated. With increased appreciation of the risk of bacteria contamination, methods have been developed to limit or potentially eliminate this risk. Among the most important methods to mitigate the risk of bacteria contamination are improved skin disinfection, initial blood draw diversion, bacteria detection, and pathogen inactivation/reduction. These technologies have been, or are now, undergoing increased use in the clinical practice of transfusion medicine. The full impact of each of these interventions has yet to be realized, but the most recent – pathogen inactivation – may herald a major step forward in the prevention of transfusion-transmitted bacterial sepsis.   ©2008 S. Karger GmbH, Freiburg i.Br.

Introduction

Contamination of platelet components with bacteria is a well-recognized risk factor for transfusion-transmitted infection [1]. Among the labile blood components, platelet components exhibit the highest prevalence of bacterial contamination due to storage at 22–24°C, a condition that facilitates bacterial proliferation [2]. More than 2 decades ago, persistent reports of platelet transfusion-associated bacterial sepsis led to widespread reduction in the storage duration for platelet components, from 7 to

5 days, in an effort to limit the extent of bacterial proliferation and to reduce the incidence of transfusion-transmitted sepsis [3]. However, the impact of a reduction in storage duration on bacteria contamination and transfusion-transmitted sepsis was never rigorously evaluated, and in recent years the introduction of more sensitive methods for the detection of bacterial contamination led to the re-institution of 7-day platelet storage in some countries. With the exception of viral epidemics in which large numbers of asymptomatic infected individuals may continue to donate blood, bacterial contamination of platelet components remains the leading risk factor for transfusion-transmitted infection [1]. This review will focus on current data regarding the prevalence of bacterial contamination, clinical outcomes as the result of transfusion of contaminated platelet components, and methods to limit or prevent bacterial contamination of platelet components and to reduce the incidence of transfusion-transmitted sepsis.

Prevalence of Bacterial Contamination of Platelet Components

Over the past decade multiple studies have been conducted to determine the prevalence of bacterial contamination of platelet components and to characterize the spectrum of bacterial species implicated in contamination [4]. These studies have identified the major sources of contamination as arising from donor skin and asymptomatic donor bacteremia resulting in contamination during blood donation. Less frequently, contamination of platelet components may occur during processing or through contamination of blood collection containers during manufacture [5]. Each of these sources may result in contamination with either gram-positive or gram-negative bacteria, although in general skin contamination is more commonly associated with gram-positive bacteria while asymptomatic donor bacteremia is more commonly associated with gram-negative organisms [6]. A very broad spectrum of organisms has been reported to contaminate blood components and specifically platelet components [6].

The prevalence of bacterial contamination of platelet components has been the subject of a large number of studies using a wide variety of methods ranging in sensitivity to detect bacteria [7]. The literature was summarized by Blajchman et al. in 2005 based on 9 prospective studies with culture of 192,053 platelet components leading to an estimate that approximately 1:3,000 platelet components was contaminated with bacteria [1].

Determination of the prevalence of contamination depends on the level of contamination and the sensitivity of the detection methods used. Across the broad spectrum of bacteria, the most sensitive methods for detection utilize culture with both aerobic and anaerobic conditions [7]. The most commonly used commercial culture system (BacT/ALERT 3D®; bioMerieux, Hazelwood, MO, USA) has been validated as a quality control assay to detect 1–10 cfu/ml. While the value of an anaerobic culture continues to be debated, most studies indicate that a second culture will increase the sensitivity of detection, either due to the increased volume sampled or the use of anaerobic conditions to facilitate growth of slow growing bacteria [8]. The recent study by the German cooperative group emphasized the importance of sampling sufficient volume and the potential value of both an aerobic and an anaerobic culture bottle [9]. While the sensitivity of culture to detect bacteria is markedly dependent on the sample volume used for culture inoculation, the concentration of bacteria in the sample withdrawn from the component depends on the time after collection of the component that a sample is taken for culture [9].

The actual level of contamination at the time of collection is theoretical, but can be assumed to be quite low based on studies demonstrating substantial differences in the frequency of positive cultures when components are sampled at varying times within 24 h after collection, and when components are re-sampled 7 days after collection [1, 10]. Theoretically, a single colony-forming unit (cfu) contaminating a platelet component (1 cfu/300 ml) is capable of growth during storage, resulting in bacteria concentrations potentially associated with clinically relevant post-transfusion events. Recently, Benjamin and Wagner [8] modeled the concentration of bacteria in platelet components sampled 24 h after collection, a common practice, based on the incidence of false-negative cultures from the clinical practice surveillance study of de Korte et al. [11]. Benjamin and Wagner estimated that, even with optimal detection methods, the levels of bacteria in false-negative cultures ranged from <0.02 to 0.15 cfu/ml (6–45 cfu in 300 ml), resulting in predicted false-negative culture rates ranging from 11 to 74%.

These estimates are consistent with the prior studies of Nussbaumer et al. that examined the sensitivity of bacterial cultures to detect low levels of contamination [12]. In their study, apheresis platelet components with a controlled volume of 285 ml were contaminated shortly after collection with 1–10 cfu, 10–100 cfu, and 100–1000 cfu using seven species of bacteria, both aerobic and anaerobic [12]. The estimated bacteria concentration levels after contamination ranged from 0.003 to 3 cfu/ml. In this study, a 10-ml sample was withdrawn from contaminated components 24, 48 and 120 h following contamination. Aliquots (4–5 ml) were inoculated into an aerobic and an anaerobic culture medium (BacT/ALERT 3D; bioMeriex, Hazelwood, MO, USA) and cultured for up to 120 h after inoculation, or until a positive culture was detected. The sample withdrawn 24 h following contamination was analogous to that obtained in commonly used bacterial detection protocols. At contamination levels of 1–10 cfu per component, 86% of cultures were false negative when sampled 24 h after collection. At contamination levels of 10–100 cfu per component, 57% of cultures were false negative [12]. These data are consistent with the false-negative rates predicted from the modeling studies of Benjamin and Wagner, confirming that bacteria detection methods, even under optimal conditions with aerobic and anaerobic cultures, result in significant false-negative rates for the detection of contamination at the low levels observed during routine practice of blood collection.

More recently, additional data to establish the prevalence of bacterial contamination in platelet components collected and tested in routine practice with optimal collection methods, including improved skin disinfection and diversion of the initial blood sample, have been reported and summarized by Dumont et al. with data from the Passport Study [13]. In this study, apheresis platelet components were sampled 24–36 h after collection (release test) and 4–5 ml were inoculated into an aerobic and an anaerobic culture using the BacT/ALERT detection system. Platelet components were held in quarantine for an additional 24 h and then, at 48–60 h after collection, components with negative culture results were available for transfusion as required. Components remaining in storage for 7 days after collection were re-cultured using methods similar to the initial culture sample (surveillance test). Both release and surveillance test cultures were monitored for 7 days. Components with negative release tests giving a positive result after release for transfusion were re-tested when available to confirm an initial positive result. Components not available for repeat testing or components with negative results on re-testing were classified as indeterminate. The Passport Study tested 193,078 components and observed a prevalence of contamination based on release test-confirmed positive samples of 0.249 components per 1,000 tested (1:4.016 components tested). This level of prevalence is within the same range for two other studies (Irish Blood Transfusion Service, IBTS, and Wales Blood Transfusion Service, WBTS) with reported prevalence of confirmed release test-positive samples of 0.312 and 0.445 per 1,000 (1:3,025 and 1:2,247 components, respectively). These observed prevalence rates are slightly greater, but consistent with the earlier bacteria contamination prevalence estimates of 1:3,000 summarized by Blajchman et al. [1].

In contrast to the prevalence rates determined from Release Tests, the results of the surveillance cultures from these three studies indicate a higher prevalence of bacterial contamination (table 1) ranging from 1:1,285 to 1:1,072 platelet components tested on day 7. The higher prevalence of contamination detected in surveillance cultures obtained 7 days after collection is due to bacterial growth during storage, resulting in increased sensitivity of detection. This is consistent with observations in the Nussbaumer study of low-level contamination in which culture of components 5 days after collection resulted in reduced false-negative cultures; the data are consistent with the models generated by Benjamin and Wagner. If one assumes all of the confirmed positive, false-positive (no growth on re-test), indeterminate (not re-tested), and false-negative samples for the interdicted components and the transfused components, 526/193,078 represents the most liberal estimate of contamination; the prevalence of contamination is 2.7/1,000 components tested (1:370) despite the use of optimal skin disinfection and diversion of the initial blood draw. Thus, the Passport Study data provide a worst-case estimate for the prevalence of contamination based on these liberal assumptions. With the addition of optimal bacteria detection, the post-initial test residual risk based on the 7-day Surveillance cultures was reduced to 1:1,250 components tested.

	Prevalence per 1,000 platelet components cultured[b]	
	release culture	7-day surveillance culture
Passport	0.249 (1:4,016)	0.778 (1:1,285)
Irish BTS	0.312 (1:3,205)	0.845 (1:1,183)
Wales BTS	0.445 (1:2,247)	0.932 (1:1,072)

Table 1. Prevalence of bacterial contamination of apheresis platelet components based on initial release and surveillance cultures[a]

[a] Adopted from [13]. Data are summarized for the U.S. Passport Study, the IBTS study, and the WBTS study. In each study, bacterial contamination was detected with a 2-culture assay system (aerobic and anaerobic) using the BacTALERT 3D system.
[b] Prevalence of bacterial contamination is expressed per 1,000 components tested and as a ratio measure per thousands of components.

Other studies, depending on the methods used, have reported prevalence for bacteria contamination similar to that of the Passport Study. A multi-center study was conducted by the collaborative GERMS group involving 15,198 apheresis platelet collections and 37,045 whole blood-derived pooled platelet concentrates [9]. The study used an improved skin disinfection method and diversion of the initial blood sample during collection. The protocol required sampling of 7.5 ml of each component for aerobic and anaerobic culture (total volume tested = 15 ml) using the BacT/ALERT system. The initial positive rate was 0.26% (1:384 components tested) with a confirmed positive rate of 0.07% (1:1,428 components tested). Similar rates have been observed in other studies with similar methodology, ranging from 0.26 to 0.65% [11, 14–16]. Considering all of the above studies, one can estimate bacteria contamination prevalence ranging from 1:150 to 1:1,500 components tested. With aerobic and anaerobic culture methods, using a total test volume of 10–15 ml, and with samples obtained 24–36 h after collection, the residual prevalence of contamination after bacterial detection remains approximately 1:1,250 components tested.

Clinical Outcomes Associated with Bacterial Contamination of Platelet Components

A considerable literature has been devoted to reporting the clinical relevance of bacterial contamination of platelet components. The range of outcomes described includes absence of clinical symptoms (asymptomatic bacteremia), immediate post-transfusion sepsis, delayed post-transfusion infection, and death due to sepsis. Another possibility that has not been widely addressed includes colonization of indwelling catheters with subsequent infection that may not be attributed to a contaminated platelet component due to delayed onset of symptoms [17]. Consistent with this possibility,

Greco et al. have reported on the potential for contaminants of platelet components to form biofilms, further increasing virulence and impairing detection [18, 19].

Detection of the clinical outcome associated with transfusion of a contaminated component is highly dependent on post-transfusion clinical surveillance methodology, and this has varied greatly among the different studies. Not only does detection of transfusion-associated sepsis require sensitive surveillance systems but more importantly awareness of primary care physicians of the potential for transfusion-transmitted sepsis [20].

The literature on transfusion-transmitted sepsis has been well summarized in several excellent reviews [1, 4]. Most of the large studies, including the recent American Red Cross study [21] and the Passport Study, were designed primarily as laboratory surveillance studies to determine the prevalence of bacteria contamination with reliance on passive reporting to determine clinical outcomes. In neither of these studies was information provided about the number of recipients, so per-patient risk during a period of platelet support cannot be estimated. The American Red Cross study used two different diversion systems and only a single bottle of aerobic cultures. In the Passport Study, which utilized an optimal skin disinfection and diversion system with an optimal detection process (aerobic and anaerobic cultures taken at 24–36 h after collection and then held in quarantine for 24 h prior to release), 120 products were released as negative but ultimately classified as confirmed positive (n = 9) or indeterminate unconfirmed cultures (n = 111), resulting in 5 reports of septic clinical outcomes. Based on the total number of components released for transfusion, the incidence of reported septic transfusion reactions was 1:38,461 components. Reporting of clinical outcomes was entirely voluntary in the Passport Study, without specific study guidance for reporting given to clinical transfusion centers. Thus, this incidence most likely represents an underestimate of the true incidence of septic post-transfusion events.

The assumption that transfusion-transmitted sepsis is underestimated is supported by many years of observation. The literature contains many case reports in which platelet transfusion-associated sepsis was only recognized as related to the platelet component some time after the transfusion [22–24]. In review of an institutional 14-year experience of surveillance of bacteria contamination and clinical outcomes, Yomtovian et al. concluded that post-transfusion surveillance underestimated the incidence of clinically relevant transfusion-transmitted bacteria [25]. Benjamin and Wagner reviewed a series of major studies using the BacT/ALERT system for detection of contaminated components and calculated, based on these reports, that for the products tested and released there was a 1:43,000 residual risk for clinical sepsis events. The fatality rate per 100,000 components tested was 0.44, and this only examined immediate fatality. They concluded that this summary provided only a minimal estimate of transfusion-associated sepsis. Others have also concluded that accurate estimation of death incidence associated with platelet transfusion-transmitted bacteria is very imprecise [26]. One important aspect of the reported deaths is that a greater proportion has been associated with gram-negative bacteria, indicating that improved skin disinfection and blood diversion may have limited efficacy to reduce severe transfusion-transmitted sepsis [27].

The study by Chiu et al. is one of the few studies that evaluated the outcome of bacterial contamination with an active surveillance design in which patients were prospectively followed for signs of sepsis after repeated platelet transfusions, and both patient and component were cultured if sepsis was suspected on a clinical basis using defined criteria [28]. They observed that a substantial proportion (27%) of febrile platelet transfusion reactions were associated with documented sepsis. They concluded that, with a patient-based analysis, 1 in 16 patients receiving multiple platelet transfusions experienced transfusion-transmitted bacteremia during a period of platelet support [28]. Synthesis of the information from these studies and others indicates that transfusion-transmitted bacterial infection is underreported [29] and underestimated [26], and the complete spectrum of the potential clinical outcomes remains to be defined.

Measures to Limit or Prevent Transfusion-Transmitted Bacterial Infection

Several interventions have been developed to limit or prevent transfusion-transmitted infection, including donor interview for recent infection, improved skin disinfection, diversion of the first aliquot of blood withdrawn, bacterial detection, and pathogen inactivation/reduction. Each of these technologies has been implemented into routine clinical practice and merits review. There are limited data with which to assess the impact of specific interview questions for detection of sub-clinical donor bacteremia, and this intervention will not be reviewed.

Skin Disinfection and Diversion

Techniques for skin disinfection have been evaluated and the preferred method utilizes a two-stage technique with isopropyl alcohol (IPA) and a tincture of iodine, which resulted in the optimal reduction of skin flora [30]. Subsequently, the impact of a two-stage IPA disinfection preparation on bacterial contamination of platelet components was evaluated and reported to slightly reduce the prevalence of contamination (0.95 to 0.85%) when components were cultured 12–22 h after collection using aerobic and anaerobic detection methods [11]. Diversion of the initial 20–30 ml of blood withdrawn with improved skin disinfection resulted in a further reduction of bacteria contamination based on initial positive cultures from 0.95 to 0.37% [11].

Testing of platelet components as a means to limit transfusion of contaminated plate-let components has been widely evaluated and various methods have been adopted in a number of countries. A large number of technologies have been developed to various stages, including visual inspection, glucose and pH levels, Gram stain, oxygen consumption, carbon dioxide production, detection of bacterial nucleic acid sequences, fluorescent cytometric detection, endotoxin detection, bacteria-specific antigen detection, and automated bacterial culture [7]. Only the bacteria culture methods have been evaluated in large-scale studies of routine practice and will be reviewed. As previously noted, a variety of different protocols have been utilized with the most sensitive culture methods [31]. There is no standard protocol in use, despite the requirement of blood transfusion accreditation agencies for use of methods to detect or limit bacteria contamination [4]. Two technologies have received approval as quality control assays, but none has been approved as a release assay sufficient to label a component as tested and considered negative for bacteria contamination. The two approved systems are the eBDS method, which relies on oxygen consumption to indicate bacteria contamination (Pall Corporation, Short Hills, NY, USA) and the BacT/ALERT culture technology with aerobic and anaerobic cultures (bioMerieux, Hazelwood, MO, USA). The eBDS system has been evaluated in relatively small-scale laboratory contamination studies in which the bacteria inocula ranged from 5 to 13 cfu/ml, relatively high levels compared to the estimated levels of contamination in clinical practice [8]. No large-scale studies with actual clinical experience in routine use have been reported using the eBDS technology. Therefore, it is not possible to fully evaluate the performance characteristics of the eBDS system under routine operating conditions with low levels of bacteria contamination.

In contrast, the performance of the BacT/ALERT system has been reviewed in a number of studies recently summarized by Benjamin and Wagner, in which they estimated false-negative rates for detection to range from 4 to more than 75%, depending on the rate of growth of the bacteria species [8]. In all of the large surveillance culture studies, the proportions of 'false-positive' and 'indeterminate' results, as defined by the AABB criteria [26], have been substantial. The classification of false-positive cultures is problematic due to the possible limitation to detect low levels of bacteria in repeat cultures, and the exclusion of indeterminate cultures from estimation of prevalence due to lack of a second specimen leaves open to question the true contamination prevalence. The review of the larger culture series by Benjamin and Wagner provides estimates for false-negative cultures of issued components per 100,000 products tested resulting in sepsis of 2.3 and a fatality incidence due to false-negative cultures of 0.44 per 100,000 products tested [8]. These data suggest that bacterial detection, even when used with optimal skin disinfection and diversion processes, results in significant residual risk for transfusion-transmitted sepsis.

Another salient aspect of bacteria culture systems is the time to detection of initial positives. In multiple studies, substantial proportions of platelet components were released prior to the observation of the initial positive culture result [15, 16, 32]. This delay in detection results in a large proportion of indeterminate culture results due to the inability to obtain a confirmation culture. Eder et al. noted that the average time to initial positive for false-positive and indeterminate culture results in the American Red Cross study was 74 ± 30 h [21]. The recent interim analysis of the Passport Study data revealed a higher prevalence of contamination than expected based on Surveillance Test cultures (1:1,285) obtained 7 days after collection compared to the rate for Release Test cultures (1:4,016). This observation is consistent with the prior observations of delayed time to a positive culture result for substantial proportions of components in routine bacteria detection operational studies, and ultimately resulted in discontinuation of 7-day platelet storage in the USA despite the use of bacteria detection with both aerobic and anaerobic cultures combined with optimal collection methods [33].

Pathogen Inactivation/Reduction

Another approach to prevent transfusion-transmitted bacterial infection is by use of pathogen inactivation/reduction technology. Two technologies have received Conformité Européenne (CE) Mark registration. Both of these processes utilize photochemical techniques, but the respective mechanisms of action are substantially different.

The INTERCEPT™ Blood System for Platelets (Cerus Europe BV, Amersfoort, The Netherlands) is registered as a Class III medical device and utilizes the synthetic psoralen, amotosalen HCl, and ultraviolet A (UVA) light ($3 J/cm^2$: 320–400 nm) to inactivate a broad spectrum of gram-positive and gram-negative bacteria associated with transfusion-transmitted sepsis (table 2) [34]. Platelet components treated with this technology have received additional national registration from AFSSaPS (French Agency of Medical Safety of Health Products) and the PEI (Paul Ehrlich Institute, Germany). This technology is designed for use within the first 24 h after collection so that treated platelet components are available for release within the same time frame as completion of serology and nucleic acid tests (fig. 1). These operational logistics avoid the inherent delay in release of components required for enhancement of bacteria detection sensitivity, and provides 4–6 days of inventory shelf life depending on whether 5- or 7-day storage is utilized.

Pathogen inactivation by amotosalen is targeted to nucleic acids and utilizes photochemistry based on the formation of covalent adducts with bacteria nucleic acids, resulting in a modification density of approximately 1 adduct per 80 base pairs [35]. The process was specifically designed to minimize the production of active oxygen species. In the absence of UVA light no pathogen inactivation occurs, and likewise, in the absence of amotosalen no inactivation occurs with UVA light [36]. This technology has

	Extent of inactivation[a] (log₁₀ reduction)

Table 2. Bacteria species inactivated by the INTERCEPT system for platelets

	Extent of inactivation[a] (log_{10} reduction)
Gram-negative bacteria	
Escherichia coli	>6.4
Serratia marcescens	>6.7
Klebsiella pneumoniae	>5.6
Pseudomonas aeruginosa	4.5
Salmonella choleraesuis	>6.2
Yersinia enterocolitica	>5.9
Enterobacter cloacae	5.9
Gram-positive bacteria	
Staphylococcus epidermidis	>6.6
Staphylococcus aureus	6.6
Streptococcus pyogenes	>6.8
Listeria monocytogenes	>6.3
Corynebacterium minutissimum	>6.3
Bacillus cereus (includes spores)	3.6
Bacillus cereus (vegetative)	>6.0
Bifidobacterium adolescentis	>6.5
Propionibacterium acnes	>6.7
Lactobacillus species	>6.9
Clostridium perfringens (vegetative form)	>7.0
Spirochete bacteria	
Treponema pallidum	≥6.8 to ≤7.0
Borrelia burgdorferi	>6.8

[a] '>' Refers to inactivation below the limit of detection of the assay. Based on previously reported data [34].

been introduced into clinical practice in multiple European countries and has replaced bacteria detection to prevent transfusion-transmitted sepsis (fig. 1). Thus far, two multi-national active hemovigilance studies involving approximately 13,000 transfusions and 2,000 patients have shown prevention of transfusion-transmitted sepsis [37, 38].

The second method of photochemical pathogen inactivation/reduction uses riboflavin (vitamin B2, 50 μg per 300 ml) in a photodynamic process (Mirasol PRT System; Navigant Biotechnologies Inc., Lakewood, CO, USA) with UVC, UVB and a portion of UVA light (265–375 nm) [39]. The final concentration of riboflavin is 50 μM and the platelets are illuminated with approximately 5 J/cm² of light [39]. This process relies on the association of riboflavin with nucleic acids and the generation of active oxygen species in proximity to nucleic acids leading to disruption [40]. In the absence of riboflavin, the UVC and UVB light create sufficient levels of active oxygen species to retain most of the bacterial inactivation capacity through non-specific dis-

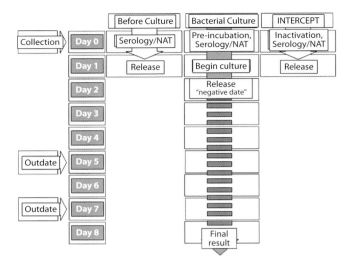

Fig. 1. Operational logistics for production and release of platelet components using three methods. Before Culture = conventional testing without bacterial culture, Bacterial Culture = conventional testing with bacterial culture, and INTERCEPT = pathogen inactivation with conventional testing.

ruption of bacterial nucleic acids and perhaps other structures [40]. This technology has received Class II CE Mark registration, but as yet no subsequent national registrations of the treated components. Laboratory studies have evaluated inactivation of a panel of gram-positive and gram-negative bacteria (table 3) [41]. To date, no studies have been reported to evaluate the efficacy of the Mirasol PRT system for prevention of transfusion-transmitted sepsis in routine clinical use.

Conclusions and Future Directions

Bacterial contamination of platelet components appears to exhibit prevalence as high as 2.7 per 1,000 components (1:370) if one includes all initial positive cultures from the studies performed with optimal detection methods. Using more conservative estimates, the prevalence appears to range from 1:1,250 to 1:3,000 components tested. Both gram-positive and gram-negative bacteria have been implicated as contaminants. The clinical consequences arising from transfusion of contaminated components range in severity from asymptomatic bacteremia to fulminant sepsis and death. The true incidence of clinically significant events arising from transfusion of contaminated platelet components is underreported and underestimated. The lack of studies with stringent active post-transfusion surveillance leaves the true incidence unknown. In the past, most studies have examined clinical outcome on the basis of the components transfused rather than on a per-patient basis of risk for patients who receive multiple platelet transfusions. The sole prospective study to examine the risk of transfusion-transmitted sepsis on a per-patient basis indicated that the risk of a platelet transfusion-associated septic event was as frequent as 1:16 patients who receive repeated exposures.

Table 3. Bacteria species inactivated by the Mirasol PRT System[a]

	Extent of inactivation[b] (log$_{10}$ reduction)
Gram-negative bacteria	
Escherichia coli (ATCC # 25922)	≥4.38
Serratia marcescens (ATCC # 43862)	4.0 ± 0.5
Pseudomonas aeruginosa (ATCC # 43088)	≥4.48
Gram-positive bacteria	
Staphylococcus epidermidis (ATCC # 12228)	≥4.15
Staphylococcus aureus (ATCC # 25923)	3.56 ± 0.35
Staphylococcus aureus (ATCC # 700787)	4.8 ± 0.8
Bacillus cereus (ATCC # 7064)	1.9 ± 0.3
Bacillus cereus (blood isolate)	2.7 ± 0.6

[a] Treatment conditions based on composite information from [41] and [39].
[b] '>' Refers to inactivation below the limit of detection of the assay. Based on previously reported data [34].

Thus far, methods to prevent transfusion-transmitted sepsis by enhanced donor history, improved skin disinfection, use of diversion, and bacteria detection have partially reduced the risk. The lack of use of these methods or some combination appears to expose transfusion recipients to a significant risk of transfusion-transmitted sepsis. However, despite the use of these measures, a substantial risk of transfusion-transmitted bacteremia remains, and the full spectrum of clinical consequences is unknown. An alternative approach to bacteria detection methods utilizes pathogen inactivation treatment of platelet components. These technologies have reached routine practice and have been implemented without adversely impacting operational logistics or platelet component inventories. They are effective against low levels of bacteria contamination, the most vulnerable aspect of detection, and against high levels of contamination. As opposed to testing, they treat the entire component and, if sufficiently robust, should provide the optimal technology to achieve an extremely low risk of transfusion-transmitted bacterial infection.

Disclosure of Conflict of Interests

Laurence Corash is an employee of Cerus Corporation, Concord, CA, USA.

Acknowledgements

The author is indebted to Lily Lin, Joseph Eiden, Morris Blajchman, and Richard Benjamin for many helpful discussions regarding bacterial contamination.

References

1 Blajchman MA, Beckers EAM, Dickmeiss E, Lin L, Moore G, Muylle L: Bacterial detection of platelets: current problems and possible resolutions. Transfus Med Rev 2005;19:259–272.

2 Braine HG, Kickler TS, Charache P, Ness PM, Davis J, Reichart C, Fuller AK: Bacteria sepsis secondary to platelet transfusion: an adverse effect of extended storage at room temperature. Transfusion 1986;26:391–393.

3 Center for Biologics Evaluation and Research (CBER): Reduction of the maximum platelet storage period to 5 days in an approved container. U.S. Food and Drug Administration [Electronic Monograph]. Available at: www.fda.gov/cber/bldmem/060286.pdf.

4 Yomtovian R: Bacterial contamination of blood: lessons from the past and road map for the future. Transfusion 2004;44:450–460.

5 Blajchman MA, Thornley JH, Richardson H, Elder D, Spiak C, Racher J: Platelet transfusion-induced *Serratia marcescens* sepsis due to vacuum tube contamination. Transfusion 1979;19:39–44.

6 Blajchman MA, Goldman M: Bacterial contamination of platelet concentrates: incidence, significance, and prevention. Semin Hematol 2001;38(suppl 11):20–26.

7 Blajchman MA, Goldman M, Baeza F: Improving the bacteriological safety of platelet transfusions. Transfus Med Rev 2004;18:11–24.

8 Benjamin RJ, Wagner SJ: The residual risk of sepsis: modeling the effect of concentration on bacterial detection in two-bottle culture systems and an estimation of false-negative culture rates. Transfusion 2007;47:1381–1389.

9 Schrezenmeier H, Walther-Wenke G, Muller TH, Weinauer F, Younis A, Holland-Letz T, Geis G, Asmus J, Bauerfeind U, Burkhart J, Deitenbeck R, Förstemann E, Gebauer W, Höchsmann B, Karakassopoulos A, Liebscher UM, Sänger W, Schmidt M, Schunter F, Sireis W, Seifried E: Bacterial contamination of platelet concentrates: results of a prospective multicenter study comparing pooled whole blood-derived platelets and apheresis platelets. Transfusion 2007;47:644–652.

10 Lee CK, Ho PL, Lee KY, Cheng WW, Chan NK, Tsoi WC, Lin CK: Estimation of bacterial risk in extending the shelf-life of PLT concentrates from 5 to 7 days. Transfusion 2003;43:1047–1052.

11 de Korte D, Cuvers J, de Kort WL: Effects of skin disinfection method, deviation bag, and bacterial screening on clinical safety of platelet transfusions in The Netherlands. Transfusion 2006;46:476–485.

12 Nussbaumer W, Allersdorfer D, Grabmer C, Rheinschmidt M, Lin L, Schönitzer D, Lass-Flörl C: Prevention of transfusion of platelet components contaminated with low levels of bacteria: a comparison of bacteria culture and pathogen inactivation methods. Transfusion 2007;47:1125–1133.

13 Dumont LJ: Gambro/Fenwal PASSPORT Post Marketing Study – 7 Day Platelets. November 29–30, 2007. Available at: www.passportstudy.com/.

14 Macauley A, Chandrasekar A, Geddis G: Operational feasibility of routine bacterial monitoring of platelets. Transfus Med 2003;13:189–195.

15 Munksgaard L, Albjerg L, Lillevang ST, Gahrn-Hansen B, Georgsen J: Detection of bacterial contamination of platelet components: six years' experience with the BactT/ALERT system. Transfusion 2004;44:1166–1173.

16 te Boekhorst PA, Beckers EA, Vos MC, Vermeij H, van Rhenen DJ: Clinical significance of bacteriologic screening in platelet concentrates. Transfusion 2005;45:514–519.

17 Hanna H, Raad I: Blood products: A significant risk factor for long-term catheter-related bloodstream infections in cancer patients. Infect Control Hosp Epidemiol 2001;22:165–166.

18 Greco C, Mastronardi C, Pagotto F, Mack D, Ramirez-Arcos S: Assessment of biofilm-forming ability of coagulase-negative staphylococci isolated from contaminated platelet preparations. Transfusion 2008;48:969–977.

19 Greco C, Martincic I, Gusinjac A, Kalab M, Yang AF, Ramirez-Arcos S: *Staphylococcus epidermidis* forms biofilms under simulated platelet storage conditions. Transfusion 2007;47:1143–1153.

20 Rao PL, Strausbaugh LJ, Liedtke LA, Srinivasan A, Kuehnert MJ, Infectious Disease Society of America Emerging Infections Network: Bacterial infections associated with blood transfusion: experience and perspective of infectious disease consultants. Transfusion 2007;47:1206–1211.

21 Eder AF, Kennedy JM, Dy B, Notari EP, Weiss JW, Fang CT, Wagner S, Dodd RY, Benjamin RJ; American Red Cross Regional Blood Centers: Bacterial screening of apheresis platelets and the residual risk of septic transfusion reactions: the American Red Cross Experience (2004–2006). Transfusion 2007;47:1134–1142.

22 Heal JM, Jones ME, Forey J, Chaudhry A, Stricof RL: Fatal *Salmonella* septicemia after platelet transfusion. Transfusion 1987;27:2–5.

23 Rhame FS, Root RK, MacLowry JD, Dadisman TA, Bennett JV: *Salmonella* septicemia from platelet transfusions: study of an outbreak traced to hematogenous carrier of *Salmonella cholerae-suis*. Ann Intern Med 1973;78:633–641.

24 Jafari M, Forsberg J, Gilcher RO, Smith JW, Crutcher JM, McDermott M, Brown BR, George JN: *Salmonella* sepsis caused by a platelet transfusion from a donor with a pet snake. N Engl J Med 2002;347:1075–1078.

25 Yomtovian RA, Palavecino EI, Dysktra AH, Downes KA, Morrissey AM, Bajaksouzian S, Pokorny MA, Lazarus HM, Jacobs MR: Evolution of surveillance methods for detection of bacterial contamination of platelets in a university hospital, 1991 through 2004. Transfusion 2006;46:719–730.

26 Yomtovian R, Tomasulo P, Jacobs MR: Platelet bacterial contamination: assessing progress and identifying quandries in a rapidly evolving field. Transfusion 2007;47:1340–1346.

27 Niu MT, Knippen M, Simmons L, Holness LG: Transfusion-transmitted *Klebsiella pneumoniae* fatalities, 1995–2004. Transfus Med Rev 2006;20:149–157.

28 Chiu EKW, Yuen KY, Lie AKW, Liang R, Lau YL, Lee AC, Kwong YL, Wong S, Ng MH, Chan TK: A prospective study of symptomatic bacteremia following platelet transfusion and of its management. Transfusion 1994;34:950–954.

29 Kuehnert M, Roth V, Haley NR, Gregory KR, Elder KV, Schreiber GB, Arduino MJ, Holt SC, Carson LA, Banerjee SN, Jarvis WR: Transfusion-transmitted bacterial infection in the United States, 1998 through 2000. Transfusion 2001;41:1493–1499.

30 McDonald CP, Lowe P, Roy A, Robbins S, Hartley S, Harrison JF, Slopecki A, Verlander N, Barbara JA: Evaluation of donor arm skin disinfection techniques. Vox Sang 2001;80:135–141.

31 Pietersz RNI, Engelfriet CP, Reesink HW: Detection of bacterial contamination of platelet concentrates. Vox Sang 2003;85:224–239.

32 Larsen CP, Ezligini F, Hermansen NO, Kjeldsen-Kragh J: Six years' experience of using the BactT/ALERT system to screen all platelet concentrates, and additional testing of outdated platelet concentrates to estimate the frequency of false-negative results. Vox Sang 2005;88:93–97.

33 Cole B, Smith T: PASSPORT: Post approval surveillance study of platelet outcomes, Release tested. Gambro BCT and Fenwal, Inc., January 29, 2008. Available at: www.passportstudy.com/.

34 Lin L, Dikeman R, Molini B, Lukehart SA, Lane R, Dupuis K, Metzel P, Corash L: Photochemical treatment of platelet concetrates with amotosalen and UVA inactivates a broad spectrum of pathogenic bacteria. Transfusion 2004;44:1496–1504.

35 Wollowitz S: Fundamentals of the psoralen-based Helinx technology for inactivation of infectious pathogens and leukocytes in platelets and plasma. Semin Hematol 2001;38(suppl 11):4–11.

36 Lin L, Cook DN, Wiesehahn GP, Alfonso R, Behrman B, Cimino GD, Corten L, Damonte PB, Dikeman R, Dupuis K, Fang YM, Hanson CV, Hearst JE, Lin CY, Londe HF, Metchette K, Nerio AT, Pu JT, Reames AA, Rheinschmidt M, Tessman J, Isaacs ST, Wollowitz S, Corash L: Photochemical inactivation of viruses and bacteria in platelet concentrates by use of a novel psoralen and long-wavelength ultraviolet light. Transfusion 1997;37:423–435.

37 Osselaer JC, Cazenave JP, Lambermont M, Garraud O, Hidajat M, Barbolla L, Tardivel R, Defoin L, Waller C, Mendel I, Raidot JP, Kandel G, De Meuter R, Fabrigli P, Dehenau D, Arroyo JL, Padrón F, Gouezec H, Corral M, Jacquet M, Sundin D, Lin L, Corash L: An active haemovigilance programme characterizing the safety profile of 7437 platelet transfusions prepared with amotosalen photochemical treatment. Vox Sang 2008;94:315–323.

38 Osselaer JC, Messe N, Hervig T, Bueno J, Castro E, Espinosa A, Accorsi P, Junge K, Jacquet M, Flament J, Corash L: A prospective observational cohort safety study of 5,106 platelet transfusions using components prepared with photochemical pathogen inactivation treatment. Transfusion 2008, in press.

39 Ruane PH, Edrich R, Gampp D, Keil SD, Leonard L, Goodrich RP: Photochemical inactivation of selected viruses and bacteria in platelet concentrates using riboflavin and light. Transfusion 2004;44:877–885.

40 Kumar V, Lockerbie O, Keil SD, Ruane PH, Platz MS, Martin CB, Ravanat JL, Cadet J, Goodrich RP: Riboflavin and UV-light based pathogen reduction: extent and consequence of DNA damage at the molecular level. Photochem Photobiol 2004;80:15–21.

41 Goodrich RP, Edrich RA, Li J, Seghatchian J: The Mirasol PRT system for pathogen reduction of platelets and plasma: An overview of current status and future trends. Transfus Apheresis Sci 2006;35:5–17.

Prof. Laurence Corash, M.D.
Cerus Corporation
2411 Stanwell Drive
Concord, CA 94520, USA
Tel. +1 925 288-6118, Fax -0194
E-Mail lcorash@cerus.com

Scharf RE (ed): Progress and Challenges in Transfusion Medicine, Hemostasis and Hemotherapy.
Freiburg i.Br., Karger, 2008, pp 248–263

Clinical Experience with Pathogen Inactivation of Platelet Components for Transfusion Support

Jean-Pierre Cazenave[a, b, c] · Chantal Waller[a] · Isabelle Mendel[a] ·
Daniel Kientz[a] · Gérard Kandel[a] · Jean-Pierre Raidot[a] ·
Marie-Louise Wiesel[a, b] · Michel Laforet[a] · Hervé Isola[a, b]

[a]EFS-Alsace, Strasbourg,
[b]INSERM U311, Strasbourg,
[c]University Louis Pasteur, Strasbourg, France

Key Words

Platelets · Transfusion · Pathogen inactivation · Amotosalen · Clinical trials

Summary

Blood transfusion is a critical supportive therapy for health care. The demand for platelet components (PCs), either derived from apheresis or from whole blood buffy coats, has continually increased as health care technology and life expectancy have increased. The public and the medical community expect that PCs for transfusion will be safe and available when needed. Pharmaceutical standards for medications to be administered intravenously to patients require sterility and absence of pyrogens. However, sterilization or inactivation of pathogens remains a major challenge for blood components. A number of physical methods (heat, light, and filtration) and chemical techniques (solvent-detergent) have been applied with success to therapeutic plasma and purified plasma proteins. However, pathogen inactivation treatment of the labile cellular blood components (platelets and red blood cells) has been much more difficult to achieve without significant loss of cell viability and cell function. The safety of labile blood products, including PCs, has previously been ensured by medical and biological donor selection measures. While these measures have improved the safety of blood transfusion, they are reactive and have not eliminated the risk of transfusion-transmitted infection. In addition to the residual risk of recognized viral, bacterial and parasitic contamination of PCs, there is the recurring risk associated with emerging pathogens as demonstrated by several recent epidemics and a continuing pattern of emergence and reemergence of transfusion-transmitted pathogens [1]. Pathogen inactivation of PCs has been implemented into routine practice and offers the potential to protect against the residual risk of known pathogens and the risk of emerging pathogens for which diagnostic tests are not available. Recently, this technology has demonstrated its utility during an epidemic of an emerging pathogen, and represents a paradigm shift in the approach to blood transfusion safety.
©2008 S. Karger GmbH, Freiburg i.Br.

Introduction

The safety of labile blood products (red blood cell concentrates, platelet components (PCs) and plasma) is currently ensured by medical and biological donor selection measures. Nonetheless, in addition to the residual risk of viral infection (window period, small number of viral copies), of bacterial contamination (in particular of PCs) and of parasitic contamination, there is the emerging danger associated with new viruses, such as West Nile virus, Chikungunya virus, Dengue virus, severe acute respiratory syndrome (SARS) corona virus, and the avian influenza virus H5N1. Pathogen inactivation based on chemical or photochemical genomic modifications is a broad-spectrum and proactive approach to reduce the risk of transfusion-transmitted infections (TTIs) [2]. These techniques have been used for more than one decade to inactivate contaminating pathogens in plasma (solvent-detergent, methylene blue) or therapeutic proteins derived from plasma or produced by recombinant technologies. Newer techniques of inactivation are being developed for application to PCs and erythrocyte concentrates.

Three techniques (UVC, riboflavin photochemistry, amotosalen and UVA) to inactivate pathogens in PCs are in various stages of clinical development and clinical practice. This review will summarize the progress made with each of these approaches. Because extensive clinical and operational experience has been obtained with pathogen inactivation of both apheresis platelet concentrates (APCs) and buffy coat platelet concentrates (BCPCs) using photochemical treatment (PCT) with amotosalen hydrochloride and UVA, it will be reported later in more detail.

Pathogen Reduction Treatment of Platelet Concentrates with UVC

A technique using illumination of PCs with UVC light under constant agitation, without addition of a chemical substance, is being developed (Theraflex-UV platelets, MacoPharma). Preclinical results demonstrate that the technique can efficiently inactivate a range of aerobic and anaerobic bacteria that can contaminate PCs. In addition, the process is active against some viruses but not against the human immunodeficiency retrovirus (HIV) [3]. Development stage clinical trials are under consideration.

Pathogen Reduction in Platelet Concentrates by Riboflavin Photochemistry: Clinical Experience

A pathogen reduction process (PRT) (Mirasol PRT; Gambro/Navigant Biotechnologies Inc., Lakewood, CO, USA) has been developed for PCs, plasma and possibly red cell concentrates, using riboflavin photochemistry (UVC, UVB and UVA light,

265–365 nm) to disrupt nucleic acids. The PRT method inactivates a wide range of pathogens including viruses, bacteria, parasites and T lymphocytes. Preclinical toxicology studies have shown acceptable safety margins [4]. In vitro platelet function and in vivo platelet recovery and survival are decreased to some extent, but acceptable for clinical use even after 5 days of storage [5]. The first phase 3 clinical trial (Miracle) has been ongoing in 6 centers in France in order to evaluate the efficacy and safety of platelet concentrates treated by Mirasol and transfused to thrombocytopenic patients. The Miracle trial was completed in December 2007; the results are under evaluation and will be reported shortly.

Pathogen Inactivation Treatment of Platelet Concentrates with Amotosalen Hydrochloride and UVA: Operational and Clinical Experience

The synthetic psoralen amotosalen hydrochloride (INTERCEPT™ Blood System for Platelets (IBSP); Cerus Europe BV, Amersfoort, The Netherlands) intercalates into nucleic acids in the dark, and with UVA light illumination (3 J/cm^2: 320–400 nm) produces multiple nucleic acid crosslinks and monoadducts preventing replication. The IBSP is a drug-device combination designed for ex vivo pathogen inactivation PCT of PCs prepared for transfusion support of patients with quantitative or qualitative platelet disorders. The PCT process is intended to reduce the risk of TTI and transfusion-associated graft-versus-host disease (TA-GVHD), because PCT inactivates a broad spectrum of clinically relevant viruses (RNA and DNA, enveloped and non-enveloped, cell-free and cell-associated), bacteria (gram-positive, gram-negative, and spirochetes), protozoa (intra- and extracellular) and T lymphocytes (without the added need for gamma irradiation to prevent TA-GVHD) which may contaminate PCs [6, 7]. Despite some limitations (ineffective against picornaviruses, bacterial spores and prions), PCT is effective against a broad spectrum of infectious agents known to cause TTI [8, 9]. The preclinical development program, conducted according to International Conference on Harmonization of Technical Requirements for Registration of Pharmaceuticals for Human Use (ICH) standards, has demonstrated the efficacy to inactivate all of the relevant blood-borne infectious pathogens, including emerging pathogens: West Nile virus, SARS, Chikungunya, Dengue virus, avian influenza virus H5N1 and *Trypanosoma cruzi*. Pre-clinical safety studies have demonstrated high safety margins [10]. The in vitro and in vivo functions of platelets are minimally affected following INTERCEPT treatment and during storage. Phase 3 clinical trials have been performed both in the USA and in Europe to demonstrate the therapeutic safety and efficacy of platelets and plasma. Based on this development program, the technology has received Conformité Européenne (CE) Mark registration as a class III drug-device combination and treated PCs have received regulatory approval in France and Germany.

Routine use of INTERCEPT-treated PC has been implemented in more than 20 blood transfusion centers in Europe, and more than 150,000 platelet and plasma components have been transfused to date. In France, INTERCEPT PC has been implemented during an epidemic of Chikungunya virus in the Ile de la Réunion and later during an epidemic of Dengue virus in the French West Indies islands of La Martinique and La Guadeloupe. In addition, a large-scale evaluation of the technology in routine use has been going on in the French region of Alsace, where all (about 12,000 units) PCs (40% APC and 60% BCPC) produced and transfused during a 1-year period, from May 2006 to April 2007, were prepared with the INTERCEPT process. An active hemovigilance post-marketing program to expand the safety profile of INTERCEPT platelets in a broader patient population, including pediatric patients and pregnant women, is being conducted in Belgium and France and is in progress throughout Europe [11, 12].

The Clinical Development Program with INTERCEPT Platelets

The potential effects of the IBSP process on platelet therapeutic efficacy and safety has been evaluated in a broad range of clinical trials in healthy subjects and in patients with transfusion-dependent thrombocytopenia (hypoproliferative thrombocytopenia, due to cytotoxic chemotherapy and hematopoietic stem cell transplantation (HSCT) for malignancy). Ten clinical trials have involved 34 healthy subjects and 886 patients. Patients aged 6 years and older were enrolled in these trials. Children younger than 6 years of age and pregnant women were not studied. All trials evaluated platelets stored for up to 5 days, the approved storage duration in the USA and most of Europe. One trial studied platelets stored for 7 days, the storage duration approved in some European countries (Belgium, Nordic countries, Spain and Ireland), provided bacterial detection or pathogen inactivation systems are used.

Platelet viability was assessed by measurement of recovery and life span of radiolabeled platelets in healthy subjects [13]. Therapeutic efficacy was evaluated in patients requiring multiple platelet transfusions as measured by correction of prolonged bleeding times [14], clinical assessment of hemostasis [15], platelet count increments [16, 17], interval between platelet transfusions, and use of red cell transfusion [15]. Safety was evaluated by assessment of adverse events (including transfusion reactions), evaluation of immunogenicity (including measurement of antibodies directed against potential amotosalen neoantigens on platelets and plasma proteins [18]), lymphocytotoxic antibodies, and clinical platelet refractoriness. Amotosalen levels in healthy subjects and patient plasma post transfusion were also measured. Evaluation of INTERCEPT platelets in this clinical trial program provided a rigorous assessment of therapeutic efficacy and safety since these patients had multiple transfusion episodes over the course of weeks to months. In addition to the clinical development program, an active post-marketing hemovigilance program has been initiated. The

IBSP received CE Mark registration in May 2002 and is approved for use in the European Union. Subsequent national marketing authorizations have been approved in France (2005) and Germany (2007).

Efficacy of Buffy Coat INTERCEPT Platelets in Patients with Platelet Transfusion-Dependent Thrombocytopenia: Phase 3 Trial euroSPRITE

Two phase 3 trials were conducted in Europe to evaluate the efficacy and safety of INTERCEPT platelets in thrombocytopenic patients requiring multiple platelet transfusions. A randomized, controlled, double-blind, pivotal phase 3 trial (euroSPRITE) of buffy coat platelets was conducted in 103 patients at sites in four European centers to evaluate the efficacy and safety of INTERCEPT platelets as prepared and transfused in clinical practice [16]. Patients with thrombocytopenia due to cytotoxic chemotherapy with or without HSCT and expected to require one or more platelet transfusions were randomized to receive all of their transfusions with either INTERCEPT platelets or control platelets for up to 56 days or until platelet independence, whichever occurred first. Patients who continued to require or had a subsequent need for platelet transfusions while the trial was still open for enrollment were eligible to receive a second cycle of study platelet transfusions of the same maximum duration (56 days), maintaining the same treatment assignment as in the first cycle.

The study design was modeled using data from the Trial to Reduce Alloimmunization to Platelets (TRAP) Study [19]. The primary endpoints were 1-h CI (count increment) and 1-h CCI (corrected count increment; i.e. adjusted for transfused platelet dose and body mass). These endpoints included only the first eight transfusions in cycle 1 to avoid confounding factors (i.e. decreased recipient response following multiple transfusions), which might render interpretation of the results more difficult [20]. Since CCI is a ratio measure that does not take into account other covariates that might affect count increment, longitudinal regression analysis of the primary endpoint including all platelet transfusions was also conducted.

This phase 3 trial was designed to characterize relevant potential differences between INTERCEPT and control platelets in 1-h post-transfusion CI and CCI. Sample size and power calculations were based on the TRAP trial. Using a 0.5 level two-sided test, a sample size of 100 was estimated to provide a power of 80% to detect a difference in CCI of 2.8×10^3 and a difference in CI of $8.0 \times 10^9/l$ between INTERCEPT and control platelets.

The overall sample size of 103 patients is relatively small for a demonstration of therapeutic efficacy. A surrogate endpoint of platelet efficacy, the post-transfusion 1-h CI and CCI, was used based on the rationale that this endpoint is used in routine clinical practice. 103 patients were transfused with 676 study transfusions in cycle 1; 54 patients were randomized to the INTERCEPT group and 52 to the control group. Only 75% of patients completed the 56-day transfusion period. More patients assigned to the INTERCEPT group completed (83%) than in the control group (67%, p = 0.05). The patients had a broad spectrum of diagnoses, treatments, and duration of platelet transfusion-dependent thrombocytopenia. Too few patients were enrolled in cycle 2 (n = 12) to draw any meaningful conclusions from these data.

One of the difficulties in conducting a trial with a labile blood product with maximum storage duration of 5 days when all platelet transfusions given to a patient need to be study transfusions is maintenance of an adequate supply of study platelets. This was evidenced in this trial by the high rate of 'off-protocol' transfusions (20% of INTERCEPT transfusions and 10% of control transfusions). It should be noted that the longitudinal regression analysis specifically excluded these off-protocol transfusions since platelet dose data were not collected for 'off-protocol' transfusions.

A proportion of transfusions (13% INTERCEPT and 7% control) did not have at least one 1-h (or 24-h) platelet count performed and therefore could not have one or more 1-h (or 24-h) CI or CCI calculated.

A total of 103 patients received one or more transfusions of INTERCEPT platelets (311 transfusions) or control platelets (256 transfusions) which were pooled, leukoreduced and stored for up to 5 days. More than 50% of PCs were stored for 4–5 days prior to transfusion. One primary endpoint was negative (1-h CI, p = 0.02) and the other was not significantly different for the first 8 transfusions (1-h CCI, p = 0.12). The planned longitudinal regression analysis demonstrated that there was an average decrease in the 1-h CI of $1.5 \times 10^9/l$ (95% confidence interval $-3.6 \times 10^9/l$); for equivalent platelet doses, INTERCEPT and control transfusions provided similar 1-h CI. INTERCEPT transfusion doses were significantly lower than control transfusion doses. These lower doses had an effect on the mean number of platelet transfusions over the entire transfusion period and the interval between platelet transfusions, although none of these reached statistical significance, perhaps due to the limited sample size. Despite the lower platelet doses, hemostasis was similar between the two groups. Despite limitations in clinical trial design to assess hemostasis and the use of surrogate endpoints, the 1-h CI and 24-h CI for comparable doses were not different to that for conventional PCs. Clinical hemostasis, hemorrhagic adverse events, and overall adverse events were not different between the two treatment groups.

To confirm the results of the pivotal phase 3 euroSPRITE trial of INTERCEPT buffy coat platelets conducted using the clinical prototype of the device, a small supplemental trial was performed as a 'bioequivalence' trial to demonstrate the comparability of the commercial prototype with the clinical prototype. The trial was appropriately designed to demonstrate non-inferiority. Processing parameters showed comparability or improvement with the commercial device.

Efficacy of Apheresis INTERCEPT Platelets in Patients with Platelet
Transfusion-Dependent Thrombocytopenia: Phase 3 Trial SPRINT

A pivotal phase 3 trial was conducted in the USA [15]. The trial was performed using apheresis platelets collected on the Amicus blood separator (Fenwal Inc., Round Lake, IL, USA) and prepared using the clinical prototype of the device. The trial was designed to evaluate the efficacy of INTERCEPT platelets assessed by prevention and treatment of clinically relevant bleeding during a period of platelet support. This study was a randomized, controlled, double-blind trial conducted at 12 study sites in the USA. INTERCEPT and control platelets were prepared at each of the 12 study site blood banks and stored under routine blood bank conditions for up to 5 days [15]. Platelet transfusion-dependent thrombocytopenic patients, 6 years and older, were randomized in a 1:1 ratio to receive INTERCEPT or control platelet transfusions, as clinically indicated for up to 28 days. Patients who continued to require or resumed the need for platelet transfusion while the trial was open for enrollment were eligible to receive a second cycle of study transfusion support, maintaining the same treatment assignment as in the first cycle. This second cycle was included to provide additional exposure to INTERCEPT platelets and to determine the incidence of any potential delayed immune response to amotosalen neoantigens on INTERCEPT platelets. The primary endpoint of the trial was the proportion of patients with grade 2 bleeding, measured using a modification of the World Health Organization (WHO) bleeding scale. The trial was designed to demonstrate non-inferiority for the primary endpoint, using a non-inferiority margin of 12.5%. The proportion of patients with grade 3 or 4 bleeding was also analyzed using non-inferiority testing, with a margin of 7%. All other endpoints were analyzed for difference at a significance level of 0.05. Based on data from the TRAP Study, a prevalence of 25% was used as an estimate of the proportion of patients with grade 2 bleeding during a typical period of platelet support [19]. A sample size of 300 patients in each treatment group provided 97% power to reject inferiority if there was no difference between treatment groups. The proportion of patients with grade 3 or 4 bleeding was estimated to be 7%.

This pivotal phase 3 trial was well designed and well conducted. It was appropriately designed as a non-inferiority trial to demonstrate that INTERCEPT platelets, when given repeatedly over up to 28 days, were not inferior to conventional control platelets for prevention or treatment of bleeding. The primary endpoint selected was clinically relevant, measuring therapeutic benefit of platelets to control bleeding in severely thrombocytopenic patients. It is the largest trial conducted to date to measure the hemostatic efficacy of platelet transfusions. Multiple secondary endpoints that are surrogate measures of platelet efficacy were also measured. A second identical period of platelet support was included to permit evaluation of patients requiring additional platelet transfusion. Margins for non-inferiority were selected based on rates of bleeding reported in the literature and seem appropriate. The modification of the WHO bleeding scale was used to provide more objective measures of bleeding at 8 anatomic sites. For both treatment groups, more than 90% of platelet transfusions were ordered as prophylactic transfusions based on the daily platelet count. There were few protocol violations for a trial of this size and complexity, and more than 90% of study platelet transfusions were prepared according to protocol. The primary endpoint of the trial was met: The proportion of patients with grade 2 bleeding in cycle 1 was not inferior for the INTERCEPT group compared to the control group, well within the pre-specified non-inferiority margin of 12.5%. The proportion of patients with grade 3 or 4 bleeding in cycle 1 was not inferior for the INTERCEPT group compared to the control group, well within the pre-specified non-inferiority margin of 7%. Numerous other secondary endpoints of hemostasis supported this conclusion, both for cycle 1 and cycle 2; however, there was a statistically significant difference (0.7 day) in mean number of days of grade 2 bleeding, favoring the control group.

Control of hemostasis by INTERCEPT platelets was notable because the 1-h and 24-h CI and CCI were significantly lower for the INTERCEPT group, primarily due to the lower dose of platelets per transfusion for the INTERCEPT group. The mean number of platelet transfusions per patient was greater for the INTERCEPT group than for the control group by an average of 2.2 transfusions, and the mean interval between transfusions was shorter by 0.5 days for the INTERCEPT group compared to the control group. These differences are all likely due to the fact that the platelet dose per transfusion was significantly lower for INTERCEPT platelets. A post-study analysis was conducted to evaluate the impact of consistency of platelet dose on the number of platelet transfusions [21]. When the number of platelet transfusions per treatment group was compared for all patients receiving PCs containing $>3.0 \times 10^{11}$ platelets, the recommended dose in the USA, no differences in the number of platelet transfusions per treatment group was detected. In this analysis, other endpoints, except for platelet count increments, were not different between the treatment groups. This analysis was not part of the planned analysis, but did demonstrate the impact of platelet dose on the number of platelet transfusions. In addition, since the longitudinal regression analysis for post-transfusion platelet counts indicated that for equal platelet doses there was still a significant effect of PCT, there seems to be some loss of viability of platelets due to the PCT process. Nevertheless, although there are some statistically significant between-group differences, the values observed are clinically acceptable and were sufficient to maintain comparable hemostasis for patients supported with INTERCEPT platelets. The impact of platelet utilization needs to be studied further in routine practice where platelet doses can be managed more consistently.

To confirm the results of the pivotal phase 3 euroSPRITE trial of INTERCEPT buffy coat conducted using the clinical prototype of the device, and to obtain data for INTERCEPT platelets collected by apheresis prepared with the commercial prototype device, a small supplemental trial with apheresis platelets was conducted in Europe. It was a randomized, controlled, double-blind phase 3 trial conducted at 3 European study sites [17]. Trial design and population closely mirrored that of previous phase 3 trials, with the same design modifications implemented in the supplemental phase

3 buffy coat trial, with a 28-day transfusion period, 7-day safety surveillance period, and a single cycle of transfusion support. Platelet transfusion-dependent thrombocytopenic patients were randomized in a 1:1 ratio to transfusion with INTERCEPT platelets prepared with the commercial prototype of the device or conventional control platelets, both collected by apheresis using the Amicus blood separator and stored for up to 5 days. As in the other European trials, 1-h CI and 1-h CCI for the first eight transfusions were selected as co-primary endpoints, and longitudinal regression analysis, using the same parameters as used in the previous euroSPRITE trial, was also performed for this endpoint. The trial was designed to characterize any potential differences between INTERCEPT and control platelets. Sample size and power estimates were based on the first 61 patients randomized in the USA phase 3 SPRINT trial with apheresis INTERCEPT platelets. Using two-sided t tests and an alpha of 0.05, a sample size of 20 patients in each group was estimated to provide 80% power to detect a difference in mean 1-h CI of $13.6 \times 10^9/l$ and a difference in mean 1-h CCI of 5.25×10^3 between INTERCEPT and control platelets. Secondary endpoints were those studied in previous trials. No statistically significant differences in either of the two co-primary endpoints were detected, although all CIs were lower for INTERCEPT platelets. No significant differences between treatment groups were observed for any of the secondary endpoints. In fact, data were somewhat better for the INTERCEPT group than the control group for most of these endpoints, perhaps because the INTERCEPT group received a slightly higher mean dose of platelets per transfusion than the control group (4.1×10^{11} vs. 3.8×10^{11} platelets per transfusion, p = 0.28). This trial met all of its primary endpoints, showing no difference between INTERCEPT platelets collected on the Amicus blood separator and prepared with the commercial prototype and conventional control platelets. However, analysis by longitudinal regression was marginally significant, showing that the 1-h platelet count was $7.2 \times 10^9/l$ lower for the INTERCEPT group than the control group (p = 0.05 for treatment difference). No differences in secondary endpoints were observed, perhaps reflecting improved INTERCEPT platelet dose in this trial. With the caveat that the statistical design was a difference rather than non-inferiority testing, this was a positive trial demonstrating no difference in efficacy between INTERCEPT platelets prepared with the commercial prototype and conventional control platelets.

Clinical Experience with Transfusion of Pathogen-Inactivated Platelet Concentrates in France

Operational Experience in Preparing INTERCEPT Platelets at EFS-Alsace

The final commercial IBSP included a closed integrated processing disposable set of the following containers: amotosalen, illumination, compound adsorption device (CAD) to remove residual amotosalen and free photo-products, and a storage container. Two processing set configurations are available: the large-volume (300–390 ml) and the small-volume set (255–325 ml). The platelet dose range for the large-volume platelet set was expanded from 2.5×10^{11} to 6.0×10^{11} platelets to 2.5×10^{11} to 7.0×10^{11} platelets.

INTERCEPT platelets can be prepared under blood bank conditions while meeting processing specifications. Processing parameters which were out of range were corrected with additional experience as the clinical trial program progressed. Although there is some loss of platelets following PCT, the loss is relatively small, should be minimized outside of the clinical trial setting where platelet unit samples were mandated, and should not compromise the clinical efficacy of transfusion with INTERCEPT platelets. Numerous process validation studies conducted at blood banks across Europe using the commercial device show that processing parameters can consistently be achieved and platelet loss can be reduced to less than 10% [22].

In France, the French National Transfusion Service (EFS) comprising 17 EFS regional centers has the responsibility for providing a safe and adequate blood supply and for preparing blood components. Over the last decade, EFS-Alsace, one of the regional centers, has gained extensive experience with pathogen inactivation of PCs and plasma. The President of EFS decided that this center should play a role as a pilot center for implementation of pathogen inactivation in France in testing new inactivation techniques, in providing resources to implement pathogen inactivation in other regional EFS centers, and as a region converted to use inactivation of PC and plasma for 100% of production.

Implementation of INTERCEPT Platelets during Epidemics in Overseas EFS Regional Centers

In May 2006, EFS implemented the IBSP for 100% of apheresis PCs in the EFS-Ile de La Réunion to provide safe PCs during the Chikungunya virus epidemic [23]. The technology was successfully introduced and enabled the provision of platelets that otherwise were unavailable because blood collection was stopped. Implementation and training of the personnel took 2 weeks. After implementation, the production of 100 APCs per month was better standardized. The average yield of platelets per APC unit was $4.2 \pm 0.4 \times 10^{11}$ and the average processing loss was 7.8%. Introduction of INTERCEPT PC had no impact on platelet utilization and reduced the incidence of acute transfusion reactions in all patients including pediatric patients [24, 25]. No cases of transfusion-transmitted Chikungunya virus were reported following more than 2,000 INTERCEPT PC transfusions.

This initial introduction of INTERCEPT PC into routine use was further extended in June 2007 to 2 other overseas regional blood transfusion centers, EFS-Guadeloupe-Guyane and EFS-Martinique, to improve safety in areas with high prevalence of Dengue virus and *Trypanosoma cruzi*.

EFS-Alsace had prior substantial experience with photochemical pathogen inactivation, and in particular with IBSP. The decision to implement IBSP was driven by medical, operational and economic considerations and made possible the following approval of the technology by AFSSAPS (Agence française de sécurité sanitaire des produits de santé) in 2005. Previously, during clinical development, randomized controlled trials were conducted in collaboration with the EFS-Alsace to evaluate IBSP. These studies demonstrated acceptable efficacy and safety of apheresis and buffy coat leukoreduced PCs when transfused to hematology-oncology patients [16, 17]. Therapeutic INTERCEPT plasma was also introduced into routine use in Alsace. A large-scale validation pilot roll-out and hemovigilance study is presently going on in the EFS-Alsace region, which provides about 15,000 doses of PCs per year to regional hospitals and clinics in the Alsace region serving approximately 2 million inhabitants. EFS-Alsace initiated implementation of IBSP for 100% of PC production starting in July 2006. The first phase of the program was to optimize the PC production process and the logistics of implementation into routine use. All components are prepared in process in the central facility of EFS-Alsace in Strasbourg. PCs derived from apheresis collections (MCS+ CSDP; Haemonetics, Braintree, MA, USA) or pooled whole blood BCPCs (Baxter Transfusion Therapies, La Châtre, France) were leukoreduced and suspended in approximately 35% plasma and 65% Intersol™, treated with IBSP, and distributed to hospitals and clinics for transfusion according to conventional medical indications. For quality control of production, residual amotosalen levels were measured by high-pressure liquid chromatography in 1% of PCs. Serologic and nucleic acid tests for HIV, hepatitis B virus (HBV), hepatitis C virus (HCV), human T lymphotrophic virus (HTLV), and *Treponema pallidum* were performed according to conventional EFS standard operating procedures. PCs treated with INTERCEPT were available for release 1 day after collection, in the same time frame as previously done for conventional components.

Since implementation, in the period from July 2006 to July 2007, more than 15,000 PCs were prepared with IBPS and issued for transfusion. 62% of the components were BCPCs and 38% were APCs. Of the components distributed, 58% were administered to hematology-oncology patients, 36% to general medical and surgical patients, and 6% to cardiovascular surgery patients. The average dose was $4.3 \pm 0.4 \times 10^{11}$ platelets. The average processing loss was 24 ± 4 ml containing $0.3 \pm 0.07 \times 10^{11}$ platelets ($7.4 \pm 1.2\%$). The average residual amotosalen level was < 0.5 µM, well below the specified threshold of 2.0 µM.

EFS-Alsace has 100% traceability for issued PCs. Longitudinal records of component use by patients is recorded and maintained in an electronic database. The platelet content of each PC is determined prior to release for transfusion. After introduction of the IBSP, the utilization of PCs was measured and compared for prior 1-year pe-

Table 1. Platelet concentrates prepared in plasma or treated by INTERCEPT transfused to all patients hospitalized in the Alsace region during 2 retrospective 1-year periods

	PC (100% plasma) 1/1/2003 – 1/2/2004 99.6%	INTERCEPT PC (35% plasma + 65% Intersol) 1/9/2006 – 1/8/2007 99%
Patients, n	2,050	2,069
Age (years), median (range)	61 (<1–94)	63 (<1–96)
Onco-hematology, cardiac surgery, general medicine and surgery, % of patients	56, 7, 37	58, 6, 36
PC transfused, n	10,629	13,241
PC transfused, mean / patient	5.2	6.4
PC transfused, median (range) / patient	2.0 (1–104)	2.0 (1–289)
PC mean dose plt × 1,011 / patient	26.9	27.0
PC median dose (range) plt × 1,011 / patient	10.4 (0.2–450)	8.4 (0.5–1149)
RBCC, mean / patient	14.4	13.5
ATR^c, % of patients	2.9%	1.7%
ATR / 1,000 PC	5.3	1.4

plt = Platelets; RBCC = red blood cell concentrates; ATR = acute transfusion reactions.

riods with conventional components. During each of the observation periods, approximately 2,000 patients received one or more PCs (table 1). Due to changes in production processes to unify the platelet dose of apheresis and whole blood PCs, the average dose of platelet per unit was slightly decreased. The mean number of inactivated PC units transfused (6.4 per patient) was comparable to that of conventional PCs (5.2 per patient). In both cases, the median number of units transfused was 2 per patient. The total INTERCEPT dose of IBSP platelets required per patient was 26.9 × 10^{11} platelets and identical to reference PCs in plasma, 27.0 × 10^{11} platelets. Thus, no increase in platelet utilization was observed during a 1-year period.

Adverse events after transfusion were monitored according to the mandatory EFS hemovigilance program [26]. Acute transfusion reactions (1.7%) attributed to IBSP PCs were less than that experienced with conventional PCs suspended in plasma (2.9%). No cases of transfusion-associated sepsis or transfusion-related mortality were reported. One case of non-fatal (grade 3) transfusion-related acute lung injury (TRALI) was associated with the transfusion of an APC treated with INTERCEPT from a multi-parous donor with high-titer human leukocyte antigen (HLA) antibodies. IBSPs were well accepted by clinicians.

The impact on logistics was evaluated after the first year of experience. IBSP was implemented in a regional blood center without impacting the time of release of PCs (median distribution between 2.3 and 2.9 days). Use of IBSP avoided implementation of bacterial detection and the use of gamma irradiation and cytomegalovirus (CMV) serology. Provided that transfusion centers are prepared to change some of their current practices based on the additional layer of safety provided by pathogen inactivation, it is possible to minimize the cost of implementing INTERCEPT in France by preparing a mix of apheresis and buffy coat PCs. This cost-based analysis is applicable to other countries. In conclusion, transfusion of PCs treated with INTERCEPT to a broad patient population for a spectrum of indications was well tolerated in routine practice. The incidence of adverse events was less than that previously reported when untreated PCs suspended in plasma or additive solution were transfused to a similar patient population. IBSP offers the potential to improve the safety and availability of PCs for transfusion and can facilitate the expansion of the donor pool. Studies have demonstrated that the technology can replace older technology, improve the supply of PCs through reduced wastage, and be implemented with minimal impact on blood center or blood donor resources.

An Active European Hemovigilance Program Characterizing the Safety Profile of INTERCEPT Platelet Transfusions

Inactivation of pathogens and leukocytes in PCs using IBSP is in routine use in some European blood centers. An active hemovigilance program (HV1) was implemented [11], as a prospective observational cohort study to document and characterize the safety profile of INTERCEPT APCs and INTERCEPT BCPCs in a broad patient population treated in hospitals located in Belgium, Norway and Spain. Blood centers were requested to complete a safety data form after each transfusion, regardless of outcome. Data for 5106 INTERCEPT PCs administered to 651 patients were monitored. A total of 5,051 (98.9%) transfusions and 609 (93.5%) patients had no reported reactions. 55 transfusions (1.1%) were associated with adverse events, and 42 (0.8%) were possibly related, probably related or related to the PC transfusion. Adverse events occurred in 42 (6.4%) patients, but in only 32 (4.9%) patients was a causal relationship to PC transfusion established. One reaction was serious, and no deaths were related to PC transfusion. Among the transfusion reactions, the most frequent clinical events in descending frequency were chills, fever, dermatologic reactions, dyspnea, nausea or vomiting, and hypotension. No episodes of TRALI were reported. In this cohort study, INTERCEPT PC exhibited a safety profile similar to that previously reported for conventional PC.

An additional hemovigilance (HV2) cohort study of 7,437 APC and BCPC leukoreduced INTERCEPT-treated transfusions was reported from centers in Belgium, France and Spain, that completed similar data forms after transfusion [12]. Although no specific time for observation was required, the focus of the study was on response to transfusion occurring within the first 24 h of transfusion. Adverse reactions occurring at any time could be reported. A total of 7,437 platelet transfusions were administered to 1,400 patients. The mean age of the patients was 57 (range 0–96) years. The majority (73.5%) of the patients had hemato-oncology disorders and required conventional chemotherapy (60.3%) or stem cell transplants (13.2%). Platelet transfusions associated with related adverse events following INTERCEPT PC transfusions were infrequent (n = 55, 0.7%) and most reactions were of grade 1 (absence of immediate or long-term life-threatening medical conditions). 45 patients (3.2%) experienced at least one event following one or more INTERCEPT PC transfusions, 39 (2.8%) of which were classified as 'related' (possibly related, probably related, or related) to the INTERCEPT platelet transfusion. The events were generally representative of the events expected with platelet transfusions. The most frequently reported signs or symptoms were chills, fever, urticaria, nausea, and vomiting. Only 5 events were considered as severe (grade 2 or more); however, no causal relationship to INTERCEPT PC transfusion was found. Furthermore, repeated exposure to INTERCEPT platelets did not appear to increase the likelihood of a transfusion reaction. No cases of TRALI and no deaths due to an INTERCEPT transfusion were reported. In this cohort study, 99.3% of INTERCEPT PC transfusions were without reported acute transfusion reactions. Only 2.8% of the patients with reported adverse reactions had a possibly related, probably related or related attribution to PC transfusions. These results are in line with those reported in the HV1 study and further suggest that transfusion of INTERCEPT PC is well tolerated, in routine use, in a wide range of patients. Adverse events following INTERCEPT platelet transfusions classified as related to transfusion were infrequent and most were of mild severity.

Conclusions and Future Directions

Technology for the inactivation of pathogens and leukocytes in PCs has been developed and approved for routine clinical practice by multiple European regulatory agencies including AFSSAPS and the Paul-Ehrlich Institute (PEI). The technology has been evaluated in a number of blood centers since 2003 to determine the impact on logistics, component utilization, patient safety, and economics. The experience with routine use in multiple centers using different methods for collection and preparation of PCs by whole blood or apheresis methods has confirmed that the technology can be deployed with minimal impact on logistics and component utilization. Prospective observational hemovigilance studies have demonstrated an excellent safety profile in broad and diverse patient populations. Importantly, the incidence of acute transfusion reactions has been further reduced with the use of PCs treated with pathogen inactivation. In addition, older technologies such as bacterial detection, gamma irradiation, and CMV serology have been replaced to reduce the cost impact of the adoption of pathogen inactivation. This technology is consistent with the prior use of pathogen inactivation of plasma components and plasma derivatives and further expands the use of proactive measures to improve the safety of platelet transfusion with improved outcomes for patients.

Disclosure of Conflict of Interests

J.-P.C. has acted as a consultant for Cerus, has been on an Advisory Board for Cerus and Gambro/Navigant and has received research grants from Cerus, Gambro/Navigant and Macopharma.

Acknowledgements

The authors are indebted to their clinical colleagues and particularly to Professor R. Herbrecht and Dr. B. Lioure from the Onco-Hematology Department at the Hôpital de Hautepierre, Strasbourg, France, for their continuous help and collaboration.

References

1 Jones KE, Patel NG, Levy MA, Storeygard A, Balk D, Gittleman JL, Daszak P: Global trends in emerging infectious diseases. Nature 2008;451:990–994.

2 Allain JP, Bianco C, Blajchman MA, Brecher ME, Busch M, Leiby D, Lin L, Stramer S: Protecting the blood supply from emerging pathogens; the role of pathogen inactivation. Transfus Med Rev 2005;19:110–126.

3 Terpstra FG, van't Wout AB, Schuitemaker H, van Engelenburg FA, Dekkers DW, Verhaar R, de Korte D, Verhoeven AJ: Potential and limitation of UVC irradiation for the inactivation of pathogens in platelet concentrates. Transfusion 2008;48:304–313.

4 Reddy HL, Dayan AD, Cavagnaro J, Gad S, Li J, Goodrich RP: Toxicity testing of a novel riboflavin-based technology for pathogen reduction and white blood cell inactivation. Transfus Med Rev 2008;22:133–153.

5 Goodrich RP, Edrich RA, Li J, Seghatchian J: The Mirasol PRT system for pathogen reduction of platelets and plasma: An overview of current status and future trends. Transfus Apheresis Sci 2006;35:5–17.

6 Wollowitz S: Fundamentals of the psoralen-based Helinx technology for inactivation of infectious pathogens and leukocytes in platelets and plasma. Semin Hematol 2001;38(suppl 11):4–11.

7 Lin L, Cook DN, Wiesehahn GP, Alfonso R, Behrman B, Cimino GD, Corten L, Damonte PB, Dikeman R, Dupuis K, Fang YM, Hanson CV, Hearst JE, Lin CY, Londe HF, Metchette K, Nerio AT, Pu JT, Reames AA, Rheinschmidt M, Tessman J, Isaacs ST, Wollowitz S, Corash L: Photochemical inactivation of viruses and bacteria in platelet concentrates by use of a novel psoralen and long-wavelength ultraviolet light. Transfusion 1997;37:423–435.

8 Lin L, Dikeman R, Molini B, Lukehart SA, Lane R, Dupuis K, Metzel P, Corash L: Photochemical treatment of platelet concentrates with amotosalen and UVA inactivates a broad spectrum of pathogenic bacteria. Transfusion 2004;44:1496–1504.

9 Lin L, Hanson CV, Alter HJ, Jauvin V, Bernard KA, Murthy KK, Metzel P, Corash L: Inactivation of viruses in platelet concentrates by photochemical treatment with amotosalen and long-wavelength ultraviolet light. Transfusion 2005;45:580–590.

10 Ciaravino V, McCullough T, Cimino G: The role of toxicology assessment in transfusion medicine. Transfusion 2003;43:1481–1492.

11 Osselaer JC, Messe N, Hervig T, Bueno J, Castro E, Espinosa A, Accorsi P, Junge K, Jacquet M, Flament J, Corash L: A prospective observational cohort safety study of 5,106 platelet transfusions using components prepared with photochemial pathogen inactivation treatment. Transfusion 2008;48:1061–1071.

12 Osselaer JC, Cazenave JP, Lambermont M, Garraud O, Hidajat M, Barbolla L, Tardivel R, Defoin L, Waller C, Mendel I, Raidot JP, Kandel G, De Meuter R, Fabrigli P, Dehenau D, Arroyo JL, Padrón F, Gouezec H, Corral M, Jacquet M, Sundin D, Lin L, Corash L: An active haemovigilance programme characterizing the safety profile of 7437 platelet transfusions prepared with amotosalen photochemical treatment. Vox Sang 2008;94:315–323.

13 Snyder E, Raife T, Lin L, Cimino G, Metzel P, Rheinschmidt M, Baril L, Davis K, Buchholz DH, Corash L, Conlan MG: Recovery and lifespan of 111indium radiolabeled platelets treated with pathogen inactivation using amotosalen HCl (S-59) and UVA light. Transfusion 2004;44:1732–1740.

14 Slichter SJ, Raife TJ, Davis K, Rheinschmidt M, Buchholz DH, Corash L, Conlan MG: Platelets photochemically treated with amotosalen HCl and ultraviolet A light correct prolonged bleeding times in patients with thrombocytopenia. Transfusion 2006;46:731–740.

15 McCullough J, Vesole DH, Benjamin RJ, Slichter SJ, Pineda A, Snyder E, Stadtmauer EA, Lopez-Plaza I, Coutre S, Strauss RG, Goodnough LT, Fridey JL, Raife T, Cable R, Murphy S, Howard F 4th, Davis K, Lin JS, Metzel P, Corash L, Koutsoukos A, Lin L, Buchholz DH, Conlan MG: Therapeutic efficacy and safety of platelets treated with a photochemical process for pathogen inactivation: the SPRINT Trial. Blood 2004;104:1534–1541.

16 van Rhenen DJ, Gulliksson H, Cazenave JP, Pamphilon D, Ljungman P, Klüter H, Vermeij H, Kappers-Klunne M, de Greef G, Laforet M, Lioure B, Davis K, Marblie S, Mayaudon V, Flament J, Conlan M, Lin L, Metzel P, Buchholz M, Corash L; euroSPRITE trial: Transfusion of pooled buffy coat platelet components prepared with photochemical pathogen inactivation treatment: the euroSPRITE trial. Blood 2003;101:2426–2433.

17 Janetzko K, Cazenave JP, Klüter H, Kientz D, Michel M, Beris P, Lioure B, Hastka J, Marblie S, Mayaudon V, Lin L, Lin JS, Conlan MG, Flament J: Therapeutic efficacy and safety of photochemically treated apheresis platelets processed with an optimized integrated set. Transfusion 2005;45:1443–1452.

18 Lin L, Conlan MG, Tessman J, Cimino G, Porter S: Amotosalen interactions with platelet and plasma components: absence of neoantigen formation after photochemical treatment. Transfusion 2005;45:1610–1620.

19 The Trial to Reduce Alloimmunization to Platelets Study Group (TRAP Study Group): Leukocyte reduction and ultraviolet B irradiation of platelets to prevent alloimmunization and refractoriness to platelet transfusions. N Engl J Med 1997;337:1861–1869.

20 Slichter SJ, Davis K, Enright H, Braine H, Gernsheimer T, Kao KJ, Kickler T, Lee E, McFarland J, McCullough J, Rodey G, Schiffer CA, Woodson R: Factors affecting post transfusion platelet increments, platelet refractoriness, and platelet transfusion intervals in thrombocytopenic patients. Blood 2005;105:4106–4114.

21 Murphy S, Snyder E, Cable R, Slichter SJ, Strauss RG, McCullough J, Lin JS, Corash L, Conlan MG; SPRINT Study Group: Platelet dose consistency and its effect on the number of platelet transfusions for support of thrombocytopenia: an analysis of the SPRINT trial of platelets photochemically treated with amotosalen HCl and ultraviolet A light. Transfusion 2006;46:24–33.

22 Webert KE, Cserti CM, Hannon J, Lin Y, Pavenski K, Pendergrast JM, Blajchman MA: Proceedings of a consensus conference: pathogen inactivation – making decisions about new technologies. Transfus Med Rev 2008;22:1–34.

23 Brouard C, Bernillon P, Quatresous I, Pillonel J, Assal A, De Valk H, Desenclos JC: Estimated risk of Chikungunya viremic blood donation during an epidemic on Reunion Island in the Indian Ocean, 2005 to 2007. Transfusion 2008, DOI: 10.1111/j.1537–2995.2008.01646.x.

24 Angelini-Tibert MF, Currie C, Slaedts M, Corash LM, Rasongles P: Safety of platelet components prepared with photochemical treatment (INTERCEPT) transfused to pediatric oncology-hematology patients. Transfusion 2007;43(S3):22A.

25 Rasongles P, Isola H, Kientz D, Cazenave JP, Sawyer L, Corash L: Rapid implementation of photochemical pathogen inactivation (INTERCEPT) for preparation of platelet components during an epidemic of Chikungunya virus. Vox Sang 2006;91(suppl 3):32.

26 Andreu G, Morel P, Forestier F, Rebibo D, Janvier G, Herve P: Hemovigilance network in France: organization and analysis of immediate transfusion incident reports from 1994–1998. Transfusion 2002;42:1356–1364.

Prof. Dr. med. Jean-Pierre Cazenave
EFS-Alsace
10, rue Spielmann, BP 36
67065 Strasbourg Cedex, France
Tel. +33 3 88212525, Fax -21
E-Mail jeanpierre.cazenave@efs-alsace.fr

Scharf RE (ed): Progress and Challenges in Transfusion Medicine, Hemostasis and Hemotherapy.
Freiburg i.Br., Karger, 2008, pp 264–273

Acute Bleeding Complications: Pathophysiology, Diagnosis and Management

Michael Spannagl

Transfusion Medicine and Hemostasis, Munich University Hospital, Munich, Germany

Key Words

Bleeding · Hemostasis · Point-of-care testing · Predictive factors · Coagulopathy · Thromboelastography · Hyperfibrinolysis

Summary

Due to its major importance for additional hospital costs but also for outcome, acute bleeding is discussed and investigated in several clinical disciplines. Significant predictive measures for bleeding complications can only be obtained by combining acute clinical signs, anamnestic information and laboratory results. Near-patient testing of whole blood coagulation and fibrinolysis has gained increasing importance. Still, global assessment of blood smear and clotting remains as a basic tool. Several hemostyptic agents and cellular and plasma products are available for treatment. Further studies should answer the question whether selective application of these compounds according to the patients' hemostatic disturbances is superior to unsighted application of cellular concentrates and fresh frozen plasma.

©2008 S. Karger GmbH, Freiburg i.Br.

Introduction

Unexpected coagulopathies still remain as a diagnostic and therapeutic challenge. Risk factors and reasons behind unexplained bleeding are heterogeneous and multifactorial. Bleeding most frequently occurs during and after surgical intervention or trauma (fig. 1), i.e. in situations where trauma and secondary alterations (e.g. hemodilution) are added to the disposition of the patient. Furthermore, it must not be forgotten that uncontrolled surgical bleeding may also lead to a dilution coagulopathy sooner or later because of the increasing loss of coagulation factors and blood cells. Today acute bleeding may also be induced by interventional procedures performed in non-surgical departments (invasive endoscopic, intravascular procedures). Therefore, prediction and, if necessary, management of acute bleeding is of general interest.

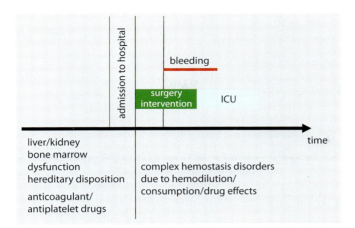

Fig. 1. Surgical intervention as the trigger for acute bleeding.

During such complex hemostasis disorders, near-patient testing and treatment algorithms have been added to unsighted therapy and need further validation.

Typically bleeding complications present in clinical routine associated with interventional procedures. This is not only because of the more frequent clinical use of established substances with antithrombotic effects (platelet inhibitors, coagulation inhibitors) but also due to the fact that indications for the transfusion of fresh frozen plasma (FFP) and platelet concentrate (PC) are being questioned more closely [1]. This is not just on medical grounds – because of the not inconsiderable adverse effects [2–4] – but also for reasons of economics [5].

Several blood components and hemostyptic agents are available for management of acute bleeding. Inappropriate polytherapy, however, is not acceptable and should be avoided. In most cases, only the right medication in the appropriate dose helps the patients. This leads to a general interest in improvement of the diagnostic and therapeutic approach to actively bleeding patients [6]. Some debate exists about suitable methods, which reflect hemostasis during these complex processes. In particular, near-patient testing is used more and more. Before discussing concepts for diagnosis and management of acute bleeding, it has to be substantiated that surgical bleeding as a major reason of perioperative and periinterventional bleeding must involve the surgeon or interventionalist in the management process.

Bleeding: Outcome, Prediction, Causes

Bleeding, as a major cause of complicated patient history, enhances transfusion requirements (costs, risk of infection or immunization), prolongs surgery (enhances costs, prolongs anesthesia, impairs outcome), causes surgical re-explorations (prolongs intensive care unit (ICU) stay, enhances costs, limits outcome) and makes surgery more difficult (poor visibility of the surgical field).

Periinterventional Bleeding and Outcome

Perioperative and periinterventional bleeding is related to patient outcome. This has been demonstrated in several surgical and interventional disciplines. Large multi-center studies have shown that postoperative bleeding is an independent risk factor for morbidity and mortality after cardiac surgery, especially when re-operation is needed to achieve hemostasis [7, 8]. Furthermore, the number of packed red blood cell units that are regularly infused because of severe surgically induced bleeding is an independent risk factor for mortality in hospital [9] and in long-term survival [10] after a cardiac surgery. The higher morbidity risk from bleeding after cardiac operations is associated with a longer postoperative hospital stay [7] and much higher treatment costs. The significantly increased mortality risk in particular requires safe and effective preventive measures, including surgical arrest of bleeding and differentiated hemostatic treatment with blood products and coagulation factors.

Acute gastrointestinal hemorrhage occurs in postoperative patients and is associated with increased length of hospital stay and mortality. In older hip fracture patients, perioperative acute gastrointestinal hemorrhage occurs in 3.9% of cases and is associated with poor outcome. Several independent risk factors for acute gastrointestinal hemorrhage have been described: pre-existing peptic ulcer, current smoking, use of an antiplatelet agent, use of non-steroidal anti-inflammatory drugs (cyclo-oxygenase-2 inhibitors) and blood group O [11]. Prophylactic use of proton pump inhibitors in patients with risk factors for acute gastrointestinal hemorrhage significantly reduced the incidence of this complication [12].

Also in interventional cardiology and radiology, acute bleeding is associated with poor outcome. Non-modifiable (age, gender, weight, renal insufficiency, anemia) and modifiable risk factors (antithrombotic therapy, percutaneous coronary intervention (PCI) procedure characteristics) have been identified [13]. In general, the traditional attitude of the physician to prefer bleeding (which can easily be substituted by blood components) vs. thromboembolism (which can hardly be detected) is more and more in debate.

Prediction of Bleeding Complications

The predictivity of the routine coagulation parameters prothrombin time (PT), activated partial thromboplastin time (aPTT) and platelet count in interventional medicine is rather weak. From a clinician's view the acute clinical signs as well as any information concerning own or family history of bleeding or thromboembolic events are of utmost importance. Is the patient at increased risk of bleeding because of a congenital or acquired (e.g. through medication) hemostatic disorder?

This question should, of course, be dealt with in the preoperative phase. Careful consideration of clinical signs as well as comprehensive information on comorbidity and comedication (fig. 2) and anamnestic information are necessary. The value of standardized bleeding history has been shown to be of great value in this respect. If there is a positive history, further investigation by a specialized hemostasis laboratory

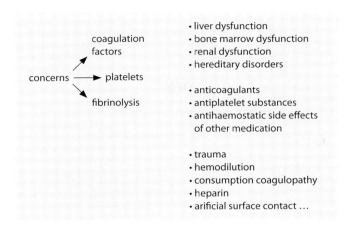

concerns → coagulation factors
- liver dysfunction
- bone marrow dysfunction
- renal dysfunction
- hereditary disorders

platelets
- anticoagulants
- antiplatelet substances
- antihaemostatic side effects of other medication

fibrinolysis
- trauma
- hemodilution
- consumption coagulopathy
- heparin
- arificial surface contact ...

Fig. 2. Comedication and co-morbidity.

should be carried out and, if necessary, specific hemostasis management prescribed in advance.

Knowledge of antiplatelet and/or anticoagulant medication of the patient is of utmost importance. Tailored recommendations for improvement of platelet function (DDAVP, PC) or antagonization of vitamin K antagonist effects (PPSB) or heparin antagonization (protamin) are available.

Causes of Hemostasis Disorders

Hemostasis disorders can have several causes. In most clinical cases, acute bleeding is a multifactorial process involving several components of plasmatic and/or cellular hemostasis (fig. 3). Chronic diseases, such as comorbidities of the hemostasis-related organs (liver, kidney, bone marrow) and hereditary diseases, can be differentiated from more acute alterations due to trauma, inflammation, hemodilution and the current treatment. The resulting alterations affect coagulation factors, platelets and fibrinolytic system. In a registry of patients with chronic subdural hematoma, anticoagulants, antiplatelets, hematologic/neoplastic disease and ethylism were identified as major risk factors [14]. Furthermore, the own and the family history of bleeding complications is of major impact.

Bleeding most frequently occurs during and after surgical interventions or injuries, i.e. in situations where trauma and secondary alterations (e.g. due to hemodilution) are added to the disposition of the patient. During such complex hemostasis disorders, the predictivity of the routine parameters PT, aPTT and platelet count is rather weak. This led to the interest in laboratory methods that better reflect hemostasis during these complex processes.

The majority of hemostasis defects that present intraoperatively and acutely as the result of massive hemorrhage in patients without relevant primary disease are caused by loss, consumption and dilution of blood and can be summarized as dilution coagulopathies. In all these cases, the results of routine tests, PT and aPTT are pathologi-

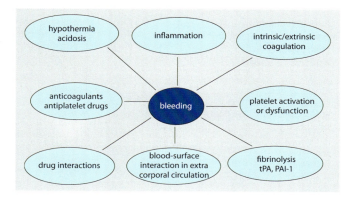

Fig. 3. Multifactorial cause for acute bleeding.

cal at an early stage. In most cases, however, specific consequences cannot be derived from the screening laboratory results.

Although these altered laboratory tests are also indicative of disseminated intravascular coagulation (DIC), the pathogenesis is different. In trauma and in perioperative blood loss, we find a consumption coagulopathy exacerbated by volume replacement, loss and possible acidosis and hypothermia and other metabolic disturbances, not primarily induced by coagulation-activating substances like in classical DIC.

The rationale for hemostasis management in acute bleeding has to be based on the understanding of the pathophysiological processes.

As distinct from a surgical problem, a disorder of hemostasis can rarely be seen directly, so that a picture has to be built up indirectly from the test results and any clinical and anamnestic pathology. Finally, rare bleeding disorders should also be mentioned in this context. Inherited rare bleeding disorders due to single-factor or platelet glycoprotein receptor deficiencies may be of importance, especially if the hemostatic system is altered by trauma or operation.

The development of acquired antibodies to coagulation factors is a typical postoperative complication. Recognition of these patients with rapidly developing bleeding signs and prolonged aPTT is still a major challenge, despite increasing awareness of acquired inhibitors as a cause of acute bleeding. Bad outcome often occurs especially in elderly patients [15]. Recombinant activated factor VII (rFVIIa) or activated prothrombin complex concentrate (FEIBA) have been applied successfully and are licensed for the management of acute bleeding in acquired hemophilia [16].

Analytical Approach

Looking at hemostasis from an analytical point of view, it makes sense to divide the hemostatic process into 4 phases: (1) primary hemostasis (platelet-vessel wall, platelet-platelet interactions), (2) thrombin generation (clotting time), (3) dynamics of clot formation (clot formation and firmness), (4) clot degradation (hyperfibrinolysis).

Primary Hemostasis

Hemostasis has been recognized as a cell-based system. Therefore, diagnostics in whole blood is of major importance. Besides thromboelastography, whole-blood platelet aggregometry is available for near-patient testing. Test systems measuring under conditions of high shear stress have also been introduced. The PFA-100® (platelet function analyzer) system is applied for pre-interventional screening for disturbances of primary hemostasis [17]. Due to a significant impact of red cell and platelet concentration, PFA measurement during acute blood loss is not recommended. Aggregometry methods can be applied to detect the effects of antiplatelet drugs.

Thrombin Generation

Conventional coagulation tests (e.g. PT, aPTT) determine the thrombin generation phase until formation of the first fibrin fibers. In addition, these conventional coagulation parameters are primarily intended to detect agents affecting coagulation (heparin, vitamin K antagonists) or reducing the activity of particular coagulation factors as sensitively as possible. As citrated plasma is generally used for modern coagulation tests, any effects of cellular elements such as platelets, leucocytes and red blood cells are lacking.

Therefore, it is no surprise that these tests mostly fail in diagnosing acute intraoperative and postoperative bleeding [18], so that alternative analytical procedures and supplementary diagnostic methods are being required in this context.

Problems of Classical Coagulation Tests with Perioperative Coagulation Disorders

A number of problems may arise when applying the classical coagulation tests (fig. 4) under conditions of perioperative coagulation disorders: On the one hand hyperfibrinolysis may not be detected, on the other hand false high fibrinogen may be measured in the presence of colloids (like hydroxyethyl starch (HES) or gelatine). Elevated fibrin(ogen) degradation products and heparin may impair clot formation and detection (avoid derived fibrinogen measurement). False long PT and aPTT may be detected in the case of hypofibrinogenemia and afibrinogenemia. In addition, platelet count does not implicate function, and clotting times (e.g. PT, aPTT and thrombin time) only determine the speed of thrombin generation, but not the mechanical stability of the clot. Furthermore, the results of coagulation tests performed in a central laboratory are usually not available before the next 30–60 min in the operating theater.

Clot Formation

Dynamics and maximum extent of clot formation can only be calculated using viscoelastic methods. Thromboelastography is extensively used in perioperative and trauma bleeding. Standard procedures applying cellular and plasma products guided by thromboelastography results have been implemented. Several data show significant cost reduction [19, 20], and the implementation of a therapeutic algorithm (together with near-patient testing) may already have a significant impact.

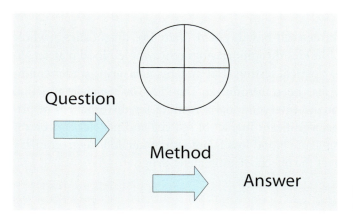

Fig. 4. Problem-related choice of laboratory method.

Hyperfibrinolysis

As a general phenomenon in serious medical conditions, hyperfibrinolysis is much more common than previously assumed. It occurs in peripartal emergencies, in cancer surgery, major trauma, hepatic trauma, and severe pelvic and brain injury. The current diagnostic deficiency to early identify hyperfibrinolysis can be explained by the absence of routine laboratory tests for fibrinolysis. The most efficient diagnostic tool to detect hyperfibrinolysis is thromboelastography. Recent studies have shown that approximately 15–20% of major trauma patients suffering from massive bleeding also present with pronounced hyperfibrinolysis. This could be supported by the observation that early administration of antifibrinolytic agents may be beneficial during hemorrhage control in severely bleeding patients [21].

Most of the above-mentioned test systems can be applied in a near-patient setting as a point-of-care testing [22]. A major advantage of this approach is to provide coagulation results in a clinically relevant time frame. As a consequence, 'sightless' ordering of blood products is prevented for severely bleeding patients. By using electronic data transfer, thrombelastography can also be used in a central lab facility, if a short turn around time is provided. Regarding the right choice of the test system, it is important firstly to identify questions derived from clinical need and thereafter to find suitable machines (fig. 4).

Targeted Treatment of Bleeding Events

The best approach to the bleeding patient is to identify and restore the hemostatic defect (fig. 5) and to monitor the therapeutic effects (see also 'Hemostasis-Navigated Hemotherapy' in this volume).

In the case of primary hemostasis defects (von Willebrand factor deficiency, platelet dysfunction), DDAVP should be administered; in order to augment thrombin

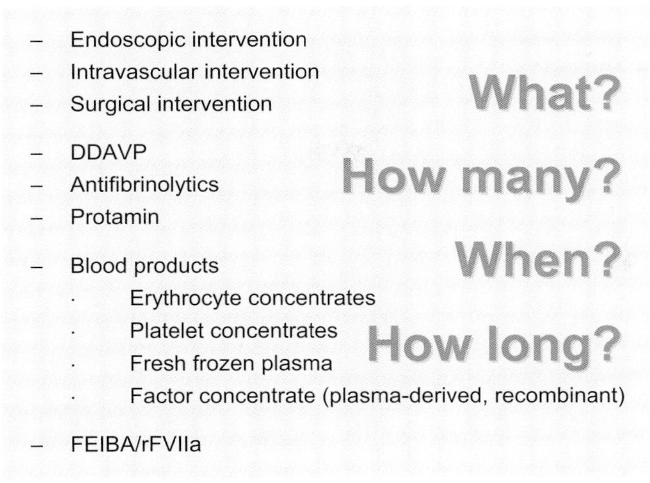

- Endoscopic intervention
- Intravascular intervention
- Surgical intervention

- DDAVP
- Antifibrinolytics
- Protamin

- Blood products
  · Erythrocyte concentrates
  · Platelet concentrates
  · Fresh frozen plasma
  · Factor concentrate (plasma-derived, recombinant)

- FEIBA/rFVIIa

What?

How many?

When?

How long?

Fig. 5. Bleeding: therapeutic options.

generation, factor concentrates, e.g. rFVIIa, should be transfused; to promote fibrin formation, fibrinogen should be administered; to enhance thrombus formation, erythrocyte or platelet concentrates should be given; and tranexamic acid may be administered as an antifibrinolytic agent.

With any hemorrhage, major efforts should be made to provide causal treatment, and here the important differences from preventive application of single-factor concentrates become apparent. The therapy of choice is a targeted application of hemostyptic agents, cellular concentrates or factor concentrates (fig. 6). Traumatic or perioperative bleeding is usually multifactorial and subject to the dynamics of the event. Beside the effects of medication (e.g. heparin) and the loss and consumption of coagulation factors, there often is a disorder of the cellular elements (e.g. platelets) to be taken into consideration. Dilution of cellular and plasma hemostatic compounds is always a concern in acute bleeding. Therefore, early and high-dose FFP application as well as red cell replacement is recommended [23, 24].

During acute bleeding, a multitude of different therapeutic options is at the disposal of the physician. The difficulty is to choose the right medication at the right time and to evaluate how much and how often the respective therapeutic option has to be applied. Typically, only the right therapy will stop the bleeding. It will hardly be of any use to the patient if he/she is transfused with FFP while he/she is bleeding because of thrombocytopenia or hyperfibrinolysis. Although this sounds self-evident, in the clinical common routine a 'blind' therapy is often applied, i.e. different medications and blood products are administered consecutively until the bleeding stops. If the cause of the bleeding is not the most obvious, unnecessary medication and blood products are administered. Thus, unnecessary costs are created and the patient is exposed to potentially harmful agents.

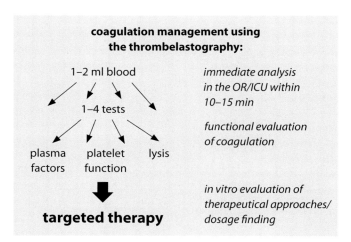

Fig. 6. Thromboelastography: guide in hemostatic therapy.

Conclusions and Future Directions

Goal-directed hemotherapy and its monitoring are recommended in acute bleeding management. A comprehensive assessment of the patient's history and acute clinical signs enable identification of specific defects of hemostasis. Near-patient testing of whole blood hemostasis contributes to therapeutic decisions. The outcome relevance of such concepts has to be proven in further studies.

Disclosure of Conflict of Interests

The author states that he has no conflict of interests.

References

1 Spahn DR: Strategies for transfusion therapy. Best Pract Res Clin Anaesthesiol 2004;18:661–673.
2 Bux J: Transfusion-related acute lung injury (TRA-LI): A serious adverse event of blood transfusion. Vox Sang 2005;89:1–10.
3 Goodnough LT: Risks of blood transfusion. Anesthesiol Clin North America 2005;23:241–252.
4 Stanworth SJ, Brunskill SJ, Hyde CJ, McClelland DB, Murphy MF: Is fresh frozen plasma clinically effective? A systematic review of randomized controlled trials. Br J Haematol 2004;126:139–152.
5 Custer B: Economic analyses of blood safety and transfusion medicine interventions: a systematic review. Transfus Med Rev. 2004;18:127–143.
6 Drews RE, Critical issues in hematology: anemia, thrombocytopenia, coagulopathy, and blood product transfusions in critically ill patients. Clin Chest Med 2003;24:607–622.
7 Dacey LJ, Munoz JJ, Baribeau YR, Johnson ER, Lahey SJ, Leavitt BJ, Quinn RD, Nugent WC, Birkmeyer JD, O'Connor GT: Reexploration for hemorrhage following coronary artery bypass grafting: incidence and risk factors. Northern England Cardiovascular Disease Study Group. Arch Surg 1998;133:442–447.
8 Moulton MJ, Creswell LL, Mackey ME, Cox JL, Rosenbloom M: Reexploration for bleeding is a risk factor for adverse outcomes after cardiac operations. J Thorac Cardiovasc Surg 1996;111:1037–1046.

9   Karkouti K, Wijeysundera DN, Yau TM, Beattie WS, Abdelnaem E, McCluskey SA, Ghannam M, Yeo E, Djaiani G, Karski J: The independent association of massive blood loss with mortality in cardiac surgery. Transfusion 2004;44:1453–1462.

10 Engoren MC, Habib RH, Zacharias A, Schwann TA, Riordan CJ, Durham SJ: Effect of blood transfusion on long-term survival after cardiac operation. Ann Thorac Surg 2002;74:1180–1186.

11 Das AM, Sood N, Hodgin K, Chang L, Carson SS: Development of a triage protocol for patient presenting with gastrointestinal hemorrhage: a prospective cohort study. Crit Care 2008;12:R57.

12 Fisher L, Fisher A, Pavli P, Davis M: Perioperative acute upper gastrointestinal haemorrhage in older patients with hip fracture: incidence, risk factors and prevention. Aliment Pharmacol Ther 2007;25:297–308.

13 Manoukian SV, Voeltz MD, Eikelboom J: Bleeding complications in acute coronary syndromes and percutaneous coronary intervention: predictors, prognostic significance, and paradigms for reducing risk. Clin Cardiol 2007;30:II24–II34.

14 König SA, Schick U, Döhnert J, Goldammer A, Vitzthum HE: Coagulopathy and outcome in patients with chronic haematoma. Acta Neurol Scand 2003;107:110–116.

15 Lambotte O, Dautremer J, Guillet B, Boutekedjiret T, Dreyfus M, Kotb R, Le Bras P, Delfraissy JF, Lambert T, Goujard C: Acquired hemophilia in older people: A poor prognosis despite intensive care. J Am Geriatr Soc 2007;55:1682–1685.

16 Collins PW: Treatment of acquired hemophilia A. J Thromb Haemost 2007;5:893–900.

17 Cammerer U, Dietrich W, Rampf T, Braun SL, Richter JA: The predictive value of modified computerized thrombelastography and platelet function analysis for postoperative blood loss in routine cardiac surgery. Anesth Analg 2003;96:51–57.

18 Gelb AB, Roth RI, Levin J, London MJ, Noall RA, Hauck WW, Cloutier M, Verrier E, Mangano DT: Changes in blood coagulation during and following cardiopulmonary bypass: Lack of correlation with clinical bleeding. Am J Clin Pathol 1996;106:87–99.

19 Anderson L, Quasim I, Soutar R, Steven M, Macfie A, Korte W: An audit of red cell and blood product use after the institution of thromboelastometry in a cardiac intensive care unit. Transfus Med 2006;16:31–39.

20 Shore-Lesserson L, Manspeizer HE, DePerio M, Francis S, Vela-Cantos F, Arisan Ergin M: Thromboelastography-guided transfusion algorithm reduces transfusions in complex surgery. Anaesth Analg 1999;88:312–319.

21 Martinowitz U, Michaelson M: Guidelines for the use of recombinant activated factor VII (rVIIa) in uncontrolled bleeding: a report by the Israeli Multidisciplinary rVIIa Task Force. J Thromb Haemost 2005;3:640–648.

22 Calatzis A, Schramm W, Spannagl M: Management of bleeding in surgery and intensive care; in: Scharrer I, Schramm W (eds): 31st Hemophilia Symposium Hamburg 2000. Berlin, Springer, 2002.

23 British Committee for Standards in Haematology, Blood Transfusion Task Force: Guidelines for the use of fresh frozen plasma, cryoprecipitate and cryosupernatant. Br J Haematol 2004;126:11–28.

24 Chowdhury P, Saayman A, Paulus U, Findlay GP, Collins PW: Efficacy of standard dose and 30 ml/kg fresh frozen plasma in correcting laboratory parameters of haemostasis in critically ill patients. Brit J Haematol 2004;125:69–73.

PD Dr. med. Michael Spannagl
Abteilung für Transfusionsmedizin und Hämostaseologie
Klinikum der Universität München
Max-Lebsche-Platz 32, 81377 München, Germany
Tel. +49 89 7095-4401, Fax -7411
E-Mail mispannagl@t-online.de

Scharf RE (ed): Progress and Challenges in Transfusion Medicine, Hemostasis and Hemotherapy.
Freiburg i.Br., Karger, 2008, pp 274–287

Challenges in Life-Threatening Hemorrhages: The Acquired Hemophilia

Marcus Stockschläder · Rüdiger E. Scharf

Department of Experimental and Clinical Hemostasis, Hemotherapy, and Transfusion Medicine, Heinrich Heine University Medical Center, Düsseldorf, Germany

Key Words

Hemophilia, acquired · Factor VIII:C · Inhibitor · Autoantibody · Bethesda units

Summary

Acquired hemophilia A is a rare immune coagulopathy causing life- or limb-threatening bleeding episodes. Responsible autoantibody inhibitors against factor VIII coagulant protein appear spontaneously in subjects with previously normal hemostatic function. Despite the fact that hemostatic efficacy of all plasmic or recombinant agents is unpredictable and that a clinically validated laboratory assay to predict successful hemostasis is still missing, bypassing agents such as recombinant factor VIIa and activated prothrombin complex concentrates lead to hemostatic control in the majority of cases. Clinical eradication of the autoantibody through immunosuppression clearly reduces the mortality rate in acquired hemophilia.   ©2008 S. Karger GmbH, Freiburg i.Br.

Introduction

Acquired hemophilia A (AH) is a clinically significant hemostatic disorder caused by development of autoimmune antibodies (inhibitors) against factor VIII coagulant protein (FVIII:C). The annual incidence of AH has been estimated at 1.34–1.48 cases per million people [1, 2]. The incidence of AH increases with age, and it is likely that AH is underdiagnosed in the elderly. AH is very uncommon in children. The incidence in males and females is similar. The age distribution of autoantibodies to FVIII:C is biphasic with a small peak in young, fertile women between 20–40 years of age (associated with pregnancy, mostly primiparous women, and the postpartum state, most often within 3 months after birth) and a major peak in the older age groups [2, 3]. There is a recognized association between development of acquired antibodies to FVIII:C and a number of diseases, especially those with an autoimmune pathogenesis such as rheumatoid arthritis, systemic lupus erythematosus, other connective tissue diseases, pemphigus, and inflammatory bowel disease. Other risk factors include chronic inflammatory and infectious states as well as malignancy, certain drugs, pregnancy and the postpartum period [4]. In about half of the cases, however, the inhibitor remains idiopathic [5].

Diagnosis

The diagnosis of AH is often difficult because the patient does not have a personal or family history of bleeding episodes. In mild cases of AH, the inhibitor may be detected incidentally because of a prolonged activated partial thromboplastin time (aPTT). Many low-titer inhibitors may remain undetected unless patients experience severe bruising or bleed after surgery or trauma. The prolongation of the aPTT with normal prothrombin time is the hallmark of laboratory diagnosis. In more severe cases, circulating inhibitors to FVIII:C may lead to an acquired hemophilic state with spontaneous, potentially life-threatening bleeding complications. Autoantibodies targeting FVIII:C often demonstrate different pharmakokinetics and binding affinities compared to alloantibodies that arise in individuals with congenital FVIII:C as a consequence of replacement therapy. The bleeding pattern, which is also different, includes bleeding into the skin (large ecchymoses) (fig. 1), mucosa (epistaxis, gingivorrhagia, metrorrhagia), muscles or retroperitoneum, hematuria, hematemesis or melena, and prolonged postpartum or postoperative bleeding. Lethality is high, reaching 22% in some series depending on age, inhibitor titer levels, and response to treatment [2, 6]. Patients in whom the inhibitor cannot be eliminated may have a mortality rate as high as 42% [7]. A recent review of 249 patients reported between 1987 and 2001 noted an overall mortality of 20%, with an 11% mortality directly related to the inhibitor despite a complete remission [7]. The high overall mortality has been attributed to

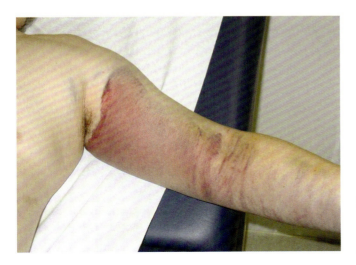

Fig. 1. A patient with acquired hemophilia A at initial clinical presentation showing a diffuse subcutaneous suggillation.

complications of therapy or to comorbidity [8]. The diagnosis of autoantibody inhibitors is based on the inability of plasma from normal individuals to correct prolonged clotting assays by patient plasma in mixing studies. The inhibitor can be quantitated using the Bethesda assay or its Nijmegen modification [9]. Both assays measure residual FVIII:C activity after incubation of patient plasma with normal plasma for 2 h at 37 °C. The inhibitors usually have complex type 2 kinetics with a rapid and nonlinear inactivation of FVIII:C, making it difficult to saturate the inhibitor by adding antigen [10]. Hence, FVIII substitution therapy is unsuccessful in the presence of high-titer inhibitors unless very high doses of FVIII are given [11]. Most FVIII inhibitors are oligo- or polyclonal IgG_4 and less frequently IgG_1 immunoglobulins, which do not fix complement and bind to the C2 and, less frequently, to the A2 domain of FVIII:C. Early recognition and rapid diagnosis of AH is important to allow treatment of bleeds, avoidance of invasive procedures and inhibitor eradication.

Treatment

The main treatment principles of AH are control of bleeding, eradication of the inhibitor, treatment of the potentially underlying disorder, and protection of the patient against trauma and invasive procedures [3, 12]. Intramuscular injections, use of aspirin, nonsteroidal antiinflammatory drugs, and anticoagulants must be avoided.

Spontaneous remissions of the autoimmune antibody inhibitor targeting FVIII:C may occur in approximately one third of cases, mostly with low-titer inhibitors and usually after months to years of involvement [6]. Up to one third of patients do not require hemostatic therapy at the time of diagnosis, but remain at risk of severe bleeding until the inhibitor has been eradicated [2, 13]. Early deaths are most often caused by uncontrolled hemorrhage within the first few weeks after presentation, while infectious complications secondary to immunosuppressive therapy account for most of the late deaths. If bleeding episodes are very severe, prompt hemostatic control is required to reduce morbidity and mortality. Hemostatic management depends on the site and severity of the bleed [3]. To prevent recurrence, hemostatic therapy often needs to be continued at a reduced dose after initial hemostasis has been achieved. Mucosal hemorrhage will benefit from concomitant therapy with antifibrinolytic agents such as topical tranexamic acid [3].

Bypassing Agents

Control of bleeding is normally achieved with FVIII-bypassing activity such as activated prothrombin complex concentrates (aPCC) or recombinant factor VIIa (rFVIIa). Both agents have been shown to be efficacious in AH [14, 15] since they are able to bypass the need for FVIII:C to generate sufficient amounts of thrombin

('thrombin burst') on the surface of activated platelets. aPCC, such as FVIII inhibitor-bypassing activity (FEIBA NF; Baxter), has been used for decades as hemostatic bypassing agent in patients with high-responding inhibitors [16]. In a recent retrospective survey of 34 patients with acquired hemophilia, an overall complete response rate of 86% with a typical dosage regime of 75 IU/kg FEIBA given every 8–12 h has been reported [15]. A dose of 200 IU/kg within a 24-h period should not be exceeded, however, to avoid thromboembolic complications. The incidence of adverse events in only 4.05 per 10^5 applications over a 10-year period indicates that thrombotic complications associated with FEIBA use are rare [17]. Furthermore, activated rFVIIa (NovoSeven, Novo Nordisk) has been introduced into clinical practice. Large amounts of administered rFVIIa may bind nonspecifically to the platelet surface and activate factor X in the absence of FVIII:C in a tissue factor-independent manner. rFVIIa is also highly effective in controlling bleeding with a reported efficacy rate of 80–90% [18, 19]. In comparison to the standard dose of rFVIIa (90 μg/kg), a single high dose (270 μg/kg) of rFVIIa appears to be as safe and effective for the home treatment of joint bleeds in hemophilia patients with inhibitors [20, 21]. High-dose regimens may reduce the number of doses required or reverse bleeding that is refractory to standard doses of rFVIIa. There are published case reports of arterial thrombosis associated with the use of rFVIIa [14], including a case of myocardial infarction in a patient with acquired hemophilia. Between 1996 and 2002 more than 600,000 doses (90 μg/kg) of rFVIIa have been given while only 21 thrombotic events occurred [22]. The recently published FEIBA 'NovoSeven Comparative Study' (FENOC) [19] demonstrated that FEIBA and NovoSeven appeared to have similar effects on joint bleeds evaluated 6 h after treatment for 96 bleeding episodes in inhibitor patients with congenital hemophilia. Patients with acquired hemophilia can develop bleeding refractory to monotherapy. The different mechanisms of action of rFVIIa and FEIBA provide a theoretic rationale for interindividual as well as intraindividual variation in the clinical efficacy between the two agents [23, 24]. Management of such bleeds is often difficult. There is, however, laboratory and clinical evidence of additive effects of FEIBA and rFVIIa. A significant shortening of the activated coagulation time (ACT) was noted when rFVIIa was added to blood from patients receiving aPCC [25, 26]. Furthermore, case reports have indicated that in FVIII inhibitor patients presenting with life-threatening bleeding complications and failing initial high-dose hemostatic treatment with rFVIIa, rebleeding was controlled by the addition of aPCC without adverse events [54]. However, treatment with a combination of these agents is not widely practiced due to concerns for the development of thromboembolic complications [27, 28]. Two such reports have been published demonstrating thrombosis in patients receiving aPCC and rFVIIa sequentially [29, 30]. Invasive procedures are associated with a significant risk of bleeding. Only essential, life-saving procedures should be considered and the benefits carefully weighed against the risks. Relatively few details are available on surgery undertaken in AH. Hemostatic efficacy with FEIBA has been reported for a bone marrow trephine and Hickman line insertion [31] while three unspecified operations were performed under rFVIIa cover with good outcome [14]. An important drawback of bypassing agents is that currently there is no validated laboratory monitoring technique that predicts or correlates with clinical efficacy. Thrombin generation [32] and thromboelastographic [33] assays are being evaluated for their correlation with clinical efficacy.

FVIII:C Concentrates

Whenever possible, optimal control of bleeding in AH should be achieved by normalizing FVIII:C activity levels in plasma. The effectiveness of FVIII:C replacement therapy depends on the inhibitor titer. Human FVIII:C concentrates should be used only if the maximum inhibitor titer, including peak anamnestic response (low responder), is consistently less than 5 Bethesda units (BU) so that the neutralizing capacity of the autoimmune inhibitor can be overwhelmed and sufficiently high plasma levels of FVIII:C can be attained. Formulae for calculating the dose are, at best, imprecise approximations due to the inaccuracies inherent in the laboratory measurement of inhibitor titers. The use of human FVIII:C in combination with immunoadsorption is more likely to result in hemostatically relevant FVIII:C levels. This treatment strategy may be useful as first line or if bypassing agents have failed [34, 35].

The practical benefits underlying the use of porcine FVIII:C include the fact that heterologous FVIII:C compared with human FVIII:C has significantly reduced cross-reactivity with antihuman FVIII:C antibody inhibitors. Therefore, neutralization of the porcine FVIII:C activity will be reduced, achieving hemostatic levels in situations where human FVIII:C is ineffective [36]. However, in vitro cross-reactivity testing with the patient's plasma before administration is strongly recommended. Porcine FVIII:C is the only one of the replacement options that will yield a measurable FVIII:C activity level in recipient plasma for clinical monitoring in the setting of high-titer inhibitors [37]. Porcine FVIII:C has been shown to have excellent hemostatic efficacy in 78% of 74 bleeds [37]. However, plasma-derived porcine FVIII is currently not available for routine clinical use. A recombinant B domain-deleted porcine FVIII is undergoing phase II clinical trials in congenital hemophilia complicated by inhibitors.

Inhibitor Eradication

Immunosuppressive therapy to eradicate the inhibitor in AH should be undertaken as soon as the diagnosis has been made [12]. Even if many patients do not have severe bleeding at presentation and some may have a spontaneous remission, fatal bleeds can occur up to 5 months after presentation if the inhibitor is not eradicated [2, 13]. Furthermore, an individual patient's presenting characteristics do not predict the risk of fatal bleeds [2]. Since almost all publications are from specialized centers [1, 34, 35], more severely affected patients may be reported preferentially. Furthermore, there may be a bias towards reporting of good outcomes. The main options for immunosuppression are steroids, cytotoxic drugs (cyclophosphamide, azathioprine, or combination therapy), cyclosporine A, intravenous immunoglobulin, the anti-CD20 antibody rituximab, plasmapheresis or immunoadsorption in combination with high-dose FVIII:C administration for immune tolerance induction. Numerous combinations of these treatments have been reported. A treatment may be considered superior if more patients achieve complete remission (CR) or if this remission is achieved more rapidly. Because autoantibodies may disappear spontaneously, the true efficacy of any given immunosuppressive regimen is difficult to assess. In one study, 4 out of 16 patients achieved a spontaneous remission [13].

Steroids and Cytotoxic Agents

One prospective randomized study is available in which 31 patients with acquired antibodies to FVIII were entered to determine the safety and efficacy of prednisone, cyclophosphamide, or their combination, in the treatment of this disorder [38]. All patients were treated initially with prednisone (1 mg/kg for 3 weeks). If the antibody persisted and there was no rise in FVIII:C activity, patients were randomized to either continue prednisone for an additional 6 weeks, to taper prednisone and begin cyclophosphamide (2 mg/kg), or to continue prednisone and add cyclophosphamide. The antibody disappeared in 10 patients during the initial prednisone therapy, and in 3 of 4 others randomized to continue on prednisone. The antibody disappeared in 3 of 6 patients treated with cyclophosphamide alone, and in 5 of 10 patients given cyclophosphamide and prednisone. There was no difference in antibody titers between those responding to prednisone and those responding to cyclophosphamide. The study provided no evidence to suggest that adding or changing to cyclophosphamide after 3 weeks was better than continuing with steroids alone [38]. A non-randomized study [2] compared patients treated with steroids versus steroids and cytotoxic agents. The 34 patients treated with steroids had 76% CR at a median of 49 (31–62) days compared with the 45 patients treated with steroids and cytotoxic agents who had 78% CR at a median of 39 (34–57) days. There was no statistically significant difference between the treatment arms and mortality was not different. A review that combined data from 20 reports [7] demonstrated that the use of steroids and cyclophosphamide resulted in more patients achieving CR compared with steroids alone. The higher CR rate was not translated into a lower mortality. The marginal advantage of cytotoxic agents over single-agent corticosteroids is mitigated in terms of neutrocytopenia and infection-induced morbidity and mortality. The combined data available from uncontrolled cohorts appears to suggest a benefit for combined steroids and cytotoxic agents. If the aggregate response rates are calculated for only those studies that included both steroids alone and combined steroid and cytotoxic therapy, the remission rates are 77 and 79%, respectively. Whichever regimen is used, 3 weeks appears to be too short a time to assess outcome because the median time to remission is 5–7 weeks.

Intravenous Immunoglobulin

Intravenous immunoglobulin (IVIG) has been suggested to be a useful agent in AH. A larger study that compared non-randomized patients who either did or did not receive IVIG [2] and a literature review [7] both showed no benefit for IVIG. At the present time, the available evidence suggests that IVIG as a single agent or in combination with steroids and cytotoxic agents is not useful in inhibitor eradication in AH.

Rituximab

Apart from the usual treatment with corticosteroids combined with cyclophosphamide, it has become clear in recent years that rituximab may be a valuable agent in managing acquired hemophilia. Rituximab, a chimeric monoclonal antibody targeting the CD20 antigen on B cells, might be a more specific agent to eliminate autoreactive B cell clones since it induces antibody-dependent cellular toxicity including apoptosis and complement-mediated lysis primarily in pre-B cell clones [39, 40]. It has been used successfully in acquired hemophilia patients leading to long-term complete clinical responses. The addition of rituximab to standard immunosuppression might permit earlier discontinuation or even avoidance of potentially toxic agents such as cyclophosphamide [41]. The blockade of B cell proliferation allows a reestablishment of an intact B cell pool after an average of 3–6 months after treatment [42]. There is now general consensus that the use of rituximab should be considered in cases where patients prove resistant to first-line therapy or in patients in whom steroids and/or cytotoxic drugs are best avoided. The largest study reported on 10 patients, 8 of whom achieved CR and the 2 non-remitters responded to subsequent intravenous cyclophosphamide [39]. This response rate of 80% is very similar to other immunosuppressive therapies. It has been suggested that rituximab may lead to more rapid remission and control of bleeding than other therapies, but without comparative patients this is difficult to ascertain [39]. Elderly patients should be carefully followed for infection. The available data support the use of rituximab as either first- or second-line therapy but do not support the assertion that rituximab is superior to other immunosuppressive agents for patients with higher-titer inhibitors as suggested by some authors [42, 43]. Rituximab is a useful option for patients who have failed first-line therapy.

Immunotolerance

For the induction of immunotolerance, treatment options include corticosteroids, immunosuppressive agents, monoclonal anti-B cell antibodies, immunoglobulins, plasmapheresis, and immunoadsorption [35, 44, 45]. The primary objective for treating patients should be the safe and rapid elimination of the inhibitor and the development of long-term immune tolerance induction (ITI). A number of different protocols have been published. The use of FVIII:C in combination with immunosuppressive agents in AH has been reported. A stated rationale for this approach is that FVIII:C may stimulate antibody-producing cells into division, making them more susceptible to cytotoxic agents. The lack of adequate controls means that a direct assessment of the role of FVIII:C cannot be made. A report of patients treated with 3-weekly infusions of FVIII:C combined with vincristine, cyclophosphamide and steroids resulted in a 92% CR rate in 12 patients after 1–3 courses [46]. The same group, however, later published a report on 6 patients who were treated with vincristine, cyclophosphamide and steroids without FVIII:C and found 83% CR after 1–7 courses [47]. The role of FVIII:C in these results is unclear because the intensity of immunosuppression was greater than for many other published protocols. Infusion of FVIII on a daily basis (30 IU/kg per day for 1 week, 20 IU/kg per day for a second week and 15 IU/kg per day for a third week) combined with intravenous cyclophosphamide and methylprednisolone resulted in a complete remission in 93% of 14 patients after a median of 4.6 weeks, compared with 67% remitting patients at a median of 28.3 weeks in 6 historical controls treated with steroids ± cyclophosphamide [43]. Taken together these reports are insufficient to conclude that immune tolerance with exogenous FVIII:C is beneficial in AH and the cost of FVIII therapy in these protocols should be taken into account. Since the successful eradication of autoantibodies appears dependent on FVIII:C 'priming', the presence of FVIII:C may be of importance in immune tolerance induction. However, since patients with acquired hemophilia have no impairment in FVIII:C production, the additional application of high-dose exogenous plasmic or recombinant FVIII is debatable [54].

Immunoadsorption

While standard plasmapheresis is not clinically useful, high-titer FVIII autoantibodies have been efficiently eliminated by intensive large-volume immunoadsorption [48]. Currently, two adsorption columns are available: Immunosorba® (sepharose-bound staphylococcal protein A) and Ig-Therasorb® (sepharose-bound polyclonal sheep antibodies to human immunoglobulin). In contrast to other extracorporeal methods such as plasma exchange, immunoadsorption has a high efficacy in removing FVIII:C antibodies (inhibitor titer reduction of 70–90%) but does not lead to significant loss of other coagulation components, which is beneficial for the achieve-

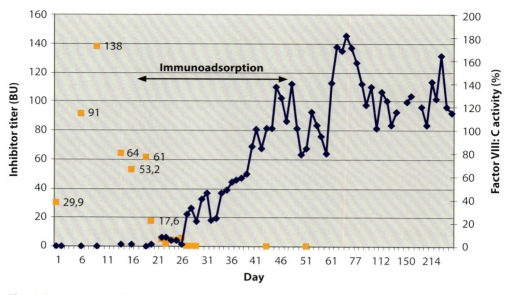

Fig. 2. Time course of FVIII:C activity (%) and Bethesda units (BU) in a patient with acquired hemophilia A who underwent immunoadsorption. The time period during which immunoadsorption was performed is indicated as black bar with arrows.

ment of adequate hemostasis [35]. The procedure is generally well tolerated and even mild side effects were reported in less than 1% of treated patients [35, 49]. Since specialized equipment and expert technical knowledge is required to perform immunoadsorption, the method is currently restricted to specialized medical centers. The role of immunoadsorption in the treatment of acquired hemophilia has not yet been standardized. In most cases, it has been used as part of multimodal immunomodulating therapeutic concepts for long-term inhibitor eradication, such as the Bonn-Malmö Protocol which also includes FVIII:C substitution, administration of intravenous immunoglobulin, and immunosuppression [35, 48]. Immunoadsorption has also been used as part of a salvage therapy of otherwise refractory bleeding due to acquired hemophilia. In this setting, immunoadsorption was reported to lead to a rapid and significant decrease of inhibitor titers, improved levels, recovery and half-life of FVIII:C and, consequently, cessation of bleeding [50, 54] (fig. 2). Thus, immunoadsorption should be considered for treatment of acquired hemophilia, particularly when a fast inhibitor titer reduction is necessary [51]. A cohort of 35 patients with AH and severe bleeding was treated with a combination of oral cyclophosphamide, prednisolone, immunoadsorption, IVIG, and FVIII:C. Rapid control of bleeding was also reported with an undetectable inhibitor at a median of 3 days and CR in 88% of patients at a median of 14 days [35]. Although the cost of FVIII:C was considerable, this treatment regimen appeared to rapidly control bleeding and induce CR. It is not possible to state what roles are played by the various components of the protocol. Furthermore, it should be remembered that unsatisfactory responses to immunoadsorption have also been reported in patients with acquired hemophilia [35].

Relapse

Relapse has been observed in 20% of 102 patients at a median of 7.5 months (range 1 week to 14 months) [2]. In this study, no underlying disease was predictive of relapse and a second CR was induced in 10 (56%) patients, and in further 4 (22%) patients the inhibitor was eradicated, FVIII:C normalized but immunosuppression could not be stopped without relapse. In 4 (22%) patients a second remission could not be achieved [2]. There is general consensus that immunosuppression aimed at eradicating the inhibitor should be started as soon as the diagnosis of AH is made. There are, at present, no convincing data to suggest that one immunosuppressive regimen is superior to any other or that the choice of regimen should be based on the inhibitor titer or FVIII:C level. Therapy is at the discretion of the clinician, based on the clinical circumstances and taking into account the potential side effects of each treatment option. If a patient does not respond to first-line steroids, then a cytotoxic agent or rituximab can be added. Similarly, if a patient fails first-line rituximab, then steroids and cytotoxic agents may be successful. Cyclosporine A is a useful second-line option. A regimen based on immunoadsorption or high-dose FVIII:C and immunoadsorption can be considered for patients with severe bleeding.

Pregnancy

There are features of pregnancy-related AH that appear to be different from other patients. AH is a rare complication of pregnancy, estimated to affect 1 in 350,000 births in the UK [2]. Patients usually present with bleeding at the time of delivery or within the first 1–4 months post partum. The reason for the late presentations is unclear; however, some patients had been symptomatic for several months and may represent delayed diagnosis rather than late onset disease. The bleeding phenotype is similar to other patients with AH, with the addition of bleeding related to vaginal delivery and Cesarean section. These patients are younger and may have a different natural history and response to inhibitor eradication therapy [52]. Retrospective reviews have reported that in pregnancy-related AH, the time to achieve remission is longer than in patients with other etiologies. A reasonable option is to treat initially with steroids alone and, if the response is not adequate, add a cytotoxic agent or rituximab after delivery. Relapse in subsequent pregnancies appears to be relatively uncommon, but women should be informed about this possibility. Since the antibody may affect the FVIII:C level of the fetus, this must be considered at the time of delivery [53].

Treatment of bleeds should follow the principles outlined for AH in general, but caution about the risk of venous thromboembolism in the postpartum period should be borne in mind.

Children

AH in children is very uncommon, with an incidence of 0.045 per million per year in one study [2]. Patients are presented with similar bleeding patterns to adults and responded to standard immunosuppression. Reported underlying disorders included juvenile rheumatoid arthritis, positive anti-nuclear antibody, infection, antibiotic use, Goodpasture's syndrome, liver disease, and gastritis.

Conclusions and Future Directions

AH is a rare autoimmune disease with the formation of antibodies against endogenous FVIII:C. Prolongation of the aPTT with normal prothrombin time is the diagnostic hallmark of the disease. Bleeding complications may be life-threatening, and the severity of bleeding complications is not proportional to the inhibitor titer. Hemorrhagic complications should be treated with a FVIII-bypassing agent such as aPCC or rFVIIa. Inhibitor eradication is accomplished in most cases with immunosuppressive therapy. Immunoadsorption may be helpful for control of bleeding complications by rapidly reducing inhibitor titers. The role of exogenous plasmic or recombinant FVIII:C remains debatable. If clinical trials show efficacy and safety, the B domain-deleted recombinant porcine FVIII molecule will be a useful addition to the treatment armamentarium. Trials that compare conventional steroid and cytotoxic agents with rituximab or investigate the role of FVIII would be useful.

Disclosure of Conflict of Interests

The authors state that they have no conflict of interests.

Acknowledgements

The authors wish to thank PD Dr. R.B. Zotz and PD Dr. A. Gerhardt for their helpful discussion and review of the manuscript.

References

1 Collins P, Macartney N, Davies R, Lees S, Giddings J, Majer R: A population based, unselected, consecutive cohort of patients with acquired haemophilia A. Br J Haematol 2004;124:86–90.

2 Collins PW, Hirsch S, Baglin TP, Dolan G, Hanley J, Makris M, Keeling DM, Liesner R, Brown SA, Hay CR: Acquired hemophilia A in the United Kingdom: a 2-year national surveillance study by the United Kingdom Haemophilia Centre Doctors' Organisation. Blood 2007;109:1870–1877.

3 Collins PW: Treatment of acquired hemophilia A. J Thromb Haemost 2007;5:893–900.

4 Sallah S, Wan JY: Inhibitors against factor VIII in patients with cancer. Analysis of 41 patients. Cancer 2001;91:1067–1074.

5 Rizza CR, Spooner RJ, Giangrande PL: Treatment of haemophilia in the United Kingdom 1981–1996. Haemophilia 2001;7:349–359.

6 Green D, Lechner K: A survey of 215 non-hemophilic patients with inhibitors to factor VIII. Thromb Haemost 1981;45:200–203.

7 Delgado J, Jimenez-Yuste V, Hernandez-Navarro F, Villar A: Acquired haemophilia: review and meta-analysis focused on therapy and prognostic factors. Br J Haematol 2003;121:21–35.

8 Delgado J, Villar A, Jimenez-Yuste V, Gago J, Quintana M, Hernandez-Navarro F: Acquired hemophilia: a single-center survey with emphasis on immunotherapy and treatment-related side-effects. Eur J Haematol 2002;69:158–164.

9 Verbruggen B, Novakova I, Wessels H, Boezeman J, van den Berg M, Mauser-Bunschoten E: The Nijmegen modification of the Bethesda assay for factor VIII:C inhibitors: improved specificity and reliability. Thromb Haemost 1995;73:247–251.

10 Biggs R, Austen DE, Denson KW, Borrett R, Rizza CR: The mode of action of antibodies which destroy factor VIII. II. Antibodies which give complex concentration graphs. Br J Haematol 1972;23:137–155.

11 Brackmann HH, Oldenburg J, Schwaab R: Immune tolerance for the treatment of factor VIII inhibitors – twenty years' 'Bonn protocol'. Vox Sang 1996;70(suppl 1):30–35.

12 Hay CR, Brown S, Collins PW, Keeling DM, Liesner R: The diagnosis and management of factor VIII and IX inhibitors: a guideline from the United Kingdom Haemophilia Centre Doctors Organisation. Br J Haematol 2006;133:591–605.

13 Lottenberg R, Kentro TB, Kitchens CS: Acquired hemophilia. A natural history study of 16 patients with factor VIII inhibitors receiving little or no therapy. Arch Intern Med 1987;147:1077–1081.

14 Hay CR, Negrier C, Ludlam CA: The treatment of bleeding in acquired haemophilia with recombinant factor VIIa: a multicentre study. Thromb Haemost 1997;78:1463–1467.

15 Sallah S: Treatment of acquired haemophilia with factor eight inhibitor bypassing activity. Haemophilia 2004;10:169–173.

16 Negrier C, Goudemand J, Sultan Y, Bertrand M, Rothschild C, Lauroua P: Multicenter retrospective study on the utilization of FEIBA in France in patients with factor VIII and factor IX inhibitors. French FEIBA Study Group. Factor eight bypassing activity. Thromb Haemost 1997;77:1113–1119.

17 Ehrlich HJ, Henzl MJ, Gomperts ED: Safety of factor VIII inhibitor bypass activity (FEIBA): 10-year compilation of thrombotic adverse events. Haemophilia 2002;8:83–90.

18 Parameswaran R, Shapiro AD, Gill JC, Kessler CM: Dose effect and efficacy of rFVIIa in the treatment of haemophilia patients with inhibitors: analysis from the Hemophilia and Thrombosis Research Society Registry. Haemophilia 2005;11:100–106.

19 Astermark J, Donfield SM, DiMichele DM, Gringeri A, Gilbert SA, Waters J, Berntorp E: A randomized comparison of bypassing agents in hemophilia complicated by an inhibitor: the FEIBA NovoSeven Comparative (FENOC) Study. Blood 2007;109:546–551.

20 Kavakli K, Makris M, Zulfikar B, Erhardtsen E, Abrams ZS, Kenet G: Home treatment of haemarthroses using a single dose regimen of recombinant activated factor VII in patients with haemophilia and inhibitors. A multi-centre, randomised, double-blind, cross-over trial. Thromb Haemost 2006;95:600–605.

21 Santagostino E, Mancuso ME, Rocino A, Mancuso G, Scaraggi F, Mannucci PM: A prospective randomized trial of high and standard dosages of recombinant factor VIIa for treatment of hemarthroses in hemophiliacs with inhibitors. J Thromb Haemost 2006;4:367–371.

22 Hedner U, Erhardtsen E: Potential role of recombinant factor VIIa as a hemostatic agent. Clin Adv Hematol Oncol 2003;1:112–119.

23 Hoffman M, Monroe DM, III: The action of high-dose factor VIIa (FVIIa) in a cell-based model of hemostasis. Dis Mon 2003;49:14–21.

24 Turecek PL, Varadi K, Gritsch H, Schwarz HP: FEIBA: mode of action. Haemophilia 2004;10(suppl 2):3–9.

25 Key NS, Christie B, Henderson N, Nelsestuen GL: Possible synergy between recombinant factor VIIa and prothrombin complex concentrate in hemophilia therapy. Thromb Haemost 2002;88:60–65.

26 Allen GA, Wolberg AS, Oliver JA, Hoffman M, Roberts HR, Monroe DM: Impact of procoagulant concentration on rate, peak and total thrombin generation in a model system. J Thromb Haemost 2004;2:402–413.

27 Schneiderman J, Nugent DJ, Young G: Sequential therapy with activated prothrombin complex concentrate and recombinant factor VIIa in patients with severe haemophilia and inhibitors. Haemophilia 2004;10:347–351.

28 Aledort LM: Comparative thrombotic event incidence after infusion of recombinant factor VIIa versus factor VIII inhibitor bypass activity. J Thromb Haemost 2004;2:1700–1708.

29 Rosenfeld SB, Watkinson KK, Thompson BH, Macfarlane DE, Lentz SR: Pulmonary embolism after sequential use of recombinant factor VIIa and activated prothrombin complex concentrate in a factor VIII inhibitor patient. Thromb Haemost 2002;87:925–926.

30 Bui JD, Despotis GD, Trulock EP, Patterson GA, Goodnough LT: Fatal thrombosis after administration of activated prothrombin complex concentrates in a patient supported by extracorporeal membrane oxygenation who had received activated recombinant factor VII. J Thorac Cardiovasc Surg 2002;124:852–854.

31 Tjonnfjord GE: Activated prothrombin complex concentrate (FEIBA) treatment during surgery in patients with inhibitors to FVIII/IX: the updated Norwegian experience. Haemophilia 2004;10(suppl 2):41–45.

32 Varadi K, Negrier C, Berntorp E, Astermark J, Bordet JC, Morfini M, Linari S, Schwarz HP, Turecek PL: Monitoring the bioavailability of FEIBA with a thrombin generation assay. J Thromb Haemost 2003;1:2374–2380.

33 Sorensen B, Ingerslev J: Whole blood clot formation phenotypes in hemophilia A and rare coagulation disorders. Patterns of response to recombinant factor VIIa. J Thromb Haemost 2004;2:102–110.

34 Guillet B, Kriaa F, Huysse MG, Proulle V, George C, Tchernia G, D'Oiron R, Laurian Y, Charpentier B, Lambert T, Dreyfus M: Protein A sepharose immunoadsorption: immunological and haemostatic effects in two cases of acquired haemophilia. Br J Haematol 2001;114:837–844.

35 Zeitler H, Ulrich-Merzenich G, Hess L, Konsek E, Unkrig C, Walger P, Vetter H, Brackmann HH: Treatment of acquired hemophilia by the Bonn-Malmo Protocol: documentation of an in vivo immunomodulating concept. Blood 2005;105:2287–2293.

36 Hay CR, Lozier JN, Lee CA, Laffan M, Tradati F, Santagostino E, Ciavarella N, Schiavoni M, Fukui H, Yoshioka A, Teitel J, Mannucci PM, Kasper CK: Safety profile of porcine factor VIII and its use as hospital and home-therapy for patients with haemophilia-A and inhibitors: the results of an international survey. Thromb Haemost 1996;75:25–29.

37 Morrison AE, Ludlam CA, Kessler C: Use of porcine factor VIII in the treatment of patients with acquired hemophilia. Blood 1993;81:1513–1520.

38 Green D, Rademaker AW, Briet E: A prospective, randomized trial of prednisone and cyclophosphamide in the treatment of patients with factor VIII autoantibodies. Thromb Haemost 1993;70:753–757.

39 Stasi R, Brunetti M, Stipa E, Amadori S: Selective B-cell depletion with rituximab for the treatment of patients with acquired hemophilia. Blood 2004;103:4424–4428.

40 Kain S, Copeland TS, Leahy MF: Treatment of refractory autoimmune (acquired) haemophilia with anti-CD20 (rituximab). Br J Haematol 2002;119:578.

41 Cartron G, Watier H, Golay J, Solal-Celigny P: From the bench to the bedside: ways to improve rituximab efficacy. Blood 2004;104:2635–2642.

42 Aggarwal A, Grewal R, Green RJ, Boggio L, Green D, Weksler BB, Wiestner A, Schechter GP: Rituximab for autoimmune haemophilia: a proposed treatment algorithm. Haemophilia 2005;11:13–19.

43 Nemes L, Pitlik E: New protocol for immune tolerance induction in acquired hemophilia. Haematologica 2000;85:64–68.

44 Brackmann HH, Schwaab R, Effenberger W, Hess L, Hanfland P, Oldenburg J: Hemophilia treatment. Side effects during immune tolerance induction. Haematologica 2000;85:75–77.

45 Nilsson IM, Freiburghaus C: Apheresis. Adv Exp Med Biol 1995;386:175–184.

46 Lian EC, Larcada AF, Chiu AY: Combination immunosuppressive therapy after factor VIII infusion for acquired factor VIII inhibitor. Ann Intern Med 1989;110:774–778.

47 Lian EC, Villar MJ, Noy LI, Ruiz-Dayao Z: Acquired factor VIII inhibitor treated with cyclophosphamide, vincristine, and prednisone. Am J Hematol 2002;69:294–295.

48 Knobl P, Derfler K: Extracorporeal immunoadsorption for the treatment of haemophilic patients with inhibitors to factor VIII or IX. Vox Sang 1999;77(suppl 1):57–64.

49 Rivard GE, St Louis J, Lacroix S, Champagne M, Rock G: Immunoadsorption for coagulation factor inhibitors: a retrospective critical appraisal of 10 consecutive cases from a single institution. Haemophilia 2003;9:711–716.

50 Jansen M, Schmaldienst S, Banyai S, Quehenberger P, Pabinger I, Derfler K, Horl WH, Knobl P: Treatment of coagulation inhibitors with extracorporeal immunoadsorption (Ig-Therasorb). Br J Haematol 2001;112:91–97.

51 Gjorstrup P, Berntorp E, Larsson L, Nilsson IM: Kinetic aspects of the removal of IgG and inhibitors in hemophiliacs using protein A immunoadsorption. Vox Sang 1991;61:244–250.

52 Hauser I, Schneider B, Lechner K: Post-partum factor VIII inhibitors. A review of the literature with special reference to the value of steroid and immunosuppressive treatment. Thromb Haemost 1995;73:1–5.

53 Ries M, Wolfel D, Maier-Brandt B: Severe intracranial hemorrhage in a newborn infant with transplacental transfer of an acquired factor VII:C inhibitor. J Pediatr 1995;127:649–650.

54 Stockschlaeder M, Ruf L, Linderer A, Schroeder T, Haas R, Gerhardt A, Sucker C, Zotz RB, Scharf RE: Induction of immunotolerance to endogenous FVIII in two high-titer FVIII inhibitor patients with acquired haemophilia. Haemophilia 2008;14:in press.

Prof. Dr. med. Marcus Stockschläder
Institut für Hämostaseologie und Transfusionsmedizin
Universitätsklinikum Düsseldorf
Heinrich-Heine-Universität Düsseldorf
Moorenstr. 5, 40225 Düsseldorf, Germany
Tel. +49 211 811 6921, Fax -6937
E-Mail stockschlaeder@med.uni-duesseldorf.de

Scharf RE (ed): Progress and Challenges in Transfusion Medicine, Hemostasis and Hemotherapy.
Freiburg i.Br., Karger, 2008, pp 288–295

The Unrecognized von Willebrand Disease: A Frequent Cause of Bleeding Complications

Reinhard Schneppenheim[a] · Ulrich Budde[b]

[a]Department of Pediatric Hematology and Oncology, Medical Center Hamburg-Eppendorf,
[b]AescuLabor Hamburg, Laboratory for Coagulation, Germany

Key Words

von Willebrand disease · von Willebrand factor · Platelets · Collagen · ADAMTS13

Summary

Quantitative and qualitative defects of von Willebrand factor (VWF) cause von Willebrand disease (VWD), the most common inborn bleeding disorder being inherited in a mainly autosomal dominant but also recessive manner. According to its modular structure characterized by distinct functional and structural domains, VWF defects correlate with considerable heterogeneity of clinical symptoms, biochemical parameters and of the underlying molecular mechanisms. This renders the diagnostic approach demanding and is also the reason for under- or misdiagnosis of VWD.　　　©2008 S. Karger GmbH, Freiburg i.Br.

Introduction

Although von Willebrand disease (VWD) occurs with a prevalence of up to 1% in the normal population, only 1:8,000 individuals come to medical attention. This is due to the lack of symptoms under normal circumstances and to the frequently unsuspicious symptoms of the mild forms of VWD. Only under special conditions, like surgery of mucous membranes, e.g. tonsillectomy, or post partum, even mild VWD may manifest unexpectedly with impressive bleedings. Responsible are quantitative and/or qualitative defects of the von Willebrand factor (VWF). VWF possesses a key role in primary hemostasis by participating in adhesion and aggregation of platelets at the injured vessel wall, by its binding sites for subendothelial matrix proteins like collagen and by its binding domains for the platelet receptors GpIb and GpIIb/IIIa, in particular under conditions of high shear in the arterial system and the microcirculation. Its second important function is the binding and stabilization of factor VIII

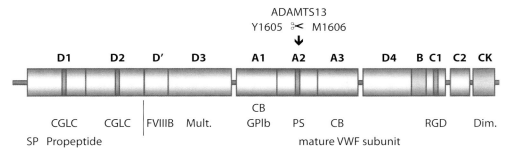

Fig. 1. Domain structure of VWF. SP = Signal peptide; CGLC = disulfide isomerase consensus sequence; Mult. = N-terminal D3 multimerization domain; Dim. = CK dimerization domain; FVIIIB, GpIb, CB, RGD = binding domains for FVIII, platelet GpIb, collagen, and platelet GpIIb/IIIa, respectively; ADAMTS13 = VWF proteolytic site in the A2 domain between Y1605 and M1606.

(FVIII), thereby preventing the rapid clearance of FVIII from the circulation. These different functions are located in distinct VWF domains (fig. 1), e.g. the FVIII binding site in the VWF D' domain, collagen binding sites in the A3 und A1 domains, platelet GpIb binding sites in the A1 domain, and the GpIIb/IIIa binding site probably in the C1 domain (RGD sequence). Furthermore, four structural domains exist: the C-terminal cysteine-rich CK domain as the site of dimerization of VWF monomers, the D1 and D2 domains with disulfide isomerase consensus sequences (CGLC) providing catalytic activity for disulfide bonding necessary for further polymerization of VWF dimers to multimers, and the N-terminal cysteine-rich D3 domain which is the putative disulfide isomerase substrate for the multimerization process [1, 2].

The functional platelet-dependent activity of VWF (binding at platelet receptors and collagen) under conditions of high shear depends solely on the presence of high-molecular-weight multimers [3], which are the largest known plasma proteins of up to 40,000 kDa.

The different functional domains and the complex post-translational biosynthesis allow a multitude of possible specific and combined defects [4]. This is the molecular basis of the impressive heterogeneity of VWF functional parameters and clinical symptoms and the reason why the diagnosis of VWD is often missed or only made after more pronounced bleeding events in many cases.

Clinical Symptoms

The leading symptoms of VWD are muco-cutaneous bleedings. Typical symptoms are therefore epistaxis, severe bleeding after tonsillectomy, adenotomy or gastrointestinal surgery as well as urogenital bleeding. In women, menorrhagia and post-partum bleedings are frequent. Hemophilia-like bleeding symptoms (joint and muscle bleeding) are almost exclusively seen in patients with severe VWD type 3 or in type 2N (see below) corresponding to very low FVIII levels.

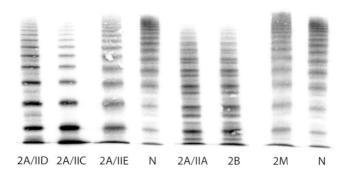

Fig. 2. VWF multimers of different VWD type 2 phenotypes. Roman numbers refer to the old nomenclature designating VWD type 2 subtypes according to their multimer structure. Note the lack of a defined triplet structure in phenotypes 2A/IID, 2A/IIC and 2A/IIE, enhanced proteolysis of phenotype 2A/IIA and subtype 2B and a 'smeary' structure in subtype 2M compared to normal plasma (N).

2A/IID 2A/IIC 2A/IIE N 2A/IIA 2B 2M N

Diagnosis

A prolonged bleeding time or a prolonged platelet function analyzer (PFA100) closure time is often detected in typical cases; however, also normal values might be observed. A prolonged activated partial thromboplastin time (APTT) may also be seen, however, only in correlation with low FVIII:C (<30%). Therefore, a normal APTT is never an exclusion criterion for VWD. The diagnosis is made in patients with a bleeding history by measuring VWF:antigen (VWF:Ag), VWF:ristocetin cofactor (VWF:RCo), VWF:collagen binding (VWF:CB) and by multimer analysis of VWF (fig. 2). Measuring VWF:FVIII binding activity (VWF:FVIIIB) is indicated in cases of 'female hemophilia' or equivocal inheritance as differential diagnosis to hemophilia A. Molecular genetic studies are indicated in difficult cases and to enable genetic counseling.

Classification

VWD is divided into 3 main types:

Type 1 is characterized by a relative reduction of VWF:Ag and a corresponding reduction of all of its functions. All multimers are present in normal concentrations. Inheritance is mostly autosomal dominant, clinical symptoms are rarely severe. This type is often not diagnosed or only after presenting with obvious bleeding symptoms. It can in many cases not clearly be distinguished from normal individuals with low VWF.

Type 3 refers to an absolute deficiency of VWF and all of its functions. Clinical symptoms are most often severe, including joint and muscle bleeding. Inheritance is autosomal recessive. This type is almost always diagnosed already in early childhood.

Type 2 represents the most heterogeneous group with varying clinical symptoms, different pathomechanisms and different traits of inheritance. This type is the most difficult to diagnose and classify. According to the current nomenclature, it is divided into 4 subtypes [5]:

1 Disregarding the molecular mechanism, subtype 2A is characterized by the lack or a significant relative decrease of large VWF multimers and the correlating decrease in platelet-dependent function (VWF:CB, VWF:RCo, GPIb binding). Different 2A phenotypes were previously designated by a Roman number and letters in alphabetical order. Inheritance is usually dominant except for the recessively inherited particular phenotype IIC. The most common 2A phenotype correlates with the previous subtype IIA, characterized by an enhanced proteolytic susceptibility of mutant VWF to the specific VWF-cleaving protease ADAMTS13 and the subsequent loss of large VWF multimers [6, 7].
2 The primary defect of subtype 2B is an enhanced affinity of mutant VWF to GpIb. The resulting partly spontaneous platelet aggregation in the circulation correlates with platelet consumption and enhanced ADAMTS13 proteolysis, with subsequent loss of large multimers undistinguishable from subtype 2A phenotype IIA [8]. Inheritance is dominant.
3 Subtype 2M is characterized by decreased platelet-dependent function (VWF:CB, VWF:RCo, GpIb binding), similar to subtype 2A, however, without significant loss of large multimers but isolated functional defects instead. Inheritance is dominant.
4 Subtype 2N (Normandy) designates an isolated VWF:FVIII binding defect. This subtype cannot reliably be distinguished from hemophilia A without the FVIII binding assay. Inheritance is autosomal recessive [9].

Problems of Classification

The correct classification is very much dependent on the results of the functional assays and VWF multimer analysis. In particular, the latter method is difficult to standardize, which may result in false classification, in particular in favor of VWD type 1 [10]. Confirmation in a reference laboratory is mandatory in equivocal cases. A synopsis of the first and the most recent classification is shown in figure 3.

Molecular Genetics

VWF is located on chromosome 12p13.1, and with its size of 178 kb and its structure of 52 exons, it is a large and complex gene. Molecular diagnosis is complicated by the presence of a pseudogene on chromosome 22 with 97% homology to exons 24–34

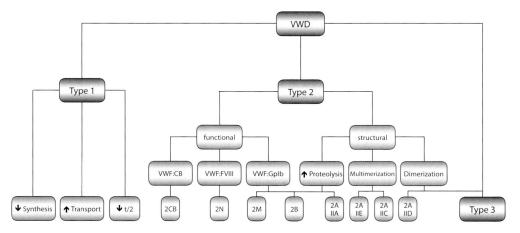

Fig. 3. Synopsis of the first and the most recent classification of VWD. Compound heterozygosity or homozygosity for some type 2 defects may result in VWD type 3.

[11]. Many of the mutations identified to date are listed in the Sheffield VWF mutation database (*www.vwf.group.shef.ac.uk/*).

VWD Type 3

A clear indication for molecular diagnosis is severe VWD type 3, because of the severity of the disease, the unreliable phenotypic diagnosis of unaffected carriers, and as a basis for genetic counseling. Unfortunately, numerous mutations are causing VWD type 3; thus, mutation screening requires covering the complete gene sequence (fig. 4). In Germany, only one single mutation (2435delC) is more frequent and is found on 20% of all type 3 chromosomes. In Sweden, this mutation was identified on 50% and in Poland even on 75% of VWD type 3 chromosomes. In other countries, this mutation is rare or not existent, suggesting a founder mutation [12]. In general, the mutation spectrum is very heterogeneous and comprises even numerous missense mutations (15–20%) and, in addition, gene conversions with the pseudogene [13]. Interestingly, this is the only known example of inter-chromosomal gene conversions.

VWD Type 1

Until recently VWD type 1 had not been studied in more detail on the molecular level. However, valuable data were obtained by a European and a Canadian multi-center study, which were just published in 2007 and 2008 [10, 14, 15]. As in VWD type 3, VWD type 1 mutations were also distributed over the gene; however, mutation clusters were identified in the D3 domain and the C-terminal region of VWF (fig. 4).

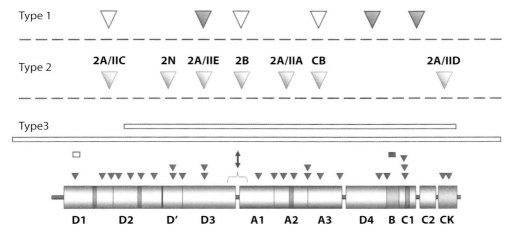

Fig. 4. Spectrum of mutations in VWD. For type 1, only the location of mutations is given. Dark triangles refer to mutation clusters. For type 2, particular phenotypes correlate with the locations of mutations. For type 3, large deletions are shown as empty bars, large insertions as filled bars, small truncating mutations and missense mutations as triangles; the double-head arrow indicates the region of gene conversions.

A more rapid clearance of VWF was identified as a novel more frequent molecular mechanism in VWD type 1.

VWD Type 2

According to its phenotypic heterogeneity, the molecular mechanisms of VWD type 2, and in particular subtype 2A, differ considerably. However, an exact phenotypic description and detailed VWF multimer analysis can define regions of interest for mutation screening [4, 16]. This is generally done by PCR of the coding exons and direct sequencing.

The particular phenotype of VWD subtype 2A, the lack or relative loss of large VWF multimers, may correlate with either primarily functional or structural abnormalities. Mutations causing the phenotype 2A/IIA were the first being identified in a qualitative VWF defect, and correlate with an enhanced susceptibility of mutant VWF for its protease ADAMTS13. The respective mutations are flanking the VWF proteolytic site in the A2 domain.

Other phenotypes of subtype 2A are due to defects of dimerization with mutations in the CK domain and defects of multimerization with mutations either in the VWF pro-peptide, i.e. the D1-D2 domain (2A/IIC), or in the D3 domain (2A/IIE) [16–19].

Gain-of-function mutations enhancing the VWF affinity to platelet GPIb can be identified in a limited region of the VWF A1 domain.

Mutations of subtype 2M are found in the A1 domain and in other regions and frequently impair VWF:GpIb binding.

Homozygous or compound-heterozygous mutations in the D' domain harboring the VWF:FVIII binding site cause VWD subtype 2N with very low FVIII:C values. All other VWF parameters may be normal in this particular subtype, which requires a FVIII binding assay to differentiate it from hemophilia A. In cases of compound heterozygosity with a null allele, VWF:Ag may also be slightly decreased. This subtype resembles closely the term 'hereditary pseudohemophilia' coined by Erik Adolf von Willebrand [20]. The locations of mutations according to the phenotype beyond the subtype level are shown in figure 4.

Conclusions and Future Directions

VWD is known since decades as one of the most heterogeneous bleeding disorders. Earlier designations as 'hereditary pseudohemophilia', 'constitutional thrombopathy von Willebrand-Juergens', or 'angiohemophilia' indicate the already earlier observed different phenotypes and the diagnostic difficulties. The up-to-date spectrum of diagnostic methods allows making a clear diagnosis in most cases; however, the whole diagnostic approach is demanding and requires prior clinical suspicion. Therefore, a higher alertness for bleeding symptoms is necessary, but also a targeted standardized record of the medical history including the patient's family.

Disclosure of Conflict of Interests

R.S. has acted as consultant to the companies CSL Behring and Siemens and has been on an Advisory Board for the company Baxter.

References

1 Sadler JE: Biochemistry and genetics of von Willebrand factor. Annu Rev Biochem 1998;67:395–424.
2 Mayadas TN, Wagner DD: Vicinal cysteines in the prosequence play a role in von Willebrand factor multimer assembly. Proc Natl Acad Sci U S A 1992;89:3531–3535.
3 Ruggeri ZM: Platelet and von Willebrand factor interactions at the vessel wall. Hämostaseologie 2004;24:1–11.
4 Schneppenheim R, Budde U, Ruggeri ZM: A molecular approach to the classification of von Willebrand disease. Best Pract Res Clin Haematol 2001;14:281–298.
5 Sadler JE, Budde U, Eikenboom JC, Favaloro EJ, Hill FG, Holmberg L, Ingerslev J, Lee CA, Lillicrap D, Mannucci PM, Mazurier C, Meyer D, Nichols WL, Nishino M, Peake IR, Rodeghiero F, Schneppenheim R, Ruggeri ZM, Srivastava A, Montgomery RR, Federici AB; Working Party on von Willebrand Disease Classification: Update on the pathophysiology and classification of von Willebrand disease: a report of the Subcommittee on von Willebrand Factor. J Thromb Haemost 2006; 4:2103–2114.

6   Zimmerman TS, Dent JA, Ruggeri ZM, Nannini LH: Subunit composition of plasma von Willebrand factor. Cleavage is present in normal individuals, increased in IIA and IIB von Willebrand disease, but minimal in variants with aberrant structure of individual oligomers (types IIC, IID, and IIE). J Clin Invest 1986;77:947–951.

7   Hassenpflug WA, Budde U, Obser T, Angerhaus D, Drewke E, Schneppenheim S, Schneppenheim R: Impact of mutations in the von Willebrand factor A2 domain on ADAMTS13-dependent proteolysis. Blood 2006;107:2339–2345.

8   Ware J, Dent JA, Azuma H, Sugimoto M, Kyrle PA, Yoshioka A, Ruggeri ZM: Identification of a point mutation in type IIB von Willebrand disease illustrating the regulation of von Willebrand factor affinity for the platelet membrane glycoprotein Ib-IX receptor. Proc Natl Acad Sci U S A 1991;88:2946–2950.

9   Nishino M, Girma JP, Rothschild C, Fressinaud E, Meyer D: New variant of von Willebrand disease with defective binding to factor VIII. Blood 1989;74:1591–1599.

10 Budde U, Schneppenheim R, Eikenboom J, Goodeve A, Will K, Drewke E, Castaman G, Rodeghiero F, Federici AB, Batlle J, Pérez A, Meyer D, Mazurier C, Goudemand J, Ingerslev J, Habart D, Vorlova Z, Holmberg L, Lethagen S, Pasi J, Hill F, Peake I: Detailed von Willebrand factor multimer analysis in patients with von Willebrand disease in the European study, molecular and clinical markers for the diagnosis and management of type 1 von Willebrand disease (MCMDM-1VWD). J Thromb Haemost 2008;6:762–771.

11 Mancuso DJ, Tuley EA, Westfield LA, Lester-Mancuso TL, Le Beau MM, Sorace JM, Sadler JE: Human von Willebrand factor gene and pseudogene: structural analysis and differentiation by polymerase chain reaction. Biochemistry 1991;30:253–269.

12 Zhang ZP, Falk G, Blomback M, Egberg N, Anvret M: A single cytosine deletion in exon 18 of the von Willebrand factor gene is the most common mutation in Swedish vWD type III patients. Hum Mol Genet 1992;1:767–768.

13 Gupta PK, Adamtziki E, Budde U, Jaiprakash M, Kumar H, Harbeck-Seu A, Kannan M, Oyen F, Obser T, Wedekind I, Saxena R, Schneppenheim R: Gene conversions are a common cause of von Willebrand disease. Br J Haematol 2005;130:752–758.

14 Goodeve A, Eikenboom J, Castaman G, Rodeghiero F, Federici AB, Batlle J, Meyer D, Mazurier C, Goudemand J, Schneppenheim R, Budde U, Ingerslev J, Habart D, Vorlova Z, Holmberg L, Lethagen S, Pasi J, Hill F, Hashemi Soteh M, Baronciani L, Hallden C, Guilliatt A, Lester W, Peake I: Phenotype and genotype of a cohort of families historically diagnosed with type 1 von Willebrand disease in the European study, Molecular and Clinical Markers for the Diagnosis and Management of Type 1 von Willebrand Disease (MCMDM-1VWD). Blood 2007;109:112–121.

15 James PD, Notley C, Hegadorn C, Leggo J, Tuttle A, Tinlin S, Brown C, Andrews C, Labelle A, Chirinian Y, O'Brien L, Othman M, Rivard G, Rapson D, Hough C, Lillicrap D: The mutational spectrum of type 1 von Willebrand disease: Results from a Canadian cohort study. Blood 2007;109:145–154.

16 Schneppenheim R, Budde U: Phenotypic and genotypic diagnosis of von Willebrand disease: a 2004 update. Semin Hematol 2005;42:15–28.

17 Schneppenheim R, Brassard J, Krey S, Budde U, Kunicki TJ, Holmberg L, Ware J, Ruggeri ZM: Defective dimerisation of von Willebrand factor subunits due to a Cys--Arg mutation in type IID von Willebrand disease. Proc Natl Acad Sci U S A 1996;93:3581–3586.

18 Gaucher C, Dieval J, Mazurier C: Characterization of von Willebrand factor gene defects in two unrelated patients with type IIC von Willebrand disease. Blood 1994;84:1024–1030.

19 Schneppenheim R, Thomas KB, Krey S, Budde U, Jessat U, Sutor AH, Zieger B: Identification of a candidate missense mutation in a family with von Willebrand disease type IIC. Hum Genet 1995;956:681–686.

20 von Willebrand EA: Hereditär pseudohemofili. Finska Läkaresällskapets Handlingar 1926;672:7–112.

Prof. Dr. rer. nat. Reinhard Schneppenheim
Universitätsklinikum Hamburg-Eppendorf
Martinistraße 52
20246 Hamburg, Germany
Tel. +49 40 42803-4270, Fax -4601
E-Mail pho@uke.de

Scharf RE (ed): Progress and Challenges in Transfusion Medicine, Hemostasis and Hemotherapy.
Freiburg i.Br., Karger, 2008, pp 296–316

Acquired Platelet Function Defects: An Underestimated but Frequent Cause of Bleeding Complications in Clinical Practice

Rüdiger E. Scharf

Department of Experimental and Clinical Hemostasis, Hemotherapy, and Transfusion Medicine, University Medical Center and Biological Medical Research Center, Heinrich Heine University Düsseldorf, Düsseldorf, Germany

Key Words

Platelet dysfunction · Antiplatelet drugs · Renal failure · Liver cirrhosis · Hematologic malignancies (acute leukemias, myelodysplastic syndromes, myeloproliferative disorders, myelomas)

Summary

Drugs represent the most common cause of platelet dysfunction in our overmedicated society. While acetylsalicylic acid, clopigogrel, and integrin αIIbβ3 (glycoprotein IIb-IIIa) receptor antagonists are well known as 'prototypes' of antiplatelet drugs, other widely used agents including nonsteroidal anti-inflammatory drugs, antibiotics, serotonin reuptake inhibitors, and volume expanders can also impair platelet function and thus cause or aggravate hemorrhages. Besides pharmacological agents, certain clinical conditions are often associated with qualitative platelet disorders and bleeding diathesis. Consequently, in contrast to inherited platelet disorders, acquired platelet function defects are much more frequent in clinical practice and therefore deserve special attention. Their pathogenesis is widespread and heterogeneous with various, sometimes overlapping abnormalities in the same clinical disorder. Moreover, acquired platelet dysfunctions can occur at any age and range in severity from mild to life-threatening hemorrhages. Due to their heterogeneity, acquired platelet function disorders will be classified and discussed according to the underlying clinical setting or disease.   ©2008 S. Karger GmbH, Freiburg i.Br.

Introduction

Antithrombotic drugs are widely used to prevent and treat thrombotic and thromboembolic events, both in the venous and arterial circulation, including the heart [1–3]. Agents that inhibit platelet function are effective for the initial management of acute coronary syndrome [4–6], for long-term management of coronary, cerebral and peripheral artery disease [4–8] and also administered for prevention of thromboembolism in atrial fibrillation [9, 10]. Percutaneous coronary interventions includ-

Fig. 1. Antiplatelet agents and their mode of action. Stimulation with agonists such as collagen, thrombin, ADP, TXA$_2$ or by physical forces such as shear stress results in platelet activation via inside-out signaling with conformational changes of GPIIb-IIIa (integrin αIIbβ3) and subsequent platelet aggregation. Inhibition of TXA$_2$ formation or antagonism of the ADP receptor P2Y$_{12}$ interrupts positive feedback loops required for sustained platelet activation. Direct pharmacological blockade of GPIIb-IIIa by specific antibodies or recep-

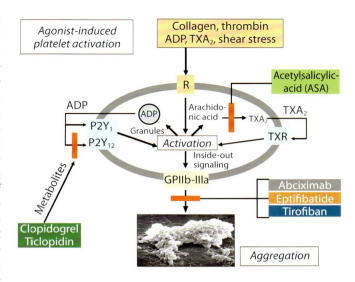

tor antagonists inhibits platelet aggregation. At approximately 15,000–20,000 intact residual GPIIb-IIIa receptor copies, platelet inhibition is sufficient to suppress occlusive platelet thrombus formation in acute settings such as percutaneous coronary intervention without inducing major bleeding [14, 66]. Modification of a figure adapted from the work of Schrör and Hohlfeld [67] and printed with permission.

ing stent placement therapy have required more intense antithrombotic strategies to prevent coronary restenosis. Thus, it has been shown that inhibiting cyclooxygenase-1 and antagonizing one of the two platelet adenosin diphosphate (ADP) receptors, P2Y$_{12}$, by combined treatment with acetylsalicylic acid (aspirin) and thienopyridines (clopidogrel) is more effective than aspirin alone for the prevention of recurrent thrombotic events in high-risk patients with acute coronary syndrome [11–13]. Moreover, blockade of platelet integrin αIIbβ3, also known as glycoprotein (GP) IIb-IIIa, by specific receptor antagonists (GPIIb-IIIa inhibitors) has been used successfully in this setting [1, 14, 15]. The mode of action of antiplatelet drugs is schematically depicted in figure 1. A major side effect of all antithrombotic regimens, however, is the induction of a potential bleeding diathesis. Consequently, treatment with antiplatelet drugs can cause or aggravate severe hemorrhage. This is especially true in patients with preexisting hemostatic defects of any kind that remain compensated, unless platelet function is not inhibited pharmacologically.

Apart from pharmacological agents, certain pathological conditions are frequently associated with platelet dysfunction(s) and clinical bleeding. These include uremia, in which small toxic compounds such as guanidinosuccinic acid and phenolic acids are produced, known to inhibit platelet aggregation; liver cirrhosis, in which severe bleeding occurs when low coagulation factor activities, dysfibrinogenemia, and thrombocytopenia are concomitantly present with platelet functional defects of multifactorial cause; myeloproliferative disorders, acute leukemias, and myeloplastic syndromes, in which dysfunctional platelet populations are being produced, resulting from clonal abnormalities of megakaryocytes; monoclonal gammopathy and antiplatelet autoantibodies frequently being associated with impaired platelet function; and cardiopulmonary bypass and hemodialysis, in which platelets are exposed to artificial surfaces, resulting in activation and degranulation ('exhausted' platelets). Acquired storage pool disease may also be observed in autoimmune thrombocytopenias, disseminated intravascular coagulation and in acute or chronic rejection following renal transplantation [16, 17]. Some of these clinical conditions listed here are discussed in more detail.

Primary Hemostasis

Human platelets are anucleated cellular fragments derived from the cytoplasma of their highly specialized precursor cells, the megakaryocytes. Upon their maturation in the bone marrow, platelets are released into the circulation by megakaryocyte fragmentation (platelet shedding), a process driven by mechanotransduction, formation of microtubule bundles and reorganization of the megakaryocytic cytoskeleton [18]. Being released into the circulation, platelets survey the integrity of the vascular system. Under physiological conditions, they reveal no interaction with the inner surface of normal vessels but adhere immediately (within milliseconds) when endothelial cells are damaged or when subendothelial matrix structures become exposed to flowing blood [19, 20]. This is a crucial initiating step both in hemostasis and thrombosis since platelet responses do not distinguish between traumatic and pathological vessel wall damage [20]. Thus, although the normal function of platelets is to contribute to the arrest of bleeding from wounds by forming a hemostatic plug, they can generate occlusive thrombi as a consequence of vascular diseases, in particular at sites of atherosclerotic lesions.

Initial Platelet-Vessel Wall Interactions (Primary Hemostasis) and Subsequent Thrombin Generation (Secondary Hemostasis)

As shown schematically in figure 2, recruitment and stimulation of circulating platelets in response to vessel wall injury follows a sequence of interactions and activation steps. The enumeration (1 through 7) corresponds to the numbers indicated in figure 2.

(1) Upon exposure of subendothelial matrix components, circulating (resting) platelets immediately adhere at sites of vascular injury. The extracelluar matrix constituents include different types of collagen and adhesive plasma proteins such as von Willebrand factor (vWF) and fibrinogen (Fg), which become immobilized onto

Fig. 2. Recruitment and activation of circulating platelets in response to vessel wall injury. Steps (1) through (7) illustrate the sequence of initial platelet responses and mechanisms leading to the formation of a platelet fibrin thrombus. (1) Exposure of subendothelial structures such as collagen and subsequent adsorption, immobilization and conformational change of adhesive plasma proteins such as vWF and Fg.

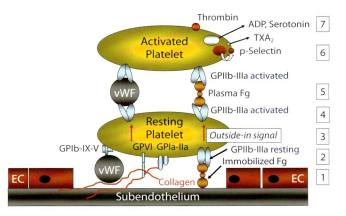

(2) Binding of circulating platelets to extracellular matrix proteins and immobilized ligands via specific receptors on the platelet surface. (3) Signal transduction of adherent platelets via outside-in pathways. (4) Platelet activation and expression of activated GPIIb-IIIa receptor copies at the luminal surface. (5) Binding of adhesive ligands from the plasma (vWF and Fg) followed by platelet aggregation. (6) Platelet secretion and release of stimulating granular constituent products or metabolites. (7) Expression of procoagulant activity on the platelet surface leading to the generation of thrombin and subsequent fibrin formation. Synergy between primary (steps 1 through 6) and secondary hemostasis (step 7) is required to arrest bleeding by forming a stable hemostatic platelet fibrin plug.

extracelluar matrices at sites of injury, thereby undergoing specific conformational changes that trigger the interaction with their corresponding receptors on the platelet surface [19]. (2) The platelet counterparts include GPIbα in the GPIb-IX-V complex, an essential binding site for vWF (bound to collagen), GPVI and GPIa-IIa (integrin α2β1), both of which directly react with collagen, and nonactivated GPIIb-IIIa (integrin αIIbβ3), which recognizes locally adsorbed (immobilized) Fg and fibrin [21]. (3) As a consequence of the multiple receptor-ligand interactions, platelets adhere and become activated by outside-in signaling. (4) While nonactivated αIIbβ3 cannot bind soluble ligands, activated receptor molecules are expressed at the luminal surface, now exhibiting high-affinity binding sites for soluble plasma proteins including Fg, vWF, thrombospondin, vitronectin, and fibronectin [22]. (5) Consequently, after a first layer of adherent and, in turn, of activated platelets is formed on the thrombogenic surface, αIIbβ3 binds adhesive ligands from the plasma (exemplified are vWF and Fg). (6) Platelet activation is directly triggered by adhesion (see step 3) but is greatly enhanced by agonists released from stimulated platelets, such as ADP, serotonin and thromboxane A_2 (TXA_2). Moreover, expression of neoepitopes (exemplified by P-selectin) occurs on the platelet surface. (7) After activation, platelets provide a catalytic membrane surface for the activation of factor X (tenase complex) and the activation of prothrombin (prothrombin complex), resulting in the circumscript generation of high concentrations of thrombin. This 'thrombin burst' induces recruitment and activation of additional circulating platelets. Thrombin also accelerates the formation of fibrin (secondary hemostasis) which is necessary to stabilize the hemostatic platelet plug or thrombus. Consolidation of the platelet-fibrin thrombus ('clot retraction') is essential to resist displacement by hemodynamic forces [19, 20, 23].

Frequency of and Screening for Defects in Primary Hemostasis

Data on the rate of primary hemostatic defects are available from a prospective analysis by Koscielny et al. [24] who studied 5,649 consecutive patients (aged 17–87 years) prior to elective surgery. Aside from history and physical examination, the investigators used a bleeding history questionnaire and a standardized test panel for hemostatic screening, including in vitro bleeding time determined by platelet function analyzer (PFA-100). Patients with preexisting hemostatic disorders or anticoagulation therapy were primarily excluded from the analysis. Of the 5,649 patients, bleeding history was negative in 5,021 (88.8%); in the remaining group (11.2%) with a bleeding history, screening for hemostatic defects was positive in 256 of the 628 patients (40.8%). Interestingly, diagnostic work-up of these 256 patients revealed platelet function defects in 73%, coagulation disorders in 0.8%, and combined hemostatic defects in 26.2% (including a predominant proportion of patients with von Willebrand disease). Among the 187 individuals with primary hemostatic defects, acquired platelet dysfunction was drug induced in 162 patients (63.3%); among them, 147 were taking aspirin, ticlopedine, clopidogrel, or other nonsteroidal anti-inflammatory agents, while in 10 patients (6.2%) antibiotic treatment appeared to be the cause of platelet dysfunction. It is conceivable that this rate of antibiotics-induced bleeding diathesis may be even higher in other patient groups. Indeed, as reported on a smaller cohort of hospitalized patients with prolonged Ivy bleeding time, 54% were receiving large doses of antibiotics and 10% were taking aspirin or other nonsteroidal anti-inflammatory agents [25].

In conclusion, the data reported by Koscielny et al. [24] convincingly illustrate several important issues: (1) Acquired platelet function defects are indeed more frequent in clinical practice than generally believed. (2) In the majority of cases, platelet dysfunction is drug induced, (3) whereby the predominant proportion of antiplatelet agents should not lead to an underestimation of given inhibitory effects by antibiotics. (4) Screening for primary hemostatic defects requires indeed appropriate laboratory techniques, as demonstrated by the PFA testing. Thus, albeit trivial, the widespread practice of platelet counting and coagulation screening (by activated partial thromboplastin time (aPTT) and prothrombin time) is entirely inappropriate to identify individuals with platelet dysfunction(s). (5) Finally, as also documented here (in 2 of 256 patients), 'pure' coagulation defects occur less frequently than generally assumed.

Antiplatelet Drugs

Acetylsalicylic acid (aspirin) and nonsteroidal anti-inflammatory agents, thienopyridines (ticlopedine, clopidogrel), and GPIIb-IIIa receptor antagonists are the most prominent causes of acquired platelet function disorders and, thus, of potential bleeding risk. Moreover, agents that increase intraplatelet cyclic adenosine monophosphate (cAMP) either by stimulation of its synthesis (prostaglandin E_1 (PGE_1), prostacyclin (PGI_2)) or by phosphodiesterase inhibition (dipyridamole, theophylline, caffeine), may also impair platelet function. Nitric oxide (NO) donors can increase the bleeding time and may contribute to hemorrhage, specifically in uremic patients. Antibiotics, particularly those of the β-lactam type such as penicillins and cephalosporins, may cause a prolongation of the bleeding time even in normal volunteers. The mechanism whereby these antibiotics impair platelet function is currently not known, although it has been proposed that they bind to the platelet membrane and inhibit the interaction of agonists and vWF or modify platelet receptors chemically [26]. Differences in the antiplatelet effect (e.g. inhibition of aggregation) of carbenicillin, penicillin G, ticarcillin, ampicillin, nafcillin, azlocillin, piperacillin, alpacillin, or mezlocillin probably relate to differences in blood levels and in drug potency. Adsorption and nonspecific binding to platelet membrane constituents are also discussed as mechanisms by which volume expanders can impair platelet aggregation; however, interference of dextran or hydroethyl starch with the interaction of GPIIb-IIIa and its plasma ligands may be relevant clinically only in patients with a preexisting hemostatic defect (e.g. von Willebrand disease).

In general, acquired platelet function defects secondary to drugs are mild and ubiquitous, considering, for example, the large number of individuals who take aspirin regularly and who therefore have impaired platelet function due to irreversible inhibition of cyclooxygenase-1-dependent TXA_2 formation. The effect of aspirin ingestion on the hemostatic competency of normal volunteers has been debated but appears to be of minor relevance. Nevertheless, individuals taking aspirin chronically report a significant increase in bruising, epistaxis, and gastrointestinal blood loss. More importantly, there was a slight, but statistically insignificant increase in hemorrhagic strokes in a group of otherwise healthy physicians who took aspirin chronically as primary prophylaxis against myocardial infarction [27].

Besides aspirin, more than 250 pharmacological agents, foods (fish oils) or diets (eicosapentaenoic acid), spices (onion, garlic), and vitamins have been reported to impair platelet function. For further information, the readers are referred to other review articles [1, 3, 26].

Taken together, for almost all agents interfering with platelet reactivity or inhibiting platelet function, data are limited to abnormal platelet aggregation studies in vitro or prolonged bleeding time, which do not necessarily reflect the true bleeding risk and therefore may have minor or questionable clinical importance. By contrast, treatment with antiplatelet agents can cause or aggravate severe hemorrhage in patients with preexisting hemostatic defects of any kind. This is particularly true for certain clinical settings (sepsis, disseminated intravascular coagulation), or conditions (cardiopulmonary bypass surgery, liver transplantation), hematologic or systemic diseases that affect platelet function or are associated frequently with bleeding disorders (renal failure, liver cirrhosis, systemic lupus erythematosus, myeloproliferative disorders, acute leukemias, myelodysplastic syndromes, and myeloma).

End-Stage Renal Disease

Bleeding may be a serious complication in patients with acute and chronic renal failure. The clinical manifestations vary from ecchymoses, epistaxis, bleeding from gums and venipuncture sites to overt hemorrhage from the gastrointestinal and genitourinary tracts and are observed in up to one third of uremic patients. The pathogenesis of uremic bleeding is multifactorial (table 1). It must be stressed that bleeding due to platelet abnormalities and other alterations involved in hemorrhagic complications is by far not the only hemostatic disorder in patients with chronic renal failure. Thus, thrombosis of vascular access is common in patients undergoing hemodialysis. Moreover, patients with uremia are highly susceptible to the development of atherosclerosis and its thrombotic complications [29].

Various platelet abnormalities, with partially conflicting results, have been reported in end-stage renal disease, including defects in platelet adhesion, aggregation, secretion, signal transduction and metabolism of arachidonic acid and NO [29–31]. The most consistent finding is prolongation of the bleeding time, which is abnormal in about 75% of uremic patients [31]. However, its value in predicting the risk of hemorrhage in uremia is not defined.

In general, uremic patients with bleeding improve upon hemodialysis and transfusion of red blood cells. In fact, reducing the serum levels of uremic toxins (table 1), which may cause or account for platelet dysfunction, and increasing the hematocrit and thereby improving blood rheology does correct several conditions that otherwise contribute to defective hemostasis. Indeed, anemia is the main determinant of the prolonged bleeding time in uremic patients, as also demonstrated by an inverse relationship of increasing the hematocrit and concomitantly decreasing the bleeding time upon treatment with recombinant human erythropoietin [29]. However, the early termination of the Normal Hematocrit Cardiac Trial [32], in which cardiac patients who had been randomly assigned to the normal hematocrit group presented with a higher mortality and a higher incidence of nonfatal myocardial infarction, raised questions about the safety of the long-term maintenance of a normal hematocrit [29].

While it is generally assumed that hemodialysis corrects platelet abnormalities and reduces bleeding, it does not eliminate the risk of hemorrhage. Thus, several studies demonstrate that platelet aggregation can be improved or even transiently worsened by hemodialysis procedures, indicating that dialysis does not only remove inhibitors

Table 1. Abnormalities and other determinants involved in the pathogenesis of bleeding associated with chronic renal failure; data from [17, 29–31, 33]

Qualitative platelet abnormalities
Reduced δ-granule content (ADP, serotonin)
Reduced α-granule content (platelet factor 4, β-thromboglobulin) with impaired secretion
    of α-granule constituents
Elevated intracellular cAMP
Abnormal mobilization of platelet Ca^{2+}
Increased generation of NO by uremic platelets
Defective cyclooxygenase activity
Abnormal platelet arachidonic acid metabolism
Abnormal platelet aggregation ex vivo in response to different stimuli
Activation and ligand binding defects of GPIIb-IIIa (integrin αIIbβ3)
Uremic toxins, including urea, creatinine, phenol, phenolic acid, guanidinosuccinic acid (GSA) and,
    in particular, parathyroid hormone (PTH)

Quantitative platelet abnormalities
Mild to moderate thrombocytopenia (due to inadequate production and/or consumption)

Anormal platelet-vessel wall interactions
Abnormal platelet adhesion
Increased formation of vascular prostacyclin
Abnormal production of NO
Quantitative and/or qualitative alterations of plasma vWF

Anemia
Altered blood rheology
Erythropoietin deficiency

Drugs
Antiplatelet agents, such as acetylsalicylic acid and clopidogrel
β-Lactam antibiotics
Third-generation cephalosporins
Nonsteroidal anti-inflammatory drugs, including indomethacin, ibuprofen, naproxen,
    phenylbutazone, and sulfinpyrazone
Serotonin and serotonin/noradrenalin reuptake inhibitors (SRI and SNRI), including clomipramin,
    amitriptylin, dibenzepin, doxein, and imipramin
Heparin (during hemodialysis)

---

of platelet function but also causes activation and granular secretion as platelets interact with the dialysis membranes [31, 33]. We have demonstrated that hemodialysis causes a transient α-granule storage pool defect leading to 'exhausted' platelets that continue to circulate and exhibit defective TXA_2 formation, a condition that favors bleeding in uremic patients [17, 33–36]. Other platelet defects in patients with chronic renal failure are related to dysfunctional GPIIb-IIIa (integrin αIIbβ3) and its defective interaction with Fg or vWF [30].

Thrombocytopenia due to inadequate production and/or consumption during regularly performed hemodialysis is also a common finding in patients with renal failure; however, the platelet count is rarely less than 80,000/µl and thus sufficient for primary hemostasis, presupposing intact platelet function. Other mechanisms that may cause a decrease in platelet concentration are related to side effects of the anticoagulation regimen for hemodialysis, in particular to heparin-induced thrombocytopenia of type I and II.

Liver Cirrhosis

Complex hemostatic defects are present in chronic hepatocellular disease, involving combined abnormalities of the megakaryocyte-platelet system, coagulation, and fibrinolysis. Mild to moderate thrombocytopenia due to increased splenic sequestration is observed in 30–50% of patients but not associated with spontaneous bleeding [16]. Apart from lienal pooling as the major mechanism, ineffective platelet production and increased platelet turnover can aggravate thrombocytopenia in individual patients with liver cirrhosis. Various functional platelet abnormalities have been described in chronic hepatocellular disease, including in vitro aggregation defects in response to ADP, epinephrine, collagen, and thrombin [31]. Some of the platelet aggregation defects can be attributed to elevated levels of Fg/fibrin degradation products and dysfibrinogenemia, which is common in chronic hepatitis and liver cirrhosis. Toxic effects of ethanol may contribute to platelet dysfunction. Other possible mechanisms are decreased availability of arachidonic acid and, consequently, reduced TXA_2 formation, increased cholesterol content of the platelet plasma membrane, impaired platelet transmembrane signaling, elevated sialic acid concentration of circulating platelets, and hypersialylated Fg [16, 31]. The diagnosis of disseminated intravascular coagulation (DIC) in patients with liver disease is often difficult to ascertain because of the multiple hemostatic alterations, as indicated above.

Cardiopulmonary Bypass and Other Extracorporeal Circulation Procedures

Open heart surgery using cardiopulmonary bypass is accompanied by significant alterations, including 'whole body inflammatory response', reduction in coagulation factors, activation of fibrinolysis, and quantitative and qualitative platelet changes. Among these alterations, triggered by the extensive contact between flowing blood and the synthetic surfaces of the extracorporeal circuit, platelet dysfunction represents the major insult to hemostasis in this setting. Thrombocytopenia secondary to bypass is caused by hemodilution and by consumption due to adherence of platelets on the bypass circuit. Bypass also results in shear stress-induced platelet activation (fig. 1), adherence onto immobilized Fg (fig. 2), formation of platelet aggregates, secretion of granular constituents, platelet fragmentation, and formation of platelet-derived microparticles. Typically, bypass causes prolonged bleeding times, reduced platelet aggregation responses to several agonists in vitro, and platelet storage pool disease involving selective α-granule secretion or depletion of both α- and δ-granules [37–39]. Circulating degranulated ('exhausted') platelets due to activation induced by the interaction between blood and artificial surfaces were also identified in patients with chronic renal failure upon hemodialysis [33, 35]. Attempts have been made to prevent platelet activation during bypass and hemodialysis by infusion of PGE_1 or PGI_2.

Antiplatelet Antibodies

The overall impact of platelet-antibody interaction may be thrombocytopenia and platelet function abnormalies, as noted in the wide range of autoimmune disorders, including idiopathic thrombocytopenic purpura (ITP), systemic lupus erythematosus (SLE), rheumatoid arthritis (RA), and acquired immunodeficiency syndrome (AIDS). Autoantibodies and alloantibodies can induce platelet dysfunction by multiple mechanisms. In some patients, the antibodies are directed against specific platelet surface glycoproteins, including GPIa, GPIIa, GPIb, GPIIb, GPIIIa, GPIV, and GPVI. In patients with ITP, autoantibodies against GPIb-IX-V and GPIIb-IIIa have been detected in 5–30% and 10–75%, respectively [40]. Several patients have been described with autoantibodies directed against GPIIb-IIIa or GIb-IX-V, blocking specifically the interaction of the receptors with their ligands, thereby producing acquired Glanzmann thrombasthenia or acquired Bernard-Soulier syndrome [28, 41–46]. Blocking autoantibodies to GPIa and GPVI have been found. Recently, a patient with ITP was identified in whom binding of the anti-GPVI autoantibody resulted in the loss of GPVI from the platelets [47]. Binding of human leukocyte antigen (HLA) alloantibodies and alloantibodies directed against human platelet antigens (HPA) may be responsible for refractory platelet transfusion in respective patients. Alloantibodies from several Glanzmann thrombasthenia individuals with a history of frequent platelet transfusions can have the same thrombasthenia-like effect on transfused platelets [48]. Management of antibody-mediated platelet dysfunction and bleeding requires identification and therapy of the underlying disease.

Myeloma

Qualitative platelet defects are observed in approximately 30% of patients with IgA myeloma or Waldenström macroglobulinemia (IgM), in 15% of patients with IgG multiple myeloma, and occasionally in patients with monoclonal gammopathy of undetermined significance. It has been suggested that some monoclonal immunoglobulins interact with the platelet surface to interfere nonspecifically with platelet adhesion or stimulus-response coupling. This contention has been also supported by the observations that platelet dysfunction is more common at high paraprotein concentrations, that platelet aggregation, secretion, clot retraction, and platelet procoagulant activity may all be affected and that normal platelets acquire these defects when incubated with patients' plasma or the purified monoclonal immunoglobulin [40]. Anecdotal cases of IgG myeloma have been described where the paraprotein bound specifically to platelet GPIIb-IIIa and blocked binding of plasma Fg, thus inducing a platelet defect of the Glanzmann thrombasthenia-like phenotype (dysfunctional αIIbβ3; see also figure 3). In addition to platelet dysfunction, other causes of bleeding must be considered in myeloma patients, including hyperviscosity syndrome, thrombocytopenia, coagulation factor deficiencies by inhibitory paraproteins, impaired fibrin polymerization, and acquired plasma vWF abnormalities. In the majority of patients, bleeding and impaired platelet function appear to correlate closely with the serum paraprotein concentration. Acute bleeding episodes can be managed by plasmapheresis, while chronic bleeding may be controlled by chemotherapy. In patients with acquired von Willebrand disease, desmopressin (DDAVP) may be transiently effective [49].

Acute Leukemias and Myelodysplastic Syndromes

The most common cause of hemorrhage in these disorders is thrombocytopenia. Acquired platelet dysfunction associated with clinical bleeding is frequently found in acute myelogenous leukemia and myeloplastic syndromes (MDS). Platelet abnormalities include reduced aggregation, storage pool defects, and reduced TXA_2 synthesis or release [40]. Bleeding in these conditions usually responds to transfusion of platelets.

Myeloproliferative Disorders

Numerous abnormalities of circulating platelets have been described in patients with myeloproliferative disorders (MPD), which include essential thrombocythemia (ET), polycythemia vera (PV), chronic idiopathic myelofibrosis, and chronic myelogenous leukemia [50]. Most likely, these alterations are the result of abnormal platelet populations derived from a diseased clone of stem cells, but some of the alterations may be secondary from enhanced platelet activation in vivo. The clinical impact of qualitative platelet defects observed in vitro is often unclear, with widely divergent findings in different studies [40, 51, 52]. Thus, platelet defects are demonstrable even in asymptomatic patients. Another unique feature of MPD is that bleeding and thrombotic events may occur in the same patient, reflecting the complexity of the pathomecha-

Fig. 3. Phenotypic characterization of dysfunctional GPIIb-IIIa (integrin αIIbβ3) in patients with MPD associated with platelet aggregation defects. Depicted are flow cytometric histograms obtained in a patient with essential thrombocythemia (solid line) as compared with a normal subject (dashed line). Citrated whole blood was incubated with anti-ligand-induced binding sites (LIBS)-1, a conformation-specific monoclonal antibody that can distinguish between the resting, activated, and lig-

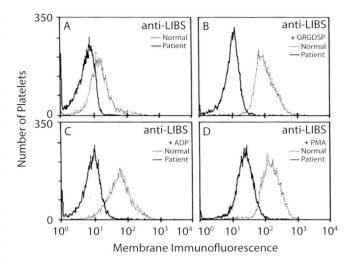

and-occupied states of GPIIb-IIIa in the absence (A) or presence (B–D) of other agents such as the GRGDSP peptide, ADP, or phorbol myristate acetate (PMA), an intracellular signal mimetic that circumvents normal agonist receptor-mediated pathways by directly activating protein kinase C. Anti-LIBS-1 selectively reacts with a ligand-induced binding site on GPIIIa. This epitope is expressed upon receptor occupancy by Fg (a process that requires platelet activation), or by Fg-mimetic small RGD-containing peptides (which bind to GPIIb-IIIa in an activation-independent manner). Immunolabeling of platelets with anti-LIBS-1 conjugated to fluorescein isothiocyanate (FITC) in the presence of GRGDSP (B) or upon stimulation with ADP (C) resulted only in a minor increase of specific membrane immunofluorescence in the patient's platelets. When platelets were stimulated with PMA (D), binding of anti-LIBS-1 increased, but still differed significantly from that in a normal volunteer. These findings are indicative of a combined defect in activation and ligand binding of GPIIb-IIIa in the patient. The conclusion was supported by the results obtained with PAC-1, a monoclonal antibody that specifically recognizes the activated GPIIb-IIIa complex (data not shown). This approach of flow cytometric analysis together with conformation-dependent and epitope-specific antibodies permits classification of platelet aggregation abnormalities as (i) defects of agonist-induced *activation* (no PAC-1 binding upon platelet stimulation with physiological agonists), (ii) defects of *ligand binding* (no LIBS expression and, consequently, no anti-LIBS-1 binding in the presence of Fg-mimetic peptides), and (iii) defects of *postoccupancy processes*. The dysfunctional postoccupancy phenotype is characterized by defective platelet aggregation despite intact binding of PAC-1 and anti-LIBS-1 in response to platelet stimulation. Adapted from Scharf et al. [54] and reprinted with permisssion.

nisms involved, and also the difficulty of interpreting laboratory findings [50]. MPD, in particular ET, are associated with microcirculatory disturbances resulting in erythromelalgia and neurologic symptoms. Aspirin effectively relieves the symptoms of erythromelalgia. Although the major mechanisms for hemorrhage in ET and chronic idiopathic myelofibrosis are the disease-related alterations in platelets (table 2), aspirin ingestion is a clinically relevant contributing cause of bleeding [53].

Bleeding time is abnormal only in approximately 15–20% of patients with MPD and appears to be more frequently prolonged in those with ET or chronic idiopathic myelofibrosis, but does not correlate with an increased risk of bleeding symptoms.

Table 2. Morphologic, metabolic and functional abnormalities in MPD; data from [40, 51, 52, 54]

Abnormalities	Specific findings
Heterogeneity in platelet size	
Morphologic abnormalities	reduction in α- and δ-granules alterations in the open canalicular and dense tubular systems reduction in number and size of mitochondria
Acquired storage pool deficiencies	decreased content of δ-granule constituents (ADP, ATP, serotonin)
Aggregation abnormalities	highly variable; enhanced responses to agonists or even spontaneous platelet aggregation in some patients, decreased aggregation responses upon stimulation with ADP (40%), collagen (35%), or epinephrine (60%)[a]; diminished or even absent epinephrine-induced platelet responses
Secretion	highly variable; elevated plasma concentrations of α-granular constituents such as platelet factor 4 and β-thromboglobulin ex vivo, indicative of platelet activation; decreased secretion of δ-granule content (ADP, ATP, serotonin) caused by platelet storage pool deficiency
Platelet plasma membrane abnormalities	
– Glycoprotein receptor defects	decreased expression of GPIIb-IIIa, GPIb-IX-V, or GPIa-IIa, increased expression of GPIV; dysfunctional GPIIb-IIIa with defective binding of soluble Fg[b]; activation defects or other ligand binding defects of GPIIb-IIIa; dysfunctional GPIa-IIa
– Agonist receptor defects	decreased number of α_2-adrenergic receptors; reduced responsiveness to TXA_2
– Alterations of Fc receptors	increased binding of IgG
– PGD_2 receptors	decreased number of PGD_2 binding sites
– Defective release of arachidonic acid	reduced conversion of arachidonic acid to prostaglandin endoperoxides (TXA_2) or 12-lipoxygenase products (see metabolic abnormalities)
Metabolic abnormalities	
– Arachidonic acid metabolism	enhanced synthesis of metabolites of the cyclooxygenase pathway (e.g. TXA_2); defective 12-lipoxygenase pathway with decreased formation of 12-hydroperoxyeicosatetraenoic acid (12-HPETE) and 12-hydroxyeicosatetraenoic acid (12-HETE)
– cAMP and cGMP metabolism	deficiency in cyclic adenylate cyclase and cyclic guanosine monophosphate (cGMP)-dependent protein kinase
Defective signaling	abnormalities in calcium mobilization; reduced Ca^{2+} fluxes across platelet membranes; impaired protein phosphorylation (see cGMP metabolism)

[a] Rates in brackets indicate percentage of patients with defective aggregation responses [50].
[b] Enhanced binding of thrombospondin to the platelet surface of MPD patients has been observed in some but not in other studies [68].

Platelet aggregation responses are also highly variable and may vary in the same patient over time [51]. Impaired responsiveness to epinephrine is a relatively frequent finding in MPD (45–57% of patients). This abnormality has been attributed to a decrease in the number of platelet α_2-adrenergic receptors [40]. Among the alterations listed in table 2, functional defects of GPIIb-IIIa (integrin αIIbβ3) have been identified resembling those observed in Glanzmann variants. Thus, by flow cytometric studies in combination with specific conformation-dependent monoclonal antibodies, platelet aggregation abnormalities in MPD can be phenotypically characterized as defects in GPIIb-IIIa activation, defects in ligand binding, or defects in post-occupancy events (fig. 3) [54]. Other platelet alterations reported in MPD include abnormal metabolism of arachidonic acid, defective signaling through the TXA_2 receptor, and impaired protein phosphorylation [40]. Abnormalities in plasma vWF documented in patients with MPD are secondary and related to the degree of thrombocytosis, as discussed below.

Acquired von Willebrand Disease

Moreover, phenotypic bleeding events of the platelet-like phenotype can be caused by acquired von Willebrand disease. Relevant pathomechanisms are increased cleavage of normal vWF multimers in aortic-valve stenosis [55, 56], due to increased susceptibility of vWF to its metalloprotease ADAMTS13 at abnormally high shear rates [57], inhibitory antibodies to vWF, binding of vWF to abnormal lymphoid cells in non-Hodgkin's lymphomas, or loss of the largest plasma vWF multimers in patients with reactive thrombocytosis following splenectomy. In this condition, high-molecular-weight plasma vWF multimers are transiently bound to the increased mass of circulating platelets and preferentially degraded [58]. The same mechanism is operating in patients with essential thrombocythemia with excessive platelet counts. Thus, acquired von Willebrand disease in these conditions may explain the apparent paradox why thrombocytosis can be associated with bleeding.

Management of Bleeding Episodes due to Impaired Platelet Function

Clinical and Laboratory Assessment
Identification of individual patients with bleeding disorders is crucial in order to manage symptoms, to minimize risk from invasive procedures, and to avoid unnecessary exposure to blood products. Thorough clinical assessment remains the cornerstone of the diagnostic strategy and the application of a staged protocol of laboratory testing. Appropriate diagnostic work-up may require meticulous laboratory investigations. As outlined above, the expanding use of antithrombotic agents and drugs interfering with platelet function has resulted in an increased proportion of patients being

at risk of unexpected bleeding. Thus, knowledge of the levels of risk associated with particular agents or combinations and of the advantages and hazards of interruption of drug use for planned interventional procedures is essential to reduce the incidence of iatrogenic hemorrhages [59].

Hemotherapy and Antifibrinolytics

Mild bleeding episodes in patients on antiplatelet agents can be managed by withdrawal of the drug(s); however, severe bleeding may require platelet transfusions. Recently, recombinant factor VIIa has been increasingly used in these cases [60]. Less specific treatments that enhance hemostasis and coagulation or inhibit fibrinolysis include DDAVP, epsilon aminocaproic acid (EACA), and tranexamic acid. Aprotinin was shown to be effective in reducing major bleeding, and thereby the need for red cell transfusions, during and following cardiac surgery. However, serious concerns regarding the safety of this drug were made. Recently, a significantly reduced long-term survival among patients who received aprotinin compared with those who received EACA, tranexamic acid, or no hemostatic medication was documented [61]. This report led to the withdrawal of aprotinin.

Desmopressin

Apart from treatment of von Willebrand disease, the evidence base for therapy with DDAVP is most developed in patients with platelet storage pool disorders [49]. However, it remains to be demonstrated that shortening of abnormal bleeding time following administration of DDAVP in patients with qualitative platelet disorders really translates into reduced clinical bleeding. For example, in patients without hereditary bleeding disorders, there is no evidence for a benefit in the use of DDAVP as prophylaxis.

Combined Treatment in Uremic Patients

Control of acute bleeding in patients with acute and chronic renal failure is probably best achieved by hemodialysis and red cell transfusion, in order to correct the hematocrit and thereby the fluid dynamic conditions that support hemostasis. Administration of DDAVP may be beneficial to shorten the bleeding time.

Therapeutic Principles in MPD

Hemorrhagic complications in patients with MPD may require rapid plateletpheresis combined with cytoreductive therapy. In addition, administration of EACA may reduce bleeding [62]. The various agents for cytoreduction include hydroxyurea, anagrelide, interferon-α, and alkylating drugs. Anagrelide is a nonmutagenic quinazoline derivative that is orally active and inhibits cAMP phosphodiesterase. More than 90% of patients with essential thrombocythemia respond to anagrelide with a decline in platelet counts.

Essential Thrombocythemia – a Special Challenge to Treat or not to Treat

Perhaps no other condition in clinical medicine has caused otherwise astute physicians to intervene inappropriately more often than in thrombocytosis, particularly if the platelet count exceeds $1 \times 10^6/\mu l$ [62]. Thus, it is commonly believed that a high platelet count must cause intravascular stasis or thrombosis. However, no controlled clinical study has ever established this association. By contrast, very high platelet concentrations are associated primarily with hemorrhage due to acquired von Willebrand disease [58], as outlined above. Therefore, administration of aspirin or other cyclooxygenase inhibitors should be limited to those patients with essential thrombocythemia who suffer from symptomatic microvascular disturbances.

Conclusions and Future Directions

The high morbidity and mortality due to cardio- and cerebrovascular complications require highly effective and safe strategies for chronic prevention of arterial thrombosis, *primary* intervention in acute vascular events, and *secondary* prophylaxis. Consequently, treatment with antiplatelet agents has been intensified over the last decade, specifically in patients at high risk [2, 14, 23, 63]. For example, blockade of ligand binding to integrin αIIbβ3 by agents such as abciximab, eptifibatide, or tirofiban (fig. 1) can completely inhibit platelet aggregation and is effective in the treatment of arterial thrombosis of *acute* coronary syndromes and intervention procedures. However, *chronic* administration of oral αIIbβ3 antagonists has not proved beneficial in preventing recurrent thrombotic events. A possible explanation for this failure is the narrow therapeutic window for these drugs, since pathological bleeding caused by complete loss of αIIbβ3 function requires maintenance treatment of less than maximal receptor blockade [14]. Therefore, we are currently facing a still unsolved problem: The agents used should be antithrombotic but not antihemostatic. In other words, we need highly effective drugs capable of preventing thrombus formation, but not at the price of a concomitant risk of increased bleeding. This demand requires innovative and highly selective therapeutic options. Thus, extensive efforts are being made to develop antiplatelet strategies that specifically block thrombotic effects without impairing or even eliminating the physiological role of platelets in hemostasis. Despite the failure of oral αIIbβ3 antagonists, this integrin remains a promising therapeutic target [15]; however, a better understanding of how this receptor functions in thrombosis at the molecular level is absolutely necessary.

Recent progress made in translational research may indeed open new therapeutic horizons. Since regulation of the affinity of αIIbβ3 for adhesive ligands is crucial to the control of platelet aggregation, the structural basis for allostery in integrins and for binding to Fg-mimetic therapeutics has been analyzed in detail [64]. Moreover, several adaptor proteins (including talin and kindlin) have been identified that interact with the cytoplasmic tail of β1 and β3 integrins, thereby having a significant impact on the conformation, signal transduction, activation status, affinity and, thus, ligand binding properties of the receptor molecules. For example, it has been shown (1) that activation of αIIbβ3 in vivo is dependent on the intact binding of talin to the β3 cytoplasmic domain and (2) that molecular modulation of β3 integrin-talin interactions can indeed provide a pharmacological target for newly designed antithrombotics [65]. More importantly, it was convincingly demonstrated in a mouse model that selective disruption of β3 integrin-talin interaction protects from thrombosis without any bleeding, since this mode of blockade leaves the ligand binding function of platelet αIIbβ3 intact [65]. These findings are indeed very promising and may offer a new antithrombotic approach by widening the therapeutic window. However, it remains to be seen whether the benefit of this selective αIIbβ3 antagonism can be really translated from mice to men.

Disclosure of Conflict of Interests

The author states that he has no conflict of interests.

Acknowledgement

The author's own work was supported by grants from the Deutsche Forschungsgemeinschaft (Scha 358/3–1 and Sonderforschungsbereich 612, Project B2). Additional support was provided by the Biological Medical Research Center, Heinrich Heine University, Düsseldorf, Germany. The assistance of Ms. U. Vandercappelle and Ms. N. Möller in preparing this manuscript is also gratefully acknowledged.

References

1 Ahrens I, Schwarz M, Peter K, Bode C: Therapeutic inhibitors of platelet aggregation – from aspirin to integrin blockers. Transf Med Hemother 2007;34:44–54.

2 Eikelboom JW, Hirsh J: Combined antiplatelet and anticoagulant therapy: clinical benefits and risks. J Thromb Haemost 2007;5(suppl 1):255–263.

3 Patrono C, Coller BS, FitzGerald GA, Hirsh J, Roth G: Platelet-active drugs: the relationship among dose, effectiveness, and side effects. The Seventh ACCP Conference on Antithrombotic and Thrombolytic Therapy. Chest 2004;126:234S–264S.

4 Antiplatelet Trialists' Collaboration: Collaborative meta-analysis of randomised trials of antiplatelet therapy for prevention of death, myocardial infarction, and stroke in high risk patients. Br Med J 2002;324:71–86.

5 Antman EM, Anbe DT, Armstrong PW, Bates ER, Green LA, Hand M, Hochman JS, Krumholz HM, Kushner FG, Lamas GA, Mullany CJ, Ornato JP, Pearle DL, Sloan MA, Smith SC Jr, Alpert JS, Anderson JL, Faxon DP, Fuster V, Gibbons RJ: ACC/AHA Guidelines update for the management of patients with unstable angina and non-ST-segment elevation myocardial infarction: A report of the American College of Cardiology/American Heart Association Task Force on Practice Guidelines (Committee to Revise the 1999 Guidelines for the Management of Patients with Acute Myocardial Infarction). J Am Coll Cardiol 2004;44:E1–E211.

6 Braunwald E, Antman E, Beasley J, Califf R, Cheitlin M, Hochman J, Jones R, Kereiakes D, Kupersmith J, Levin TN, Pepper CJ, Schaeffer JW, Smith III EE, Stewart DE, Theroux P, Gibbons RJ, Antman EM, Alpert JS, Faxon DP, Fuster V: ACC/AHA Guideline update for the management of patients with unstable angina and non-ST-segment elevation myocardial infarction – 2002: Summary article: A report of the American College of Cardiology/American Heart Association Task Force on Practice Guidelines (Committee on the Management of Patients with Unstable Angina). Circulation 2002;106:1893–1900.

7 Hirsch AT, Haskal ZJ, Hertzer NR, Bakal CW, Creager MA, Halperin JL, Hiratzka LF, Murphy WR, Olin JW, Puschett JB, Rosenfield KA, Sacks D, Stanley JC, Taylor Jr LM, White CJ, White J, White RA, Antman EM, Smith Jr SC, Adams CD: ACC/AHA 2005 Practice Guidelines for the management of patients with peripheral arterial disease (lower extremity, renal, mensenteric, and abdominal aortic): a collaborative report from the American Association for Vascular Surgery/Society for Vascular Surgery, Society for Cardiovascular Angiography and Interventions, Society for Vascular Medicine and Biology, Society for Interventional Radiology, and the ACC/AHA Task Force on Practice Guidelines (Writing Committee to Develop Guidelines for the Management of Patients with Peripheral Arterial Disease) endorsed by the American Association of Cardiovascular and Pulmonary Rehabilitation; National Heart, Lung, and Blood Institute; Society for Vascular Nursing; TransAtlantic Inter-Society Consensus; and Vascular Disease Foundation. Circulation 2006;113:e463–e654.

8 Sacco RL, Adams R, Albers G, Alberts MJ, Benavente O, Furie K, Goldstein LB, Gorelick P, Halperin R, Johnston SC, Katzan I, Kelly-Hayes M, Kenton EJ, Marks M, Schwamm LH, Tomsick T: Guidelines for prevention of stroke in patients with ischemic stroke or transient ischemic attack: a statement for healthcare professionals from the American Heart Association/American Stroke Association Council on Stroke: co-sponsored by the Council on Cardiovascular Radiology and Intervention: the American Academy of Neurology affirms the value of this guideline. Circulation 2006;113:e409–e449.

9 Aguilar M, Hart R: Antiplatelet therapy for preventing stroke in patients with non-valvular atrial fibrillation and no previous history of stroke or transient ischemic attacks. Cochrane Database Syst Rev 2005;4:CD001925.

10 Fuster V, Ryden LE, Cannon DS, Crijns HJ, Curtis AB, Ellenbogen KA, Halperin JL, Le Heuzey JY, Kay GN, Lowe JE, Olsson SB, Prystowsky EN, Tamargo JL, Wann S, Smith Jr SC, Jacobs AK, Adams CD, Anderson JL, Antman EM, Helperin JL: ACC/AHA/ESC 2006 Guidelines for the management of patients with atrial fibrillation: a report of the American College of Cardiology/American Heart Association Task Force on Practice Guidelines and the European Society for Cardiology Committee for Practice Guidelines (Writing Committee to Revise the 2001 Guidelines for the Management of Patients with Atrial Fibrillation) developed in collaboration with the European Heart Rhythm Association and the Heart Rhythm Society. Circulation 2006;114:c257–c354.

11 Chen ZM, Jiang LX, Chen YP, Xie JX, Pan HC, Peto R, Collins R, Liu LS: Addition of clopidogrel to aspirin in 45,852 patients with acute myocardial infarction: randomised placebo-controlled trial. Lancet 2005;366:1607–1621.

12 Sabatine MS, Cannon CP, Gibson CM, Lopez-Sendon JL, Montalescot MS, Theroux P, Claeys MJ, Cools F, Hill KA, Skene AM, McCabe CH, Braunwald E, CLARITY-TIMI 28 Investigators: Addition of clopidogrel to aspirin and fibrinolytic therapy for myocardial infarction with ST-segment elevation. N Engl J Med 2005;352:1179–1189.

13 Yusuf S, Zhao F, Mehta SR, Chrolavicius S, Tognoni G, Fox KK: Effects of clopidogrel in addition to aspirin in patients with acute coronary syndromes without ST-segment elevation. N Engl J Med 2001;345:494–502.

14 Bhatt DL, Topol EJ: Scientific and therapeutic advances in antiplatelet therapy. Nat Rev Drug Discov 2003;2:15–28.

15 Coller BS: Anti-GPIIb-IIIa drugs: current strategies and future directions. Thromb Haemost 2001;86:427–443.

16 Scharf RE: Thrombozyten und Mikrozirkulationsstörungen. Klinische und experimentelle Untersuchungen zum Sekretionsverhalten und Arachidonsäurestoffwechsel der Blutplättchen. Stuttgart, Schattauer, 1986.

17 Scharf RE: In vitro thromboxane synthesis of depleted platelets following renal transplantation. Thromb Haemost 1990;64:161–164.

18 Italiano JE, Patell-Hett S, Hartwig JH: Mechanics of proplatelet elaboration. J Thromb Haemost 5(suppl 1):18–23.

19 Ruggeri ZM: Platelet interactions with vessel wall components during thrombogenesis. Blood Cell Mol Dis 2006;47:1903–1910.

20 Ruggeri ZM, Mendolicchio GL: Adhesion mechanisms in platelet function. Circ Res 2007;100:1673–1685.

21 Savage B, Ruggeri ZM: Selective recognition of adhesive sites in surface-bound fibrinogen by glycoprotein IIb-IIIa on nonactivated platelets. J Biol Chem 1991;266:11227–11233.

22 Savage B, Almus-Jacobs F, Ruggeri ZM: Specific synergy of multiple substrate-receptor interactions in platelet thrombus formation under flow. Cell 1998;94:657–666.

23 Scharf RE, Zotz RB: Blood platelets and myocardial infarction: do hyperactive platelets really exist? Transf Med Hemother 2006;33:189–199.

24 Koscielny J, Ziemer S, Radtke H, Schmutzler M, Pruss A, Sinha P, Salama A, Kiesewetter H, Latza R: A practical concept for preoperative identification of patients with impaired primary hemostasis. Clin Appl Thromb 2004;10:195–204.

25 Wisloff F, Godal HC: Prolonged bleeding time with adequate platelet count in hospital patients. Scand J Haematol 1981;27:45–50.

26 George JN, Shattil SJ: The clinical importance of acquired abnormalities of platelet function. N Engl J Med 1991;324:27–39.

27 Steering Committee of the Physicians' Health Study Research Group: Final report on the aspirin component of the ongoing Physicians' Health Study. N Engl J Med 1989;321:129–135.

28 Scharf RE: Molecular basis and clinical aspects of hereditary megakaryocyte and platelet membrane glycoprotein disorders. Hämostaseologie 1996;16:114–138.

29 Boccardo P, Remuzzi G, Galbusera M: Platelet dysfunction in renal failure. Semin Thromb Hemost 2004;30:578–589.

30 Gawaz MP, Dobos G, Spath M, Schollmeyer G, Gurland HJ, Mujais SK: Impaired function of platelet membrane glycoprotein IIb-IIIa in end stage renal disease. J Am Soc Nephrol 1994;5:36–46.

31 Joist JH, George JN: Hemostatic abnormalities in liver and renal disease; in: Colman RW, Hirsh J, Marder VJ, Clowes AW, George JN (eds): Hemostasis and Thrombosis. Basic Principles and Clinical Practice. Philadelphia, Lippincott, Williams and Wilkins, 2004, pp 955–973.

32 Besarab A, Bolton WK, Brown JK, Egrie JC, Nissenson AR, Okamoto DM, Schwab SJ, Goodkin DA: The effects of normal as compared with low hematocrit values in patients with cardiac disease who are receiving hemodialysis and epoetin. N Engl J Med 1998;339:584–590.

33 Scharf RE, Schneider W: Evaluation of platelet secretion and thrombin generation in patients with chronic renal failure. Thromb Haemost 1985;50:10.

34 Reimers HJ, Scharf RE, Baker RK: Thrombin pretreatment of human platelets impairs thromboxane A2 synthesis from endogenous precursors in the presence of normal cyclooxygenase activity. Blood 1984;63:858–865.

35 Scharf RE: Erworbene Plättchen-Speichergranula-Defekte: Klinische und experimentelle Betrachtungen. Alexander-Schmidt-Gedächtnis-Vorlesung; in: Wenzel E, Hellstern P, Morgenstern E, Köhler M, von Blohn G (Hrsg): Rationelle Therapie und Diagnostik von hämorrhagischen und thrombotischen Diathesen. Stuttgart, Schattauer, 1986, pp 1.27–1.44.

36 Stockschläder M, Scharf RE: Failure of preactivated human blood platelets to restore defective thromboxane synthesis despite prolonged incubation in plasma. Thromb Haemost 1989;62:16–22.

37 Bick RL: Hemostasis defects associated with cardiac surgery, prosthetic devices, and other extracorporeal circuits. Semin Thromb Hemost 1985;11:249–280.

38 Harker LA: Bleeding after cardiopulmonary bypass. N Engl J Med 1986;314:1446–1448.

39 Harker LA, Malpass TW, Branson HE, Hessel EA, Slicher SJ: Mechanism of abnormal bleeding in patients undergoing cardiopulmonary bypass: acquired transient platelet dysfunction associated with selective α-granule release. Blood 1980;56:824–834.

40 Rao AK: Acquired qualitative platelet defects; in: Colman RW, Hirsh J, Marder VJ, Clowes AW, George JN (eds): Hemostasis and Thrombosis. Basic Principles and Clinical Practice. Philadelphia, Lippincott, Williams and Wilkins, 2004, pp 905–919.

41 Di Minno G, Coraggio F, Cerbone AM, Capitanio AM, Manzo C, Spina M, Scarpato P, Dattoli GM, Mattioli PL, Mancini M: A myeloma paraprotein with specifity for platelet glycoprotein IIIa in a patient with a fatal bleeding disorder. J Clin Invest 1986;77:157–164.

42 Morath C, Hoffmann T, Kirchhoff EM, Sis J, Zeier M, Scharf RE, Andrassy K: Acquired Glanzmann's thrombasthenia variant and immune thrombocytopenia in a renal transplant recipient receiving tacrolimus. Thromb Haemost 2005;94:879–880.

43 Niessner H, Clemetson KJ, Panzer S, Mueller-Eckhardt C, Santoso S, Bettelheim P: Acquired thrombasthenia due to GPIIb-IIIa specific autoantibodies. Blood 1986;68:571–576.

44 Nurden P, Nurden AT: Congenital disorders associated with platelet dysfunctions. Thromb Haemost 2008;99:253–263.

45 Scharf RE: Congenital and acquired platelet function disorders. Hämostaseologie 2003;23:170–180.

46 Varon D, Gitel SN, Varon N, Lahav J, Dardik R, Klepfish A, Berribi A: Immune Bernard-Soulier-like syndrome with an anti-glycoprotein-IX antibody. Am J Hematol 1992;41:67–68.

47 Boylan B, Chen H, Rathore V, Paddock C, Salacz M, Friedman KD, Curtis BR, Stapleton M, Newman DK, Kahn ML, Newman PJ: Anti-GPVI-associated ITP: an acquired platelet disorder caused by autoantibody-mediated clearance of the GPVI/FcRγ-chain from the human platelet surface. Blood 2004;104:1350–1355.

48 Coller BS, Peerschke EJ, Seligsohn U, Scudder LE, Nurden AT, Rosa JP: Studies on the binding of an alloimmune and two murine monoclonal antibodies to the platelet glycoprotein IIb-IIIa complex receptor. J Lab Clin Med 1986;107:384–392.

49 Mannuci PM: Desmopressin (DDAVP) in the treatment of bleeding disorders: the first 20 years. Blood 1997;90:2515–2521.

50 Schafer AI: Bleeding and thrombosis in myeloproliferative disorders. Blood 1984;64:1–12.

51 Wehmeier A, Fricke S, Scharf RE, Schneider W: A prospective study of haemostatic parameters in relation to the clinical course of myeloproliferative disorders. Eur J Haematol 1990;45:191–197.

52 Wehmeier A, Daum I, Jamin H, Schneider W: Incidence and clinical risk factors for bleeding and thrombotic complications in myeloproliferative disorders. A retrospective analysis of 260 patients. Ann Hematol 1991;63:101–106.

53 Cortelazzo S, Viero P, Finazzi O, D'Emilio A, Rodeghiero F, Barbui T: Incidence and risk factors for thrombotic complications in a historical cohort of 100 patients with essential thrombocythemia. J Clin Oncol 1990;8:556–562.

54 Scharf RE, Suhijar D, Del Zoppo GJ: Analysis of platelet aggregation defects: characterization of dysfunctional GPIIb-IIIa using conformation-specific antibodies. Thromb Haemost 1993;69:1018.

55 Sucker C, Feindt P, Scharf RE: Aortic stenosis, von Willebrand factor, and bleeding. N Engl J Med 2003;349:1773–1774.

56 Vincentelli A, Susen S, Le Torneau T, Six I, Fabre O, Juthier F, Bauters A, Decoene C, Goudmand J, Prat A, Jude B: Acquired von Willebrand syndrome in aortic stenosis. N Engl J Med 2003;349:343–349.

57 Sadler JE: Aortic stenosis, von Willebrand factor, and bleeding. N Engl J Med 2003;349:323–325.

58 Budde U, Scharf RE, Franke P, Hartmann-Budde K, Dent J, Ruggeri ZM: Elevated platelet count as a cause of abnormal von Willebrand factor multimer distribution in plasma. Blood 1994;82:475–482.

59 Greaves M, Watson HG: Approach to the diagnosis and management of mild bleeding disorders. J Thromb Haemost 2007;5(suppl 1):167–174.

60 Zotz RB, Scharf RE: Recombinant factor VIIa in patients with platelet function disorders or thrombocytopenia. Hämosteologie 2007;27:251–262.

61 Mangano DT, Miao Y, Vuylsteke A, Tudor IC, Juneja R, Filipescu D, Hoeft A, Fontes ML, Hillel Z, Ott E, Titov T, Dietzl C, Levin J: Mortality associated with aprotinin during five years following coronary artery bypass graft surgery. JAMA 2007;297:527–529.

62 Spivak JL: Polycythemia vera and other myeloproliferative diseases; in: Kasper DL, Braunwald E, Fauci AS, Hauser SL, Longo DL, Jameson JL (eds): Harrison's Principles of Internal Medicine, ed 16. New York, McGraw-Hill, 2005, pp 626–631.

63 May AE, Geisler T, Gawaz MP: Individualized antithrombotic therapy in high risk patients after coronary stenting. A double-edged sword between thrombosis and bleeding. Thromb Haemost 2008;99:487–493.

64 Xiao T, Takagi J, Coller BS, Wang J-H, Springer TA: Structural basis for allostery in integrins and binding to fibrinogen-mimetic therapeutics. Nature 2004;432:59–67.

65 Petrich BG, Fogelstrand P, Partridge AW, Yousefi N, Ablooglu AJ, Shattil SJ, Ginsberg MH: The antithrombotic potential of selective blockade of talin-dependent integrin αIIbβ3 (platelet GPIIb-IIIa) activation. J Clin Invest 2007;117:2250–2259.

66 Tcheng JE, Ellis SG, George BS, Kereiakes DJ, Kleiman NS, Talley JD, Wang AL, Weosman HF, Califf RM, Topol EJ: Pharmacodynamics of chimeric glycoprotein IIb/IIIa integrin antiplatelet antibody Fab 7E3 in high-risk angioplasty. Circulation 1994;90:1757–1764.

67 Schrör K, Hohlfeld T: Acetylsalicylic acid. Weinheim, Wiley-VCH, 2008, p 109.

68 Wehmeier A, Tschöpe D, Esser I, Menzel C, Nieuwenhuis HK, Schneider W: Circulating activated platelets in myeloproliferative disorders. Thromb Res 1991;61:271–278.

Prof. Dr. med. Rüdiger E. Scharf, F.A.H.A.
Institut für Hämostaseologie und Transfusionsmedizin
Universitätsklinikum Düsseldorf
Heinrich-Heine-Universität
Moorenstraße 5, 40225 Düsseldorf, Germany
Tel. +49 211 81-17344/17345, Fax -16221
E-Mail rscharf@uni-duesseldorf.de

Scharf RE (ed): Progress and Challenges in Transfusion Medicine, Hemostasis and Hemotherapy.
Freiburg i.Br., Karger, 2008, pp 317–325

Past, Presence, and Future of Genetics in Thrombophilia

Pieter H. Reitsma

Einthoven Laboratory for Experimental Vascular Medicine, Leiden University Medical Center, The Netherlands

Key Words

Venous thrombosis · Genetics · Risk factors · Mutation · Factor V Leiden · Single-nucleotide polymorphism

Summary

Venous thrombosis is a disease with an annual incidence of about 1:1,000 that is associated with a flexible combination of acquired and genetic risk factors. During the past 25 years, rare and common genetic risk factors have been identified, like deficiencies of protein C, protein S, antithrombin and factor V Leiden. More recently, attention has shifted to frequent single-nucleotide polymorphisms (SNPs) in coagulation genes. First, SNPs in candidate genes were tested in case-control studies and documented the associated risk. For several SNPs the intermediate phenotype, in the form of the plasma level of a coagulation protein, has been examined to document a biological explanation for the association between SNP and thrombotic risk. Genome-wide family and case-control studies were recently finished which searched for new candidate risk factors. These studies indeed revealed SNPs that are associated with an intermediate phenotype and confer thrombotic risk. The risk versions of these SNPs are frequent in the population, but the associated risks are quite modest (~1.5-fold increased). In conclusion, much progress has been made in the identification of genetic risk factors for venous thrombosis, and we now have a comprehensive view of the genetic architecture of this disease.   ©2008 S. Karger GmbH, Freiburg i.Br.

Introduction

The blood coagulation system consists of an intricate set of reactions that protect the body from bleeding and thrombosis. In general, the system is well balanced and excessive bleeding or runaway coagulation in an individual are not daily events. Only in cases with profound inherited or acquired imbalances in the coagulation system (e.g. hemophilia, complete deficiencies of natural anti-coagulants, auto-antibodies against coagulation proteins, severe acute infection, etc.) bleeding or thrombosis is an immediate threat. Despite this, the life-time risk of a single event of, e.g., venous thrombosis is high and difficult to predict. Therefore, much effort has been put into discovering acquired and genetic causes of episodic venous thrombosis in order to improve our understanding of the disease and to tailor prognosis and treatment. This short review will focus on the search for genetic causes of venous thrombosis.

Venous Thrombosis

Venous thrombosis has an annual incidence of about 1:1,000 per year [1, 2]. There is a steep age gradient, with younger people being at a very low risk whereas the risk rises to 6:1,000 in old age [2]. Acquired and genetic risk factors play an important role in determining the individual risk of a patient. Acquired risk factors include surgery, prolonged bed rest, and oral contraceptive use, but also life-style factors such as obesity, sports, and travel by airplane [3]. In addition, acquired antibodies against key components of the coagulation system like lupus anti-coagulants may increase thrombotic risk considerably.

Deficiencies of Natural Anti-Coagulants

Based on the familial occurrence of venous thrombosis, already in the early 1950's it was postulated that inherited variation in clotting factor genes might influence thrombotic risk. This indeed appeared to be the case. Chronologically, the first genetic defect that was identified was antithrombin deficiency [4]. Antithrombin is a circulating inhibitor of serine proteases with high specificity for the pro-coagulant proteins thrombin, factor IXa and factor Xa. Based on careful studies of the plasma levels of antithrombin it became clear that an inherited deficiency, in heterozygous form, led to familial clustering of venous thrombosis. Please remember that, at the time of the discovery of antithrombin deficiency, genes had not yet been cloned nor was it possible to do meaningful DNA sequencing.

It was not until about 20 years later that protein C deficiency was discovered as a strong risk factor for venous thrombosis [5, 6]. Again, the identification of this inherited risk factor followed after careful analysis of plasma for the level of protein C. Shortly thereafter, several laboratories documented families with multiple members affected by heterozygous protein C deficiency. These heterozygous deficiency states increase the risk for thrombosis about 10-fold and usually are not symptomatic in the young.

Protein C is the zymogen of a serine protease that becomes activated by thrombin when the latter is complexed with an endothelial receptor called thrombomodulin. Activated protein C is capable of inactivating, by proteolytic cleavage, the pro-coagulant co-factors factor Va and factor VIII. This inactivation leads to down-regulation of the coagulation cascade and, as is evident from the clinical features of homozygous deficiency, this inhibiting activity is crucial for a proper hemostatic balance. Protein C, in isolation, is a poor inactivator of factors Va and VIIIa, and only becomes effective in the presence of the co-factor protein S. Deficiencies of this co-factor lead to a clinical phenotype that is very similar to that of protein C deficiency. Homozygotes are severely affected with life-threatening thrombotic episodes in the perinatal period, whereas heterozygotes are often without symptoms into adulthood [7–11]. Protein S deficiency was discovered about a year after protein C deficiency.

Other components of the protein C anti-coagulant system, i.e. thrombomodulin and the endothelial protein C receptor (EPCR), are more difficult to implicate as causes of venous thrombosis. Mouse studies suggest that homozygous deficiencies of these endothelial cell membrane proteins interfere with normal embryogenesis and are not compatible with life, which would explain that homozygous deficiencies have not been documented [12, 13]. Heterozygous deficiencies have also not been found with certainty. A possible reason for this is that it is difficult, if not impossible, to get a good reading of the level of thrombomodulin or EPCR on endothelial cell membranes. Surrogate assays that measure soluble forms of thrombomodulin and EPCR are available, but these have not been helpful in identifying potential deficiency states, either because such states do not exist or because these surrogate assays are not reflective of what is present or active on the endothelial membrane. There are reports of rare mutations in thrombomodulin, but their association with thrombomodulin levels or function is unclear at best [14]. In addition, these mutations are so rare that the relationship with venous thrombosis can not be established with certainty.

While the discovery of deficiencies of the natural anti-coagulants unrolled, a revolution took place in the field of molecular biology and genetics. This allowed, from the mid-1980's onwards, the cloning and sequencing of all coagulation genes, including those for antithrombin, protein C, and protein S. In the wake of these discoveries, more and more genetic defects were documented in individuals with deficiencies in natural anti-coagulants. The main take-home message from these genetic studies is that there is an infinite number of different mutations that underlie these deficiency states [15–17]. This is not surprising from the perspective that the mutations involved can be classified as loss-of-function mutations. Since there are many possibilities to destruct the function of a gene, each family that carries a deficiency may have a private mutation that arose independently. By the same token, the prevalence of these loss-of-function mutations, which have all arisen independently, is quite similar between different ethnic groups, and it is therefore assumed that deficiencies of natural anti-coagulants are evenly spread over all populations.

Pro-Coagulant Proteins

As we have seen above, a (partial) deficiency of coagulation inhibitors tips the hemostatic balance in the direction of venous thrombosis. Alternatively, an excess of procoagulant factors may tip the balance in the same direction. The first example of such a pro-coagulant factor is factor V Leiden. The discovery of this mutation was based on seminal findings of Dahlbäck et al. in a family with what is now called APC resistance [18]. The plasma phenotype in this family became evident in assays where the activated partial thromboplastin time (APTT) was measured in the absence and presence of activated protein C (APC). In most individuals the addition of APC markedly prolonged the APTT, but in some the prolongation was much less. Later studies showed that this is due to a mutation in coagulation factor V within one of the cleavage sites for APC, and this mutation was named factor V Leiden [19]. From the perspective of gene function, this mutation is a gain-of-function mutation because the pro-coagulant potential of factor V Leiden is stronger than that for normal factor V. Since there are fewer options to improve gene function, there is little or no heterogeneity in the genetic basis of APC resistance; in other words, the plasma phenotype almost always goes with the same mutation. Although this mutation may have arisen multiple times in the past, the majority of mutation carriers in the population seem to have inherited the mutation from a common ancestor of Caucasians who lived about 50,000 years ago [20]. By consequence, in those populations that diverged before this point in the history of the human race, like the Chinese, Blacks, and Indians, factor V Leiden is rare.

Homozygotes for factor V Leiden have a relatively mild phenotype, at least compared to the very severe phenotype of homozygotes for deficiencies of natural anticoagulants [21]. From the viewpoint of population genetics, this implies that there is little negative selective pressure on the prevalence of factor V Leiden in the population, and on account of this, it is not surprising that the prevalence in the Caucasian population is quite high, ranging from 3–15%.

At about the same time when APC resistance and factor V Leiden were discovered, a second unique mutation in a pro-coagulant protein was found. This mutation involved prothrombin, also called factor II. The reasoning behind the identification of this mutation was quite different. From the dual role in coagulation, i.e. the pro-coagulant conversion of fibrinogen to fibrin and the anti-coagulant conversion of protein C to APC, it was argued that there perhaps would exist mutations that interfere with the activation of APC, thus tipping the hemostatic balance towards thrombosis. In a search for such a mutation, DNA from a relatively small panel of individuals from thrombophilic families was put together with the purpose of sequencing all exons and splice junctions of the factor II gene. A mutation that could interfere with APC generation was never found, but one nucleotide change caught attention [22]. This was a G-to-A transition of the final nucleotide of the factor II mRNA, i.e. the nucleotide to which the poly A tail is added when mRNA matures. Interestingly, this mutation was associated with mildly increased levels of prothrombin and with thrombotic risk. This mutation, called FII G20210A, was later shown to influence the level of prothrombin mRNA by improving 3' end formation of mature mRNA [23]. By analogy with factor V Leiden, the thrombotic tendency in homozygotes is relatively modest, the prevalence in the general population is quite high, and the mutation is present primarily in Caucasians and not in other races. The latter is again due to a common founder who lived at about the same time when factor V Leiden arose [24].

Single-Nucleotide Polymorphisms in Candidate Genes

As research into the genetics of thrombosis progressed and advances in DNA analysis technology were made, we witnessed a gradual shift from studies in families to population-based case-control studies. Such studies also allowed estimating the risk for weaker genetic risk factors [25]. In fact, the relationship between thrombotic disease and the deficiency of natural anti-coagulants is much more difficult to study in a case-control setting than in families, whereas the reverse is the case for weaker genetic risk factors like factor V Leiden and prothrombin G20210A. Ongoing sequencing efforts yielded more and more genetic variations in coagulation genes, and these were invariably studied in many different case-control studies like the Leiden Thrombophilia Study (LETS) [26]. This has led to a confusing literature on the relationship between common genetic variation in coagulation genes and venous thrombotic risk. For the same variation, some studies would report a risk whereas other studies were negative. The main reason for this was that the risk involved was quite low or non-existent, and that many studies were grossly underpowered to provide good risk estimates. As studies are growing larger now and since more and more studies are combined in collaborative efforts, the data become more reliable [26]. It is still too early to list all common genetic variants for which there is good evidence for thrombotic risk, but this certainly will be possible in the near future.

Modern Family Studies

In parallel projects, researchers are trying to discover new genetic variants that cause venous thrombosis. On the one hand, there are extensions of the well-established family-based studies like the GAIT in Spain, GENES in The Netherlands, and protein C Vermont in the USA [27, 28]. Such studies have a large set of, preferably, thrombophilic families as a starting point and use whole genome linkage studies in an attempt to identify novel loci in the genome that influence thrombotic risk. The main advantage of such studies is that no assumption is made with regard to the candidate genes involved, an assumption that is implicit in the studies described above. In principle, such genetic studies thus offer the possibility to discover completely new players in the coagulation system, a prospect that is indeed very exiting. Although it is still much too early for a verdict, it should be noted that up to now no such new candidate genes have been identified and that much still needs to be done in this area. The same family studies have been much more successful from the perspective of identifying quantitative trait loci (QTLs) for coagulation factor levels [28, 29]. Natural variation in coagulation factor levels has turned out to be strongly influenced by genetic factors, and numerous loci have been discovered in the genome that govern this variation. Further study of the genetic variation in these loci almost certainly will yield novel genetic risk factors for venous thrombosis.

Whole-Genome Association Studies

As said, the family studies described above do not make assumptions regarding the candidate gene in which to search for genetic variation that goes with thrombotic risk. An alternative approach, again driven by technological advances in the field of DNA analysis, is to do whole-genome association studies within the context of a case-control study. The concept of these studies is quite simple. First, assays for a large set of genetic markers are set up. The current sets use microarray chips and identify up to several hundreds of thousands of SNPs in a single reading. These SNPs are chosen so that they cover most of the common genetic variation in the human genome. Second, a large case-control study is taken in which the microarray analyses are done. Comparing allele frequencies between cases and controls yields candidate risk factors for disease. Such studies are now under way for a host of complex diseases. A recent publication in JAMA yielded the first results for venous thrombosis [30, 31]. In this study, a so-called gene centric approach was taken. This means that SNPs were selected from the list of then known variations that were located within a gene, and not in the gene 'deserts' between genes, and that preference was given to those SNPs that were most likely to have an effect on gene function. This could be because they were causing a missense or nonsense mutation, or because they were located in a splice junction or gene promoter. In total, almost 20,000 SNPs were selected and tested.

Straight testing of so many SNPs in a single case-control study would lead to many false-positive results. Therefore, a staged approach was chosen that takes care of this problem of false discoveries that is plaguing genome-wide association studies in which the number of measurements is much larger than the number of samples. In fact, a triplication approach was taken. This approach brought down the number of candidate SNPs from 1,206 in the first step to only 18 after triplication. There are several lessons that can be learned from this study [31]. The first lesson is that indeed novel risk factors can be uncovered in this approach, which have a good chance of being replicated in further studies in other laboratories. Secondly, the risk for venous thrombosis that goes with these risk factors is relatively low, i.e. in the order of 1.5-fold. At the same time, the prevalence of the risk factors is quite high, and in one example is even affecting the majority of the population. Thirdly, the risk factors – for which there was the best evidence for involvement in venous thrombosis – were mostly in coagulation factor genes and not in genes that have never been implicated in the coagulation system. This may mean that the coagulation system is quite well characterized and that genetic studies contribute little to the further advancement in our understanding of the functioning of this system. A cautionary note here is that a gene-centric approach was used and that a large proportion of common genetic variation was not assayed. Additional studies using the newest generation of microarrays may further refine our knowledge of the genetic architecture of venous thrombosis, and in particular define in more detail the role that is played by common genetic variation.

Conclusions and Future Directions

In this review, we have shown how research into the genetic background of venous thrombosis slowly shifted from discovering proteins and genes based on plasma assays to whole-genome studies aimed at determining the risk associated with common genetic variation. At the same time, we have seen attention shift from genetic abnormalities that go with high risk, e.g. 20-fold for antithrombin deficiency, to those with very small risk. This shift was mostly driven by technological advances and limitations. One should note that none of the high-tech approaches that are currently undertaken to find new risk factors would even come close to identifying deficiencies in natural anti-coagulants. The reasons for this are varied but include the fact that these deficiencies are associated with a private mutation in each family and thus by definition will not show up on the microarrays that visualize common genetic variation. Family studies are also prone to failure because the genetic background of venous thrombosis differs from family to family. Such heterogeneity dictates that one cannot safely aggregate multiple families into a single study. In fact, aggregation of families may result in dilution of linkage signals rather than a strengthening thereof. This can be solved by including very large families only, but this is often not practical. A possible solution to these dilemmas is probably provided by a large-scale DNA sequencing strategy. Such strategies will allow deep resequencing of large portions of the genome in large case-control or family studies. This will yield unprecedented insight into rare genetic variation in and outside of coagulation genes and into the role these variations play in determining the risk for disease. It is expected that these insights will finally make stratification of risk for venous thrombosis possible in a clinical meaningful way so that treatment can be better tailored based on patient characteristics.

Disclosure of Conflict of Interests

The author states that he has no conflict of interests.

References

1 Oger E: Incidence of venous thromboembolism: a community-based study in Western France. EPI-GETBP Study Group. Groupe d'Etude de la Thrombose de Bretagne Occidentale. Thromb Haemost 2000;83:657–660.

2 Naess IA, Christiansen SC, Romundstad P, Cannegieter SC, Rosendaal FR, Hammerstrom J: Incidence and mortality of venous thrombosis: a population-based study. J Thromb Haemost 2007;5:692–699.

3 Rosendaal FR: Venous thrombosis: a multicausal disease. Lancet 1999;353:1167–1173.

4 Egeberg O: Inherited antithrombin III deficiency causing thrombophilia. Thromb Diath Haemorrh 1965;13:516–530.

5 Griffin JH, Evatt B, Zimmerman TS, Kleiss AJ, Wideman C: Deficiency of protein C in congenital thrombotic disease. J Clin Invest 1981;68:1370–1373.

6 Bertina RM, Broekmans AW, van der Linden IK, Mertens K: Protein C deficiency in a Dutch family with thrombotic disease. Thromb Haemost 1982;48:1–5.

7 Comp PC, Nixon RR, Cooper MR, Esmon CT: Familial protein S deficiency is associated with recurrent thrombosis. J Clin Invest 1984;74:2082–2088.

8 Schwarz HP, Fischer M, Hopmeier P: Plasma protein S deficiency in familial thrombotic disease. Blood 1984;64:1297–1300.

9 Long GL, Tomczak JA, Rainville IR, Dreyfus M, Schramm W, Schwarz HP: Homozygous protein C deficiency in two unrelated families exhibiting thrombophilia related to Ala136Pro or Arg286His mutations. Thromb Haemost 1994;72:526–533.

10 Estelles A, Garcia Plaza I, Dasi A, Aznar J, Duart M, Sanz G, Perez Requejo JL, Espana F, Jimenez C, Abeledo G: Severe inherited „homozygous" protein C deficiency in a newborn infant. Thromb Haemost 1984;52:53–56.

11 Gómez E, Ledford MR, Pegelow CH, Reitsma PH, Bertina RM: Homozygous protein S deficiency due to a one base pair deletion that leads to a stop codon in exon III of the protein S gene. Thromb Haemost 1994;71:723–726.

12 Weiler H, Lindner V, Kerlin B, Isermann BH, Hendrickson SB, Cooley BC, Meh DA, Mosesson MW, Shworak NW, Post MJ, Conway EM, Ulfman LH, von Andrian UH, Weitz JI: Characterization of a mouse model for thrombomodulin deficiency. Arterioscler Thromb Vasc Biol 2001;21:1531–1537.

13 Gu JM, Crawley JT, Ferrell G, Zhang F, Li W, Esmon NL, Esmon CT: Disruption of the endothelial cell protein C receptor gene in mice causes placental thrombosis and early embryonic lethality. J Biol Chem 2002;277:43335–43343.

14 Öhlin AK, Marlar RA: The first mutation identified in the thrombomodulin gene in a 45-year-old man presenting with thromboembolic disease. Blood 1995;85:330–336.

15 Lane DA, Bayston T, Olds RJ, Fitches AC, Cooper DN, Millar DS, Jochmans K, Perry DJ, Okajima K, Thein SL, Emmerich J: Antithrombin mutation database: 2nd (1997) update. For the Plasma Coagulation Inhibitors Subcommittee of the Scientific and Standardization Committee of the International Society on Thrombosis and Haemostasis. Thromb Haemost 1997;77:197–211.

16 Gandrille S, Borgel D, Ireland H, Lane DA, Simmonds R, Reitsma PH, Mannhalter C, Pabinger I, Saito H, Suzuki K, Formstone C, Cooper DN, Espinosa Y, Sala N, Bernardi F, Aiach M: Protein S deficiency: a database of mutations. For the Plasma Coagulation Inhibitors Subcommittee of the Scientific and Standardization Committee of the International Society on Thrombosis and Haemostasis. Thromb Haemost 1997;77:1201–1214.

17 Reitsma PH: Protein C deficiency: summary of the 1995 database update. Nucleic Acids Res 1996;24:157–159.

18 Dahlbäck B, Carlsson M, Svensson PJ: Familial thrombophilia due to a previously unrecognized mechanism characterized by poor anticoagulant response to activated protein C: prediction of a cofactor to activated protein C. Proc Natl Acad Sci U S A 1993;90:1004–1008.

19 Bertina RM, Koeleman BP, Koster T, Rosendaal FR, Dirven RJ, de Ronde H, van der Velden PH, Reitsma PH: Mutation in blood coagulation factor V associated with resistance to activated protein C. Nature 1994;369:64–67.

20 Zivelin A, Griffin JH, Xu X, Pabinger I, Samama M, Conard J, Brenner B, Eldor A, Seligsohn U: A single genetic origin for a common Caucasian risk factor for venous thrombosis. Blood 1997;89:397–402.

21 Rosendaal FR, Koster T, Vandenbroucke JP, Reitsma PH: High risk of thrombosis in patients homozygous for factor V Leiden (activated protein C resistance). Blood 1995;85:1504–1508.

22 Poort SR, Rosendaal FR, Reitsma PH, Bertina RM: A common genetic variation in the 3'-untranslated region of the prothrombin gene is associated with elevated plasma prothrombin levels and an increase in venous thrombosis. Blood 1996;88:3698–3703.

23 Gehring NH, Frede U, Neu-Yilik G, Hundsdoerfer P, Vetter B, Hentze MW, Kulozik AE: Increased efficiency of mRNA 3' end formation: a new genetic mechanism contributing to hereditary thrombophilia. Nat Genet 2001;28:389–392.

24 Rosendaal FR, Doggen CJ, Zivelin A, Arruda VR, Aiach M, Siscovick DS, Hillarp A, Watzke HH, Bernardi F, Cumming AM, Preston FE, Reitsma PH: Geographic distribution of the 20210 G to A prothrombin variant. Thromb Haemost 1998;79:706–708.

25 Franco RF, Reitsma PH: Genetic risk factors of venous thrombosis. Hum Genet 2001;109:369–384.

26 Koster T, Rosendaal FR: Activated protein C resistance in venous thrombosis. Lancet 1994;343:541.

27 Soria JM, Almasy L, Souto JC, Tirado I, Borell M, Mateo J, Slifer S, Stone W, Blangero J, Fontcuberta J: Linkage analysis demonstrates that the prothrombin G20210A mutation jointly influences plasma prothrombin levels and risk of thrombosis. Blood 2000;95:2780–2785.

28 Souto JC, Almasy L, Soria JM, Buil A, Stone W, Lathrop M, Blangero J, Fontcuberta J: Genome-wide linkage analysis of von Willebrand factor plasma levels: results from the GAIT project. Thromb Haemost 2003;89:468–474.

29 Esparza-Gordillo J, Soria JM, Buil A, Souto AC, Almasy L, Blangero J, Fontcuberta J, de Cordoba SR: Genetic determinants of variation in the plasma levels of the C4b-binding protein (C4BP) in Spanish families. Immunogenetics 2003;54:862–866.

30 Bezemer ID, Bare LA, Doggen CJ, Arellano AR, Tong C, Rowland CM, Catanese J, Young BA, Reitsma PH, Devlin JJ, Rosendaal FR: Gene variants associated with deep vein thrombosis. JAMA 2008;299:1306–1314.

31 Bovill EG: Gene discovery in venous thrombosis: progress and promise. JAMA 2008;299:1362–1363.

Prof. Dr. Pieter H. Reitsma
Einthoven Laboratory for Experimental Vascular Medicine
Leiden University Medical Center
Albinusdreef 2, P.O. Box 9600, 2300 RC Leiden, The Netherlands
Tel. + 31 71 526-6985, Fax -6994
E-Mail p.h.reitsma@lumc.nl

Scharf RE (ed): Progress and Challenges in Transfusion Medicine, Hemostasis and Hemotherapy.
Freiburg i.Br., Karger, 2008, pp 326–343

Thrombophilia and Vascular Complications in Pregnancy

Andrea Gerhardt · Rüdiger E. Scharf

Department of Experimental and Clinical Hemostasis, Hemotherapy, and Transfusion Medicine,
Heinrich Heine University Medical Center, Düsseldorf, Germany

Key Words

Pregnancy · Thrombophilia · Venous thromboembolism · Fetal loss · Preeclampsia · Intrauterine growth
restriction

Summary

Women with acquired and hereditary thrombophilia are at increased risk of developing venous thromboembolism (VTE) and other associated gestational vascular complications like fetal loss, preeclampsia,
intrauterine growth restriction, and placental abruption during pregnancy. These complications are a
major cause of maternal and fetal morbidity and mortality. In view of the data documenting an association between thrombophilia and these adverse pregnancy outcomes, clinicians are increasingly using
antithrombotic therapy in women at risk of these complications. Aside from recurrent pregnancy loss in
antiphospholipid syndrome and prevention of VTE, there is limited evidence on the benefit of antithrombotic interventions to guide therapy. The data in favor of antithrombotic therapy in women with hereditable thrombophilia and vascular placental complications consist predominantly of small uncontrolled
trials or observational studies. Randomized, placebo-controlled trials are lacking as most patients do not
accept placebo. Further randomized controlled trials are urgently required to explore the efficacy and
safety in this clinical setting.   ©2008 S. Karger GmbH, Freiburg i.Br.

Introduction

Pregnancy is recognized as a 'thrombogenic state' and thromboembolic disease is
a leading cause of maternal morbidity and mortality during pregnancy and the puerperium. Several studies suggest that there is a link between thrombophilia and
adverse pregnancy outcomes as well as venous thromboembolism (VTE) [1]. This
article reviews the association, management, and prevention of VTE and other as-

sociated gestational vascular complications related to thrombophilia. Therapeutic modalities to prevent these gestational complications are discussed. Because of the potential regarding anticoagulant-related fetal and maternal complications and the paucity of good-quality data upon which to base clinical decisions, this issue remains particularly challenging.

Thrombophilia and Venous Thromboembolism during Pregnancy

The incidence of VTE associated with pregnancy and the puerperium is approximately 1 per 1,000 to 1 per 2,000 deliveries [2–5]. The overall incidence of fatal pulmonary embolism in pregnancy has decreased dramatically since the 1950s until today; however, pulmonary embolism remains a leading cause of maternal mortality in the Western world [6]. Bearing this in mind, it is important to develop strategies, firstly, to estimate the *individual* risk of thrombosis during pregnancy and, secondly, to be able to carry out specific, risk-adapted prophylaxis (e.g. anticoagulation with heparins), in cases where there is danger of thrombosis. However, this requires the most possibly exact, statistically based knowledge about the relative and absolute risks of all possible hereditary and acquired risk factors for venous thromboembolic events.

Pregnancy as an Expositional Risk Determinant

In 1847, Virchow postulated three main causes of thrombosis, including alterations of the vessel wall, venous stasis, and changes in the composition of blood [7]. These abnormalities leading to VTE all occur in pregnancy and the puerperium.

Pregnancy is an acquired and also independent risk condition for VTE. During normal pregnancy, there is a change in the plasma concentrations and activities of several proteins involved in platelet adhesion and aggregation, blood coagulation and fibrinolysis. These alterations can promote platelet function, coagulation, or both (e.g. increase in fibrinogen, factor VIII:C, and von Willebrand factor), reduce anticoagulation (decrease in protein S and antithrombin), and inhibit fibrinolysis (increase in plasminogen activator inhibitors 1 and 2), representing the 'physiological preparation' for the hemostatic challenge of delivery [8].

The venous system of the lower extremities is particularly vulnerable to thrombosis as a result of the compression by the gravid uterus [9, 10]. Endothelial damage to pelvic vessels can occur during vaginal or abdominal delivery [11]. Further acquired risk determinants, which in the course of pregnancy and the puerperium do significantly increase the thrombotic risk, include maternal age (women >35 years), obesity (weight >80 kg), high parity (≥4), infection, personal or family history of VTE, and cesarean section (particularly emergency cesarean section) [11].

Pregnancy and Hereditary Risk Determinants of Venous Thrombosis

Even 20 years ago, the relevance of familial disposition to thrombosis, i.e. hereditary thrombophilia, as origin of venous pregnancy-associated thromboembolism was unknown or underestimated. Evidently, at that point in time, only the antithrombin deficiency was known as the most important hereditary risk factor for thrombophilia [12]. Due to the rarity of this defect in the population, antithrombin deficiency was only diagnosed in few women with thrombophilic diathesis during pregnancy and the puerperium. This situation has changed fundamentally in the past 15 years. Since 1994 further genetically determined risk factors for thrombophilia have been identified. Among them are, besides the already known deficiencies of protein C and S, the G1691A mutation of the factor V gene (factor V Leiden) [13] and the G20210A mutation of factor II (prothrombin) gene [14].

About 50% of all women with VTE during pregnancy and the puerperium and about 15% of the average population are carriers of these genetically determined markers of thrombophilia [12]. The prevalence of the hereditary risk factors is relatively high in the general population (e.g. factor V Leiden up to 8%, prothrombin mutation G20210A about 2%). The presence of a hereditary risk factor alone, however, does on no account presuppose deep venous thrombosis. Based on Virchow's triad (alterations of the vessel wall, stasis, and changes in the composition of blood) [7], which is still valid in its main features, the etiology of venous thromboembolic events by today's understanding originates from the multifactorial interaction of both acquired and genetic risk determinants and the resulting risk constellations [15].

We provided positive predictive values for each thrombophilic risk determinant assuming an underlying rate of VTE of 1:1,500 pregnancies, consistent with estimates from Western populations [16, 17]. These values were 1:500 for individuals heterozygous for the factor V Leiden mutation, 1:200 for those heterozygous for the prothrombin 20210A allele, 1:20 for double heterozygotes, and 1:80 for those homozygous for factor V Leiden [16, 17]. In a further analysis, a retrospective study of 72,000 pregnancies, in which women with venous thrombosis were assessed for thrombophilia and where the underlying prevalence of these defects in the population was known, showed that the risk of thrombosis was 1:437 for women with the factor V Leiden mutation, 1:113 for those with protein C deficiency, 1:2.8 for women with type 1 antithrombin deficiency, and 1:42 for those with type 2 antithrombin deficiency [18].

A recent systematic review of 9 studies that assessed the risk of VTE in pregnant women with hereditary thrombophilia, all congenital thrombophilias with the exception of the thermolabile methylene tetrahydrofolate reductase variant (MTHFR 677TT) were found to be associated with a statistically significant increase in the risk of pregnancy-related VTE (table 1) [19]. Although not systematically examined in any of these studies, persistent antiphospholipid antibodies (APLAs) [20, 21] are probably also associated with an increased risk of VTE during pregnancy and the puerperium.

Table 1. Risk of pregnancy-associated VTE in thrombophilic women without prior disease [1, 19]

Thrombophilia	Relative risk of VTE OR (95 % CI)	Estimated absolute risk of VTE events per 1,000 patients[a]
Factor V Leiden (heterozygous)	8.32 (5.44–12.70)	8
Prothrombin gene variant (heterozygous)	6.80 (2.46–18.77)	6
Factor V Leiden (homozygous)	34.40 (9.86–120.05)	34
Prothrombin gene variant (homozygous)	26.36 (1.24–559.20)	26
Antithrombin deficiency	4.69 (1.30–16.96)	4
Protein C deficiency	4.76 (2.15–10.57)	4
Protein S deficiency	3.19 (1.48–6.88)	3
MTHFR C677T (homozygous, 677TT)	0.74 (0.22–2.48)	1

[a] Assuming a baseline risk of 1 event per 1,000 pregnant patients without a known thrombophilia.
CI = Confidence interval; OR = odds ratio; MTHFR = methylene tetrahydrate folate reductase;
VTE = venous thromboembolism.

Given that the background rate of VTE during pregnancy is approximately 1:1,000 [10], the absolute risk of VTE remains modest for the majority of these thrombophilias, except homozygosity for the factor V Leiden mutation and combined defects. We believe, however, that the risk associated with protein C deficiency, and particularly with antithrombin deficiency, is probably much higher than indicated in table 1. We could previously demonstrate that mild antithrombin deficiencies (≤80% activity) were associated with a rather low risk for thrombosis, whereas antithrombin activities of 60% or lower had a considerably higher risk (odds ratio 64, 95% confidence interval 10.3–208). A further analysis of women with antithrombin activities between 60 and 81% showed an odds ratio of 5.1 (95% confidence interval 0.6–44). Likewise, decreasing activities of protein C were associated with an increasing risk for VTE. Women with protein C activities below 68% showed an odds ratio of 3.6 (95% confidence interval 0.7–17.8), and women with protein C activities of 50% or lower had a considerably higher risk (odds ratio 7.3, 95% confidence interval 2.3–22.5) [22].

Identification of Patients at Risk

Bearing in mind the high rates of morbidity and mortality in pregnancy-related thromboembolic complications, it is necessary to estimate the *individual* risk of thrombosis based on statistically evaluated risk stratification in order to reduce VTE. The results on thromboses probability can be consulted for this and these can form the basis for an *individualized* risk-adapted thromboembolic prophylaxis.

VTE during pregnancy is of multicausal origin and results from the interaction of different risk determinants. The absolute thrombosis risk is decisively determined by the presence of a positive patient and/or family history of venous thromboembolic events and evidence of hereditary and/or acquired thrombophilic risk factors. About 70% of all women with VTE during pregnancy and the puerperium have acquired and/or hereditary thrombophilic risk factors and a positive patient and/or family history of venous thromboembolic events [12]. This emphasizes the necessity to develop and implement concepts and treatment strategies for primary and secondary prevention, to be able to use an individual risk stratification for a scientifically based anticoagulation therapy of endangered women during pregnancy and the postpartal phase [23, 24]. The history of venous thromboembolic events is of considerable importance for the assessment of the individual thrombosis risk.

A prior thromboembolism is an important risk indicator for a future thrombosis during pregnancy. Thus, women with a prior thromboembolic event are at an increased risk for recurrent venous thrombosis during a future pregnancy [25–27]. Here, especially the type of prior thromboembolism (idiopathic vs. transient risk situation) is defining for the thrombosis risk. In assessing the individual thrombosis risk, a positive family history of venous thromboembolic events is of substantial significance. Thus, members of families with hereditary thrombophilia show a higher prevalence of genetic risk factors and a higher relative risk of venous thrombosis than consecutive patients with the same deficiencies or mutations [24]. Independent of particular genetic risk markers, the age of members of thrombophilic families at the time of the initial thromboembolic event is considerably lower than the age at which venous thromboses occur in consecutively examined patients [28]. The same is true for thrombophilic families without identifiable risk markers. These findings indicate the presence of further, to date unknown, hereditary risk factors. One can therefore assume that the combination of a positive family history and a defined genetic defect is associated with a higher risk of thrombosis during pregnancy, than evidence of a hereditary risk factor alone.

Anticoagulation during Pregnancy

In 2004, updated recommendations were published by the American College of Chest Physicians (ACCP) for risk-adapted therapy and prophylaxis of thrombosis during pregnancy [29] (table 2). The use of anticoagulant therapy during pregnancy is challenging because of the potential for fetal as well as maternal complications. Anticoagulation during pregnancy and the puerperium is indicated for the prevention and treatment of VTE, and for the prevention and therapy of systemic embolisms in patients with mechanic valvular transplants. As well as this, procoagulatory changes due to hereditary thrombophilia also have a prothrombotic influence on utero-placentary circulation. Thrombosis prophylaxis can be given as unfractionated heparin (UFH) and as low-

Table 2. Dosage recommendations for risk-adapted prophylaxis and therapy with heparin during pregnancy and the puerperium [29]

Dose: ACCP recommendations	Risk group
No medical treatment required	*Women with prior VTE:* Women with a singular thrombotic event associated with a transient risk factor no longer persisting; no thrombophilic risk factor: low/moderate risk[a]
	Women without prior VTE: Women without relevant thrombophilia (laboratory-approved anomaly[b]) including APLA (no abortion): low/moderate risk
Prophylactic dose	*Women with prior VTE:* Prior event was associated with pregnancy or use of oral contraceptives or existence of additional risk factors (e.g. adipositas): moderate risk
	Women without prior VTE[c]: Women with antithrombin deficiency, combined heterozygous or homozygous prothrombin G20210A mutation/factor V Leiden G1691A: intermediate risk
Prophylactic or intermediate dose	*Women with prior VTE:* Women with a singular thrombotic event and thrombophilia (defect verified by laboratory) or familial thrombophilia, not receiving long-term anticoagulation: moderate/intermediate risk Women with a singular idiopathic thrombotic event, not receiving long-term anticoagulation: moderate risk
Intermediate 'half therapeutic' dose	*Women with prior VTE:* Women with history of thrombosis, antithrombin deficiency, combined heterozygous or homozygous prothrombin G20210A mutation/factor V Leiden G1691A: high/intermediate risk
Therapeutic dose	*Women with prior VTE:* Thrombosis in current pregnancy: high risk Women with recurrent (two or more) thrombotic events and/or long-term anticoagulation (e.g. singular thrombotic event – idiopathic or associated with thrombophilia incl. antiphospholipid syndrome): high risk

[a] The authors prefer prophylactic dose in this setting.
[b] Relevant thrombophilia: antithrombin deficiency, combined heterozygous or homozygous prothrombin G20210A mutation/factor V Leiden G1691A.
[c] In patients with antithrombin deficiency < 60%, the authors prefer an intermediate dose.

molecular-weight heparin (LMWH) (for dosages, see table 3). Advantages of LMWH are a low rate of heparin-induced thrombocytopenia type II, a lower osteoporosis rate and a lower rate of allergic skin reactions, while of the same prophylactic antithrombotic efficacy [30, 31]. Pre-existing oral anticoagulation, e.g. due to prior thromboembolic events, should be completed by the 6th week of pregnancy to prevent embryopathies.

Table 3. Dosage recommendations for risk-adapted prophylaxis and therapy with heparin during pregnancy and the puerperium[a]

LMWH	UFH[b]
	Minidose 5000 IU s/c q12h
Prophylactic dose, e.g. Enoxaparin 40 mg (4,000 IU) s/c q24h Dalteparin 5,000 IU s/c q24h Nadroparin 4,000 IU s/c q24h	*Prophylaxis adjusted (moderate dose)* anti-Xa activity 0.1–0.3 U/ml (3 h after s/c administration) e.g. 2 × 10,000 IU s/c q24h
Intermediate 'half therapeutic' dose, e.g. Enoxaparin 40 mg (4000 IU) s/c q12h Dalteparin 5,000 IU s/c q12h	
Therapeutic dose[c], weight-adapted *as recommended 1–2 × s/c q24, e.g.* Enoxaparin 1 mg/kg s/c q12h or 1.5 mg/kg s/c q24h Dalteparin 100 IU/kg s/c q12h or 200 IU/kg s/c q24h Tinzaparin 175 mg/kg s/c q24h	*Therapeutic dose adjusted[c]* aPTT 6 h after s/c administration in the therapeutic range (e.g. 60–80 s) e.g. 2 × 15,000–30,000 IU s/c q24h

[a] LMWH is predominantly in use in Europe because of the lower rate of side effects.
[b] According to ACCP recommendations. Anti-Xa activity is lower with UFH than with LMWH, but comparable in its anticoagulatory efficacy.
[c] As the half-life of LMWH is shorter in pregnancy, twice-daily dosing is preferable, at least in the initial treatment phase.
aPTT = Activated partial thromboplastin time.

Thrombophilia and Vascular Placental Complications

Adverse pregnancy outcomes are rather frequent. Thus, 25% of human conceptions end in miscarriage. Of those, 5% of women at the reproductive age experience 2 or more fetal losses and 1–2% have 3 or more consecutive losses [32]. Several etiologies have been implicated to cause recurrent fetal loss, including chromosomal translocations and inversions, anatomic alterations of the uterus, endocrinological abnormalities and autoimmune disorders. However, most recurrent fetal losses remain unexplained. Preeclampsia, a leading cause of both fetal and maternal morbidity and mortality, is seen in 3–7% of pregnancies, while placental abruption is uncommon (0.5% of gestations) but carries a high risk of fetal mortality [33].

Association of Vascular Placental Complications with Thrombophilia

In pregnancy, a successful outcome is highly dependent on appropriate placental development and sustained placental function. These processes, in turn, require the formation of an adequate feto-maternal circulatory system [34]. Adverse pregnancy outcomes are associated with abnormal placental vasculature and inadequate placental maternal-fetal circulation [35–38]. The hemostatic pathways are intimately involved in ovulation, implantation and placentation [39]. Both acquired and inherited thrombophilia are associated with an increased risk of pregnancy failure, as well as hypertensive pregnancy complications such as preeclampsia and HELLP syndrome (= hemolysis, elevated liver function tests, and low platelet count).

The most compelling data for a link between thrombophilia and pregnancy complications derive from studies in women with APLAs. The association of acquired thrombophilia such as APLAs with recurrent fetal loss is well established [40]. There is substantial interest in examining whether heritable thrombophilias are also associated with adverse pregnancy outcomes, and whether this can be improved by antithrombotic therapy. Several studies have examined the association between thrombophilia and pregnancy complications, often with differing results, likely reflecting heterogeneity of study design, sample size, inclusion criteria, population studied, outcome definition, and thrombophilias studied [19, 41–43]. In table 4 the associations between various forms of pregnancy failure and preeclampsia are listed.

Pregnancy Loss
The data presented are obtained from meta-analyses from case-control studies [19, 40, 41]. It should be noted that significant heterogeneity between studies was found [19, 41]. In the meta-analysis by Robertson et al. [19], women homozygous for factor V Leiden or with hyperhomocysteinemia were at a significantly higher risk of suffering an early pregnancy loss compared to women with other thrombophilias. Moreover, the risk of early pregnancy loss with hyperhomocysteinemia was greater than the risk of any other pregnancy complication with this condition. The acquired thrombophilias, including elevated anticardiolipin antibodies, lupus anticoagulants and acquired activated protein C resistance, were also significantly associated with pregnancy loss before 24-week gestation. The magnitude of risk was modest; however, early pregnancy loss is a very heterogeneous condition, and only a proportion of these losses will be related to thrombophilia. A stronger association was found with recurrent miscarriage, which is likely to be more specific for an underlying thrombophilia. When early pregnancy loss was classified according to recurrent loss in the first trimester and non-recurrent loss in the second trimester, a higher risk of second-trimester loss for both factor V Leiden and prothrombin G20210A heterozygotes was calculated [19]. This is consistent with a further analysis on thrombophilia and recurrent pregnancy loss by Rey et al. [41]. They have shown that factor V Leiden was

Table 4. Association between various forms of thrombophilia and pregnancy failure and complications [67]: meta-analyses from case-control studies [19, 40, 41]

Thrombophilia defect	Sporadic miscarriage OR (95% CI)	Recurrent miscarriage[a] OR (95% CI)	Intrauterine fetal death[a] OR (95% CI)	Preeclampsia OR (95% CI)
Lupus anticoagulant	3.0 (1.0–8.6)	7.8 (2.3–26.5)	2.4 (0.8–7.0)	1.5 (0.8–2.8)
Anticardiolipin antibodies	3.4 (1.3–8.7) 3.6 (2.3–5.7)	5.1 (1.8–14.0)	3.3 (1.6–6.7)	2.7 (1.7–4.5)
Antithrombin deficiency	1.5 (1.0–2.5)	0.9 (0.2–4.5)	7.6 (0.3–196)	3.9 (0.2–97.2)
Protein C deficiency	1.4 (1.0–2.1)	1.6 (0.2–10.5)	3.1 (0.2–38.5)	5.2 (0.3–102.2)
Protein S deficiency	heterogeneous data	14.7 (1.0–218.0) 20.1 (3.7–109.2)	7.4 (1.3–42.8)	2.8 (0.8–10.6)
Factor V Leiden mutation	1.7 (1.2–2.5) 1.7 (1.1–2.6)	2.0 (1.1–3.6) 1.9 (1.0–3.6)	3.3 (1.8–5.8) 2.1 (1.1–3.9)	2.2 (1.5–3.3)
Prothrombin 20210A mutation	2.1 (1.2–3.5) 2.5 (1.2–5.0)	2.3 (1.1–4.8) 2.7 (1.4–5.3)	2.3 (1.1–4.9) 2.7 (1.3–5.5)	2.5 (1.5–4.2)
Homozygous defects or combinations of defects	2.7 (1.3–5.6)	–	–	1.9 (0.4–7.9)
Mild hyperhomocysteinemia	6.3 (1.4–28.4)	2.7 (1.4–5.2) 4.2 (1.3–13.9)	1.0 (0.2–5.6)	3.5 (1.2–10.1)

[a] Definition varies across studies.

associated with early and late recurrent fetal loss, and late non-recurrent fetal loss. Exclusion of women with other pathologies that could explain fetal loss strengthened the association between factor V Leiden and recurrent fetal loss. The prothrombin G20210A mutation and protein S deficiency were also associated with early recurrent and late non-recurrent fetal loss. Methylene tetrahydrofolate reductase mutation, protein C, and antithrombin deficiencies were not significantly associated with fetal loss. In women with late pregnancy loss, significant associations were observed in carriers of heterozygous factor V Leiden, heterozygous prothrombin mutation, protein S deficiency, and anticardiolipin antibodies. No evidence of heterogeneity was documented [19].

Preeclampsia
Preeclampsia has been associated with both acquired and inherited thrombophilia [19, 44]. However, the contribution of thrombophilia is less well established, and recent studies did not confirm earlier data suggesting an association between hereditary thrombophilia and this vascular gestational complication [43, 45, 46].

With regard to preeclampsia, significant associations with hyperhomocysteinemia, elevated anticardiolipin antibodies, heterozygosity for factor V Leiden and pro-thrombin G20210A were found. Evidence of heterogeneity was present in the analysis on heterozygous factor V Leiden (p = 0.04). The studies included in the meta-analysis consisted of diagnoses of both mild and severe preeclampsia [19]. Sensitivity analysis was performed by analyzing the studies reporting mild and severe preeclampsia independently. When restricting the analysis to mild preeclampsia only, an odds ratio of 2.3 (95% confidence interval 1.27–4.16) was obtained, but heterogeneity remained (p = 0.01). However, when restricting the analysis to severe preeclampsia only, an odds ratio of 2.04 (95% confidence interval 1.23–3.36) was obtained and evidence of heterogeneity was removed (p = 0.31). Preeclampsia was the only outcome for which a significant association with homozygosity for MTHFR C677T (i.e. 677TT) was found. However, the increase in risk of preeclampsia with thrombophilia is modest [19]. Thrombophilia may contribute to the severity and onset of preeclampsia because of an exaggerated effect of thrombophilia on the disorder [43, 45]. For example, women who are carriers of the G20210A prothrombin gene mutation and the PAI-1 5G/5G genotype are at risk *for early onset* of severe preeclampsia [43]. It appears that these risk factors do not induce the pathomechanism but accelerate the course of preeclampsia. The pathomechanism of preeclampsia comprises placental vascular alterations, imposing primarily as endothelial inflammation, and thrombotic occlusion of the placental vasculature [35–37]. Since endothelial dysfunction is a major stimulus of hemostasis, it is likely that a risk determinant of hypercoagulability remains without consequence in normal blood vessels. In case of predisposing vascular alterations, a prothrombotic risk factor such as the G20210A mutation of the prothrombin gene may modulate the disease process by induction of a premature onset [43]. As a consequence, a mild increase in risk due to the thrombophilic risk factor may be simulated when late-onset preeclampsia at term in contrast to early-onset preeclampsia is not diagnosed.

Placental Abruption and Intrauterine Growth Restriction
Several studies evaluated the association between thrombophilia and placental abruption [19]. Overall, thrombophilia was associated with an increased risk of placental abruption, but significant associations were only observed with heterozygous factor V Leiden (odds ratio 4.7; 95% confidence interval 1.13–19.59) and heterozygous prothrombin gene mutation (odds ratio 4.7; 95% confidence interval 1.13–19.59). There was a general trend of increased intrauterine growth restriction risk in pregnant women with thrombophilia [19]. However, based on data from one study [47], a significant association was observed only with anticardiolipin antibodies (odds ratio 6.9; 95% confidence interval 2.7–17.9) [19].

Role of Hemostasis in Fetal and Placental Development

Nevertheless, it is unlikely that hypercoagulability with thrombosis of placental vasculature is to be the sole mechanism by which acquired and hereditary thrombophilia increases the risk for adverse pregnancy outcomes, most notably early losses.

In women with recurrent fetal loss, an association with risk factors of thrombophilia has been demonstrated [19, 41]. However, the risk of fetal loss is only mildly increased (odds ratio 2 for early fetal loss) in carriers of a heterozygous G1691A mutation in the factor V gene or a heterozygous G20210A mutation in the prothrombin gene. Since recurrent pregnancy loss affects approximately 1–2% of women at the reproductive age, the positive predictive value of factor V Leiden for recurrent fetal loss is only 2.9% (assuming a 5% prevalence of heterozygous factor V Leiden in the general population, a 1% rate of recurrent pregnancy loss, and an odds ratio of 3). Thus, 97.1% of women who are carriers of factor V Leiden will not experience recurrent fetal loss, a reason not to screen for thrombophilic risk factors in women without prior abortion. The low positive predictive value of factor V Leiden and other hereditary thrombophilic risk factors for recurrent early fetal loss is an additional indicator for the multifactorial origin of the underlying disorder, which is not caused but aggravated or modulated by thrombophilic risk factors. If heparin prophylaxis in pregnancy in fact contributes to an increased birth rate, a positive effect independent of the presence of known thrombophilic risk factors can be hypothesized.

Effects on trophoblast differentiation and early placentation may be involved through yet unknown mechanisms. The vast majority of women with recurrent fetal loss have early losses. Contact of maternal spiral arteries with the placental intervillous space cannot be recognized until the 8th week [48]. The placenta replaces the yolk sac as the source of blood supply to the embryo during the 8th or 9th week of gestation [49]. Maternal hemostatic defects are unlikely to play a role before this period. Experimental models to study trophoblast differentiation and early placentation in women with inherited thrombophilia are lacking. However, as shown by Isermann et al. [50], disruption of the mouse gene encoding the blood coagulation inhibitor thrombomodulin leads to embryonic lethality prior to the 8th or 9th week of gestation caused by an unknown defect in the placenta. The abortion of thrombomodulin-deficient embryos is caused by tissue factor-initiated activation of the blood coagulation cascade at the feto-maternal interface. Activated coagulation factors induce cell death and growth inhibition of placental trophoblast cells by two distinct mechanisms. The death of giant trophoblast cells is caused by conversion of the thrombin substrate fibrinogen to fibrin and subsequent formation of fibrin degradation products. In contrast, the growth arrest of trophoblast cells is not mediated by fibrin, but is a likely result of engagement of protease-activated receptors (PAR)-2 and PAR-4 by coagulation factors. These findings show a new function for the thrombomodulin-protein C system in controlling the growth and survival of trophoblast cells in the placenta. The described function is essential for the maintenance of pregnancy. Administration of heparin or aspirin to the mice was unable to restore trophoblast differentiation and overcome the growth defect of these thrombomodulin-deficient embryos.

Evidence on Anticoagulant Therapy in Placental Vascular Complications

Pregnancy Loss

In view of the data showing an association between *hereditary thrombophilia* and adverse pregnancy outcomes, clinicians are increasingly using antithrombotic therapy in women at risk of these complications. However, the data surrounding the use of antithrombotics in women with hereditable thrombophilia and pregnancy loss are less convincing than those in women with APLAs, and consist predominantly of small uncontrolled trials or observational studies [51–55]. Randomized, placebo-controlled trials are lacking as most patients do not accept placebo. LMWH was approved in open, non-placebo-controlled studies in which outcomes were compared with either the spontaneous previous pregnancies [51–53], with outcomes in a parallel non-treated group [54], or with outcomes in a parallel group treated differently [55].

The studies by Brenner et al. [51, 52] (women with three miscarriages in the first trimester, two in the second, one in the third; any thrombophilia) documented that enoxaparin was associated with improvement in live birth rates (from 20 to 75–80%), 40 mg once a day being equivalent to 80 mg. However, there has been considerable debate about this trial, focusing on its limitations, particularly the absence of an untreated control group, the heterogeneous entry criteria, and the risk of regression toward the mean with the use of a historic control group. In the study by Carp et al. (three miscarriages before 20 weeks and thrombophilia), 70% of the enoxaparin-treated women, vs. 44% of the non-treated women, had a live birth [54]. Gris et al. reported that treatment with enoxaparin in pregnant women (40 mg daily from the beginning of the 8th week) with thrombophilia (factor V Leiden, prothrombin gene mutation, or protein S deficiency) and one previous pregnancy loss after 10 weeks of gestation results in a significantly higher live birth rate (86% of the 80 LMWH-treated women) compared with low-dose aspirin (100 mg daily) alone (29% of the 80 aspirin-treated women) [55]. The superiority of enoxaparin was apparent for each thrombophilia. This trial has some limitations, such as small sample size, absence of an untreated control group, and inadequate concealment of allocation. Given the relatively high success rate of subsequent pregnancies after a single miscarriage, it is difficult to assess the implications of these results.

In view of these data, some circumstantial evidence is provided that LMWH may improve the pregnancy outcome in women with hereditable thrombophilia and recurrent pregnancy loss or loss after 10 weeks; however, available studies have important methodological limitations, and firm recommendations cannot be made regarding the use of antithrombotics in these women.

In 2004, updated recommendations were published by the ACCP for risk-adapted prophylaxis of gestational vascular complications [29]. Depending on the quality of the underlying data, the recommendations are classified as 'grade 1' or 'grade 2'. 'Grade 1' indicates that the benefits of the recommendation are superior to the accompanying disadvantages (risk, burdens, and cost). 'Grade 2' is an indication that individual patient characteristics may necessitate a different decision for therapy to the recommendations. Most recommendations are only 'grade 2', owing to inadequate data, i.e. a different therapy decision may be necessary due to the individual risk constellation of the particular patient.

The ACCP recommendations [29] suggest for women with recurrent pregnancy loss (three or more miscarriages) that screening for congenital thrombophilia and APLAs should be performed. For women with a congenital thrombophilia and recurrent miscarriages, a second-trimester or later loss, low-dose aspirin therapy plus either minidose heparin or prophylactic LMWH (grade 2C) is suggested. However, since adding aspirin is speculative, many experts do not administer heparin and aspirin in combination. Postpartum anticoagulants can be administered to these women (grade 2C).

Antiphospholipid Syndrome: A Special Case

There is convincing evidence that the presence of APLAs is associated with an increased risk of thrombosis [20] and pregnancy loss [56, 57]. Thus, pregnant women with APLAs should be considered at risk for both of these complications. In addition, women with recurrent pregnancy loss should be screened for the presence of APLAs prior to or during the early part of pregnancy.

In women with recurrent miscarriage based on the antiphospholipid syndrome, two randomized trials documented an improved fetal survival with the use of a combination of low-dose UFH and low-dose aspirin, compared with aspirin alone [58, 59]. A further randomized trial in which LMWH was added to aspirin did not demonstrate any benefit of this combination therapy, with live birth rates of 72 and 78% in both treatment arms [59]. This study has been criticized because of the inclusion of women with low antibody titers, at a relatively late gestational age, and cross-over effects between treatment groups [60]. Results of published case series [61, 62] suggest that LMWH is efficacious in pregnant women with APLAs and fetal loss, and a recent pilot study in which UFH was compared directly with LMWH showed an improved fetal outcome in subsequent pregnancies in both treatment groups of 80 and 85% [63].

The ACCP guidelines [29] suggest for pregnant patients with APLAs and a history of multiple (two or more) early pregnancy losses or one or more late pregnancy losses, preeclampsia, intrauterine growth restriction (IUGR), or abruption, administration of antepartum aspirin plus minidose or moderate-dose UFH or prophylactic LMWH (grade 2B). Patients with APLAs and a history of venous thrombosis are usually receiving long-term oral anticoagulation therapy because of the high risk of recurrence. During pregnancy, adjusted-dose LMWH or UFH therapy plus low-dose aspirin and resumption of long-term oral anticoagulation therapy postpartum is recommended (grade 1C). Patients with APLAs and no prior VTE or pregnancy loss are considered to have an increased risk for the development of venous thrombosis and, perhaps, pregnancy loss. One of the following approaches is suggested: surveillance, minidose heparin, prophylactic LMWH, and/or low-dose aspirin, 75–160 mg daily (all grade 2C).

Preeclampsia, Placental Abruption, and Intrauterine Growth Restriction

While large interventional trials have studied the effect of aspirin on the recurrence rate of preeclampsia, only limited data are available regarding LMWH. When used for prevention of preeclampsia, low-dose aspirin has minimal benefits [64]: 51–109 patients must be treated for only one success, 50–238 women for preventing one premature delivery, and 128–909 patients for preventing the death of one infant. In two prospective trials, no benefit in pregnancy outcome was observed following treatment with aspirin compared to placebo in women with a history of preeclampsia [65, 66]. Experience in the prevention of preeclampsia by prophylactic heparin is very limited. Uncontrolled series suggest improved outcomes in subsequent pregnancies, with a lower rate of preeclampsia [52, 53]. Ongoing prospective studies are investigating the recurrence rate of preeclampsia in women receiving LMWH.

In summary, there is limited evidence to support anticoagulant therapy in this setting. It remains to be established whether intervention with LMWH is of benefit in women with thrombophilia and these underlying pregnancy complications. Further randomized controlled trials are needed to explore this possibility. This supports the very low-grade recommendation for LMWH given by the ACCP [29] which suggests, for women with prior severe or recurrent preeclampsia, abruptions, or otherwise unexplained intrauterine death, screening for congenital thrombophilia and APLAs (grade 2C). Furthermore, for women with a congenital thrombophilic deficit and severe or recurrent preeclampsia, or abruption, low-dose aspirin therapy plus either minidose heparin or prophylactic LMWH therapy (grade 2C) is suggested and postpartum anticoagulants can be administered to these women (grade 2C).

Conclusions and Future Directions

Whether universal screening for thrombophilia should be performed prior to pregnancy is still a matter of debate. Women with thrombophilia are at increased risk of developing complications during pregnancy. However, despite the increase in relative risk, the absolute risk of VTE and adverse outcomes in pregnancy remain low. Furthermore, aside from recurrent pregnancy loss in antiphospholipid syndrome and prevention of VTE, there is limited evidence on the benefit of antithrombotic interventions to guide therapy. The data in favor of antithrombotic therapy in women with hereditable thrombophilia and vascular placental complications consist predominantly of small uncontrolled trials or observational studies. Randomized, placebo-controlled trials are lacking as most patients do not accept placebo. Further randomized controlled trials are urgently required to explore the efficacy and safety in this clinical setting. Decisions on screening for thrombophilia should be made after reviewing with the patient the limitations of the available data, along with the potential benefits, harms, and costs of any intervention.

Acknowledgements

The authors wish to thank PD Dr. R. B. Zotz for reviewing this manuscript. We are also grateful to our colleagues, Prof. H. G. Bender and associates, Dept. of Obstetrics and Gynecology, and Prof. W. Sandmann, Dept. of Surgery, Division of Vascular Surgery and Renal Transplantation, Heinrich Heine University Medical Center, for long-standing collaboration. Our own work was supported by an institutional grant (no. 9772153) of the Faculty of Medicine, Heinrich Heine University, Düsseldorf.

Disclosure of Conflict of Interests

The authors state that they have no conflict of interests.

References

1 Bates SM: Management of pregnant women with thrombophilia or a history of venous thromboembolism. Hematology Am Soc Hematol Educ Program 2007;2007:143–150.

2 National Institute of Health Consensus Development Conference: Prevention of venous thrombosis and pulmonary embolism. JAMA 1986;256:744–749.

3 Kierkegaard A: Incidence and diagnosis of deep-vein thrombosis associated with pregnancy. Acta Obstet Gynecol Scand 1983;62:239–243.

4 Treffers PE, Huidekoper BL, Weenink GH, Kloosterman GJ: Epidemiological observations of thromboembolic disease during pregnancy and in the puerperium, in 56,022 women. Int J Gynaecol Obstet 1983;21:327–331.

5 Bergqvist A, Bergqvist D, Hallbook T: Deep-vein thrombosis during pregnancy – a prospective-study. Acta Obstet Gynecol Scand 1983;62:443–448.

6 Greer IA: The special case of venous thromboembolism in pregnancy. Haemostasis 1998;28:22–34.

7 Virchow R: Phlogose und Thrombose im Gefäßsystem; in Virchow R (Hrsg): Gesammelte Abhandlungen zur Wissenschaftlichen Medicin. Frankfurt, 1856, pp 458–636.

8 Greer IA: Haemostasis and thrombosis in pregnancy; in Bloom AL, Forbes CD, Thomas DP, Tuddenham EGD (eds): Haemostasis and Thrombosis. London, Churchill Livingstone, 1994, pp 987–1015.

9 Bates SM, Ginsberg JS: Thrombosis in pregnancy. Curr Opin Hematol 1997;4:335–343.

10 Ikard RW, Ueland K, Folse R: Lower limb venous dynamics in pregnant women. Surg Gynecol Obstet 1971;132:483–488.

11 Greer IA: Thrombosis in pregnancy: maternal and fetal issues. Lancet 1999;353:1258–1265.

12 Greer IA: The challenge of thrombophilia in maternal-fetal medicine. N Engl J Med 2000;342:424–425.

13 Bertina RM, Koeleman BPC, Koster T, Rosendaal FR, Dirven RJ, deRonde H, Vandervelden PA, Reitsma PH: Mutation in blood-coagulation factor-V associated with resistance to activated protein-C. Nature 1994;369:64–67.

14 Poort SR, Rosendaal FR, Reitsma PH, Bertina RM: A common genetic variation in the 3'-untranslated region of the prothrombin gene is associated with elevated plasma prothrombin levels and an increase in venous thrombosis. Blood 1996;88:3698–3703.

15 Rosendaal FR: Venous thrombosis: a multicausal disease. Lancet 1999;353:1453–1457.

16 Gerhardt A, Scharf RE, Beckmann MW, Struve S, Bender HG, Pillny M, Sandmann W, Zotz RB: Prothrombin and factor V mutations in women with a history of thrombosis during pregnancy and the puerperium. N Engl J Med 2000;342:374–380.

17 Zotz RB, Gerhardt A, Scharf RE: A rebuttal: Inherited thrombophilia and first venous thromboembolism during pregnancy and puerperium. Thromb Haemost 2003;89:769–770.

18 McColl MD, Ramsay JE, Tait RC, Walker ID, McCall F, Conkie JA, Carty MJ, Greer IA: Risk factors for pregnancy associated venous thromboembolism. Thromb Haemost 1997;78:1183–1188.

19 Robertson L, Wu O, Langhorne P, Twaddle S, Clark P, Lowe GDO, Walker ID, Greaves M, Brenkel I, Regan L, Greer IA: Thrombophilia in pregnancy: a systematic review. Br J Haematol 2006;132:171–196.

20 Long AA, Ginsberg JS, Brill-Edwards P, Johnston M, Turner C, Denburg JA, Bensen WG, Cividino A, Andrew M, Hirsh J: The relationship of antiphospholipid antibodies to thromboembolic disease in systemic lupus-erythematosus – a cross-sectional study. Thromb Haemost 1991;66:520–524.

21 Khamashta MA, Cuadrado MJ, Mujic F, Taub NA, Hunt BJ, Hughes GRV: The management of thrombosis in the antiphospholipid-antibody syndrome. N Engl J Med 1995;332:993–997.

22 Gerhardt A, Scharf RE, Zotz RB: Effect of hemostatic risk factors on the individual probability of thrombosis during pregnancy and the puerperium. Thromb Haemost 2003;90:77–85.

23 Zotz RB, Gerhardt A, Scharf RE: Prediction, prevention, and treatment of venous thromboembolic disease in pregnancy. Semin Thromb Hemost 2003;29:143–153.

24 Zotz RB, Gerhardt A, Scharf RE: Inherited thrombophilia and gestational venous thromboembolism. Best Pract Clin Haematol 2003;16:243–259.

25 Brill-Edwards P, Ginsberg JS, Gent M, Hirsh J, Burrows R, Kearon C, Geerts W, Kovacs M, Weitz JI, Robinson KS, Whittom R, Couture G: Safety of withholding heparin in pregnant women with a history of venous thromboembolism. N Engl J Med 2000;343:1439–1444.

26 Pabinger I, Grafenhofer H, Kaider A, Kyrle PA, Quehenberger P, Mannhalter C, Lechner K: Risk of pregnancy-associated recurrent venous thromboembolism in women with a history of venous thrombosis. J Thromb Haemost 2005;3:949–954.

27 Zotz RB, Gerhardt A, Scharf RE: Venöse Thrombose in der Schwangerschaft. Hamostaseologie 2006;26:63–71.

28 DeStefano V, Leone G, Mastrangelo S, Tripodi A, Rodeghiero F, Castaman G, Barbui T, Finazzi G, Bizzi B, Mannucci PM: Thrombosis during pregnancy and surgery in patients with congenital deficiency of antithrombin III, protein C, protein S. Thromb Haemost 1994;71:799–800.

29 Bates SA, Greer IA, Hirsh J, Ginsberg JS: Use of antithrombotic agents during pregnancy. Chest 2004;126:627S–644S.

30 Sanson BJ, Lensing AWA, Prins MH, Ginsberg JS, Barkagan ZS, Lavenne-Pardonge E, Brenner B, Dulitzky M, Nielsen JD, Boda Z, Turi S, MacGillavry MR, Hamulyak K, Theunissen IM, Hunt BJ, Buller HR: Safety of low-molecular-weight heparin in pregnancy: A systematic review. Thromb Haemost 1999;81:668–672.

31 Douketis JD, Ginsberg JS, Burrows RF, Duku EK, Webber CE, Brill-Edwards P: The effects of long-term heparin therapy during pregnancy on bone density – A prospective matched cohort study. Thromb Haemost 1996;75:254–257.

32 Hatasaka HH: Recurrent miscarriage – epidemiologic factors, definitions, and incidence. Clin Obstet Gynecol 1994;37:625–634.

33 Brenner B: Clinical management of thrombophilia-related placental vascular complications. Blood 2004;103:4003–4009.

34 Preston FE, Rosendaal FR, Walker ID, Briet E, Berntorp E, Conard J, Fontcuberta J, Makris M, Mariani G, Noteboom W, Pabinger I, Legnani C, Scharrer I, Schulman S, van der Meer FJM: Increased fetal loss in women with heritable thrombophilia. Lancet 1996;348:913–916.

35 Roberts JM, Taylor RN, Musci TJ, Rodgers GM, Hubel CA, McLaughlin MK: Preeclampsia – an endothelial-cell disorder. Am J Obstet Gynecol 1989;161:1200–1204.

36 Salafia CM, Pezzullo JC, Lopezzeno JA, Simmens S, Minior VK, Vintzileos AM: Placental pathological features of preterm preeclampsia. Am J Obstet Gynecol 1995;173:1097–1105.

37 Shanklin DR, Sibai BM: Ultrastructural aspects of preeclampsia. 1. Placental bed and uterine boundary vessels. Am J Obstet Gynecol 1989;161:735–741.

38 Khong TY, Pearce JM, Robertson WB: Acute atherosis in preeclampsia – maternal determinants and fetal-outcome in the presence of the lesion. Am J Obstet Gynecol 1987;157:360–363.

39 Rai R: Is miscarriage a coagulopathy? Curr Opin Obstet Gynecol 2003;15:265–268.

40 Opatrny L, David M, Kahn SR, Shrier I, Rey E: Association between antiphospholipid antibodies and recurrent fetal loss in women without autoimmune disease: A metaanalysis. J Rheumatol 2006;33:2214–2221.

41 Rey E, Kahn SR, David M, Shrier I: Thrombophilic disorders and fetal loss: a meta-analysis. Lancet 2003;361:901–908.

42 Gerhardt A, Scharf RE, Mikat-Drozdzynski B, Krussel JS, Bender HG, Zotz RB: The polymorphism of platelet membrane integrin alpha 2 beta(1) (alpha(2)807TT) is associated with premature onset of fetal loss. Thromb Haemost 2005;93:124–129.

43 Gerhardt A, Goecke TW, Beckmann MW, Wagner KJ, Tutschek B, Willers R, Bender HG, Scharf RE, Zotz RB: The G20210A prothrombin-gene mutation and the plasminogen activator inhibitor (PAI-1) 5G/5G genotype are associated with early onset of severe preeclampsia. J Thromb Haemost 2005;3:686–691.

44 Kupferminc MJ, Eldor A, Steinman N, Many A, Bar-Am A, Jaffa A, Fait G, Lessing JB: Increased frequency of genetic thrombophilia in women with complications of pregnancy. N Engl J Med 1999;340:9–13.

45 Morrison ER, Miedzybrodzka ZH, Campbell DM, Haites NE, Wilson BJ, Watson MS, Greaves M, Vickers MA: Prothrombotic genotypes are not associated with pre-eclampsia and gestational hypertension: Results from a large population-based study and systematic review. Thromb Haemost 2002;87:779–785.

46 De Maat MPM, Jansen MWJC, Hille ETM, Vos HL, Bloemenkamp WM, Buitendijk S, Helmerhorst FM, Wladimiroff JW, Bertina RM, de Groot CJM: Preeclampsia and its interaction with common variants in thrombophilia genes. J Thromb Haemost 2004;2:1588–1593.

47 Yasuda M, Takakuwa K, Tokunaga A, Tanaka K: Prospective studies of the association between anticardiolipin antibody and outcome of pregnancy. Obstet Gynecol 1995;86:555–559.

48 Hamilton WJ, Boyd JD: Development of the human placenta in the 1st 3 months of gestation. J Anat 1960;94:297–324.

49 Makikallio K, Tekay A, Jouppila P: Yolk sac and umbilicoplacental hemodynamics during early human embryonic development. Ultrasound Obstet Gynecol 1999;14:175–179.

50 Isermann B, Sood R, Pawlinski R, Zogg M, Kalloway S, Degen JL, Mackman N, Weiler H: The thrombomodulin-protein C system is essential for the maintenance of pregnancy. Nat Med 2003;9:331–337.

51 Brenner B, Hoffman R, Blumenfeld Z, Weiner Z, Younis JS: Gestational outcome in thrombophilic women with recurrent pregnancy loss treated by enoxaparin. Thromb Haemost 2000;83:693–697.

52 Brenner B, Hoffman R, Carp H, Dulitsky M, Younis J: Efficacy and safety of two doses of enoxaparin in women with thrombophilia and recurrent pregnancy loss: the LIVE-ENOX study. J Thromb Haemost 2005;3:227–229.

53 Grandone E, Brancaccio V, Colaizzo D, Scianname N, Pavone G, Di Minno G, Margaglione M: Preventing adverse obstetric outcomes in women with genetic thrombophilia. Fertil Steril 2002;78:371–375.

54 Carp H, Dolitzky M, Inbal A: Thromboprophylaxis improves the live birth rate in women with consecutive recurrent miscarriages and hereditary thrombophilia. J Thromb Haemost 2003;1:433–438.

55 Gris JC, Mercier E, Quere I, Lavigne-Lissalde G, Cochery-Nouvellon E, Hoffet M, Ripart-Neveu S, Tailland ML, Dauzat M, Mares P: Low-molecular-weight heparin versus low-dose aspirin in women with one fetal loss and a constitutional thrombophilic disorder. Blood 2004;103:3695–3699.

56 Ginsberg JS, Brill-Edwards P, Johnston M, Denburg JA, Andrew M, Burrows RF, Bensen W, Cividino A, Long AA: Relationship of antiphospholipid antibodies to pregnancy loss in patients with systemic lupus-erythematosus – a cross-sectional study. Blood 1992;80:975–980.

57 Laskin CA, Bombardier C, Hannah ME, Mandel FP, Ritchie JWK, Farewell V, Farine D, Spitzer K, Fielding L, Soloninka CA, Yeung M: Prednisone and aspirin in women with autoantibodies and unexplained recurrent fetal loss. N Engl J Med 1997;337:148–153.

58 Rai R, Cohen H, Dave M, Regan L: Randomised controlled trial of aspirin and aspirin plus heparin in pregnant women with recurrent miscarriage associated with phospholipid antibodies (or antiphospholipid antibodies). Br Med J 1997;314:253–257.

59 Kutteh WH: Antiphospholipid antibody-associated recurrent pregnancy loss. Treatment with heparin and low-dose aspirin is superior to low-dose aspirin alone. Am J Obstet Gynecol 1996;174:1584–1589.

60 Rai R, Regan L: Recurrent miscarriage. Lancet 2006;368:601–611.

61 Lima F, Khamashta MA, Buchanan NMM, Kerslake S, Hunt BJ, Hughes GRV: A study of sixty pregnancies in patients with the antiphospholipid syndrome. Clin Exp Rheumatol 1996;14:131–136.

62 Backos M, Rai R, Baxter N, Chilcott IT, Cohen H, Regan L: Pregnancy complications in women with recurrent miscarriage associated with antiphospholipid antibodies treated with low dose aspirin and heparin. Br J Obstet Gynaecol 1999;106:102–107.

63 Noble LS, Kutteh WH, Lashey N, Franklin RD, Herrada J: Antiphospholipid antibodies associated with recurrent pregnancy loss: prospective, multicenter, controlled pilot study comparing treatment with low-molecular-weight heparin versus unfractionated heparin. Fertil Steril 2005;83:684–690.

64 Duley L, Henderson-Smart DJ, Knight M, King JF: Antiplatelet agents for preventing preeclampsia and its complications. Cochrane Database Syst Rev 2004;CD004659.

65 Caritis S, Sibai B, Hauth J, Lindheimer MD, Klebanoff M, Thom E, VanDorsten P, Landon M, Paul R, Miodovnik M, Meis P, Thurnau G: Low-dose aspirin to prevent preeclampsia in women at high risk. N Engl J Med 1998;338:701–705.

66 Beroyz G, Casale R, Farreiros A, et al.: Clasp – a randomized trial of low-dose aspirin for the prevention and treatment of preeclampsia among 9364 pregnant-women. Lancet 1994;343:619–629.

67 Middeldorp S: Thrombophilia and pregnancy complications: cause or association? J Thromb Haemost 2007;5:276–282.

Prof. Dr. med. Rüdiger E. Scharf, F.A.H.A.
Institut für Hämostaseologie und Transfusionsmedizin
Universitätsklinikum Düsseldorf
Heinrich-Heine-Universität
Moorenstraße 5, 40225 Düsseldorf, Germany
Tel. +49 211 81-17345, Fax -16221
E-Mail rscharf@uni-duesseldorf.de

Scharf RE (ed): Progress and Challenges in Transfusion Medicine, Hemostasis and Hemotherapy.
Freiburg i.Br., Karger, 2008, pp 344–351

Prevention and Therapy of Pregnancy-Associated Thromboembolic Events

Ingrid Pabinger

Clinical Division of Haematology and Haemostasis, Department of Internal Medicine I,
General Hospital of Vienna, Medical University of Vienna, Austria

Key Words

Pregnancy · Thrombophilia · Venous thromboembolism · Abortion · Foetal loss · Pre-eclampsia

Summary

Pregnancy is associated with increased morbidity and mortality due to venous thromboembolism (VTE).
The incidence of VTE is around 1 in 1000 pregnancies; the risk is highest during the first 3–6 weeks after
delivery. Heparin can safely be used during pregnancy, whereas vitamin K antagonists have a teratogenic
effect when given between the 6th and 12th week of gestation. Acute venous thromboembolic events
are treated with therapeutic doses of low-molecular-weight heparin (LMWH); treatment is continued
until 6 weeks to 3 months after delivery. Lower doses of LMWH may be considered after 4–6 weeks on
therapeutic doses. Prevention of VTE is recommended for women with a history of major VTE and for
those with antithrombin deficiency type I, homozygous factor V Leiden and the lupus anti-coagulant.
Although almost no controlled trials on anti-coagulation in pregnant women are available, treatment
and prophylaxis of VTE in pregnancy can nowadays be regarded as highly effective and safe.

©2008 S. Karger GmbH, Freiburg i.Br.

Introduction

Pregnancy is associated with an increased risk for venous thromboembolism (VTE).
Anti-coagulant therapy is used for prevention and treatment, but it also bears the
potential of foetal complications. Since controlled clinical trials are lacking, recommendations about the use of anti-coagulants in pregnant women are largely based
on data obtained from non-pregnant patients and from case series of pregnant patients.

Heparin, including low-molecular-weight heparin (LMWH), does not cross the
placental barrier and is thus non-teratogenic, whereas vitamin K antagonists cross

the placental barrier and may cause coumarin embryopathy, which is characterised by nose deformation and other deformations of the skeletal structure (stippled epiphysis) [1]. Furthermore, bleeding might occur in the anti-coagulated foetus, leading to severe and life-threatening clinical situations, such as cerebral bleeding. Chan and colleagues found that the use of vitamin K antagonists during pregnancy was associated with congenital foetal anomalies in 35 of 549 live births [2]. The dimension of the teratogenic risk remains controversial ranging from 0 up to 29.6% [1]. This risk is only present when vitamin K antagonists are taken between the 6th and 12th week of gestation. Coumarins have also been associated with anomalies of the central nervous system after exposure to them during any trimester. Moreover, vitamin K antagonists have been associated with abortion [2, 3].

Women receiving vitamin K antagonist therapy have to be clearly informed about the risks of oral anti-coagulant therapy. The use of danaparoid treatment has been reviewed recently. 51 pregnancies occurred in 49 patients, 3 foetal deaths were reported, but all of them were associated with maternal complications antedating danaparoid use [4]. Although not licensed, danaparoid seems to be an alternative in case of allergic reactions to LMWH. Reports on the successful use of fondaparinux in pregnant women [5, 6] have been published; however, potential adverse effects on the foetus cannot be excluded. Thrombolytic agents should only be used in life-threatening situations. There are still concerns about the use of vitamin K antagonists in nursing mothers; however, many experts in the field agree on the potential use of these agents in nursing mothers [7]. It is suggested to substitute vitamin K orally in the child (e.g. 1 mg of vitamin K once a week). The use of heparin including LMWH, danaparoid and fondaparinux in the lactating woman is regarded as safe for the child [1, 8].

The risk for VTE after caesarean delivery has been described to be around 0.5 per 1,000 deliveries and is higher when the intervention is performed as an emergency procedure compared to an elective procedure [1]. Pulmonary embolism (PE) is more frequent after caesarean delivery and complicates around 0.4/1,000 of caesarean deliveries. Caesarean section is a risk factor for VTE; this risk may be augmented by other risk factors. Such risk factors are pre-eclampsia and eclampsia, thrombophilia or infection, probably also prolonged labour, immobilisation, lower limb paresis and other clinical or medical conditions, such as obesity or heart failure. Whereas thromboprophylaxis may not be justified on the basis of caesarean section alone, it is clearly recommended in women with one or more of the above-mentioned additional risk factors [1].

No adequately powered trials have been performed in women undergoing caesarean section [9–12]. Usually, based on experience from clinical trials in high-risk patients, thrombosis prophylaxis with LMWH may be recommended the way it is used in general surgery in high-risk patients. There are also no data concerning the duration of prophylaxis; experts suggest a minimum duration of 5 days.

Acute Venous Thromboembolism during Pregnancy

VTE is an important and frequent complication of pregnancy, and PE is nowadays the most frequent cause of maternal mortality in the developed countries [13]. The incidence of VTE is around 1 episode per 1,000 deliveries [14], and is thus much higher than in non-pregnant women of comparable age. About two-thirds of DVT occur ante partum; VTE may occur at any trimester and is more or less equally distributed throughout all three trimesters [15]. Approximately 50% of pregnancy-related episodes of PE occur in the first 6 weeks after delivery [16].

When an acute event of VTE occurs in a pregnant woman, LMWH is the treatment of choice. The dose is adapted to the body weight of the woman [17]. It has been shown that during the course of pregnancy the dosage of LMWH that is needed to reach a therapeutic anti-Xa level increases [18–20]. However, experts do not agree as to whether measurement of anti-Xa levels is mandatory in pregnant women with acute VTE or whether it is sufficient to adapt the dosage of LMWH to the weight of the pregnant woman. Since vitamin K antagonists are contra-indicated during pregnancy due to their potential of causing embryopathy, secondary prophylaxis with LMWH is used in pregnant women. LMWH has a lower risk for development of osteoporosis and, also for this reason, is the preferred option for these women [21]. Whether or not dose adjustments are necessary during the course of pregnancy is still seen controversially. Whereas some experts suggest increasing the dosage according to the increase of weight, others prefer adjustment of dosage of LMWH to the actual anti-Xa level. A target level of 0.5–1.2 U/ml is recommended when a twice-daily regimen is used and up to 1.5 U/ml are recommended if a once-daily regimen is chosen. Measurement is performed approximately 4 h after the administration of LMWH.

Yet, it still remains unclear whether the dose of LMWH can be safely reduced after the acute thromboembolic event after an initial phase of therapeutic anti-coagulation. Several suggestions have been made: either the maintenance of therapeutic doses of anti-coagulation throughout pregnancy or the reduction of LMWH to prophylactic levels or to 50–75% of the full dose of LMWH after 4–6 weeks of full therapeutic anti-coagulation. Such an approach may reduce the risks of anti-coagulant-related bleeding and heparin-induced osteoporosis.

A dangerous complication of anti-coagulation is bleeding during labour [22]. When induction of labour or elective caesarean section is planned, the doses of LMWH are reduced 24 h before the planned intervention and anti-coagulation is re-installed after delivery. In women planning to have a spontaneous delivery, the doses of heparin might be reduced to prophylactic levels after the 37th week of gestation. When the thromboembolic event has occurred shortly before delivery, the insertion of a caval filter has to be suggested. The filters can be removed after the therapeutic anti-coagulation has been reinduced after delivery (3–10 days after delivery). Women with a very high risk for recurrent VTE could also be switched to therapeutic intravenous unfractionated heparin (UFH), which is then discontinued 4–6 h prior to the expected time of delivery.

No studies clarifying the duration of anti-coagulation after delivery are available. It is accepted by most experts that a minimum of 6 weeks of anti-coagulation after delivery should be recommended, allowing for a duration of up to 3–6 months in women in whom VTE had occurred shortly before delivery or in those who still have an increased risk, e.g. due to infection, immobilisation or other predisposing factors.

Prevention of Venous Thromboembolism in Pregnant Women with a History of Venous Thromboembolism

Women with a history of VTE are at increased risk for recurrence during the pregnancy period [23]. There are no sufficiently powered studies examining the incidence of VTE in pregnant women with and without heparin. From observational studies, the risk for recurrence can be deduced to be between 5–10% during pregnancy [24–26]. In a prospective study designed to estimate the true incidence of recurrence in 125 women with prior VTE, Brill-Edwards [23] found a risk of 2.4% of recurrence (95% confidence interval (CI) 0.2–6.9%). In a retrospective study of 159 women without thromboprophylaxis, the probability of developing ante-partum VTE was 6.2% (95% CI, 0.2–6.9%), while that for post-partum VTE was 6.5% (95% CI, 3.5–11.9%) [25]. The magnitude of the risk is similar throughout the whole period of pregnancy and thus is already increased during the first trimester. The risk of recurrence has been balanced against the risk of treatment, inconvenience and costs. The risk of prophylaxis is heparin-induced thrombocytopenia and bleeding; when higher (therapeutic) doses are administered, there is also a risk of developing osteoporosis and osteoporotic fractures, which has been observed in prospective studies [21, 27–29]. At the site of injection, allergic reactions and bleeding might occur, which causes itching and pain and a small risk of heparin-induced skin necrosis. Since LMWH is administered during very long time periods (up to or even more than 9 months), there is also a cost issue that has to be taken into account. An important task would be to identify women with a high risk of recurrence. Up to now, several factors have been found that are clearly associated with an increased risk of recurrence, such as presence of antithrombin deficiency or homozygous factor V Leiden [30]. There is ongoing discussion whether milder risk factors, such as factor V Leiden or the prothrombin variation in heterozygous form, can be regarded as risk factors for an increased risk for pregnancy-associated recurrence. There is a clear recommendation for prophylaxis after delivery in comparison to ante-partum prophylaxis because of the shorter duration of required treatment (i.e. 6 weeks) and the higher average daily risk of VTE in the post-partum period. There are no controlled studies available with regard to the dosage of LMWH and the avoidance of thrombosis. Prophylactic doses, such as 40 mg enoxaparin or 5,000 U dalteparin, prevent the occurrence of thrombosis. During this treatment, only 2 thrombotic events out of 86 pregnancies occurred [31]. It is not yet clear which women need higher doses of LMWH to prevent thrombosis. During prophylaxis with LMWH, the rate of thrombosis (primary and recurrent) is very low; rates of 1–3% have been described [21, 31, 32]. The risk of heparin-induced thrombocytopenia and osteoporosis is also very low [21].

Risk of Pregnancy-Associated Venous Thromboembolism and Prevention in Women with Thrombophilia

There are several risk factors for thromboembolism ('thrombophilia') causing a considerable increase of the risk for VTE [33]. The most important one is antithrombin deficiency type I [34]. Rates of VTE of 20–40% have been described in women with antithrombin deficiency, sometimes occurring very early during the course of pregnancy [35]. Women with homozygous factor V Leiden are as well at a high risk for VTE during pregnancy [30]; there are only very scarce data on patients with homozygous prothrombin variation. The risk for VTE in women with factor V Leiden in heterozygous form is slightly increased (1 in 430 women) [34]. There is also an increased risk in women with protein C deficiency and, to a lesser extent, in women with protein S deficiency [34].

There is ongoing discussion as to which women should receive primary prophylaxis. The author of this manuscript suggests thrombosis prophylaxis in women with antithrombin deficiency and in those with homozygous factor V Leiden. Additionally, women who fulfil the criteria for an anti-phospholipid syndrome would most probably benefit from thrombosis prophylaxis with LMWH including aspirin with a better outcome for the foetus [36]. In all other women, the recommendation is rather against thrombosis prophylaxis, but it seems mandatory to provide profound information for these women on the symptoms of VTE and, if symptoms compatible with VTE occur, to immediately and objectively verify or exclude a thrombotic event. Also in this case there is no unanimity among experts on the dose of prophylaxis. Usually 4,000–5,000 anti-Xa units per day are recommended for these women.

It can be concluded that pregnancy indeed is a risk factor for VTE. Although controlled trials have not been performed so far, recommendations for treatment and prophylaxis rely vastly on experience. Thrombosis prophylaxis has to be given to high-risk women.

Conclusions and Future Directions

VTE has become one of the most important complications of pregnancy. Although systematic clinical studies have been performed only rarely, the knowledge on prophylaxis and management of VTE has increased considerably within the last 10–20 years.

Specifically LMWHs play an important role, as in cohort studies they have been shown to be safe for the woman and the foetus, and to be effective. Other direct anti-coagulants will be available in the future and have to find their place in the management of pregnant women. Further advances might be reached by defining more clearly women at risk for VTE and by defining more precisely the dosage of anti-coagulants.

Disclosure of Conflict of Interests

The author has received unrestricted grants from Pfizer, CSL Behring and Bayer and furthermore honoraria for lectures at various events from different pharmaceutical companies.

Acknowledgements

Special thanks to T. Altreiter for her efficient editorial work.

References

1 Bates SM, Greer IA, Pabinger I, Sofaer S, Hirsh J: Venous thromboembolism, trombophilia, antithrombotic therapy, and pregnancy; American College of Chevt Physicians evidence-based clinical practice guidelines. Chest 2008;133:844S-886S.

2 Chan WS, Anand S, Ginsberg JS: Anticoagulation of pregnant women with mechanical heart valves: A systematic review of the literature. Arch Intern Med 2000;160:191–196.

3 Schaefer C, Hannemann D, Meister R, Eléfant E, Paulus W, Vial T, Reuvers M, Robert-Gnansia E, Arnon J, De Santis M, Clementi M, Rodriguez-Pinilla E, Dolivo A, Merlob P: Vitamin K antagonists and pregnancy outcome. A multi-centre prospective study. Thromb Haemost 2006;95:949–957.

4 Lindhoff-Last E, Kreutzenbeck H-J, Magnani HN: Treatment of 51 pregnancies with danaparoid because of heparin intolerance. Thromb Haemost 2005;93:63–69.

5 Harenberg J: Treatment of a woman with lupus and thromboembolism and cutaneous intolerance of heparins using fonaparinux during pregnancy. Thromb Res 2007;119:385–388.

6 Mazzolai L, Hohlfeld P, Spertini F, Hayoz D, Schapira M, Duchosal MA: Fondaparinux is a safe alternative in case of heparin intolerance during pregnancy. Blood 2006;108:1569–1570.

7 Clark S, Porter F, West FG: Coumarin derivatives and breast-feeding. Obstet Gynecol 2000;95:938–940.

8 Lindhoff-Last E, Willeke A, Thalhammer C, Nowak G, Bauersachs R: Hirudin treatment in a breastfeeding woman. Lancet 2000;355:467–468.

9 Gates S, Brocklehurst P, Davis LJ: Prophylaxis for venous thromboembolic disease in pregnancy and the early postnatal period. Cochrane Database Syst Rev 2002;2:CD001689.

10 Ellison J, Thomson AJ, Conkie JA, McCall F, Walker ID, Greer IA: Thromboprophylaxis following caesarean section. A comparison of the antithrombotic properties of three low molecular weight heparins – dalteparin, enoxaparin, and tinzaparin. Thromb Haemost 2001;86:1374–1378.

11 Burrows RF, Gan ET, Gallus AS, Wallace EM, Burrows EA: A randomised double-blind placebo controlled trial of low molecular weight heparin as prophylaxis in preventing venous thrombolic events after caesarean section: a pilot study. BJOG 2001;108:835–839.

12 Heilmann L, Heitz R, Koch FU, Ose C: Perioperative thrombosis prophylaxis at the time of caesarean section: results of a randomized prospective comparative study. With 6% hydroxyethyl starch 0.62 and low-dose heparin. Z Geburtshilfe Perinatol 1991;195:10–15.

13 Confidential Enquiries into Maternal and Child Health. 'Why Mothers Die: 2000–02'. The Sixth Report of the UK Confidential Enquiries into Maternal Deaths. London, The Royal College of Obstetricians and Gynaecologists Press, November 2004. www.cemach.org.uk.

14 Chang J, Elam-Evans LD, Berg CJ, Herndon J, Flowers L, Seed KA, Syverson CJ: Pregnancy-related mortality surveillance – United States, 1991–1999. MMWR Surveill Summ 2003;62:1–88.

15 Ray JG, Chan WS: Deep vein thrombosis during pregnancy and the puerperium: a meta-analysis of the period of risk and leg of presentation. Obstet Gynecol Surv 1999;54:254–271.

16 Gherman RB, Goodwin TM, Leung B, Byrne JD, Hethumumi R, Montoro M: Incidence, clinical characteristics, and timing of objectively diagnosed venous thromboembolism during pregnancy. Obstet Gynecol 1999;94:730–734.

17 Macklon NS, Greer IA: Venous thromboembolic disease in obstetrics and gynaecology: the Scottish experience. Scott Med J 1996;41:83–86.

18 Crowther MA, Spitzer K, Julian J, Ginsberg J, Johnston M, Crowther R, Laskin C: Pharmacokinetic profile of a low-molecular weight heparin (Reviparin) in pregnant patients: a prospective cohort study. Thromb Res 2000;98:133–138.

19 Barbour LA, Oja JL, Schultz LK: A prospective trial that demonstrates that dalteparin requirements increase in pregnancy to maintain therapeutic levels of anticoagulation. Am J Obstet Gynecol 2004;191:1024–1029.

20 Ellison J, Walker ID, Greer IA: Antifactor Xa profiles in pregnant women receiving antenatal thromboprophylaxis with enoxaparin for prevention and treatment of thromboembolism in pregnancy. Br J Obstet Gynaecol 2000;107:1116–1121.

21 Greer IA, Nelson Piercy C: Low molecular weight heparins for thromboprophylaxis and treatment of venous thromboembolism in pregnancy: a systematic review of safety and efficacy. Blood 2005;106:401–407.

22 Anderson DR, Ginsberg JS, Burrows R, Brill-Edwards P: Subcutaneous heparin therapy during pregnancy: a need for concern at the time of delivery. Thromb Haemost 1991;65:248–250.

23 Pabinger I, Grafenhofer H, Kyrle PA, Quehenberger P, Mannhalter C, Lechner K, Kaider A: Temporary increase in the risk for recurrence during pregnancy in women with a history of venous thromboembolism. Blood 2002;100:1060–1062.

24 Brill-Edwards P, Ginsberg JS, Gent M, Hirsh J, Burrows R, Kearon C, Geerts W, Kovacs M, Weitz JI, Robinson KS, Whittom R, Couture G; Recurrence of Clot in this Pregnancy (ROCIT) Study Group: Safety of withholding antepartum heparin in women with a previous episode of venous thromboembolism. Recurrence of Clot in this Pregnancy Study Group. N Engl J Med 2000;343:1439–1444.

25 Pabinger I, Grafenhofer H, Kaider A, Kyrle PA, Quehenberger P, Mannhalter C, Lechner K: Risk of pregnancy-associated recurrent venous thromboembolism in women with a history of venous thrombosis. J Thromb Haemost 2005;3:949–954.

26 Tengborn L: Recurrent thromboembolism in pregnancy and puerperium: Is there a need for thromboprophylaxis? Am J Obstet Gynecol 1989;160:90–94.

27 Sanson BJ, Lensing AW, Prins MH, Ginsberg JS, Barkagan ZS, Lavenne-Pardonge E, Brenner B, Dulitzky M, Nielsen JD, Boda Z, Turi S, Mac Gillavry MR, Hamulyák K, Theunissen IM, Hunt BJ, Büller HR: Safety of low-molecular-weight heparin in pregnancy: a systematic review. Thromb Haemost 1999;81:668–672.

28 Hunt BJ, Doughty HA, Majumdar G, Copplestone A, Kerslake S, Buchanan N, Hughes G, Khamashta M: Thromboprophylaxis with low molecular weight heparin (Fragmin) in high risk pregnancies. Thromb Haemost 1997;77:39–43.

29 Greer IA: Thrombosis in pregnancy: maternal and fetal issues. Lancet 1999;353:1258–1265.

30 Pabinger I, Nemes L, Rintelen C, Koder S, Lechler E, Loreth RM, Kyrle PA, Scharrer I, Sas G, Lechner K, Mannhalter C, Ehrenforth S: Pregnancy-associated risk for venous thromboembolism and pregnancy outcome in women homozygous for factor V Leiden. Hematol J 2000;1:37–41.

31 Alguel G, Vormittag R, Simanek R, Kyrle PA, Quehenberger P, Mannhalter C, Husslein P, Pabinger I: Preeclampsia and pregnancy loss in women with a history of venous thromboembolism and prophylactic low-molecular-weight heparin (LMWH) during pregnancy. Thromb Haemost 2006;96:285–289.

32 Bauersachs RM, Dudenhausen J, Faridi A, Fischer T, Fung S, Geisen U, Harenberg J, Herchenhan E, Keller F, Kemkes-Matthes B, Schinzel H, Spannagl M, Thaler CJ; EThIG Investigators: Risk stratification and heparin prophylaxis to prevent venous thromboembolism in pregnant women. Thromb Haemost 2007;98:1237–1245.

33 Gerhardt A, Scharf RE, Beckmann MW, Struve S, Bender HG, Pillny M, Sandmann W, Zotz RB: Prothrombin and factor V mutations in women with a history of thrombosis during pregnancy and the puerperium. N Eng J Med 2000;342:374–380.

34 McColl MD, Ramsay JE, Tait RC, Walker ID, Mc-Call F, Conkie JA, Carty MJ, Greer IA: Risk factors for pregnancy associated venous thromboembolism. Thromb Haemost 1997;8:1183–1188.

35 Pabinger I, Schneider B and GTH Study Group on Natural Inhibitors: Thrombotic risk in hereditary antithrombin III-, protein C- and protein S-deficiency: a cooperative retrospective study. Arterioscler Thromb Vasc Biol 1996;16:742–748.

36 Pabinger I, Vormittag R: Thrombophilia and pregnancy outcomes. J Thromb Haemost 2005;3:1603–1610.

Prof. Dr. med. Ingrid Pabinger
Clinical Division of Haematology and Haemostasis
Department of Internal Medicine I, Medical University of Vienna
Waehringer Guertel 18–20, 1090 Vienna, Austria
Tel. +43 1 40400 4448, Fax -4030
E-Mail ingrid.pabinger@meduniwien.ac.at

Scharf RE (ed): Progress and Challenges in Transfusion Medicine, Hemostasis and Hemotherapy.
Freiburg i.Br., Karger, 2008, pp 352–362

The Potential Role of Natural Killer Cells in the Treatment of Malignant Disease

Rupert Handgretinger · Matthias Pfeiffer · Heiko-Manuel Teltschik ·
Tobias Feuchtinger · Ingo Mueller · Peter Lang

Children's University Hospital, Department of Hematology / Oncology and General Pediatrics,
University of Tübingen, Germany

Key Words

Natural killer (NK) cells · Leukemia · Solid tumors · Killer Ig-like receptor (KIR) · Cytotoxicity · Adoptive transfer

Summary

Since their discovery natural killer (NK) cells have been implicated in the control of tumor growth and metastasis in vivo. Originally described as large granular lymphocytes, NK cells are a heterogeneous population of lymphocytes with functional differences in terms of cytokine production and cytotoxicity. They express a variety of receptors which regulate their function and which allow them to recognize and eliminate tumor cells. Especially the discovery of inhibitory and activatory receptors for certain human leukocyte antigens has tremendously added insight into the role of NK cells in tumor surveillance, and the anti-tumor effect of alloreactive NK cells has been demonstrated in killer Ig-like receptor-mismatched allogeneic stem cell transplantion. The possibility to manipulate the balancing receptors and their ligands offers new perspectives of NK cell-based therapies, and the possibility to isolate NK cells in large numbers for clinical use allows the ex vivo activation and adoptive transfer of NK cells for treatment of various malignant diseases.   ©2008 S. Karger GmbH, Freiburg i.Br.

Introduction

Natural killer (NK) cells have been identified as a subpopulation comprising 10–20% of lymphocytes that are able to lyse human leukocyte antigen (HLA)-negative tumor and virus-infected cells. Extensive research over the years has revealed that NK cells are a heterogeneous population of cells with various functions in terms of cytokine production and cytotoxicity. Especially the expression of the CD56 antigens on NK cells has widely facilitated the identification of subsets of NK cells and, moreover, allows their large-scale clinical isolation for ex vivo activation and subsequent adoptive

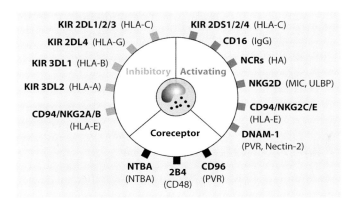

Fig. 1. Schematic overview on the expression of inhibitory and activatory receptors and co-receptors expressed on NK cells.

transfer into patients [1, 2]. NK cells express a variety of surface receptors with inhibitory and activatory functions which play a role in various diseases including cancer [3]. The final functional response of NK cells is determined by the response of these receptors in combination with the signaling of various co-receptors and other surface structures upon binding to their cognate ligands [4].

In figure 1, a schematic overview over the inhibitory, activatory and co-receptors and the various ligands is shown. The inhibitory receptors include different specificities for HLA class I molecules. The two main groups are the killer Ig-like receptors (KIRs) which are receptors for HLA class I ligands [5] and the CD94-NKG2A/B which recognize HLA-E [6]. Since NK cells exert spontaneous cytotoxicity in the absence of inhibition, the lack of single HLA alleles on target cells, as often seen in tumor cells, renders them susceptible to NK cell-mediated lysis. Based on the observation that NK cells lyse lymphohematopoietic target cells that express HLA class I molecules for which they do not express the corresponding inhibitory receptor, the concept of alloreactive NK cells (KIR mismatch) has been introduced in allogeneic stem cell transplantation [7]. Killer activatory Ig-like receptors (KARs) are also triggered by HLA class I alleles [4], but additional activatory receptors exist, such as NKG2D, the leukocyte adhesion molecule DNAX accessory molecule (DNAM-1; CD226) and the natural cytotoxicity receptors (NCR) NKp46, NKp30 and NKp44 for which so far -unknown ligands are expressed on hematopoietic cells [4, 5, 8]. The Fc receptor CD16, binding the Fc portion of immunoglobulin G (IgG), mediates the antibody-dependent cellular cytotoxicity (ADCC) of NK cells. NKD2D and DNAM-1 are receptors for stress-induced ligands, such as the MHC class I-related chains A and B (MIC A/B), UL16-binding proteins (ULBP) and poliovirus receptor (CD155) and Nectin-2 (CD112), respectively [9–11]. Other surface molecules contribute to the functional status of NK cells, among them the 2B4, NK-T-B-antigen (NTB-A) and NKp80 co-receptors, CD18/CD11, CD2 adhesion molecules, and Toll-like receptors (TLRs) [8, 12].

Incubation of NK cells with various cytokines leads to their stimulation; they are then named lymphokine-activated killer (LAK) cells. LAK cells express additional surface and intracellular molecules such as perforin, granzymes, Fas ligand and TNF-related apoptosis-inducing ligand (TRAIL), which enables them to effectively kill a wide spectrum of various tumor cells via induction of necrosis or apoptosis [13].

The important role of NK cells in tumor surveillance has further been demonstrated in a long-term follow-up study, in which the NK activity of 3625 individuals was measured longitudinally and the results were compared with the incidence of cancer. And indeed, individuals who had a high spontaneous NK activity had a lower risk to develop cancer whereas individuals with lower activity had a higher incidence of malignant disease [14].

Therefore, strategies to augment the anti-tumor activity of the NK cell system in the autologous or allogeneic setting could be beneficial in the treatment of patients with cancer.

Natural Killer Cell-Based Therapies in Cancer

The first clinical trials exploiting NK cells in the treatment of cancer used infusions of autologous ex vivo interleukin (IL)-2-activated NK cells and subsequent application of IL-2 in patients with various tumors. While some clinical responses have been observed, this treatment was limited by severe side effects, such a capillary leak syndrome and others [15]. With the discovery of inhibitory receptors on NK cells, the introduction of the concept of alloreactive NK cells, and with more insights into their iology, NK cell-based immunotherapeutic strategies have regained a wide interest, not only in the treatment of patients with hematological malignancies but also in the treatment of patients with solid metastasized tumors.

The Concept of Alloreactive Natural Killer Cells

Based on the concept of the interaction of inhibitory receptors with HLA class I molecules, various clinical situations can be envisioned, which are summarized in figure 2: NK cells can express KIRs for which the tumor cells have the corresponding ligands (fig. 2A). This leads to inhibition of the killing machinery of the NK cells and the tumor cells will not be attacked. In figure 2B, the NK cells express KIRs for which the tumor cells do not have the corresponding inhibitory ligands (lack of inhibition), resulting therefore in the activation of the NK cells and thus killing of the tumor cells. Another situation is the reduced expression or complete lack of HLA class I molecules, which can be encountered in leukemic blasts or certain tumors, such as neuroblastoma (fig. 2C). This constellation leads to killing of the tumor cells, and the intensity of killing is dependent on the amount of HLA molecules expressed on the

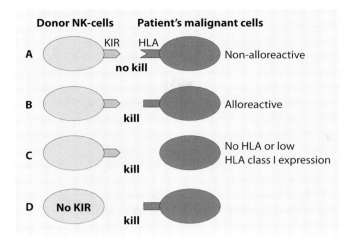

Fig. 2. Possible constellations of the expression of inhibitory receptors (KIR) on NK cells and the expression of KIR-binding or KIR-nonbinding HLA class I molecules on tumor target cells, all of which influence the overall cytotoxic activity of an NK cell.

surface of the target cells [16]. Another situation seen clinically in the phase of immunoreconstitution of NK cells after haploidentical transplantation is the absence of KIRs on the NK cells [17], and this situation allows the NK cells to kill their target independently of the amount or the specificity of the HLA class I molecules on the tumor target cells (fig. 2D).

Do 'Autoreactive' Natural Killer Cells Exist?

While the concept of alloreactive NK cells has been described in the setting of allogeneic stem cell transplantation between a KIR mismatch donor and recipient, recent published data have shown that NK cells lacking inhibitory receptors for self HLA class I molecules exist in healthy individuals and that these NK cells can exert cytotoxic functions against normal hematopoietic precursors from the same individual [18]. In addition, a similar mechanism has been implied in the cause of pure red cell aplasia in a patient with a clonal expansion of cytotoxic granular lymphocytes expressing killer cell inhibitory receptors and lack of self HLA class I molecules [19].

Based on these observations, the KIR repertoire of patients with solid tumors or lymphomas who received an autologous transplant was analyzed and compared with the patients' HLA class I molecules. And indeed, those patients with a KIR repertoire for which they had no inhibitory HLA class I molecules had a significantly lower risk of relapse than patients who expressed the inhibitory HLA ligands [20]. In addition, the number of KIR-HLA mismatches further influenced the risk of relapse, and patients with two mismatches had a lower risk of relapse than patients with one mismatch. In this setting, the pronounced expansion of NK cells as often seen after autologous transplantation and their lack of inhibition might have contributed to the anti-tumor effect of the NK cells observed in these patients.

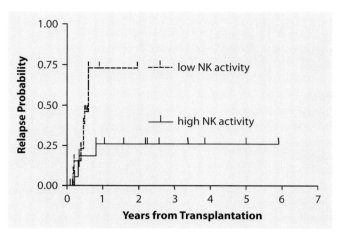

Fig. 3. The NK activity against the standard target cell line K 562 was measured in 46 patients with hematological malignancies at various time points after allogeneic transplantation. Patients with a persistent high NK activity over the observation period had a lower risk of relapse whereas patients with a persistent low NK activity had a high risk of relapse.

The Role of KIR-Mismatched Natural Killer Cells in Allogeneic Stem Cell Transplantion for Leukemia

Impressive clinical effects of alloreactive NK cells have been reported especially in the context of haploidentical transplantation in adults with acute myeloid leukemia [21] as well as in children with acute myeloid and lymphoblastic leukemia [22]. Patients who received a graft from a haploidentical KIR-mismatched donor (NK-alloreactive donor) had a significantly lower risk of relapse. In the HLA-matched allogeneic transplantation situation, the influence of KIR mismatch on relapse is less clear [23].

More recently, a decreased incidence of relapse and improved disease-free survival for patients with acute leukemia has been described in inhibitory KIR-ligand-mismatched transplantations from unrelated umbilical cord blood [24]. However, there are a number of factors that might interfere with the cytotoxic activity of NK cells in this setting, such as graft-versus-host disease and others [25].

In addition, there are a number of other factors that influence the NK cell function post-transplant, such as the number of surface HLA class I molecules on the blasts [16], the KIR repertoire of the reconstituting NK cells and the functional activity of the NK cells. Serial measurements of the NK activity against the standard target cell line K 562 in 46 patients with leukemia for up to 3 years post-allogeneic transplant have further documented the importance of the functional status of the NK cells (own unpublished data). While patients with a persistent low NK activity had a higher risk of relapse, patients with a high spontaneous NK activity during the first year after transplant had a lower risk of relapse (fig. 3).

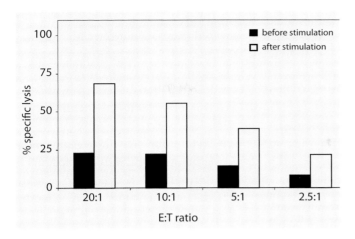

Fig. 4. NK activity against K 562 cells of G-CSF-mobilized CD3/19-depleted mononuclear cells from 7 haploidentical donors before and after overnight incubation with IL-15 (10 ng/ml) at various effector-to-target (E:T) ratios.

Clinical Application of Alloreactive Natural Killer Cells

Hematological Malignancies

It is foreseeable that alloreactive NK cells will play a major role in the KIR mismatch setting after haploidentical transplantation in the treatment of patients with leukemia. The possibility to better identify KIR mismatch donors [26] and further research will hopefully result in the selection of the 'best' mismatched donor in the future. In this setting, it has been demonstrated in mouse models that alloreactive NK cells not only have an anti-leukemic effect but also facilitate engraftment by the elimination of residual host hematopoiesis [27], thus allowing the use of reduced intensity conditioning (RIC) regimens in allogeneic and especially in haploidentical transplantation [28, 29]. In addition, recent advances in T cell depletion technologies from mobilized peripheral stem cells allow the co-infusion of large numbers of NK cells [30]. This technology in combination with RIC regimens is associated with a much lower transplant-related mortality (TRM) than seen with previous methods [28]. In addition, T cell-depleted and NK cell-enriched grafts can be further activated ex vivo prior to infusion with cytokines. An important cytokine for NK cell activation is IL-15. This cytokine appears to be more efficient than IL-2 in expanding the NK cell compartment due to its effects on promotion of survival and protection of NK cells from activation-induced cell death [31]. Overnight incubation of T cell-depleted mobilized grafts from haploidentical donors led to an increase of their cytotoxicity (fig. 4), and the infusion of these IL-15-activated NK cells was well tolerated in 5 patients so far [32]. In the presence of suitable monoclonal antibodies, such as anti-CD19 or anti-CD20, the ADCC of NK cells overrides the KIR-mediated inhibition, and the concurrent treatment of patients with such antibodies post-transplant should further increase the anti-leukemic activity of NK cells [33].

In another setting, purified alloreactive haploidentical NK cells were given several days after a myeloablative conditioning regimen and transplantation with purified CD34+ stem cells from the same haploidentical donor [34]. This approach resulted in a long-term remission in a patient who relapsed after a standard myeloablative allogeneic transplantation and presented with refractory leukemia at the time of haploidentical second transplantation. Based on this observation, clinical studies using this approach have been initiated.

Most of the clinical data obtained so far have been collected in the transplant setting with full sustained engraftment of donor hematopoiesis. Another approach for the exploitation of the anti-tumor effect of alloreactive NK cells is in a non-transplant setting [35]. With this therapy, patients receive a moderate chemotherapy to induce homeostatic lymphocyte proliferation after infusion of alloreactive IL-2-activated NK cells from an allogeneic KIR-mismatched donor. Additional low-dose IL-2 is administered to the patients to induce and maintain in vivo proliferation of donor NK cells. And indeed, transient proliferation of donor NK cells for several weeks has been observed in the patients and some impressive tumor responses have been reported. However, this approach does not result in a long-term engraftment of donor hematopoiesis and further long-term follow-up studies are needed.

Solid Tumors

The concept of alloreactive NK cells might also apply for the treatment of solid metastasized tumors. It has been shown that KIR-ligand-mismatched alloreactive NK cells effectively lyse primary solid tumors obtained from different cancers [36] as well as tumor cell lines established from melanoma or renal cell carcinoma [37]. In addition, some pediatric tumors, such as neuroblastoma, express low or only low amounts of HLA class I molecules on their surface and are therefore susceptible target cells for NK cells [38]. Tumor cell lines obtained from rhabdomyosarcoma and Ewing sarcoma show a variable susceptibility to NK cell-mediated lysis (own unpublished observations). Based on this concept, clinical protocols using the RIC approach and haploidentical transplantation of CD3/19-depleted and NK cell-enriched stem cell grafts have been initiated in patients with advanced and refractory pediatric malignant solid tumors including neuroblastoma, rhabdomyosarcoma and Ewing sarcoma [39]. Up to date (February 2008), 18 patients have been included in this protocol. The engraftment was rapid in 17 patients with a median of 10 days to reach $>1 \times 10^9$/l leukocytes and 8 days to independence of platelet substitution (own unpublished results). One patient rejected and was successfully regrafted with a second haploidentical graft. In figure 5, the Kaplan-Meier estimate for the event-free survival (EFS) of these 18 patients is shown. The sole cause of death was disease progression and none of the patients died from transplant-related toxicity.

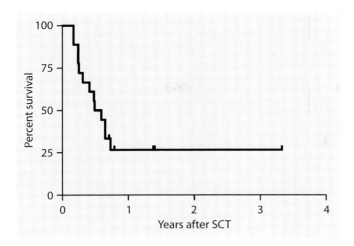

Fig. 5. Kaplan-Meier estimate of the event-free survival of 18 patients with various advanced metastasized tumors (neuroblastoma 10, Ewing sarcoma 5, rhabdomyosarcoma 2, synovial sarcoma 1) after haploidentical transplantation; SCT = stem cell transplantation.

Conclusions and Further Directions

New insights into the biology of NK cells have attracted significant interest of researchers and clinicians to exploit this lymphocyte subpopulation for the treatment of patients with malignancies. In the autologous setting, ex vivo induced NK cells have been used with some clinical responses. More convincing evidence exists in the allogeneic transplant setting where alloreactive NK cells have been shown to exert an anti-leukemic effect especially after KIR-ligand-mismatched haploidentical transplantation. Increasing insights into the biology of NK cells, such as into their ontogeny, the development of the KIR repertoire especially after transplantation, the cross-talk of NK cells with other cells of the immune system and the interaction of their multiple surface receptors with tumor cells, will enable to more effectively harness this cell population in cancer treatment. Mouse models such as the recently described humanized mouse system will be crucial to elucidate how NK cells can be directed in vivo to exert more efficient anti-tumor responses [40, 41] and will allow the translation of these results into clinical protocols. The further development of methods for T cell depletion retaining the bulk of NK cells and other effector cells [42] and of methods for large-scale clinical isolation of NK cells and their ex vivo activation with various cytokines and subsequent reinfusion will further lead to a broader clinical use of this lymphocyte subset. Based on the current observations, further prospective clinical trials using adoptive therapy with NK cells are warranted.

However, more insights into the biological role of NK cells will be needed before their potential anti-tumor properties can be exploited to the full extent.

Disclosure of Conflict of Interests

The authors state that they have no conflict of interests.

References

1 Lang P, Pfeiffer M, Handgretinger R, Schumm M, Demirdelen B, Stanojevic S, Klingebiel T, Kohl U, Kuci S, Niethammer D: Clinical scale isolation of T cell-depleted CD56+ donor lymphocytes in children. Bone Marrow Transplant 2002;29:497–502.

2 Iyengar R, Handgretinger R, Babarin-Dorner A, Leimig T, Otto M, Geiger TL, Holladay MS, Houston J, Leung W: Purification of human natural killer cells using a clinical-scale immunomagnetic method. Cytotherapy 2003;5:479–484.

3 Boyton RJ, Altmann DM: Natural killer cells, killer immunoglobulin-like receptors and human leucocyte antigen class I in disease. Clin Exp Immunol 2007;149:1–8.

4 Moretta L, Bottino C, Pende D, Vitale M, Mingari MC, Moretta A: Different checkpoints in human NK-cell activation. Trends Immunol 2004;25:670–676.

5 Bottino C, Moretta L, Pende D, Vitale M, Moretta A: Learning how to discriminate between friends and enemies, a lesson from natural killer cells. Mol Immunol 2004;41:569–575.

6 Braud VM, Allan DS, O'Callaghan CA, Soderstrom K, D'Andrea A, Ogg GS, Lazetic S, Young NT, Bell JI, Phillips JH, Lanier LL, McMichael AJ: HLA-E binds to natural killer cell receptors CD94/NKG2A, B and C. Nature 1998;391:795–799.

7 Ruggeri L, Mancusi A, Burchielli E, Aversa F, Martelli MF, Velardi A: Natural killer cell alloreactivity in allogeneic hematopoietic transplantation. Curr Opin Oncol 2007;19:142–147.

8 Trinchieri G: Biology of natural killer cells. Adv Immunol 1989;47:187–376.

9 Pende D, Rivera P, Marcenaro S, Chang CC, Biassoni R, Conte R, Kubin M, Cosman D, Ferrone S, Moretta L, Moretta A: Major histocompatibility complex class I-related chain A and UL16-binding protein expression on tumor cell lines of different histotypes: analysis of tumor susceptibility to NKG2D-dependent natural killer cell cytotoxicity. Cancer Res 2002;62:6178–6186.

10 Cerwenka A, Lanier LL: NKG2D ligands: unconventional MHC class I-like molecules exploited by viruses and cancer. Tissue Antigens 2003;61:335–343.

11 Pende D, Bottino C, Castriconi R, Cantoni C, Marcenaro S, Rivera P, Spaggiari GM, Dondero A, Carnemolla B, Reymond N, Mingari MC, Lopez M, Moretta L, Moretta A: PVR (CD155) and Nectin-2 (CD112) as ligands of the human DNAM-1 (CD226) activating receptor: involvement in tumor cell lysis. Mol Immunol 2005;42:463–469.

12 Sivori S, Carlomagno S, Moretta L, Moretta A: Comparison of different CpG oligodeoxynucleotide classes for their capability to stimulate human NK cells. Eur J Immunol 2006;36:961–967.

13 Zamai L, Ponti C, Mirandola P, Gobbi G, Papa S, Galeotti L, Cocco L, Vitale M: NK cells and cancer. J Immunol 2007;178:4011–4016.

14 Imai K, Matsuyama S, Miyake S, Suga K, Nakachi K: Natural cytotoxic activity of peripheral-blood lymphocytes and cancer incidence: an 11-year follow-up study of a general population. Lancet 2000;356:1795–1799.

15 Rosenberg SA, Lotze MT, Yang JC, Topalian SL, Chang AE, Schwartzentruber DJ, Aebersold P, Leitman S, Linehan WM, Seipp CA: Prospective randomized trial of high-dose interleukin-2 alone or in conjunction with lymphokine-activated killer cells for the treatment of patients with advanced cancer. J Natl Cancer Inst 1993;85:622–632.

16 Pfeiffer M, Schumm M, Feuchtinger T, Dietz K, Handgretinger R, Lang P: Intensity of HLA class I expression and KIR-mismatch determine NK-cell mediated lysis of leukaemic blasts from children with acute lymphatic leukaemia. Br J Haematol 2007;138:97–100.

17 Handgretinger R, Lang P, Schumm M, Pfeiffer M, Gottschling S, Demirdelen B, Bader P, Kuci S, Klingebiel T, Niethammer D: Immunological aspects of haploidentical stem cell transplantation in children. Ann N Y Acad Sci 2001;938:340–357.

18 Grau R, Lang KS, Wernet D, Lang P, Niethammer D, Pusch CM, Handgretinger R: Cytotoxic activity of natural killer cells lacking killer-inhibitory receptors for self-HLA class I molecules against autologous hematopoietic stem cells in healthy individuals. Exp Mol Pathol 2004;76:90–98.

19 Handgretinger R, Geiselhart A, Moris A, Grau R, Teuffel O, Bethge W, Kanz L, Fisch P: Pure red-cell aplasia associated with clonal expansion of granular lymphocytes expressing killer-cell inhibitory receptors. N Engl J Med 1999;340:278–284.

20 Leung W, Handgretinger R, Iyengar R, Turner V, Holladay MS, Hale GA: Inhibitory KIR-HLA receptor-ligand mismatch in autologous haematopoietic stem cell transplantation for solid tumour and lymphoma. Br J Cancer 2007;97:539–542.

21 Ruggeri L, Mancusi A, Capanni M, Urbani E, Carotti A, Aloisi T, Stern M, Pende D, Perruccio K, Burchielli E, Topini F, Bianchi E, Aversa F, Martelli MF, Velardi A: Donor natural killer cell allorecognition of missing self in haploidentical hematopoietic transplantation for acute myeloid leukemia: challenging its predictive value. Blood 2007;110:433–440.

22 Leung W, Iyengar R, Turner V, Lang P, Bader P, Conn P, Niethammer D, Handgretinger R: Determinants of antileukemia effects of allogeneic NK cells. J Immunol 2004;172:644–650.

23 Farag SS, Bacigalupo A, Eapen M, Hurley C, Dupont B, Caligiuri MA, Boudreau C, Nelson G, Oudshoorn M, van Rood J, Velardi A, Maiers M, Setterholm M, Confer D, Posch PE, Anasetti C, Kamani N, Miller JS, Weisdorf D, Davies SM: The effect of KIR ligand incompatibility on the outcome of unrelated donor transplantation: a report from the center for international blood and marrow transplant research, the European blood and marrow transplant registry, and the Dutch registry. Biol Blood Marrow Transplant 2006;12:876–884.

24 Willemze R, Arrais-Rodriguez C, Lapobin M, Ionescu I, Boudjedir K, Sanz G, Michel G, Socie G, Rio B, Garcia J, Koegler L, Lecchi L, Loseau P, Gluckman E, Rocha V: Inhibitory KIR-ligand mismatching is associated with decreased incidence of relapse and improved disease-free survival after unrelated cord blood stem cell transplantation for patients with acute leukemia. Bone Marrow Transplant 2008;41(suppl 1):S1(abstr).

25 Lowe EJ, Turner V, Handgretinger R, Horwitz EM, Benaim E, Hale GA, Woodard P, Leung W: T-cell alloreactivity dominates natural killer cell alloreactivity in minimally T-cell-depleted HLA-non-identical paediatric bone marrow transplantation. Br J Haematol 2003;123:323–326.

26 Leung W, Iyengar R, Triplett B, Turner V, Behm FG, Holladay MS, Houston J, Handgretinger R: Comparison of killer Ig-like receptor genotyping and phenotyping for selection of allogeneic blood stem cell donors. J Immunol 2005;174:6540–6545.

27 Ruggeri L, Capanni M, Urbani E, Perruccio K, Shlomchik WD, Tosti A, Posati S, Rogaia D, Frassoni F, Aversa F, Martelli MF, Velardi A: Effectiveness of donor natural killer cell alloreactivity in mismatched hematopoietic transplants. Science 2002;295:2097–2100.

28 Handgretinger R, Chen X, Pfeiffer M, Mueller I, Feuchtinger T, Hale GA, Lang P: Feasibility and outcome of reduced-intensity conditioning in haploidentical transplantation. Ann N Y Acad Sci 2007;1106:279–289.

29 Bethge WA, Faul C, Bornhauser M, Stuhler G, Beelen DW, Lang P, Stelljes M, Vogel W, Hagele M, Handgretinger R, Kanz L: Haploidentical allogeneic hematopoietic cell transplantation in adults using CD3/CD19 depletion and reduced intensity conditioning: an update. Blood Cells Mol Dis 2008;40:13–19.

30 Barfield RC, Otto M, Houston J, Holladay M, Geiger T, Martin J, Leimig T, Gordon P, Chen X, Handgretinger R: A one-step large-scale method for T- and B-cell depletion of mobilized PBSC for allogeneic transplantation. Cytotherapy 2004;6:1–6.

31 Rodella L, Zamai L, Rezzani R, Artico M, Peri G, Falconi M, Facchini A, Pelusi G, Vitale M: Interleukin 2 and interleukin 15 differentially predispose natural killer cells to apoptosis mediated by endothelial and tumour cells. Br J Haematol 2001;115:442–450.

32 Pfeiffer M, Lang P, Schumm M, Mueller I, Feuchtinger T, Handgretinger R: IL-15 activated CD3/19 depleted grafts for haploidentical transplantation in children: strongly increased NK activity in vitro and excellent tolerability in vivo. Bone Marrow Transplant 2008;41(suppl 1):S51(abstr).

33 Lang P, Barbin K, Feuchtinger T, Greil J, Peipp M, Zunino SJ, Pfeiffer M, Handgretinger R, Niethammer D, Fey GH: Chimeric CD19 antibody mediates cytotoxic activity against leukemic blasts with effector cells from pediatric patients who received T-cell-depleted allografts. Blood 2004;103:3982–3985.

34 Triplett B, Handgretinger R, Pui CH, Leung W: KIR-incompatible hematopoietic-cell transplantation for poor prognosis infant acute lymphoblastic leukemia. Blood 2006;107:1238–1239.

35 Miller JS, Soignier Y, Panoskaltsis-Mortari A, McNearney SA, Yun GH, Fautsch SK, McKenna D, Le C, Defor TE, Burns LJ, Orchard PJ, Blazar BR, Wagner JE, Slungaard A, Weisdorf DJ, Okazaki IJ, McGlave PB: Successful adoptive transfer and in vivo expansion of human haploidentical NK cells in patients with cancer. Blood 2005;105:3051–3057.

36 Re F, Staudacher C, Zamai L, Vecchio V, Bregni M: Killer cell Ig-like receptors ligand-mismatched, alloreactive natural killer cells lyse primary solid tumors. Cancer 2006;107:640–648.

37 Igarashi T, Wynberg J, Srinivasan R, Becknell B, McCoy JP Jr, Takahashi Y, Suffredini DA, Linehan WM, Caligiuri MA, Childs RW: Enhanced cytotoxicity of allogeneic NK cells with killer immunoglobulin-like receptor ligand incompatibility against melanoma and renal cell carcinoma cells. Blood 2004;104:170–177.

38 Prigione I, Corrias MV, Airoldi I, Raffaghello L, Morandi F, Bocca P, Cocco C, Ferrone S, Pistoia V: Immunogenicity of human neuroblastoma. Ann N Y Acad Sci 2004;1028:69–80.

39 Lang P, Pfeiffer M, Muller I, Schumm M, Ebinger M, Koscielniak E, Feuchtinger T, Foll J, Martin D, Handgretinger R: Haploidentical stem cell transplantation in patients with pediatric solid tumors: preliminary results of a pilot study and analysis of graft versus tumor effects. Klin Padiatr 2006;218:321–326.

40 Shultz LD, Lyons BL, Burzenski LM, Gott B, Chen X, Chaleff S, Kotb M, Gillies SD, King M, Mangada J, Greiner DL, Handgretinger R: Human lymphoid and myeloid cell development in NOD/LtSz-scid IL2R gamma null mice engrafted with mobilized human hemopoietic stem cells. J Immunol 2005;174:6477–6489.

41 Traggiai E, Chicha L, Mazzucchelli L, Bronz L, Piffaretti JC, Lanzavecchia A, Manz MG: Development of a human adaptive immune system in cord blood cell-transplanted mice. Science 2004;304:104–107.

42 Chaleff S, Otto M, Barfield RC, Leimig T, Iyengar R, Martin J, Holiday M, Houston J, Geiger T, Huppert V, Handgretinger R: A large-scale method for the selective depletion of alphabeta T lymphocytes from PBSC for allogeneic transplantation. Cytotherapy 2007;9:746–754.

Prof. Dr. med. Rupert Handgretinger
Abteilung I, Universitätskinderklinik
Eberhard-Karls-Universität Tübingen
Hoppe-Seyler-Str. 1, 72076 Tübingen, Germany
Tel. +49 7071 2984744, Fax 294713
E-Mail Rupert.Handgretinger@med.uni-tuebingen.de

Scharf RE (ed): Progress and Challenges in Transfusion Medicine, Hemostasis and Hemotherapy.
Freiburg i.Br., Karger, 2008, pp 363–372

Current and Future Use of Dendritic Cells for Tolerance Induction

Holger Hackstein

Institute for Clinical Immunology and Transfusion Medicine, University Hospital Giessen and Marburg,
Giessen, Germany

Key Words

Dendritic cells · Tolerance · Organ rejection · Autoimmunity · Immunoregulation · Transplantation

Summary

Dendritic cells (DCs) are in the focus of interest as regulators of immune responses because it is now clear that DCs can be manipulated in the laboratory and in vivo to promote their tolerogenicity. DCs can promote T cell anergy, T cell hyporesponsiveness and T cell deletion. Recent evidence has indicated that DCs can promote the differentiation and expansion of both naturally occurring CD4+ CD25+ and adaptive type 1 regulatory T cells. The purpose of this review is to summarize current insights and strategies to promote the tolerogenic potential of these professional antigen-presenting cells with a focus on pharmacologically modulated DCs. This knowledge may provide the basis for the development of novel clinical concepts for the therapy of transplant rejection, graft-versus-host disease and autoimmunity.

©2008 S. Karger GmbH, Freiburg i.Br.

Introduction

In the 1980's and 90's interest in dentritic cells (DCs) was focused primarily on their unsurpassed immunostimulatory activity, leading to the definition that DCs represent 'Nature's adjuvant' [1]. This definition still has to be considered as true since DCs represent the most potent immunostimulatory professional antigen-presenting cells (APC) and are unique with respect to their capability to stimulate the proliferation of naive T effector cells [2]. However, within the recent years it has become evident that DCs play a dualistic role in the regulation of immune responses. DCs initiate adaptive immunity by the activation of naive lymphocytes and they represent powerful stimulators of natural killer cells, the crucial cellular instigators of the innate

Table 1. Key features of tolerogenic dendritic cells

Low production of bioactive IL-12p70 and TNF-α
Production of IL-10 or indoleamine 2,3-dioxygenase
Low expression of MHC class II and costimulatory molecules (i.e. immature DCs)
High ratio of MHC class II, costimulatory molecule expression versus low IL-12p70 and TNF-α
Ability to migrate to regional lymph nodes
Maturation resistance after interaction with danger signals

immune system. However, in addition to their immunostimulatory capacities, DCs induce central and peripheral tolerance by mechanisms that include T cell deletion, T cell anergy and induction of regulatory lymphocytes [3–8]. DCs are extremely well equipped for their dual role in immunostimulation and immunoregulation: They are unrivalled in their ability to capture macromolecules via macropinocytosis and mannose receptor-mediated endocytosis into major histocompatibility complex (MHC) class II-rich intracellular compartments [9]. Following antigen (Ag) uptake and activation, DCs migrate from the periphery to secondary lymphoid tissues, redistribute MHC-Ag complexes to the cell surface and up-regulate surface expression of costimulatory (CD80, CD86) and other molecules that promote DC survival and DC-T cell clustering (CD40, receptor activator of NF-κB (RANK), CD54, CD58) [10]. The process of maturation includes also the production of high amounts of the pro-inflammatory cytokines interleukin (IL)-12 and tumor necrosis factor (TNF)-α, converting DC into very powerful T cell-priming APC. Alternatively, an increasing number of publications have described the immunoregulatory capacity of immature and semi-mature DCs [11, 12]. Immature DCs induce T cell anergy and are characterized by low surface expression of MHC class II/costimulatory molecules and the pro-inflammatory cytokines IL-12 and TNF-α [3, 10, 13]. In contrast, so-called semi-mature or alternatively activated DCs are characterized by high expression of MHC class II and costimulatory molecules and low or negative production of IL-12 and TNF-α [11]. Semi-mature DCs have been suggested to have important immunoregulatory functions and to induce CD4+ regulatory T cells in vitro and in vivo [11, 14]. Additionally, immunoregulatory DCs are able to release immunosuppressive molecules such as IL-10 or indoleamine 2,3-dioxygenase (table 1).

Manipulation of Dendritic Cells for Tolerance Induction

Three different types of DCs have been utilized so far to promote tolerance induction: immature DCs, maturation-resistant DCs, and alternatively activated DCs. Based on the finding that modulation of DC maturation is critical for the tolerogen-

Hackstein

ic or immunogenic capacity of DCs, one strategy to promote the tolerogenicity of DCs is the use of drugs that modulate DC maturation. Within the recent years, the strategies to modulate DC maturation have become more sophisticated [12, 15]. In the beginning, many groups simply applied agents that grossly impaired all aspects of DC maturation, i.e. surface expression of MHC class II molecules, costimulatory molecules, chemokine receptors, and cytokine production. This strategy seemed reasonable since Jonuleit et al. have shown that repetitive in vitro stimulation of allogeneic T cells with immature DCs leads to the generation of non-proliferating, IL-10-producing T regulatory (Treg) cells [16]. Proliferation of these T cells could not be restored by exogenous IL-2 and the proliferation of T helper (Th)1 cells was inhibited in a contact-dependent but not Ag-specific manner. In agreement with these findings, Dhodapkara et al. injected immature autologous monocyte-derived DCs pulsed with influenza matrix peptide and keyhole limpet hemocyanin subcutaneously into two human volunteers [17]. They reported an Ag-specific inhibition of CD8+ T cell killing activity and the appearance of peptide-specific IL-10-producing T cells, accompanied by a decrease in interferon (IFN)-γ-producing T cells. However, the strategy to utilize immature DCs for tolerance induction exhibits two important drawbacks that limit clinical application: (i) Immature DCs are impaired with respect to their capacity to migrate into regional lymph nodes, but in order to induce active immunoregulation, interaction with T cells in the lymphoid tissue is required. (ii) Immature DCs are not necessarily maturation resistant; i.e. if the immature phenotype is not stable after in vivo injection it is difficult to control the immunological effects of these DCs after application. These observations have stimulated a more differentiated search for pharmacological agents that are able to promote alternatively activated DCs that can be characterized to exhibit a relative high ratio of MHC class II versus costimulatory molecule expression and relatively low expression of the pro-inflammatory cytokines IL-12p70 and TNF-α. Furthermore, maturation-resistant DCs can be generated in the laboratory after culture of bone marrow cells with low-dose granulocyte/macrophage colony-stimulating factor (GM-CSF) [18].

Experimental Tolerance Induction with Dendritic Cells

Evidence for the tolerogenic ability of DCs, either as immature cells or as alternatively activated cells, comes from studies where DCs have been administered to non-immunosuppressed recipients before transplantation or in models of autoimmune disease. These studies have demonstrated that DCs of donor or recipient origin can prolong heart [18–22], kidney [23] or pancreatic islet allograft survival [24]. Autologous DCs, with or without autoantigen pulsing, inhibit the development of experimental allergic encephalomyelitis (EAE) [25] or type-1 diabetes [26, 27]. A growing number of reports have described the immunoregulatory capacity of alternatively activated DCs.

Menges et al. demonstrated that repetitive injections of DCs matured with TNF-α, but not immature DCs or DCs matured with lipopolysaccharide (LPS) and CD40 ligand (CD40L), induced IL-10-producing peptide-specific T cells in vivo and Ag-specific protection from experimental autoimmune encephalomyelitis [28]. The tolerogenic DCs were characterized as MHC class II[high] and costimulatory molecule[high], but they were weak producers of pro-inflammatory IL-12p70 in comparison to LPS/CD40L-matured DCs. A similar approach was successfully employed by Sato et al. who expanded DCs in the presence of IL-10 and transforming growth factor (TGF)-β and 'matured' these APCs with either LPS or TNF-α [29, 30]. These semi-mature DCs expressed high levels of MHC class II and low levels of costimulatory molecules, and it is conceivable, although it was not directly investigated, that these DCs were low producers of pro-inflammatory cytokines. By using a murine model for graft-versus-host disease (GVHD) and leukemia relapse, it was demonstrated that host-matched semi-mature DCs protected mice in an Ag-specific manner from GVHD lethality and induced the expansion of IL-10-producing CD4+ CD25+ suppressor T cells [29]. Treatment with semi-mature DCs retained the graft-versus-leukemia (GVL) effect in recipients of allogeneic bone marrow and spleen mononuclear cells. However, the underlying mechanism for protection from GVHD without abrogating GVL efficacy remains to be elucidated.

Pharmacological Generation of Tolerogenic Dendritic Cells

Mammalian Target of Rapamycin Inhibitors

Rapamycin is a bacterial macrolide antibiotic with potent immunosuppressive action introduced in recent years as anti-rejection therapy in organ transplantation [31]. Rapamycin, like FK506, binds intracellularly to FK506-binding proteins (FKBP) but, unlike FK506, inhibits the function of the serine/threonine kinase mammalian target of rapamycin (mTOR) [32]. mTOR is a common effector protein shared by many signaling pathways. Inhibition of mTOR results in suppression of cytokine-driven cell proliferation, ribosomal protein synthesis, translation initiation and cell cycle arrest at the G1 phase [32, 33]. In addition to its suppressive effects on lymphocytes, rapamycin suppresses the generation of GM-CSF-expanded human monocyte-derived DCs in vitro and the generation of fms-like tyrosine 3 kinase ligand (Flt3L)-expanded DCs in mice in vivo [34–36]. Moreover, we identified rapamycin as the first clinically relevant substance that inhibits DC Ag uptake in a maturation-independent manner [37]. At low concentrations, rapamycin impairs macropinocytosis and mannose receptor-mediated endocytosis of murine bone marrow-derived DCs and human monocyte-derived DCs. Furthermore, inhibition of DC Ag uptake by rapamycin was confirmed with human monocyte-derived DCs and after in vivo administration of the drug [37, 38]. Recently, it has been demonstrated that rapamycin-conditioned DCs are maturation resistant and can enrich for naturally occurring CD4+ CD25+ Foxp3+ Treg cells but have reduced capacity to expand CD4+ effector T cells [39]. Application of recipient-derived, rapamycin-exposed DCs pulsed with alloantigen significantly prolonged allograft survival in different experimental models [22, 39]. Furthermore, a short course of post-/perioperative tacrolimus or rapamycin prolonged graft survival indefinitely [22, 39]. Given the fact that rapamycin also currently represents the most potent pharmacological agent that promotes the direct expansion CD4+ CD25+ Foxp3+ Treg cells [8], it is conceivable that this agent will be very likely to be included into future clinical trials aiming to promote tolerance induction.

Aspirin, Corticosteroids and Vitamin D3

Two independent studies provided recent evidence that aspirin (the most commonly used analgetic and anti-inflammatory drug) profoundly suppresses the maturation and T cell stimulatory function of human monocyte- [40] and mouse bone marrow-derived DCs [41]. Aspirin-treated DCs failed to induce cell-mediated contact hypersensitivity reactions in vivo [41], indicating that exposure to aspirin is a highly effective and inexpensive approach to manipulation of the immunostimulatory potential of DCs, which may find clinical application. However, with respect to immunostimulatory TNF-α, one study suggested that aspirin-exposed DCs exhibit higher TNF-α production capacity [42]. In contrast to salicylates, corticosteroids not only suppress DC maturation but also potently inhibit DC differentiation both in vitro [43, 44] and in vivo [45]. Corticosteroid-treated human monocyte-derived or mouse bone marrow-derived DCs promote the generation of IL-5- and IL-10-producing T cells while inhibiting IFN-γ secretion and therefore favor Th2/Treg immune responses [46, 47]. Future studies are necessary to determine whether ex vivo treatment of DCs with corticosteroids and subsequent injection facilitate the expansion of Th2/Treg cells in vivo. $1,25(OH)_2D_3$, the biologically active metabolite of vitamin D3, or its analog $1\alpha,25(OH)_2$-16-ene-23-yne-26,27-hexafluoro-19-nor-vitamin D3 (D3-analog) inhibits the maturation of human monocyte-derived DCs [48–50] and mouse bone marrow-derived DCs in vitro [51]. $1,25(OH)_2D_3$- or D3-analog-treated DCs are poor stimulators of allogeneic T cells, show impaired IL-12 but increased IL-10 secretion and exhibit enhanced endocytic activity [48–51]. In vitamin D receptor (VDR) knockout (KO) mice, the inhibitory effects of $1,25(OH)_2D_3$ and the D3-analog on DC maturation and T cell stimulatory function were absent [51]. Interestingly, VDR KO mice show hypertrophy of subcutaneous lymph nodes, as well as increased numbers of mature DC in lymph nodes, suggesting the physiological importance of the $1,25(OH)_2D_3$-VDR loop in DC homeostasis and maturation in vivo [52]. Pretreatment of mice with vitamin D3-exposed donor DCs prolongs skin graft survival [52].

Calcineurin Inhibitors and Mycophenolate Mofetil

The effects of the calcineurin inhibitors cyclosporine A (CsA) and tacrolimus (FK506) have been investigated by many groups with conflicting results. Whereas Lee et al. suggested that CsA interfered with DC maturation via NF-κB inhibition [53], other studies have failed to demonstrate significant effects of CsA on the maturation of monocyte-derived DCs [44] and on epidermal Langerhans cell function [54]. Future studies analyzing the effects of CsA on DC maturation and function in vivo are necessary to clarify this issue. Interestingly, Chen et al. reported that CsA inhibits DC migration through inhibition of CC-chemokine receptor 7 expression [55]. With respect to the calcineurin inhibitor tacrolimus (FK506), two studies have indicated no significant effects on DC maturation [44, 56]. However, since tacrolimus suppresses TNF-α production by DC [44] and DC T cell stimulatory capacity [57, 58], it is reasonable to believe that this substance also targets functional DC maturation, but the precise molecular mechanism remains elusive. Mycophenolate mofetil (MMF) is a reversible inhibitor of inosine monophosphate dehydrogenase (IMPD) that is critical for the de novo synthesis of guanosine and deoxyguanosine molecules necessary for the generation of RNA and DNA [59]. MMF is thought to selectively target the proliferation of B and T cells which depend to a greater extent than other cells on the de novo synthesis of purines [60]. Mehling et al. [61] reported that MMF directly affects DC maturation and impairs their capacity to induce a cell-mediated immune response in vivo. This study indicates a novel role of the enzyme IMPD in DC activation and the findings have been confirmed recently by another group [62].

Sanglifehrin A

Sanglifehrin A (SFA), originally described by Sanglier and Fehr, is produced by the actinomycetes strain *Streptomyces* A92-308110 and belongs to a novel family of immunophilin-binding ligands [63, 64]. Although SFA, like CsA, binds with high affinity to cyclophilin, unlike the latter, SFA does not inhibit the activity of the calcineurin phosphatase [65]. Competitive experiments with a non-immunosuppressive cyclophilin-binding derivative of CsA have suggested that the immunosuppressive activity of SFA is not dependent on cyclophilin binding [65]. In addition, SFA does not bind to FKBP12 and does not inhibit the enzymatic activity of $p70^{s6k}$ kinase, a major downstream target of mTOR [65, 66]. These results suggest that SFA represents a novel class of immunophilin-binding immunosuppressants with a new, yet undefined mode of action. Studies of the immunosuppressive effects of SFA have been focused on T and B lymphocytes. SFA has been reported to exhibit a lower immunosuppressive activity in the mixed leukocyte reaction (MLR) when compared with CsA [63]. We have reported that SFA rapidly blocks bioactive IL-12 production by human DCs. In direct comparison to the related agents CsA and rapamycin, we found that SFA acts uniquely within 1 h to inhibit 80–95% of the IL-12p70 production by DCs [67]. Additionally, Woltman et al. reported that SFA potently inhibits DC Ag uptake receptor expression and DC endocytosis [68]. With respect to the in vivo relevance of these findings, we have found that SFA potently inhibits DC endocytosis in vivo as well as bioactive IL-12p70 production, indicating that SFA targets key DC functions in vitro and in vivo [69].

Conclusions and Future Directions

Experimental and clinical studies indicate the potential of DCs for regulation of allo- and autoimmunity. Pharmacological agents can be used to generate tolerogenic DCs and regulatory T cells in vitro and in vivo. The challenge within the next 10 years lies in the translation of experimental studies into feasible, safe and efficient novel clinical therapies.

Disclosure of Conflict of Interests

The author states that he has no conflict of interests.

Acknowledgements

The author's work is supported by grants from the 'Stiftung Hämotherapie Forschung', Bonn, Germany, the Roche Organ Transplantation Research Foundation, Switzerland, the German Research Foundation (DFG, Sonderforschungsbereich 547-A5), and the Excellence Cluster Cardiopulmonary System (EC-CPS), Giessen.

References

1 Banchereau J, Steinman RM: Dendritic cells and the control of immunity. Nature 1998;392:245–252.
2 Vulink A, Radford KJ, Melief C, Hart DN: Dendritic cells in cancer immunotherapy. Adv Cancer Res 2008;99:363–407.
3 Steinman RM, Hawiger D, Nussenzweig MC: Tolerogenic dendritic cells. Annu Rev Immunol 2003;21:685–711.
4 Hackstein H, Morelli AE, Thomson AW: Designer dendritic cells for tolerance induction: guided not misguided missiles. Trends Immunol 2001;22:437–442.
5 Roncarolo MG, Levings MK, Traversari C: Differentiation of T regulatory cells by immature dendritic cells. J Exp Med 2001;193:F5–9.
6 Raimondi G, Thomson AW: Dendritic cells, tolerance and therapy of organ allograft rejection. Contrib Nephrol 2005;146:105–120.
7 Morelli AE, Thomson AW: Dendritic cells: regulators of alloimmunity and opportunities for tolerance induction. Immunol Rev 2003;196:125–146.
8 Roncarolo MG, Battaglia M: Regulatory T-cell immunotherapy for tolerance to self antigens and alloantigens in humans. Nat Rev Immunol 2007;7:585–598.

9 Sallusto F, Cella M, Danieli C, Lanzavecchia A: Dendritic cells use macropinocytosis and the mannose receptor to concentrate macromolecules in the major histocompatibility complex class II compartment: downregulation by cytokines and bacterial products. J Exp Med 1995;182:389–400.

10 Banchereau J, Briere F, Caux C, Davoust J, Lebecque S, Liu YJ, Pulendran B, Palucka K: Immunobiology of dendritic cells. Annu Rev Immunol 2000;18:767–811.

11 Lutz MB, Schuler G: Immature, semi-mature and fully mature dendritic cells: which signals induce tolerance or immunity? Trends Immunol 2002;23:445–449.

12 Hackstein H, Thomson AW: Dendritic cells: emerging pharmacological targets of immunosuppressive drugs. Nat Rev Immunol 2004;4:24–34.

13 Jonuleit H, Schmitt E, Steinbrink K, Enk AH: Dendritic cells as a tool to induce anergic and regulatory T cells. Trends Immunol 2001;22:394–400.

14 Morelli AE, Thomson AW: Tolerogenic dendritic cells and the quest for transplant tolerance. Nat Rev Immunol 2007;7:610–621.

15 Adler HS, Steinbrink K: Tolerogenic dendritic cells in health and disease: friend and foe! Eur J Dermatol 2007;17:476–491.

16 Jonuleit H, Schmitt E, Schuler G, Knop J, Enk AH: Induction of interleukin 10-producing, nonproliferating CD4(+) T cells with regulatory properties by repetitive stimulation with allogeneic immature human dendritic cells. J Exp Med 2000;192:1213–1222.

17 Dhodapkar MV, Steinman RM, Krasovsky J, Munz C, Bhardwaj N: Antigen-specific inhibition of effector T cell function in humans after injection of immature dendritic cells. J Exp Med 2001;193:233–238.

18 Lutz MB, Suri RM, Niimi M, Ogilvie AL, Kukutsch NA, Rossner S, Schuler G, Austyn JM: Immature dendritic cells generated with low doses of GM-CSF in the absence of IL-4 are maturation resistant and prolong allograft survival in vivo. Eur J Immunol 2000;30:1813–1822.

19. Giannoukakis N, Bonham CA, Qian S, Zhou Z, Peng L, Harnaha J, Li W, Thomson AW, Fung JJ, Robbins PD, Lu L: Prolongation of cardiac allograft survival using dendritic cells treated with NF-κB decoy oligodeoxyribonucleotides. Mol Ther 2000;1:430–477.

20 Min WP, Gorczynski R, Huang XY, Kushida M, Kim P, Obataki M, Lei J, Suri RM, Cattral MS: Dendritic cells genetically engineered to express Fas ligand induce donor-specific hyporesponsiveness and prolong allograft survival. J Immunol 2000;164:161–167.

21 Fu F, Li Y, Qian S, Lu L, Chambers F, Starzl TE, Fung JJ, Thomson AW: Costimulatory molecule-deficient dendritic cell progenitors (MHC class II+, CD-80dim, CD86–) prolong cardiac allograft survival in nonimmunosuppressed recipients. Transplantation 1996;62:659–665.

22 Taner T, Hackstein H, Wang Z, Morelli AE, Thomson AW: Rapamycin-treated, alloantigen-pulsed host dendritic cells induce Ag-specific T cell regulation and prolong graft survival. Am J Transplant 2005;5:228–236.

23 Gorczynski RM, Bransom J, Cattral M, Huang X, Lei J, Xiaorong L, Min WP, Wan Y, Gauldie J: Synergy in induction of increased renal allograft survival after portal vein infusion of dendritic cells transduced to express TGFbeta and IL-10, along with administration of CHO cells expressing the regulatory molecule OX-2. Clin Immunol 2000;95:182–189.

24 O'Rourke RW, Kang SM, Lower JA, Feng S, Ascher NL, Baekkeskov S, Stock PG: A dendritic cell line genetically modified to express CTLA4-Ig as a means to prolong islet allograft survival. Transplantation 2000;69:1440–1446.

25 Huang YM, Yang JS, Xu LY, Link H, Xiao BG: Autoantigen-pulsed dendritic cells induce tolerance to experimental allergic encephalomyelitis (EAE) in Lewis rats. Clin Exp Immunol 2000;122:437–444.

26 Feili-Hariri M, Dong X, Alber SM, Watkins SC, Salter RD, Morel PA: Immunotherapy of NOD mice with bone marrow-derived dendritic cells. Diabetes 1999;48:2300–2308.

27 Shinomiya M, Fazle Akbar SM, Shinomiya H, Onji M: Transfer of dendritic cells (DC) ex vivo stimulated with interferon-gamma (IFN-gamma) downmodulates autoimmune diabetes in non-obese diabetic (NOD) mice. Clin Exp Immunol 1999;117:38–43.

28 Menges M, Rossner S, Voigtlander C, Schindler H, Kukutsch NA, Bogdan C, Erb K, Schuler G, Lutz MB: Repetitive injections of dendritic cells matured with tumor necrosis factor alpha induce antigen-specific protection of mice from autoimmunity. J Exp Med 2002;195:15–21.

29 Sato K, Yamashita N, Baba M, Matsuyama T: Regulatory dendritic cells protect mice from murine acute graft-versus-host disease and leukemia relapse. Immunity 2003;18:367–379.

30 Sato K, Yamashita N, Baba M, Matsuyama T: Modified myeloid dendritic cells act as regulatory dendritic cells to induce anergic and regulatory T cells. Blood 2003;101:3581–3589.

31 Kahan BD, Camardo JS: Rapamycin: clinical results and future opportunities. Transplantation 2001;72:1181–1193.

32 Sehgal SN: Rapamune (RAPA, rapamycin, sirolimus): mechanism of action immunosuppressive effect results from blockade of signal transduction and inhibition of cell cycle progression. Clin Biochem 1998;31:335–340.

33 Raught B, Gingras AC, Sonenberg N: The target of rapamycin (TOR) proteins. Proc Natl Acad Sci U S A 2001;98:7037–7044.

34 Woltmann AM, de Fijter JW, Kamerling SW, van Der Kooij SW, Paul LC, Daha MR, van Kooten C: Rapamycin induces apoptosis in monocyte- and CD34-derived dendritic cells but not in monocytes and macrophages. Blood 2001;98:174–180.

35 Monti P, Mercalli A, Leone E, DiCarlo V, Allavena P, Piemonti L: Rapamycin impairs antigen uptake of human dendritic cells. Transplantation 2003;75:137–145.

36 Hackstein H, Taner T, Zahorchak AF, Morelli AE, Logar AJ, Gessner A, Thomson AW: Rapamycin inhibits IL-4-induced dendritic cell maturation in vitro and dendritic cell mobilization and function in vivo. Blood 2003;101:4457–4463.

37 Hackstein H, Taner T, Logar AJ, Thomson AW: Rapamycin inhibits macropinocytosis and mannose receptor-mediated endocytosis by bone marrow-derived dendritic cells. Blood 2002;100:1084–1087.

38 Monti P, Mercalli A, Leone E, DiCarlo V, Allavena P, Piemonti L: Rapamycin impairs antigen uptake of human dendritic cells. Transplantation 2003;75:137–145.

39 Turnquist HR, Raimondi G, Zahorchak AF, Fischer RT, Wang Z, Thomson AW: Rapamycin-conditioned dendritic cells are poor stimulators of allogeneic CD4+ T cells, but enrich for antigen-specific Foxp3+ T regulatory cells and promote organ transplant tolerance. J Immunol 2007;178:7018–7031.

40 Matasic R, Dietz AB, Vuk-Pavlovic S: Cyclooxygenase-independent inhibition of dendritic cell maturation by aspirin. Immunology 2000;101:53–60.

41 Hackstein H, Morelli AE, Larregina AT, Ganster RW, Papworth GD, Logar AJ, Watkins SC, Falo LD, Thomson AW: Aspirin inhibits in vitro maturation and in vivo immunostimulatory function of murine myeloid dendritic cells. J Immunol 2001;166:7053–7062.

42 Ho LJ, Chang DM, Shiau HY, Chen CH, Hsieh TY, Hsu YL, Wong CS, Lai JH: Aspirin differentially regulates endotoxin-induced IL-12 and TNF-alpha production in human dendritic cells. Scand J Rheumatol 2001;30:346–352.

43 Matasic R, Dietz AB, Vuk-Pavlovic S: Dexamethasone inhibits dendritic cell maturation by redirecting differentiation of a subset of cells. J Leukoc Biol 1999;66:909–914.

44 Woltman AM, de Fijter JW, Kamerling SW, Paul LC, Daha MR, van Kooten C: The effect of calcineurin inhibitors and corticosteroids on the differentiation of human dendritic cells. Eur J Immunol 2000;30:1807–1812.

45 Moser M, De Smedt T, Sornasse T, Tielemans F, Chentoufi AA, Muraille E, Van Mechelen M, Urbain J, Leo O: Glucocorticoids down-regulate dendritic cell function in vitro and in vivo. Eur J Immunol 1995;25:2818–2824.

46 Vieira PL, Kalinski P, Wierenga EA, Kapsenberg ML, de Jong EC: Glucocorticoids inhibit bioactive IL-12p70 production by in vitro-generated human dendritic cells without affecting their T cell stimulatory potential. J Immunol 1998;161:5245–5251.

47 Matyszak MK, Citterio S, Rescigno M, Ricciardi-Castagnoli P: Differential effects of corticosteroids during different stages of dendritic cell maturation. Eur J Immunol 2000;30:1233–1242.

48 Penna G, Adorini L: 1 Alpha,25-dihydroxyvitamin D3 inhibits differentiation, maturation, activation, and survival of dendritic cells leading to impaired alloreactive T cell activation. J Immunol 2000;164:2405–2411.

49 Berer A, Stockl J, Majdic O, Wagner T, Kollars M, Lechner K, Geissler K, Oehler L: 1,25-Dihydroxyvitamin D(3) inhibits dendritic cell differentiation and maturation in vitro. Exp Hematol 2000;28:575–583.

50 Piemonti L, Monti P, Sironi M, Fraticelli P, Leone BE, Dal Cin E, Allavena P, Di Carlo V: Vitamin D3 affects differentiation, maturation, and function of human monocyte-derived dendritic cells. J Immunol 2000;164:4443–4451.

51 Griffin MD, Lutz WH, Phan VA, Bachman LA, McKean DJ, Kumar R: Potent inhibition of dendritic cell differentiation and maturation by vitamin D analogs. Biochem Biophys Res Commun 2000;270:701–708.

52 Griffin MD, Lutz W, Phan VA, Bachman LA, McKean DJ, Kumar R: Dendritic cell modulation by 1alpha,25 dihydroxyvitamin D3 and its analogs: a vitamin D receptor-dependent pathway that promotes a persistent state of immaturity in vitro and in vivo. Proc Natl Acad Sci U S A 2001;98:6800–6805.

53 Lee JI, Ganster RW, Geller DA, Burckart GJ, Thomson AW, Lu L: Cyclosporine A inhibits the expression of costimulatory molecules on in vitro-generated dendritic cells: association with reduced nuclear translocation of nuclear factor kappa B. Transplantation 1999;68:1255–1263.

54 Peguet-Navarro J, Slaats M, Thivolet J: Lack of demonstrable effect of cyclosporin A on human epidermal Langerhans cell function. Arch Dermatol Res 1991;283:198–202.

55 Chen T, Guo J, Yang M, Han C, Zhang M, Chen W, Liu Q, Wang J, Cao X: Cyclosporin A impairs dendritic cell migration by regulating chemokine receptor expression and inhibiting cyclooxygenase-2 expression. Blood 2004;103:413–421.

56 Morelli AE, Antonysamy MA, Takayama T, Hackstein H, Chen Z, Qian S, Zurowski NB, Thomson AW: Microchimerism, donor dendritic cells, and alloimmune reactivity in recipients of Flt3 ligand-mobilized hemopoietic cells: modulation by tacrolimus. J Immunol 2000;165:226–237.

57 Duperrier K, Velten FW, Bohlender J, Demory A, Metharom P, Goerdt S: Immunosuppressive agents mediate reduced allostimulatory properties of myeloid-derived dendritic cells despite induction of divergent molecular phenotypes. Mol Immunol 2005;42:1531–1540.

58 Tiefenthaler M, Hofer S, Ebner S, Ivarsson L, Neyer S, Herold M, Mayer G, Fritsch P, Heufler C: In vitro treatment of dendritic cells with tacrolimus: impaired T-cell activation and IP-10 expression. Nephrol Dial Transplant 2004;19:553–560.

59 Sintchak MD, Fleming MA, Futer O, Raybuck SA, Chambers SP, Caron PR, Murcko MA, Wilson KP: Structure and mechanism of inosine monophosphate dehydrogenase in complex with the immunosuppressant mycophenolic acid. Cell 1996;85:921–930.

60 Suthanthiran M, Morris RE, Strom TB: Immunosuppressants: cellular and molecular mechanisms of action. Am J Kidney Dis 1996;28:159–172.

61 Mehling A, Grabbe S, Voskort M, Schwarz T, Luger TA, Beissert S: Mycophenolate mofetil impairs the maturation and function of murine dendritic cells. J Immunol 2000;165:2374–2381.

62 Colic M, Stojic-Vukanic Z, Pavlovic B, Jandric D, Stefanoska I: Mycophenolate mofetil inhibits differentiation, maturation and allostimulatory function of human monocyte-derived dendritic cells. Clin Exp Immunol 2003;134:63–69.

63 Sanglier JJ, Quesniaux V, Fehr T, Hofmann H, Mahnke M, Memmert K, Schuler W, Zenke G, Gschwind L, Maurer C, Schilling W: Sanglifehrins A, B, C and D, novel cyclophilin-binding compounds isolated from Streptomyces sp. A92–308110. I. Taxonomy, fermentation, isolation and biological activity. J Antibiot 1999;52:466–473.

64 Fehr T, Kallen J, Oberer L, Sanglier JJ, Schilling W: Sanglifehrins A, B, C and D, novel cyclophilin-binding compounds isolated from Streptomyces sp. A92–308110. II. Structure elucidation, stereochemistry and physico-chemical properties. J Antibiot 1999;52:474–479.

65 Zenke G, Strittmatter U, Fuchs S, Quesniaux VF, Brinkmann V, Schuler W, Zurini M, Enz A, Billich A, Sanglier JJ, Fehr T: Sanglifehrin a, a novel cyclophilin-binding compound showing immunosuppressive activity with a new mechanism of action. J Immunol 2001;166:7165–7171.

66 Zhang LH, Liu JO: Sanglifehrin a, a novel cyclophilin-binding immunosuppressant, inhibits IL-2-dependent T cell proliferation at the G1 phase of the cell cycle. J Immunol 2001;166:5611–5618.

67 Steinschulte C, Taner T, Thomson AW, Bein G, Hackstein H: Cutting edge: Sanglifehrin a, a novel cyclophilin-binding immunosuppressant blocks bioactive IL-12 production by human dendritic cells. J Immunol 2003;171:542–546.

68 Woltman AM, Schlagwein N, van der Koij SW, van Kooten C: The novel cyclophilin-binding drug Sanglifehrin A specifically affects antigen uptake receptor expression and endocytic capacity of human dendritic cells. J Immunol 2004;172:6482–6489.

69 Hackstein H, Steinschulte C, Fiedel S, Eisele A, Rathke V, Stadlbauer T, Taner T, Thomson AW, Tillmanns H, Bein G, Holschermann H: Sanglifehrin a blocks key dendritic cell functions in vivo and promotes long-term allograft survival together with low-dose CsA. Am J Transplant 2007;7:789–798.

Prof. Dr. med. Holger Hackstein
Institut für Klinische Immunologie und Transfusionsmedizin
Universitätsklinikum Gießen und Marburg
Langhansstr. 7, 35385 Gießen, Germany
Tel. + 49 641 9941-511, Fax -519
E-Mail Holger.Hackstein@immunologie.med.uni-giessen.de

Scharf RE (ed): Progress and Challenges in Transfusion Medicine, Hemostasis and Hemotherapy.
Freiburg i.Br., Karger, 2008, pp 373–384

Adult and Embryonic Stem Cell Therapy

Jürgen Hescheler · Dimitry Spitkovsky

Institute of Neurophysiology, University of Cologne, Germany

Key Words

Embryonic stem cells · Adult stem cells · Differentiation · Cardiomyocytes · Transplantation · Cell therapy

Summary

A number of experiments have demonstrated that embryonic stem (ES) cells can give rise to a broad range of specialized cells, such as cardiomyocytes, insulin-producing beta cells, dopaminergic neurons and others. These differentiated cells exhibit phenotypic properties comparable to corresponding adult cells and can be successfully used for the replacement of damaged cells in several disease animal models including heart infarction, diabetes and Parkinson's disease. The results of the animal transplantation studies have raised hopes that ES cell-based tissue regeneration could become a useful treatment for a number of diseases also in humans. Very promising results have also been obtained with adult stem cells as stromal mesenchymal stem cells (MSC). MSC can be found in almost any adult organ. They can be isolated and expanded to up to hundreds of millions of cells within several weeks. New cell isolation methods may significantly enrich for the desired cell population and reduce the time required for cell expansion. MSC have got both unique biological properties and a unique molecular signature, which clearly discriminate them from other stem cell types. They express a strong immunomodulatory activity and secrete a variety of growth factors and cytokines. MSC can be differentiated into cells of several lineages. The therapeutic potential of MSC has been evaluated and they were found to be useful in both preclinical animal models and clinical trials. Future and ongoing study will further define the utility of both ES cells and adult stem cells for regenerative medicine. ©2008 S. Karger GmbH, Freiburg i.Br.

Introduction

Cell transplantation is an emerging innovative approach for the treatment of many degenerative diseases like myocardial infarction, Parkinson's disease, diabetes, and others. These disorders result in irreversible cell and tissue loss due to cell/tissue injury or ageing. Cell therapy aims to reverse, improve or prevent further decline in the normal functions of the tissues or organs. The practical utility of cell transplantation significantly depends upon defining an optimal stem cell source, the stem cell availability, and the logistics to preserve and expand the cells into sufficient cell doses under clinically compliant conditions as well as the ability to differentiate the stem cells into the desired cell population if required. Embryonic stem (ES) cells appear to be an important source of cells with multiple differentiation potential. After differentiation, ES cells may acquire properties of adult specialized cells. Therefore, ES cell applications for regenerative medicine are very promising. For example, human ES cell-derived cardiomyocytes should be considered as candidate donor cells in heart diseases. However, many critical obstacles associated with ES cell derivation, propagation, differentiation and application still need to be solved.

Adult mesenchymal stem cells (MSC) represent an ethically acceptable source of cells for therapeutic applications. MSC can be isolated from different tissues and organs. These cells have a broad differentiation potential in vitro and can be differentiated into bone, cartilage, adipocytes, neuronal cells and some other cell types. It is possible to expand MSC from a single donor to up to hundreds of millions of cells, the amount suitable for many downstream applications. Potential therapeutic applications of the MSC have been demonstrated in small animal models, and the cells are able to support bone reconstitution, chondrogenesis as well as neuronal differentiation in injured brain tissue. Moreover, a great potential of the cells for cell therapy applications has been revealed in preclinical models of myocardial infarction. In this review, we evaluate the progress made towards both ES and MSC cell replacement therapy as well as examples of the clinical MSC applications and the obstacles to be resolved in the near future.

Embryonic and Other Stem Cells Types as Candidates for Therapeutic Applications

ES cells can be isolated as a result of in vitro manipulation of the undifferentiated inner cell mass of blastocysts. ES cells are pluripotent, and they can develop into all cell types of the embryo proper derived from endoderm, ectoderm and mesoderm. The first isolation of mouse ES cells has been reported in the early 1980's by two independent groups [1, 2]. Mouse ES cells and associated technologies utilizing transgenic, knock-out and knock-in animals have been essential in defining the functions of many disease-associated genes. It took another 16 years until human ES cells were first isolated and described [3, 4]. Similarly to their mouse counterparts, human ES cells have the capacity to differentiate into a wide range of specialized cells, including those of particular interest for regenerative medicine like cardiomyocytes, neurons, beta cells of the pancreas, hepatic cells and others [5]. So far, multiple human ES cell isolates have been generated and 78 of them have been listed in the Registry of the National Institute of Health. Utilization of human embryos for ES cell generation meets ethical controversies that hinder the application of these cells. Alternative techniques producing cells with ES-like properties while not associated with the destruction of a viable human blastocyst have been proposed. Somatic cell nuclear transfer has been used for the generation of pluripotent stem cells. The method requires that the nucleus isolated from an adult somatic cell be injected into an enucleated oocyte. The factors contained within the oocyte cytoplasm have been shown to be sufficient to reprogram the genetic material of somatic cells to the pluripotent cell stage. However, only recently the feasibility to generate human pluripotent cells via nuclear transfer has finally been demonstrated [6]. Similarly to ES cell technology, the nuclear transfer method remains highly controversial due to ethical concerns regarding the utilization of human oocytes. Cell fusion methodology represents another way of human adult somatic cell reprogramming. Thereby, human ES cells have been fused with human fibroblasts to generate pluripotent cells [7]. However, the generated cell hybrids are polyploid and therefore abnormal. Extracts of ES cells have been shown to be able to reprogram somatic cells into stem cells with multilineage potential, as reviewed in [8]. Pluripotent cells can be generated as a result of cell explantation when lineage-restricted cells become multipotent in a process of cell adaptation during in vitro cultivation. It has been demonstrated that cells isolated from mouse testis could acquire ES-like cell properties [9]. Lastly, the possibility to create pluripotent ES-like cells from human somatic cells via direct reprogramming after viral-mediated transduction of defined transcription factors has been demonstrated. Human fibroblasts have been reprogrammed into induced pluripotent (iPS) cells after simultaneous transduction of Oct3/4, Sox2, c-Myc, and Klf4 genes [10]. This technology has opened a broad avenue to create ES-like cells from somatic cells of genetically diverse donors, including donors with genetic diseases. In this way, the ethical controversy associated with ES cells seems to be resolved because iPS cell generation does not require the destruction of either human blastocysts or human oocytes. However, while iPS cells have a broad differentiation potential similar to ES cells, they may still differ significantly from ES cells. It is worth mentioning that even ES cell lines isolated by a single experimental group via a similar technique have very diverse differentiation propensities. More than 100-fold differences in lineage-specific gene expression have been found after in vitro differentiation of 17 human ES cell lines [11]. Additionally, the iPS cells may be less safe than ES cells due to the possibility of insertion mutagenesis after genomic integration of the viral genome, as well as potential reactivation of the integrated genes in iPS cell derivatives, leading to their malignant transformation. Therefore, research implementing both human ES cells and human iPS cells must continue.

Tissue compatibility still remains one of the major obstacles while considering stem cell transplantation in regenerative medicine. Differentiated cells derived from ES cells have been suggested to be less susceptible to immune attack. Furthermore, MSC have been shown to be negative modulators of immune responses (see below). The interaction of transplanted stem cells or their derivatives with the host immune system still requires intense research and better understanding. Generation of patient-specific stem cell lines could prevent the imminent immune attack associated with transplantation of cells obtained from donors with partial HLA mismatch. However, the costs and logistics in the generation of customized patient-specific stem cell lines may not be affordable. Homozygous ES cells would help to solve this problem as only limited numbers of haplotypes would be sufficient to cover the majority of potential recipients within a given population. Computer simulation analysis has shown that, for the Japanese population, it is possible to find at least one donor with complete matching at the three HLA loci if homozygous ES cell lines could be established from 55 randomly selected donated oocytes [12]. Four HLA-homozygous parthenogenetic stem cell lines with properties resembling those of ES cell have been created from both HLA-homozygous and HLA-heterozygous activated unfertilized oocytes. Humans with homozygous HLA haplotypes are very rare among the total population. Additionally, the proposed protocol for HLA-homozygous stem cell line generation minimizes the use of animal-derived components and therefore is more applicable to potential clinical utilization of the cells [13]. Furthermore, this approach is considered to be less ethically controversial as compared to ES cell generation from viable blastocysts, due to the fact that mammalian embryos generated in the process of parthenogenesis are not able to complete the normal development.

Derivation of stromal cells from bone marrow or MSC has been first described in the 1960's. The cells were derived via plastic adhesion and have been shown to manifest a fibroblast-like morphology and differentiation potential into osteogenic, chondrogenic and adipogenic lineages in vitro and osteogenic potential in vivo [14]. Later, bone marrow-derived stromal cells were isolated in numerous labs, although different cell generation, expansion and characterization methods were used. Additionally, other types of fetal and adult stem cells were isolated from human tissues. Some of them have been found to be highly proliferative and pluripotent and therefore very interesting for potential therapeutic applications. Among the most interesting stem cell candidates, there are bone marrow-derived multipotent adult progenitor cells (MAPC) [15], adult multilineage-inducible cells from bone marrow (MIAMI) [16], tissue-committed stem cells (TCSC) [17], unrestricted somatic stem cells (USSC) from umbilical cord blood [18] and amniotic fluid-derived stem cells (AFS) [19]. MIAMI cells can proliferate extensively without evidence of senescence, and they have been shown to express two ES cell markers, Oct-4 and Rex-1. MAPC can differentiate into adipocytes, chondroblasts, and osteoblasts, neuronal and pancreatic cells. USSC may also differentiate into a variety of tissues in vitro and in vivo. USSC constitutively produce multiple cytokines and growth factors as stem cell factor (SCF), leukemia inhibitory factor (LIF), transforming growth factor (TGF)-1β, macrophage colony-stimulating factor (M-CSF), granulocyte/macrophage CSF (GM-CSF), vascular endothelial growth factor (VEGF), interleukin (IL)-1β, IL-6, IL-8, IL-11, IL-12, IL-15, stromal cell-derived factor (SDF)-1a, and hepatocyte growth factor (HGF). Production of both SCF and LIF is significantly higher in USSC as compared to bone marrow-derived MSC, with 278-fold compared to 5-fold [20]. AFS cells express some ES cell markers such as Oct-4 and SSEA-4, while they do not express other ES markers such as SSEA-3, TRA-1–60 and TRA-1–81; they also express adult stem cell markers as CD73, CD90 and CD105. AFS may proliferate extensively over 250 population doublings (PD) without any feeder support, and they can differentiate into cells of all three embryonic germ layers representing mesoderm, ectoderm and endoderm. MAPC, USSC and AFS appear to be less versatile as ES cells, but they are clearly very proliferative, more immature and have broader differentiation potential as compared to MSC. Nevertheless, reproducibility of the generation and differentiation of these stem cells has to be confirmed by other groups. Future clinical relevance of these cells depends on the ability to reproduce isolation of these cells and to confirm a truly pluripotent status of the cells and their ability to differentiate into specific mature cell types relevant for clinical indications.

Safety of Embryonic and Adult Stem Cell Transplantation

Potential applications of ES cells and other stem cells in clinical settings require thorough investigation of their safety. One of the major concerns in cell therapy is based on potential tumor growth after stem cell application. Not only ES cells but also their differentiated derivatives are able to produce tumors. Human ES cells differentiated into the neural lineage are still fully capable of tumor generation even after intense in vitro selection [21], whereby the teratoma formation assay is a standard test to demonstrate the pluripotency of ES cells. In a highly sensitive biosafety model of stem cell-derived grafts, it has been demonstrated that as few as 2 ES cells could form tumors after injection into immunodeficient mice [22].

MSC may play an important role in both tumor development and growth. Donor cells may contribute to tumorigenesis after bone marrow transplantation either as a source of tumor cells [23] or as modulator cells affecting tumor growth [24]. Interactions between normal cells and tumor components may be very complex and so far different outcomes have been reported. The immunosuppressive effects of MSC may favor tumor growth in allogeneic settings [25]. MSC can significantly inhibit the proliferation of tumor cells of various hematopoietic origin in vitro while in vivo they rather accelerate tumor growth. Therefore, clinical use of MSC in patients with malignant diseases must be handled with extreme caution [26]. Contradictory to tumor-promoting properties in Kaposi's sarcoma, MSC may also manifest antitumorigenic effects. The in vivo antitumor effects of MSC correlate with their ability to home to sites of tumorigenesis, to make direct cell-cell contacts and inhibit the target cell Akt protein kinase activity [27]. Concern has been raised that MSC may acquire significant genetic alterations as a result of long-term in vitro cultivation, leading to a malignant phenotype before or after cell transplantation. Few examples of malignant transformation of MSC have been demonstrated in rodent systems. Human cells, which are generally less susceptible to malignant transformation than rodent cells, nevertheless also can be transformed, and fat tissue-derived MSC have been shown to undergo spontaneous transformation after long-term (4–5 months) in vitro cell cultivation [28]. MSC can be transformed in culture after transduction with the telomerase gene (hTERT) but require additional genetic alterations leading to Ki-ras oncogene activation [29]. Nevertheless, another study has demonstrated that bone marrow-derived MSC from 10 donors can be safely expanded in vitro for up to 44 weeks, and the cells maintain a normal karyotype and are not susceptible to malignant transformation [30]. These concerns must be addressed in future studies.

Mechanisms of Stem Cell Action and Animal Models

Due to the significant tumorigenic potential of non-differentiated ES cells, it is considered that only fully differentiated and highly purified ES cell derivatives must be used for the purposes of regenerative medicine. So far, ES cell derivatives have been shown in several human disease-relevant animal models. Transplantation of ES cell-derived progenitors could improve behavior in rats with Parkinson's disease, and the grafted cells differentiated into dopamine-producing neurons [31]. In a mouse model, it has been demonstrated that cardiomyocytes derived from mouse ES cells but not other stem cells could restore the contractile function in the infarcted myocardium [32]. Human ES cell-derived cardiomyocytes have also been shown to be able to functionally engraft in a porcine model [33]. Retinal epithelium derived from human ES cells could preserve visual function in rats with macular dystrophy [34].

Paracrine signaling has been shown to be an important mediator of MSC biological activity in several experimental models. MSC promoted proliferation and migration of both endothelial and smooth muscle cells in a dose-dependent manner in vitro. Several important cytokines and growth factors have been expressed by MSC and the expression can be further increased under hypoxic conditions [35]. Immunomodulatory activity is one of the most striking properties of MSC [36]. The immunomodulatory activity of MSC has been shown to be mediated via different mechanisms. MSC inhibit T cell responses both in vitro and in vivo. MSC may also inhibit the differentiation and function of dendritic cells. It has been found that the enzyme indoleamine 2,3-dioxygenase (IDO) is expressed in human MSC. IDO activity results in tryptophan depletion and in inhibition of T cell responses, while tryptophan readdition can restore T cell function [37].

The feasibility of MSC transplantation in diverse animal models has been a matter of intense studies by numerous research groups. Some in vivo studies have suggested that MSC can differentiate not only into cells of 3 lineages (adipocytes, chondrocytes and osteoblasts) but also into cells of other lineages at the sites where they have been transplanted. However, the broad differentiation abilities of MSC have been questioned, and in several publications it has been demonstrated that MSC do not undergo real trans-differentiation but rather fuse with specialized differentiated cells in the tissue where the MSC have been transplanted. For example, it has been shown that the bone marrow-derived cells fuse spontaneously with neurons and cardiomyocytes, resulting in the formation of multinucleated cells [38]. Nevertheless, there is also evidence supporting fusion-independent trans-differentiation mechanisms, as cord blood cells can repopulate the NOD-SCID mouse liver and become mature hepatocytes without any detectable cell fusions between donor and host cells. This suggests that human cord blood cells can truly trans-differentiate into hepatocytes in vivo [39].

Fat tissue-derived MSC have been shown to restore expression of dystrophin when transplanted into a mouse model of Duchenne muscular dystrophy (mdx mice) [40]. MSC may also acquire a neuronal fate and differentiate into neurons and astrocytes after implantation into neonatal mouse brain [41]. MSC implanted into the brain can restore sensorimotor function after experimental stroke in rats [42]. A very promising approach is a potential application of MSC as genetically modified vehicles to travel and to deliver defined genes into the site of injury. MSC with the human insulin transgene can reverse streptozotocin-induced diabetes in mice [43]. Overexpression of Akt1 in bone marrow-derived MSC has been proposed as a strategy to accelerate cardiac repair after myocardial infarction. MSC with exogenously introduced Akt1 have been shown to regenerate 80–90% of the lost myocardial volume in a rat model of heart infarction [44].

Application of Mesenchymal Stem Cells in Clinical Settings

So far, MSC have been tested in multiple clinical indications. MSC have been applied to support hematopoietic stem cell engraftment, as immune modulators and in regenerative medicine. The studies have shown the feasibility and safety of MSC applications. Allogeneic MSC have been used to repair skeletal defects in 6 children with osteogenesis imperfecta (OI) caused by a genetic defect in the collagen type I gene. In 5 of 6 patients, engraftment of MSC at one or more sites has been found and sustained acceleration of patient bone mineral density and growth velocity during a 6-month follow-up period has been reported [45]. This phase I trial demonstrates the feasibility of MSC intravenous infusion. In another safety study, MSC were isolated from 15 patients with hematologic malignancies in complete remission phase. The cells were expanded for 28 to 49 days. In separate patient groups, the cell escalating dose was evaluated as 1, 10 and 50 million cells [46]. Furthermore, the safety of the application of culture-expanded MSC has been demonstrated in 28 breast cancer patients receiving MSC infusion simultaneously with autologous peripheral blood progenitor cell transplantation after chemotherapy. The patients received intravenously between 1 and 2.2 million cells [47m associated toxicity has also been shown [48]. Furthermore, the same groups have presented evidence of the feasibility and safety of allogeneic MSC infusion in patients with Hurler syndrome and metachromatic leukodystrophy (MLD) who previously underwent bone marrow transplantation. In several patients, significant improvements in nerve conduction velocities were detected and bone mineral density was maintained or slightly improved in all patients [49]. Gastrointestinal tract Crohn's disease has been successfully treated with autologous MSC derived from adipose tissue. 9 fistulas in 4 patients were inoculated with MSC. The treatment demonstrated no adverse effects, while 6 out of 8 fistulas (75%) were closed as demonstrated in a 2-month follow-up [50]. A first case of treatment with MSC of terminal-stage graft-versus-host disease (GVHD) has been reported [51]. The patient had improved significantly due to the immunosuppressive effect invoked by the MSC. Further clinical benefits of MSC transplantation for steroid-resistant GVHD have been confirmed with 9 additional patients who had received allogeneic MSC. The survival rates were significantly better than in the control group [52]. Preliminary evaluations of MSC efficacy have also been performed in patients with amyotrophic lateral sclerosis (ALS). The cells were transplanted into the spinal cord of the patients. The safety of the procedure has been demonstrated, and no major adverse events have been reported. However, it is too early to conclude on any clinical benefits [53]. Moreover, the safety and efficacy of autologous MSC intravenous infusion have been evaluated in 5 patients with ischemic stroke. The clinical outcome of the MSC group was improved significantly during the 12-month follow-up compared with the control group, while no adverse cell-associated effects were detected [54].

There are 2 studies describing the application of autologous MSC in acute myocardial infarction patients. The left ventricular ejection fraction was improved and the area of perfusion defects was significantly reduced in a group of 34 patients after intra-coronary injections of MSC as compared to the control group in the 3-month follow-up period [55]. A second study has demonstrated a significant improvement of the myocardial contractility of significantly affected heart segments in 5 out of 11 patients who had received a mixture of MSC and endothelial precursor cells (EPC) [56]. Unfortunately, the MSC isolation procedure that was utilized in both studies does not allow production of sufficiently pure MSC populations.

There are several ongoing clinical trials with autologous bone marrow-derived MSC application to patients with chronic myocardial ischemia or with heart failure. Osiris Therapeutics (*www.osiris.com*) has initiated a phase I clinical study with fully mismatched allogeneic MSC transplantation into myocardial infarction patients. The MSC were isolated and expanded from healthy volunteers. The results of these studies have not been published so far.

Conclusions and Future Directions

Transplantation of either specialized cells derived from ES cells or adult stem cells opens a new avenue in treatment of diseases where current therapy reaches its limits.

The cell therapy holds great promise and may be potentially used for multiple clinical indications. However, in spite of the fact that the ES cells apparently have got the broadest differentiation potential, exploitation and practical therapeutic application of human ES cells is still at the beginning and several key issues must be resolved before the initiation of any clinical trial. Important milestones still have to be achieved including ethical issues, overcoming the high tumorigenic potential of non-differentiated ES cells, and the ability to generate clinically relevant amounts of cells of the desired lineages under clinically compliant conditions. Another issue is the immune compatibility of ES lines suitable for therapy with the immune system of potential donors. There are rapidly emerging new tools to generate pluripotent cells with ES cell-like properties. However, newly derived pluripotent stem cells would still require more basic research and advanced knowledge based on the ongoing ES cell research. Contrary to ES cells, MSC have got a relatively narrow proven differentiation potential. Nevertheless, due to a range of unique biological properties, the clinical applications of MSC can be very broad. MSC represent an easily accessible and highly proliferative cell source. MSC can be used to support hematopoietic stem cell engraftment, to inhibit non-desirable immune responses during organ transplantation, to reduce manifestation of GVHD, and to treat different autoimmune conditions. They can be applied systemically or locally, can be used as vehicles to deliver specific genes to target tissue and can be utilized as building blocks for artificially engineered tissues. It has to be defined in a comprehensive study whether MSC isolated from different tissues may have any particular therapeutic advantages. Significant and not resolved challenges represent a possibility to apply MSC in either autologous or allogeneic settings. Ongoing and emerging basic research and clinical trials will finally define the potential value of MSC for therapeutic applications.

Disclosure of Conflict of Interests

The authors state that they have no conflict of interests.

Acknowledgements

Funding for this work has been provided in part by Cryo Save Group, Mechelen, Belgium, and by EC grant LSHB-CT-2006-037261.

References

1 Evans MJ, Kaufman MH: Establishment in culture of pluripotential cells from mouse embryos. Nature 1981;292:154–156.
2 Martin GR: Isolation of a pluripotent cell line from early mouse embryos cultured in medium conditioned by teratocarcinoma stem cells. Proc Natl Acad Sci U S A 1981;78:7634–7638.
3 Thomson JA, Itskovitz-Eldor J, Shapiro SS, Waknitz MA, Swiergiel JJ, Marshall VS, Jones JM: Embryonic stem cell lines derived from human blastocysts. Science 1998;282:1145–1147.
4 Shamblott MJ, Axelman J, Wang S, Bugg EM, Littlefield JW, Donovan PJ, Blumenthal PD, Huggins GR, Gearhart JD: Derivation of pluripotent stem cells from cultured human primordial germ cells. Proc Natl Acad Sci U S A 1998;95:13726–13731.

5   Trounson A: The production and directed differentiation of human embryonic stem cells. Endocr Rev 2006;27:208–219.

6   French AJ, Adams CA, Anderson LS, Kitchen JR, Hughes MR, Wood SH: Development of human cloned blastocysts following somatic cell nuclear transfer with adult fibroblasts. Stem Cells 2008;26:485–493.

7   Cowan CA, Atienza J, Melton DA, Eggan K: Nuclear reprogramming of somatic cells after fusion with human embryonic stem cells. Science 2005;309:1369–1373.

8   Collas P, Taranger CK: Epigenetic reprogramming of nuclei using cell extracts. Stem Cell Rev 2006;2:309–317.

9   Kanatsu-Shinohara M, Inoue K, Lee J, Yoshimoto M, Ogonuki N, Miki H, Baba S, Kato T, Kazuki Y, Toyokuni S, Toyoshima M, Niwa O, Oshimura M, Heike T, Nakahata T, Ishino F, Ogura A, Shinohara T: Generation of pluripotent stem cells from neonatal mouse testis. Cell 2004;119:1001–1012.

10 Takahashi K, Tanabe K, Ohnuki M, Narita M, Ichisaka T, Tomoda K, Yamanaka S: Induction of pluripotent stem cells from adult human fibroblasts by defined factors. Cell 2007;131:861–872.

11 Osafune K, Caron L, Borowiak M, Martinez RJ, Fitz-Gerald CS, Sato Y, Cowan CA, Chien KR, Melton DA: Marked differences in differentiation propensity among human embryonic stem cell lines. Nat Biotechnol 2008;26:313–315.

12 Nakajima F, Tokunaga K, Nakatsuji N: Human leukocyte antigen matching estimations in a hypothetical bank of human embryonic stem cell lines in the Japanese population for use in cell transplantation therapy. Stem Cells 2007;25:983–985.

13 Revazova ES, Turovets NA, Kochetkova OD, Agapova LS, Sebastian JL, Pryzhkova MV, Smolnikova V, Kuzmichev LN, Janus JD: HLA homozygous stem cell lines derived from human parthenogenetic blastocysts. Cloning Stem Cells 2008;10:11–24.

14 Friedenstein AJ, Piatetzky S, II, Petrakova KV: Osteogenesis in transplants of bone marrow cells. J Embryol Exp Morphol 1966;16:381–390.

15 Schwartz RE, Reyes M, Koodie L, Jiang Y, Blackstad M, Lund T, Lenvik T, Johnson S, Hu WS, Verfaillie CM: Multipotent adult progenitor cells from bone marrow differentiate into functional hepatocyte-like cells. J Clin Invest 2002;109:1291–1302.

16 D'Ippolito G, Diabira S, Howard GA, Menei P, Roos BA, Schiller PC: Marrow-isolated adult multilineage inducible (MIAMI) cells, a unique population of postnatal young and old human cells with extensive expansion and differentiation potential. J Cell Sci 2004;117:2971–2981.

17 Ratajczak MZ, Kucia M, Reca R, Majka M, Janowska-Wieczorek A, Ratajczak J: Stem cell plasticity revisited: CXCR4-positive cells expressing mRNA for early muscle, liver and neural cells 'hide out' in the bone marrow. Leukemia 2004;18:29–40.

18 Kogler G, Sensken S, Airey JA, Trapp T, Muschen M, Feldhahn N, Liedtke S, Sorg RV, Fischer J, Rosenbaum C, Greschat S, Knipper A, Bender J, Degistirici O, Gao J, Caplan AI, Colletti EJ, Almeida-Porada G, Muller HW, Zanjani E, Wernet P: A new human somatic stem cell from placental cord blood with intrinsic pluripotent differentiation potential. J Exp Med 2004;200:123–135.

19 De Coppi P, Bartsch G, Jr., Siddiqui MM, Xu T, Santos CC, Perin L, Mostoslavsky G, Serre AC, Snyder EY, Yoo JJ, Furth ME, Soker S, Atala A: Isolation of amniotic stem cell lines with potential for therapy. Nat Biotechnol 2007;25:100–106.

20 Kogler G, Radke TF, Lefort A, Sensken S, Fischer J, Sorg RV, Wernet P: Cytokine production and hematopoiesis supporting activity of cord blood-derived unrestricted somatic stem cells. Exp Hematol 2005;33:573–583.

21 Roy NS, Cleren C, Singh SK, Yang L, Beal MF, Goldman SA: Functional engraftment of human ES cell-derived dopaminergic neurons enriched by coculture with telomerase-immortalized midbrain astrocytes. Nat Med 2006;12:1259–1268.

22 Lawrenz B, Schiller H, Willbold E, Ruediger M, Muhs A, Esser S: Highly sensitive biosafety model for stem-cell-derived grafts. Cytotherapy 2004;6:212–222.

23 Barozzi P, Luppi M, Facchetti F, Mecucci C, Alu M, Sarid R, Rasini V, Ravazzini L, Rossi E, Festa S, Crescenzi B, Wolf DG, Schulz TF, Torelli G: Posttransplant Kaposi sarcoma originates from the seeding of donor-derived progenitors. Nat Med 2003;9:554–561.

24 Peters BA, Diaz LA, Polyak K, Meszler L, Romans K, Guinan EC, Antin JH, Myerson D, Hamilton SR, Vogelstein B, Kinzler KW, Lengauer C: Contribution of bone marrow-derived endothelial cells to human tumor vasculature. Nat Med 2005;11:261–262.

25 Djouad F, Plence P, Bony C, Tropel P, Apparailly F, Sany J, Noel D, Jorgensen C: Immunosuppressive effect of mesenchymal stem cells favors tumor growth in allogeneic animals. Blood 2003;102:3837–3844.

26 Ramasamy R, Lam EW, Soeiro I, Tisato V, Bonnet D, Dazzi F: Mesenchymal stem cells inhibit proliferation and apoptosis of tumor cells: impact on in vivo tumor growth. Leukemia 2007;21:304–310.

27 Khakoo AY, Pati S, Anderson SA, Reid W, Elshal MF, Rovira, II, Nguyen AT, Malide D, Combs CA, Hall G, Zhang J, Raffeld M, Rogers TB, Stetler-Stevenson W, Frank JA, Reitz M, Finkel T: Human mesenchymal stem cells exert potent antitumorigenic effects in a model of Kaposi's sarcoma. J Exp Med 2006;203:1235–1247.

28 Rubio D, Garcia-Castro J, Martin MC, de la Fuente R, Cigudosa JC, Lloyd AC, Bernad A: Spontaneous human adult stem cell transformation. Cancer Res 2005;65:3035–3039.

29 Serakinci N, Guldberg P, Burns JS, Abdallah B, Schrodder H, Jensen T, Kassem M: Adult human mesenchymal stem cell as a target for neoplastic transformation. Oncogene 2004;23:5095–5098.

30 Bernardo ME, Zaffaroni N, Novara F, Cometa AM, Avanzini MA, Moretta A, Montagna D, Maccario R, Villa R, Daidone MG, Zuffardi O, Locatelli F: Human bone marrow derived mesenchymal stem cells do not undergo transformation after long-term in vitro culture and do not exhibit telomere maintenance mechanisms. Cancer Res 2007;67:9142–9149.

31 Ben-Hur T, Idelson M, Khaner H, Pera M, Reinhartz E, Itzik A, Reubinoff BE: Transplantation of human embryonic stem cell-derived neural progenitors improves behavioral deficit in Parkinsonian rats. Stem Cells 2004;22:1246–1255.

32 Kolossov E, Bostani T, Roell W, Breitbach M, Pillekamp F, Nygren JM, Sasse P, Rubenchik O, Fries JW, Wenzel D, Geisen C, Xia Y, Lu Z, Duan Y, Kettenhofen R, Jovinge S, Bloch W, Bohlen H, Welz A, Hescheler J, Jacobsen SE, Fleischmann BK: Engraftment of engineered ES cell-derived cardiomyocytes but not BM cells restores contractile function to the infarcted myocardium. J Exp Med 2006;203:2315–2327.

33 Kehat I, Khimovich L, Caspi O, Gepstein A, Shofti R, Arbel G, Huber I, Satin J, Itskovitz-Eldor J, Gepstein L: Electromechanical integration of cardiomyocytes derived from human embryonic stem cells. Nat Biotechnol 2004;22:1282–1289.

34 Lund RD, Wang S, Klimanskaya I, Holmes T, Ramos-Kelsey R, Lu B, Girman S, Bischoff N, Sauve Y, Lanza R: Human embryonic stem cell-derived cells rescue visual function in dystrophic RCS rats. Cloning Stem Cells 2006;8:189–199.

35 Kinnaird T, Stabile E, Burnett MS, Lee CW, Barr S, Fuchs S, Epstein SE: Marrow-derived stromal cells express genes encoding a broad spectrum of arteriogenic cytokines and promote in vitro and in vivo arteriogenesis through paracrine mechanisms. Circ Res 2004;94:678–685.

36 Le Blanc K: Immunomodulatory effects of fetal and adult mesenchymal stem cells. Cytotherapy 2003;5:485–489.

37 Meisel R, Zibert A, Laryea M, Gobel U, Daubener W, Dilloo D: Human bone marrow stromal cells inhibit allogeneic T-cell responses by indoleamine 2.3-dioxygenase-mediated tryptophan degradation. Blood 2004;103:4619–4621.

38 Alvarez-Dolado M, Pardal R, Garcia-Verdugo JM, Fike JR, Lee HO, Pfeffer K, Lois C, Morrison SJ, Alvarez-Buylla A: Fusion of bone-marrow-derived cells with Purkinje neurons, cardiomyocytes and hepatocytes. Nature 2003;425:968–973.

39 Newsome PN, Johannessen I, Boyle S, Dalakas E, McAulay KA, Samuel K, Rae F, Forrester L, Turner ML, Hayes PC, Harrison DJ, Bickmore WA, Plevris JN: Human cord blood-derived cells can differentiate into hepatocytes in the mouse liver with no evidence of cellular fusion. Gastroenterology 2003;124:1891–1900.

40 Rodriguez AM, Pisani D, Dechesne CA, Turc-Carel C, Kurzenne JY, Wdziekonski B, Villageois A, Bagnis C, Breittmayer JP, Groux H, Ailhaud G, Dani C: Transplantation of a multipotent cell population from human adipose tissue induces dystrophin expression in the immunocompetent mdx mouse. J Exp Med 2005;201:1397–1405.

41 Kopen GC, Prockop DJ, Phinney DG: Marrow stromal cells migrate throughout forebrain and cerebellum, and they differentiate into astrocytes after injection into neonatal mouse brains. Proc Natl Acad Sci U S A 1999;96:10711–10716.

42 Zhao LR, Duan WM, Reyes M, Keene CD, Verfaillie CM, Low WC: Human bone marrow stem cells exhibit neural phenotypes and ameliorate neurological deficits after grafting into the ischemic brain of rats. Exp Neurol 2002;174:11–20.

43 Xu J, Lu Y, Ding F, Zhan X, Zhu M, Wang Z: Reversal of diabetes in mice by intrahepatic injection of bone-derived GFP-murine mesenchymal stem cells infected with the recombinant retrovirus-carrying human insulin gene. World J Surg 2007;31:1872–1882.

44 Mangi AA, Noiseux N, Kong D, He H, Rezvani M, Ingwall JS, Dzau VJ: Mesenchymal stem cells modified with Akt prevent remodeling and restore performance of infarcted hearts. Nat Med 2003;9:1195–1201.

45 Horwitz EM, Gordon PL, Koo WK, Marx JC, Neel MD, McNall RY, Muul L, Hofmann T: Isolated allogeneic bone marrow-derived mesenchymal cells engraft and stimulate growth in children with osteogenesis imperfecta: Implications for cell therapy of bone. Proc Natl Acad Sci U S A 2002;99:8932–8937.

46 Lazarus HM, Haynesworth SE, Gerson SL, Rosenthal NS, Caplan AI: Ex vivo expansion and subsequent infusion of human bone marrow-derived stromal progenitor cells (mesenchymal progenitor cells): implications for therapeutic use. Bone Marrow Transplant 1995;16:557–564.

Adult and Embryonic Stem Cell Therapy

47 Koc ON, Gerson SL, Cooper BW, Dyhouse SM, Haynesworth SE, Caplan AI, Lazarus HM: Rapid hematopoietic recovery after coinfusion of autologous-blood stem cells and culture-expanded marrow mesenchymal stem cells in advanced breast cancer patients receiving high-dose chemotherapy. J Clin Oncol 2000;18:307–316.

48 Lazarus HM, Koc ON, Devine SM, Curtin P, Maziarz RT, Holland HK, Shpall EJ, McCarthy P, Atkinson K, Cooper BW, Gerson SL, Laughlin MJ, Loberiza FR, Jr., Moseley AB, Bacigalupo A: Cotransplantation of HLA-identical sibling culture-expanded mesenchymal stem cells and hematopoietic stem cells in hematologic malignancy patients. Biol Blood Marrow Transplant 2005;11:389–398.

49 Koc ON, Day J, Nieder M, Gerson SL, Lazarus HM, Krivit W: Allogeneic mesenchymal stem cell infusion for treatment of metachromatic leukodystrophy (MLD) and Hurler syndrome (MPS-IH). Bone Marrow Transplant 2002;30:215–222.

50 Garcia-Olmo D, Garcia-Arranz M, Herreros D, Pascual I, Peiro C, Rodriguez-Montes JA: A phase I clinical trial of the treatment of Crohn's fistula by adipose mesenchymal stem cell transplantation. Dis Colon Rectum 2005;48:1416–1423.

51 Le Blanc K, Rasmusson I, Sundberg B, Gotherstrom C, Hassan M, Uzunel M, Ringden O: Treatment of severe acute graft-versus-host disease with third party haploidentical mesenchymal stem cells. Lancet 2004;363:1439–1441.

52 Ringden O, Uzunel M, Rasmusson I, Remberger M, Sundberg B, Lonnies H, Marschall HU, Dlugosz A, Szakos A, Hassan Z, Omazic B, Aschan J, Barkholt L, Le Blanc K: Mesenchymal stem cells for treatment of therapy-resistant graft-versus-host disease. Transplantation 2006;81:1390–1397.

53 Mazzini L, Fagioli F, Boccaletti R, Mareschi K, Oliveri G, Olivieri C, Pastore I, Marasso R, Madon E: Stem cell therapy in amyotrophic lateral sclerosis: a methodological approach in humans. Amyotroph Lateral Scler Other Motor Neuron Disord 2003;4:158–161.

54 Bang OY, Lee JS, Lee PH, Lee G: Autologous mesenchymal stem cell transplantation in stroke patients. Ann Neurol 2005;57:874–882.

55 Chen SL, Fang WW, Qian J, Ye F, Liu YH, Shan SJ, Zhang JJ, Lin S, Liao LM, Zhao RC: Improvement of cardiac function after transplantation of autologous bone marrow mesenchymal stem cells in patients with acute myocardial infarction. Chin Med J 2004;117:1443–1448.

56 Katritsis DG, Sotiropoulou PA, Karvouni E, Karabinos I, Korovesis S, Perez SA, Voridis EM, Papamichail M: Transcoronary transplantation of autologous mesenchymal stem cells and endothelial progenitors into infarcted human myocardium. Catheter Cardiovasc Interv 2005;65:321–329.

Prof. Dr. med. Jürgen Hescheler
Institut für Neurophysiologie
Universität zu Köln
50931 Köln, Germany
Tel. +49 221 478 6960, Fax -3834
E-Mail J.Hescheler@uni-koeln.de

Scharf RE (ed): Progress and Challenges in Transfusion Medicine, Hemostasis and Hemotherapy.
Freiburg i.Br., Karger, 2008, pp 385–393

Hemostasis-Navigated Hemotherapy: Diagnosis, Management, and Monitoring of Patients with Active Bleeding

Bernd Pötzsch[a]   Rüdiger E. Scharf[b]

[a]Institute for Experimental Hematology and Transfusion Medicine, University Medical Center Bonn,
[b]Department of Experimental and Clinical Hemostasis, Hemotherapy, and Transfusion Medicine,
 Heinrich Heine University Medical Center, Düsseldorf, Germany

Key Words

Bleeding · Diagnostic work-up · Hemostasis monitoring · Point-of-care testing · Coagulation factor concentrates · Platelet concentrates · Transfusion triggers

Summary

The management of patients with active bleeding starts with a comprehensive clinical assessment in order to determine the likelihood of a hemorrhagic disorder. Typically, such disorders are characterized by spontaneous bleeding, excessive or prolonged bleeding following trauma or minor surgery, and/or bleeding from more than one site. If there is evidence for an acquired or inherited hemorrhagic disorder, laboratory investigation should be performed to identify and classify the underlying defect. Starting with some very basic hemostasis assays, such as the screening tests, several specific coagulation and platelet assays will be performed. After the diagnosis is established, specific hemotherapy is initiated. Treatment strategies involve pharmacological enhancement of hemostasis using desmopressin (DDAVP), administration of antifibrinolytics, substitution of coagulation factors and/or platelets and the use of recombinant activated factor VII, all of which require close monitoring by appropriate laboratory assessment. In patients with a life-threatening hemorrhage or bleeding at a critical site who need urgent therapeutic interventions, point-of-care testing is useful to guide hemotherapy.   ©2008 S. Karger GmbH, Freiburg i.Br.

Introduction

The diagnostic and therapeutic approach to the patient with bleeding depends on the severity and type of bleeding and on the clinical situation. Patients showing a life-threatening hemorrhage or bleeding at a critical site require urgent therapeutic interventions. Laboratory evaluations are initially restricted to those hemostasis assays that are rapidly performable and that are useful to guide the therapeutic interventions.

In relation to the given situation, a thorough clinical assessment should precede the laboratory investigation. A hemostasis screen is performed if clinical evaluation determines the likelihood that a bleeding disorder is present. Based on the results of the hemostasis screen, specific tests will be performed to identify the underlying hemostasis defect. A normal hemostasis screen should be interpreted in light of the pretest diagnosis, since not all abnormalities can be ruled out by the screening assays routinely used. When the level of clinical suspicion is high, a staged protocol of laboratory investigations is appropriate, independent of the results of the screen.

What Is Hemostasis-Navigated Hemotherapy?

Appropriate treatment of bleeding patients with hemostatic defects requires both, adequate transfusion of hemotherapeutics and close monitoring of their effects. While improvement or restoration of oxygen transport upon replacement therapy with packed red blood cells (RBC) is easy to examine in anemic patients, administration of fresh frozen plasma (FFP), prothrombin complex and/or other coagulation factor concentrates, and platelet units requires close monitoring. This is best achieved by longitudinal laboratory assessment within short-term intervals. Screening tests of coagulation, i.e. prothrombin time (PT), activated partial thromboplastine time (APTT), fibrinogen, and as measure of fibrin cross-linking such as D-dimer/fibrin degradation product should be performed together with platelet counting. In addition, evaluation of platelet responses using the platelet function analyzer (PFA)-100 will provide valuable information to guide hemotherapy and document its effects. Thus, instead of 'empirical' substitution, simply controlled by clinical observation, such as cessation of bleeding, a rational, efficient, and also economic hemotherapy can be achieved, replacing specifically those components that are depleted in the individual patient. This procedural approach has several advantages: (1) It strictly follows the guidelines of modern hemotherapy by administrating cellular or plasma products targeted and adjusted to the individual needs of a given patient ('as much as required, as less as needed'), (2) prevents from overtreatment, (3) indicates therapeutic failure, and (4) allows detection of imminent side-effects or complications, e.g. disseminated intravascular coagulation (DIC) in due time.

Hemostasis-navigated hemotherapy also requires an ongoing synopsis of laboratory and clinical findings. Thus, a comprehensive clinical follow-up is mandatory. The best way to achieve this requirement is that a clinically experienced hemostasis consultant examines the patient at the bedside and discusses clinical and laboratory results along with the therapeutic consequences directly with the physicians primarily responsible.

Component	Critical level	Blood loss, % (range)
Fibrinogen	100 mg/dl	142 (117–169)
Prothrombin	20%	201 (160–244)
Factor V	25%	229 (167–300)
Factor VII	20%	236 (198–277)
Platelets	50,000/μl	230 (169–294)

Table 1. Critical level of hemostatic components correlated with the calculated volume of blood loss according to Hippala et al. [5]

Life-Threatening and Critical-Site Bleeding

A life-threatening hemorrhage is defined as one that either results in a significant volume loss or bleeding into a critical site, such as the intracranial space [1, 2]. Accidental or surgical trauma and antithrombotic treatment are the leading causes of life-threatening and critical-site bleeding, although platelet and/or coagulation disorders may also induce these types of bleeding.

Coagulopathy of the Massively Transfused Patient

Massive transfusion is commonly defined as the replacement of 1 blood volume over a period of 24 h or transfusion of at least 4 units of packed RBC within 1 h when ongoing need is predictable [3]. Massively transfused patients show evidence of coagulopathy in a high percentage of cases. Occurrence of coagulopathy is associated with an increase in overall mortality [3, 4].

Uncontrolled bleeding initially leads to loss of coagulation factors and platelets. Studies on the change of hemostatic components when major surgical blood loss was replaced using RBC and colloids indicate that a deficiency of fibrinogen develops earlier than any other hemostatic abnormality [5]. A critical platelet count of 50,000/μl was reached at a blood loss matching approximately twice the calculated blood volume (table 1). In addition to the loss of coagulation factors and platelets, trauma-induced exposure of the thromboplastin-rich subendothelial tissue to flowing blood induces the activation of coagulation, which may trigger consumptive coagulation, including DIC.

Based on the definition of the critical levels of the hemostatic components, as outlined in table 1, the laboratory diagnosis of coagulopathy in the massive transfusion setting can be established by a simple hemostasis screen including the following tests: platelet count, fibrinogen, APTT, and PT. However, laboratory analysis of the APTT, the PT and of the fibrinogen level may take more than 30 min in most surgical and trauma centers. A major problem with this delay in obtaining results is that the tests may not reflect the actual hemostasis of the patient. Near-patient screens such as point-of-care testing of the PT and the APTT and thrombelastography (TEG) might

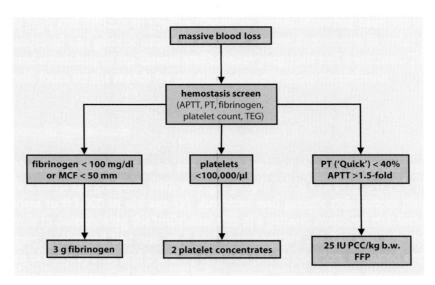

Fig. 1. Management algorithm for the treatment of massive blood loss-associated coagulopathy. The diagnosis of coagulopathy is established by a hemostasis screen that includes testing for APTT, PT, fibrinogen level, platelet count and TEG. The results obtained guide the transfusion of platelets, plasma (fresh frozen plasma, FFP), prothrombin complex concentrates (PCC), and fibrinogen.

be helpful to overcome these limitations. TEG measures the viscoelastic properties of whole blood after induction of clotting under low shear conditions. The pattern of changes in viscoelasticity reflects the kinetics of all stages of thrombus formation (reaction, r-time) and coagulation time (CT) and maximum clot firmness (MCF) [6]. Because of the dynamic changes of hemostasis in massive bleeding, testing should be performed repeatedly.

Aims of the hemotherapy in the massively transfused patients are (1) the correction of the hemostatic defect(s) to stop bleeding and (2) to prevent coagulopathy. Correction of the defect(s) requires substitution of plasma, platelets, and purified coagulation factors. A management algorithm is shown in figure 1.

To prevent bleeding, a fixed ratio of FFP to transfused RBC of 1:2, and of 1:1 after 10 units of RBC have been transfused, is recommended [7]. Platelet concentrates should be administered when the platelet count is below 100,000/µl.

Recombinant activated factor VII (rFVIIa) should not be used routinely for the treatment of coagulopathic bleeding in massively transfused patients [8], since the results of several studies indicate that rFVIIa does not significantly affect mortality rates. The use of rFVIIa should be restricted to those patients who failed to respond to standard hemotherapy. Recommended dosing for this 'last-ditch hemotherapy' is 100 µg/kg body weight (b.w.) given by intravenous (i.v.) bolus injection [8, 9].

Pötzsch/Scharf

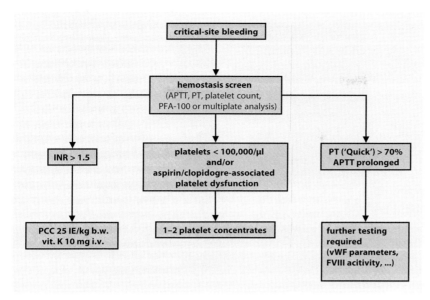

Fig. 2. Algorithm for the management of critical-site bleeding. Depending on the results of the hemostasis screen, patients are treated with PCC or platelet concentrates.

Antithrombotic Treatment Associated with Bleeding

Bleeding is the main complication of long-term anticoagulant and long-term antiplatelet treatment. The annual incidence of major hemorrhage induced by vitamin K antagonist (VKA) treatment is ~2%, and ~10% of major bleeds are lethal, yielding a 0.2% annual rate of fatal bleeding in such patients [10–12].

Once a patient is presenting with a bleeding at a critical site, immediate laboratory evaluation should be initiated in order to identify an underlying hemostatic defect, especially a drug-induced defect. The following screening tests should be performed: platelet count, whole-blood platelet function testing, and the APTT and PT. A prolonged closure time of the collagen/epinephrin cartridge of the platelet function analyzer (PFA)-100 is highly indicative of aspirin-induced platelet dysfunction, if the platelet count lies within the normal range. Similarly, an impaired adenosin diphosphate (ADP) response of the whole blood platelet aggregation testing is compatible with clopidogrel-induced platelet inhibition.

In patients who experience critical-site bleeding while on VKA treatment, prothrombin complex concentrates (PCC) should be immediately administered using an initial bolus of 25 IE PCC/kg b.w. [13]. Additionally, 10 mg vitamin K should be administered to neutralize the remaining VKA activity. After stopping of the bleeding, alternative anticoagulation considering the strength of indications for anticoagulant treatment should be initiated. A treatment algorithm based on the results of the hemostasis screen is shown in figure 2.

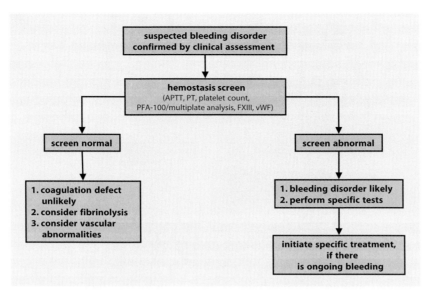

Fig. 3. Management algorithm for patients with a suspected bleeding disorder. APTT, activated partial thromboplastin time; PT, prothrombin time; PFA-100, platelet function analyzer; FXIII, factor XIII activity; vWF, von Willebrand factor parameters.

Management of Abnormal but not Critical Bleeding

When faced with a patient with abnormal bleeding that is not life threatening, the clinical probability of a bleeding disorder and the nature of the disorder, either coagulation or platelet/vascular and either congenital or acquired, should be determined (fig. 3). Evidence that increases the likelihood of a bleeding disorder includes a previous history of abnormal bleeding, a predisposing medical background, and a positive family history.

In obtaining a history of bleeding, it is important to question a patient carefully regarding the frequency of bleeding and to ascertain whether episodes of bleeding are spontaneous or occur in risk situations such as minor trauma. Topics that should be questioned are listed in table 2.

Indicative of the presence of a bleeding disorder are spontaneous bleeding, bleeding from multiple sites, excessive bleeding after minimal trauma or transfusion requirements after minor surgery. Although spontaneous skin bleeding is a common finding in patients with bleeding disorders, it is not usually due to a hemostatic defect. This is because skin bleeding occurs very commonly in women and children. In women, it is usually a manifestation of the benign 'easy bruising' syndrome; in children, bruises are mostly due to trauma caused by the rough and tumble of play. In either case, bruises larger than 2–3 cm, more than two to three at once, and bruises away from usual sites of trauma should lead to a consideration of a bleeding disorder

Main category	Details
Spontaneous bleeding	age at onset bruising hematoma formation bleeding in muscles joint bleeding mucous membrane bleeding
Prolonged bleeding after minor trauma	duration of bleeding transfusion requirements healing of wound (scar formation)
Prolonged bleeding after surgery	dental work transfusions after minor surgery
Drugs interfering with the hemostatic system	anticoagulants antiplatelet agents antibiotics
Family history	

Table 2. Obtaining a bleeding history

Test	Screens positive for ...
Platelet count and blood smear	thrombocytopenia, inherited platelet dysfunctions associated with abnormal platelet morphology, acquired platelet dysfunctions
PFA-100 or multiplate testing	platelet dysfunctions, drug-induced platelet dysfunctions
APTT and PT	coagulation factor deficiencies except for factor XIII deficiency
Factor XIII activity	factor XIII deficiency
von Willebrand factor assays	inherited or acquired von Willebrand disease

Table 3. Hemostasis screen for evaluation of abnormal bleeding

or a beaten child syndrome. Bruises due to atrophy of subcutaneous tissue, occurring on the forearms of older individuals, should be readily recognized as not being due to a bleeding disorder.

Once a positive clinical history has been obtained, laboratory evaluation should be performed starting with a hemostasis screen. This hemostasis screen should include procedures that are helpful to identify the vast majority of bleeding disorders. Tests that fulfill these criteria are listed in table 3.

If the hemostasis screen is normal, disorders of platelets and coagulation are unlikely. Hyperfibrinolysis and vascular abnormalities of bleeding should be considered. At present there is no single test available that specifically identifies hyperfibrinolysis.

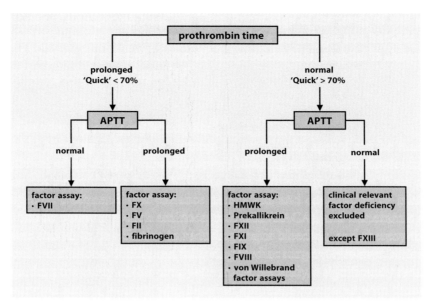

Fig. 4. Laboratory evaluation of prolonged APTT/PT values. This decision path defines the need for extra testing based on the APTT and PT values measured in the initial hemostasis screen.

However, a predisposing underlying disorder, decreased plasma levels of fibrinogen, and increased levels of D-dimer support the diagnosis of hyperfibrinolysis. Such a clinical and laboratory feature warrants the 'diagnostic' treatment with tranexamic acid. The antifibrinolytic agent tranexamic acid is administered either orally (3×1 g) or intravenously (50–100 mg/kg b.w./24 h). The i.v. route is preferred in critically ill patients or in patients with ongoing severe bleeding. The diagnosis of a vascular cause of bleeding can be established only on the clinical feature.

If the hemostasis screen is abnormal, the results should be interpreted in synopsis with the clinical situation. Extra testing is often required to confirm the diagnosis and to identify the hemostatic abnormality on the molecular level. For example, prolonged APTT/PT values require factor assays in order to identify the underlying factor deficiency (fig. 4). If the diagnosis of a bleeding disorder has been established in a patient with ongoing bleeding, specific hemotherapy should be initiated and monitored.

Conclusions and Future Directions

Hemostasis-navigated hemotherapy provides a rational, efficient and economic concept for the clinical management of patients with active bleeding. Currently available screening assays of platelet function and coagulation have several limitations. Thus, technical innovations in point-of-care testing may also improve monitoring of hemotherapy.

Disclosure of Conflict of Interests

The authors state that they have no conflict of interests.

References

1 Kozek-Langenecker S: Management of massive operative blood loss. Minerva Anestesiol 2007;73:1–15.
2 Asdaghi N, Manawadu D, Butcher K: Therapeutic management of acute intracerebral haemorrhage. Expert Opin Pharmacother 2007;8:3097–3116.
3 MacLeod JB, Lynn M, McKenney MG, Cohn SM, Murtha M: Early coagulopathy predicts mortality in trauma. J Trauma 2003;55:39–44.
4 Sauaia A, Moore FA, Moore EE, Moser KS, Brennan R, Read RA, Pons PT: Epidemiology of trauma deaths: a reassessment. J Trauma 1995;38:185–193.
5 Hippala ST, Myllylä GJ, Vahtera EM: Hemostatic factors and replacement of major blood loss with plasma-poor red cell concentrates. Anesth Analg 1995;81:360–365.
6 Lang T, Bauters A, Braun SL, Potzsch B, von Pape KW, Kolde HJ: Multi-centre investigation on reference ranges for ROTEM thromboelastometry. Blood Coagul Fibrinolysis 2005;16:301–310.
7 Tieu BH, Holcomb JB, Schreiber MA: Coagulopathy: Its pathophysiology and treatment in the injured patient. World J Surg 2007;31:1055–1064.
8 Mittal S, Watson HG: A critical appraisal of the use of recombinant factor VIIa in acquired bleeding conditions. Br J Haematol 2006;133:355–363.
9 Goodnough LT, Shander AS: Recombinant factor VIIa: safety and efficacy. Curr Opin Hematol 2007;14:504–509.
10 Büller HR, Prins MH: Secondary prophylaxis with warfarin for venous thromboembolism. N Engl J Med 2003;349:702–704.
11 Kearon C: Long-term management of patients after venous thromboembolism. Circulation 2004;110(suppl I):I10–I18.
12 Linkins L, Choi PT, Douketis JD: Clinical impact of bleeding in patients taking oral anticoagulant therapy for venous thromboembolism: a meta-analysis. Ann Intern Med 2003;139:893–900.
13 Freeman WD, Aguilar MI: Management of warfarin-induced intracerebral hemorrhage. Expert Rev Neurother 2008;8:271–290.

Prof. Dr. med. Bernd Pötzsch
Institut für Experimentelle Hämatologie und Transfusionsmedizin
Universitätsklinikum Bonn
Sigmund-Freud-Str. 25
53105 Bonn, Germany
Tel. +49 228 287-16745, Fax -19090
E-Mail bernd.poetzsch@ukb.uni-bonn.de

Scharf RE (ed): Progress and Challenges in Transfusion Medicine, Hemostasis and Hemotherapy.
Freiburg i.Br., Karger, 2008, pp 394–402

The Impact of Demographic Changes on Transfusion Demand and Blood Supply: Need for Systematic Blood Donor Research

Andreas Greinacher[a] · Uwe Konerding[b] · Konstanze Fendrich[b] ·
Ulf Alpen[a] · Wolfgang Hoffmann[b]

[a]Institute for Immunology and Transfusion Medicine, Greifswald,
[b]Institute for Community Medicine, Ernst-Moritz-Arndt-University of Greifswald, Germany

Key Words

Demographic changes · Blood supply · Donor research · Transfusion · Red blood cell concentrates ·
Epidemiology

Summary

The population structure in most European countries is currently changing, with a shift from younger to older age groups. We recently determined the impact of these demographic changes on future blood demand and supply in a well-characterized region in North-East Germany. This indicates two developments. One is the well-known increase in the older population, resulting in an increased demand for blood transfusions of about 12%. The second is the decrease in the number of the younger population due to the decreased birth rate in most of the countries of the former East European block after 1990. This may account for a decrease in blood donations of 25%. We further discuss the reasons for the over-proportional increase in blood demand during the next decades. Prevention of blood shortages will need an increase in the percentage of the population donating blood. To approach new blood donors most efficiently, information about the background of blood donors in comparison to those who do not donate is required. The methodology for performing this type of donor research is presented. As the demographic trends will affect many regions in Europe concomitantly within the next 15 years, coordinated efforts are urgently required to prevent blood shortages.   ©2008 S. Karger GmbH, Freiburg i.Br.

Introduction

Blood supply is the transfer of blood from the population of donors to the population of recipients. These two groups differ considerably in their demographic characteristics. The donor population consists primarily of young, healthy individuals. In contrast, most patients requiring blood transfusion are considerably older. Therefore, blood supply is influenced by the demographic changes in the main age groups of blood donors, while blood demand is influenced by the demographic changes in the age groups of blood recipients.

Blood requirements have steadily increased over the past two decades in Germany and other countries in Europe and North America. This was mainly caused by major therapeutic advances in hematology-oncology and a constant increase in the numbers of major surgical procedures. For example, allogeneic stem cell transplantation in Europe increased by a factor of 4.5 between 1990 and 2000 (from 4,234 to 19,136 procedures) [1], and open heart surgery in Germany increased by a factor of 2.5 between 1990 and 2002 (from 38,712 to 96,194 procedures) [2]. Probably even more important is the extension of the eligibility of older patients for major surgical procedures and the improved (but often still transfusion-dependent) survival following chemotherapy. In Germany, 12% of patients requiring open heart surgery in 1990 were between 70 and 80 years of age, and only 1% was above 80 years. By 2002, however, 39% of patients were 70–80 years old, and 6% were older than 80 years [2]. A less well known factor influencing the number of older patients potentially needing blood transfusions is the sharp increase in life expectancy following the reunification in Germany (mean of 5.1 and 4.8 years for men and women, respectively, since 1989) [3, 4]. The gain in life expectancy was predominantly due to decreases in mortality in men aged 40–64 years and women aged 65 years and older. A variety of reasons for this decrease in mortality after the reunification are assumed: changes in diet with easy access to fresh fruit and vegetables, the modernization of the health care system, the higher availability of modern pharmaceutical drugs and medical technology, a better emergency health care, an increased availability of nursing care, and improvements in overall living conditions especially for the older people [5, 6].

Impact of Demographic Changes on Blood Supply and Blood Demand

Recently, we analyzed how demographic factors will determine future blood demand in Mecklenburg-West Pomerania, a region in Eastern Germany where the demographic change is particularly dynamic, and where detailed donor and recipient data are available from the database of the Department of Transfusion Medicine and the database of the Institute for Community Medicine of the University of Greifswald [7]. This study indicates the potential for a major shortfall of blood supply in the area beginning by the end of this decade, if current age-specific blood donation and demand patterns remain unchanged. The magnitude of this shortfall was calculated to be in the order of 32–35% of red blood cell concentrates (RBCs) required, and is primarily driven by demographics. A major finding of the study was that the expected decrease in blood donations resulting from a relative decrease in the younger donor population has a higher impact than the increase of blood demand. Thus, the impact of demographic changes on transfusion medicine is particularly striking as blood donors and recipients belong to different age groups and demographic changes affect these populations in the opposite direction. During the next decades, the absolute number of the older age groups will increase. At the same time, the younger adults who donate considerably more blood will decrease by more than 50% by 2015 as compared to the population numbers of 2004, at least in the eastern parts of Germany. The same trend as in Greifswald has been found in Magdeburg, the capital of Saxonia-Anhalt. In this city, the percentage of the population in the age group of 18–68 years, which is the age group of potential blood donors, will decrease from 72 to 65% within 10 years [8]. Thus, the sharply reduced number of potential blood donors, together with increasing demand for blood transfusions in the older population, will result in a growing shortage of RBC units from 2008 onwards.

The shift in the older age groups of the population will have a much more pronounced effect on blood demand than implied by the numbers. This is because malignancies and other diseases, which typically require supportive therapy by blood components, will increase overproportionally in this age group. As a consequence, the incident number of patients with colon cancer will increase by 24.4% until 2012 (+30.9% in 2020), and with myocardial infarction by 27.5% until 2012 (+40.9% in 2020) [9]. Thus, it is very likely that the overall need for blood products will constantly increase although the total population will decrease by 10.5% in Mecklenburg-West Pomerania until 2012.

These demographic changes occur more rapidly in the eastern regions of Germany than in other parts of the country, in which, however, similar demographic changes will manifest with a delay of only a few years. Comparing the demographic data in Germany of 2007 and of 2028 (fig. 1) shows that the peak of the demographic changes that cause the imbalance between blood supply and demand will occur when the 'baby boomer' generation will enter their 7th decade of age. This population group is currently the largest age group in the country and consists of those being between 40 and 50 years of age and therefore currently in the age group primarily donating blood. Thus, the transfusion medicine community has about 15 years to develop strategies to secure blood supply.

As in Mecklenburg-West Pomerania several parameters together have an impact on population numbers, the region may constitute a model region to assess how different approaches may influence blood donation frequency. This may then be transferred to other regions in Germany and Europe which expect similar changes with a delay of just a few years.

Medical advances may reduce RBC demand. However, recent trends indicate the opposite (fig. 2) and indicate that we most likely even underestimate the true need for RBCs in future.

It will be difficult for transfusion medicine specialists to directly achieve a reduction in the transfusion rates, as this is the predominant area of the clinical specialists who are directly involved in patient care. While clinical transfusion medicine can contribute to a reduction in RBC consumption by appropriate clinical trials and on-

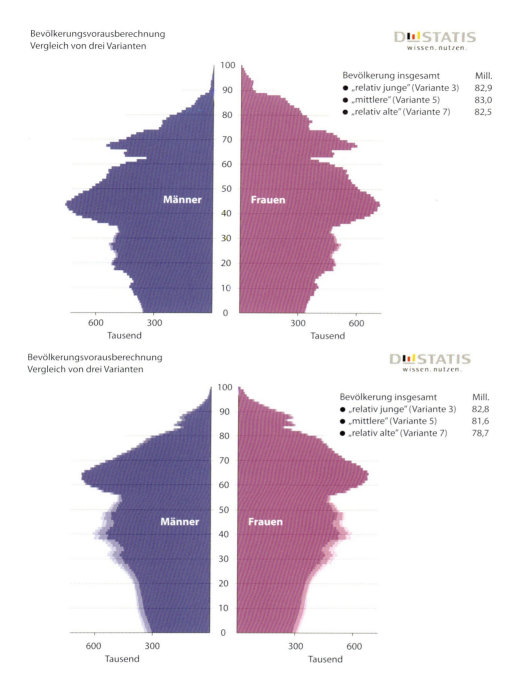

Fig. 1. Demographic pattern of the population in Germany **a** in 2007 and **b** in 2028. The decrease in the younger age group as seen in figure 1a for those up to 20 years of age will continue over the next 20 years. The baby boomer generation will remain the biggest age group for the next 20 years. However, they will change from the age group still representing the biggest group of blood donors to the age group with the highest blood demand. This will result in a major shortfall in blood supply if the percentage of blood donors in the younger age group will not be considerably increased within the next 15 years. (©Statistisches Bundesamt)

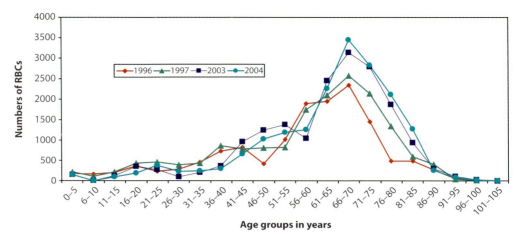

Fig. 2. The figure gives the number of RBCs transfused per age group and year at the University Hospital Greifswald for the years 1996, 1997, and 2003, 2004. While the relative distribution of the age groups of blood recipients remained very similar over the years, the absolute number of transfusions constantly increased. As the University Hospital is the only hospital in the city, these numbers very likely reflect the overall trend of blood demand. It is noteworthy that, during the same time period, major efforts were made to reduce unnecessary RBC transfusions as seen by the reduction of blood transfusions in the younger age groups.

going education on the optimal use of blood products, most blood donation services will have a more important role in obtaining sufficient amounts of blood.

Blood Donor Research: Potential Use and Possible Methods

One approach to counterbalance the threat of a shortfall in blood supply is to increase the percentage of those who donate blood per age group. This will require motivation campaigns, specific advertisement, and identification of those groups in the population who might be addressed most efficiently. However, very little is currently known about the social background and motivation of blood donors. Even more striking is the nearly complete lack of information on the reasons why those who would be eligible for blood donation do not donate.

Such type of studies requires the knowledge and expertise developed in social sciences. Well-planned and scientifically valid donor studies have the potential to provide meaningful data, based on which future activities can be planned and donor recruitment strategies can be designed. 'Self-made' questionnaires are very unlikely to be able to fulfill these requirements. The following section does address how a representative analysis of the blood donor population with regard to their social background and motivation could be designed and analyzed in the context of the regional population. The regional context is of major importance as it is very unlikely that the same criteria and strategies apply for those living in a major city as for those living in a small village.

Greinacher/Konerding/Fendrich/Alpen/Hoffmann

Methods for Blood Donor Research

Designing interventions for increasing the number of blood donors requires information about the characteristics of those who donate blood and those who do not. The most accurate approach would be a population-representative survey in the region in question. This survey should address the blood donating behavior and, additionally, those variables which are supposed to be relevant to the design of interventions for gaining blood donors. However, if the proportion of blood donors in the population is low, then the sample investigated in such a survey must be very large to have sufficient power. Therefore, population-representative surveys that are specifically designed for assessing the differences between people who donate blood and those who do not are too costly. Alternative approaches are needed. In the following, two possible alternative approaches are discussed. Both rely upon questioning blood donors in the context of the blood donating procedure. The first approach is restricted only to data obtained in this context; the second is based upon additionally applying data from a general population-representative survey performed in the region where the respective blood donating center is located.

Applying Data only from Blood Donors

The survey performed with the blood donors in the course of the blood donating process should fulfill three conditions:

1 The survey should last 1 year. This is important because there might be seasonal variations in the behavior of the blood donors as well as in the behavior of the blood donation center. With a survey interval of 1 year, most of these variations will level out.
2 People enrolling for donating blood should be approached for study participation in constant intervals over the whole time the donation center is open. The counting should start at the first day of the survey and should be continued from one day to the next. This is important because different groups of people might prefer different times for donating blood, e.g. those donating during morning hours might consist of a totally different group of the population than those donating after regular working hours. It is therefore important that everybody has the same chance of participating in the study.
3 For each participant, the number of blood donations given within the study year must be recorded. This is important because this is the central information for determining those features that are associated with the tendency of donating blood.

The data obtained from the blood donors do not contain information about those people who do not donate. They contain, however, information about frequent donors and about sporadic donors. This information, in turn, might be very valuable because there are good reasons to assume that those characteristics that discriminate between people who donate often and those who donate only once or twice also discriminate between people who donate and those who do not. Therefore, the relation between the number of blood donations per year and the characteristics in question should be investigated. If the prevalence of a certain feature increases constantly with the number of blood donations per year, then there is good reason to assume that this feature is underrepresented in people who do not donate at all. If, in contrast, the prevalence of a certain feature decreases constantly with the number of blood donations, then there is good reason to assume that this feature is overrepresented in people who do not donate at all.

Additionally Applying Data from a Population-Representative Survey
in the Same Region

Inferring characteristics of people who do not donate blood from characteristics of people who do is associated with a certain degree of uncertainty. This uncertainty can only be reduced by applying data from people who actually do not donate blood. These data can be obtained if there has been a population-representative survey in the region of the blood donating center.

If data of the population-representative survey are to be analyzed together with the data from the blood donor survey, then the latter survey must fulfill three further conditions in addition to the three conditions described above:

1 The blood donor survey must contain, at least partly, the same questions as the population-representative survey.
2 The information that was relevant to the recruitment procedure of the population-representative survey must also be obtained for the blood donors. In most cases, this is information concerning gender, age and residence. Gender and age are usually registered anyhow. For the residence, in most cases, the postal code will be sufficient.
3 Participants of the blood donor survey should be asked whether they have also participated in the population-representative survey.

In most cases, age and residence will be distributed very differently in both data sets merely because of differences in the recruitment procedures. Therefore, those age groups and those residence areas that are represented in only one of the two data sets should be removed before both data sets are merged. Even after removing non-matching groups, there will still be differences between data from the blood donor and the population-representative survey that are merely produced by differences in the recruitment procedures. Usually, these differences will refer to the distribution of gender, age and residence. These differences should be controlled when both samples are compared in order to identify characteristics that distinguish people who donate blood from those who do not. For this purpose, the comparisons should be performed using multivariate regression analyses with the characteristic in question as dependent variable and gender, age and residence as control variables. Dummy variables for all different frequencies of donating blood per year should be applied as independent variables belonging to the population-representative survey as reference category. Analyses of this kind reveal, specified for each number of donations per year, how blood donors differ from participants of the population-representative survey. Ideally, participants of the population survey who are also blood donors should be excluded to avoid any bias.

Conclusions and Future Directions

Analysis of demographic data indicates increased future demand for blood and blood products that coincides with reduction in blood donations. This process will begin in 2008 in East Germany as in this year the generation affected by the 'post reunification' birth decrease will become 18 and therefore enter the age for blood donation. From now on in the east of Germany, each year the age group of the younger population will be decreased by 50%. In other words, in 2008 the donor population of those being 18 years of age is only half as big as in previous years. In 2009, the donor population of those being 18 and 19 years of age will be reduced by 50%; in 2010 this will affect those being 18, 19, and 20 years of age, and so on. This will inevitably cause shortfalls in blood supply if the transfusion medicine community will not be able to increase the percentage of blood donors in all age groups. Despite some uncertainties in several parameters used in our projection, the threat of major blood shortages is evident. Although these shortfalls might initially be compensated by importing blood from other regions within Germany, this will become increasingly difficult as these demographic trends begin to affect virtually all regions in Europe simultaneously, although to varying degrees. While demographic changes are more pronounced in the eastern states of Germany than in most other areas of Europe, their overall profile resembles that seen elsewhere to various degrees. In Italy and in East European countries, the younger populations decreased markedly during the past decades, whereas in countries like France and England/Wales, the situation is more favorable. Nevertheless, even in the latter countries, the absolute number of the elderly will increase in the future, leading to an increase in blood demand. This has been estimated to be about 30% in Scotland until 2026 [10] and 64% in the USA until 2030 [11, 12]. The latter study also identified the overall population growth, particularly those over 65 years of age as the main cause of the increased demand and also predicted a shortfall between number of donations and number of transfusions required, as the younger age group population will increase less than the one of the older age groups.

It will be increasingly important to motivate younger people to donate blood and to increase the proportion of those who become permanent donors. This needs systematic donor research. We propose that this is an ideal area for a joint approach of experts in social sciences and experts in transfusion medicine. The methodology outlined above might improve the efficacy of donor motivation campaigns. The second major approach to counteract shortfalls in blood supply, which has not been addressed here, is to decrease unnecessary blood transfusion whenever possible.

Disclosure of Conflict of Interests

The authors state that they have no conflict of interests.

References

1 Gratwohl A for the European Group for Blood Marrow Transplantation: The role of the EBMT activity survey in the management of hematopoietic stem cell transplantation. Int J Hematol 2002;76(suppl 1):386–392.

2 Bruckenberger E: 16. Herzbericht 2003 mit Transplantationschirurgie. Hannover, Bruckenberger, 2004.

3 Statistisches Landesamt Mecklenburg-Vorpommern: Statistisches Jahrbuch Mecklenburg-Vorpommern 2004. Schwerin, cw Obotritendruck GmbH, 2004.

4 Fischer H, Karpinski J, Kück U: Bevölkerungsentwicklung in Mecklenburg-Vorpommern seit der Wende – Bilanz und Ausblick. Statistisches Monatsheft Mecklenburg-Vorpommern 2002;249–262.

5 Luy M: A tempo-based hypothesis for converging mortality in West and East Germany. Extended abstract at the IUSSP XXV International Population Conference. Tours, France, 2005.

6 Nolte E, Shkolnikov V, McKee M: Changing mortality patterns in East and West Germany and Poland. II: Short-term trends during transition and in the 1990s. J Epidemiol Community Health 2000;54:899–906.

7 Greinacher A, Fendrich K, Alpen U, Hoffmann W: Impact of demographic changes on the blood supply – Mecklenburg-West Pomerania as a model region for Europe. Transfusion 2007;47:395–401.

8 Schulze S, Ludwig S, Heim MU: Age structure of the blood donors at the University Clinic of Magdeburg and the residential district of the local institute of transfusion medicine. Transfus Med Hemother 2003;30(Sonderheft 1):56 (Abstract).

9 Fendrich K, Hoffmann W: More than just ageing societies: The demographic change has an impact on actual numbers of patients. J Public Health 2007;15:345–351.

10 Currie CJ, Patel TC, McEwan P, Dixon S: Evaluation of the future supply and demand for blood products in the United Kingdom National Health Service. Transfus Med 2004;14:19–24.

11 Vamvakas EC: Epidemiology of blood transfusion and forecasts of the demand for blood; in Vamvakas EC (ed): Evidence-based practice of transfusion medicine. Bethesda, AABB Press, 2001, pp 177–199.

12 Vamvakas EC, Taswell HF: Epidemiology of blood transfusion. Transfusion 1994;34:464–470.

Prof. Dr. Andreas Greinacher
Institute for Immunology and Transfusion Medicine
Ernst-Moritz-Arndt-Universität Greifswald
Sauerbruchstraße, 17489 Greifswald, Germany
Tel. +49 3834 865482, Fax -489
E-Mail greinach@uni-greifswald.de

Author Index

Key Word Index